N.J. NORRISS.

A SHORT TEXTBOOK OF MEDICINE

UNIVERSITY MEDICAL TEXTS

General Editors

SELWYN TAYLOR DM, MCh(OXON), FRCS, Hon FRCS (Ed), HON FCS(SA)

H. J. ROGERS MA, MB, BChir, PhD, MRCP

A complete list of titles in the series is available from the publishers.

A Short Textbook of Surgery
SELWYN TAYLOR DM, MCh(Oxon), FRCS

L. T. COTTON MCh(Oxon), FRCS

A Short Textbook of Medical Microbiology
D. C. TURK DM, MRCP, MRCPath

I. A. PORTER MD, FRCPath

A Short Textbook of Chemical Pathology
D. N. BARON MD, DSc, MRCP, FRCPath

A Short Textbook of Clinical Oncology
R. D. RUBENS MD, BSc, MRCP

R. K. KNIGHT MB, FRCP

A Short Textbook of Psychiatry
W. L. LINFORD REES BSc, MD, FRCP, DPM

A SHORT TEXTBOOK OF

MEDICINE

Eighth Edition

J. C. HOUSTON

MD, FRCP

Physician Emeritus, Guy's Hospital, formerly Dean, United Medical and Dental Schools, Guy's and St. Thomas' Hospitals, London

C. L. JOINER

MD, FRCP

Physician, Guy's Hospital, London
Honorary Consultant Physician to the British Army

J. R. TROUNCE

MD, FRCP

Professor Emeritus of Clinical Pharmacology, United Medical and Dental Schools, Guy's and St. Thomas' Hospitals, London

HODDER AND STOUGHTON

LONDON SYDNEY AUCKLAND TORONTO

Cover illustration: showing an electronmicrograph of a longitudinal section through three vertebrate cardiac muscle cells. Courtesy of Y. Uehara, G. R. Campbell and G. Burnstock, Department of Anatomy, University College, London.

British Library Cataloguing in Publication Data

Houston, J. C.
A short textbook of medicine.—8th ed.
—(University medical texts)
1. Pathology
I. Title II. Joiner, C. L.
III. Trounce, J. R. IV. Series
616 RB111

ISBN 0 340 35271 X

First Edition 1962. Reprinted 1964
Second Edition 1966. Reprinted 1967
Third Edition 1968. Reprinted 1970, 1971 (with revisions)
Fourth Edition 1972. Reprinted with revisions 1973
Fifth Edition 1975. Reprinted with revisions 1977, 1978
Sixth Edition 1979
Seventh Edition 1982
Eighth edition 1985

Typeset in 10/11 pt Times (Monophoto) by Macmillan India Ltd. Bangalore.

Printed in Great Britain for
Hodder and Stoughton Educational,
a division of Hodder and Stoughton Ltd,
Mill Road, Dunton Green, Sevenoaks, Kent
by Richard Clay (The Chaucer Press) Ltd,
Bungay, Suffolk

EDITOR'S FOREWORD

'Books must follow sciences, and not sciences books.'
Francis Bacon

Houston, Joiner and Trounce is the corner-stone of this series of Short Textbooks, one of the first to appear over twenty years ago, it has been rewritten and revised repeatedly.

Despite rewriting and revision it remains a reasonable size by dint of its conciseness, its greatest attraction being the clarity of presentation without lapse into the cryptic and synoptic style of most books of this scope. Textbooks of medicine which contain a similar amount of information are usually multivolume works.

A Short Textbook of Medicine remains a delight to read and contains within its covers all that the clinical apprentice needs in his early years. Indeed many of us also use it as a refresher course in this rapidly expanding subject, since the text is always being so rigorously updated.

It is a great compliment to the authors that it has become prescribed reading not only in many medical schools in Great Britain but throughout the Commonwealth and in European countries as well. Translation into Italian and Spanish testify to its wide appeal. The addition of a chapter on tropical diseases and infestations has now become a necessity with world travel introducing a new dimension to differential diagnosis.

I am confident that the eighth edition will add even further distinction to the book's enviable reputation.

Selwyn Taylor

PREFACE

In this edition Professor Woodruff has been responsible for writing the whole of the chapter on Tropical Diseases and Helminthic Infections. We are grateful to Dr G. C. Cook for his valuable contributions to previous editions.

Every chapter has again been subjected to careful revision and although a good deal of new material has been added judicious pruning has prevented more than a modest increase in size. It is hoped the new format will make the book easier and more convenient to handle.

The Editors believe *A Short Textbook of Medicine* continues to provide a clear, accurate, up-to-date and inexpensive account of the essentials of the subject.

CONTRIBUTORS

SIR JOHN BUTTERFIELD, OBE, MD, FRCP
Regius Professor of Physic, University of Cambridge, formerly Professor of Medicine, Guy's Hospital Medical School, London.

S. COHEN, CBE, PHD, FRC PATH, MD, FRS
Professor of Chemical Pathology, United Medical and Dental Schools, Guy's and St. Thomas' Hospitals, London.

R. GRAHAME, MD, FRCP
Consulting Rheumatologist, Guy's Hospital, London

B. H. HICKS, MD, FRCP
Consultant Endocrinologist, Guy's Hospital, and Senior Lecturer in Medicine, United Medical and Dental Schools, Guy's and St. Thomas' Hospitals, London.

M. D. O'BRIEN, MD, MRCP
Consulting Neurologist, Guy's Hospital, London, and to Maidstone Health District.

M. E. PEMBREY, MD, MRCP
Senior Lecturer in Paediatric Genetics, The Institute of Child Health, London.

G. W. SCOTT, MD, FRCP
Physician, Guy's Hospital, London.
Physician to the Chest Clinic, Guy's Hospital, London.

J. P. WATSON, MD, FRCP, FRC PSYCH, DPH, DCH
Professor of Psychiatry, United Medical and Dental Schools, Guy's and St. Thomas' Hospitals, London.

R. S. WELLS, MD, FRCP
Consulting Dermatologist, Guy's Hospital, London.
Senior Lecturer in Clinical Dermatology, Institute of Dermatology, St. John's Hospital, London.

A. W. WOODRUFF, CMG, MD, PHD, FRCP (Ed), DTM & H
Professor of Medicine, University of Juba, Southern Region, Sudan.
Emeritus Professor of Tropical Medicine, University of London, London School of Hygiene and Tropical Medicine.

CONTENTS

CHAPTER 1

MEDICAL GENETICS

There are some people whose failing health in early life is determined at conception. All the intrauterine influences, the dietary, infectious and toxic factors that contribute to the child's environment after birth, including at present the efforts of his doctors, do little to alter the course of *Duchenne muscular dystrophy*. At his conception his single X chromosome is carrying the Duchenne muscular dystrophy gene, either inherited from his mother or arriving as a new mutation in the ovum before fertilisation; and this alone is sufficient to cause him to be chairbound by the end of his first decade and dead by the end of his second. The tragedy for the family is compounded by the fear that subsequent boys will also be affected. The actual risk of this may be very high or low depending on the relative probability of either his mother being a carrier or his disease being the result of a new mutation. As with other genetic disorders clinical geneticists are likely to become involved in estimating this risk of recurrence, and then discussing this risk and the various options available to the couple involved. Certain principles of human genetics assist the doctor in this task. This chapter recalls some of these principles and describes their application in clinical medicine.

GENETIC VARIATION

In a sense genetically determined disease like Duchenne muscular dystrophy are just the tip of the iceberg of genetic variation in human populations. With the exception of identical (monozygotic) twins, we all differ genetically and not only do these differences account for much of the variation in physical attributes like height, but also for some of the differences in the susceptibility to disease. Most common diseases are the result of a complex interaction between environmental and genetic influences, the latter being the result of many genes each having a small effect. Most of these genes cannot be regarded as abnormal in the sense that the gene for blood group O is no more abnormal than for blood group A. Here we are dealing with specific alternative genes which in most circumstances provide for adequate health. By contrast much of what follows in this chapter concerns alternative genes that are harmful, their effect generally overriding all other genetic and environmental influences; so-called monogenic inheritance.

Now that so much is known about the actual structure of genes and how they are encoded in the chromosomal DNA (deoxyribonucleic acid), it is helpful to explain some of the classic genetic concepts (derived from the study of the pattern of inheritance of characters) in simple structural terms. In females the 46 chromosomes are present in homologous pairs and thus there are two copies of every gene, one maternal and the other paternal in origin. It is the same in males except for the difference in the sex chromosome pair X and Y.

A structural gene is made up of the DNA nucleotide sequences that code for a single polypeptide chain synthesised at the ribosomes in the cell cytoplasm. The polypeptide chain may subsequently be modified, or more than one type of polypeptide chain may associate to make a macromolecule; α globin and β globin chains go to make up adult haemoglobin, Hb A. Each structural gene has a specific site on the DNA of a particular chromosome; there is one β globin gene on each of the pair of chromosomes 11. The two β globin genes together constitute the β globin gene *locus*. Alternative genes at a single locus are called *alleles*. One of the nucleotides in one of the two β globin genes is altered in people with the sickle-cell trait, and therefore the sickle, or β^s, gene and the normal β gene are alleles. Obviously with only two DNA sites any one individual can only have two alleles at any one locus. However, in the population there may be numerous alleles and indeed over a hundred β globin chain variants have been described.

An individual with two different alleles at a particular locus is *heterozygous* for that locus. Where both alleles are the usual ones, we refer to *normal homozygous*, and where both are the same harmful alleles, the term *abnormal homozygous* can be used. Genes on the X chromosome are not one of a pair in males, and when such a gene is abnormal in a male, the term *hemizygous* is sometimes used.

MONOGENIC INHERITANCE

Autosomal Dominant Disorders

In medical genetics the term autosomal dominant refers to the situation where a monogenic disorder is manifest clinically in the heterozygous state. In Britain the overall incidence of autosomal dominant disorders is about 7 per 1000 live births; some of the more common conditions being *polycystic kidney disease*, *monogenic hypercholesterolaemia*, *neurofibromatosis*, and *Huntington's chorea*. Appreciating that each parent passes on only one chromosome of each pair to the child it can be simply deduced that any child of a person with an autosomal dominant disorder has a 1 in 2 chance of being affected. On average half will inherit the chromosome carrying the abnormal gene, and half the chromosome carrying the normal gene. Thus given enough offspring the condition can manifest in each generation and in both sexes, with only affected individuals able to pass it on.

Unfortunately in clinical practice the matter is complicated by two things, variation in the expression of the gene and new mutation. Both points are illustrated by neurofibromatosis, which has an incidence of about 1 in 3000. The manifestations in someone carrying the gene vary from just a few characteristic pigmented patches on the skin, so-called 'café au lait' spots, to gross disfigurement with a mass of cutaneous and subcutaneous tumours, and mental handicap. In neurofibromatosis as in many autosomal dominant disorders, a mildly affected person has to be warned that any child inheriting the gene may not be so lucky as they have been. It can also be seen that a person with minimal manifestations may be regarded as normal, and give rise to the view that the condition has 'skipped a generation'. Taking variation in the expression of the gene one stage further, one can argue that in some situations there will be no manifestation of the gene carried by some family members; that is, the gene has less than 100% penetrance. Reduced penetrance as a concept distinct from variable gene expression is not very helpful in practice. The important message is that you cannot advise someone until you have performed a careful physical examination, a general rule in clinical medicine. If they are clear one may be reassuring about risks to their children, but you can never give an absolute guarantee.

It is important, of course, to know the usual age of onset of the disease because quite a proportion of autosomal dominant disorders only manifest later in life, often after the carrier of the gene has completed his family. Huntington's chorea is a degenerative disorder of the brain, particularly of the basal ganglia, with an average age of onset of about 42 years. In the absence of any test to detect the gene early, people at risk (and their offspring) can only be reassured once they have reached the age of about 70 years with no manifestations of the disease.

All dominant disorders have to start at some time as new mutations in the ovum or sperm, and obviously the more severe the type of disease, the less likely the patient is to reproduce, and the greater proportion of affected individuals will be the result of a new mutation. In the mild dominant disorders, or those of late onset, the vast majority of patients have inherited it from an affected parent. New mutations and the variable gene expression can combine to create difficult clinical decisions. If a single child in the family has overt neurofibromatosis, the apparently healthy parents will want to know the risk to further children. If it is decided the child is the result of a new mutation, then the risk of recurrence is very low. However, if an examination reveals convincing minimal signs of neurofibromatosis in one parent, then the couple face a 1 in 2 risk with each pregnancy. This demonstrates the importance of knowing what are the minimal signs of the disorder, and the difficulties that could arise in doubtful cases.

It is estimated that about half the cases of neurofibromatosis are due to new mutations and this represents an estimated mutation rate of about 10^{-4}; that is, 1 in 10 000 germ cells mutate per generation, or 1 in 5000 babies have neurofibromatosis as a result of a new mutation. This is one of the highest mutation rates in man, and estimated mutation rates for dominant (and X-linked conditions) usually lie between 10^{-5} and 10^{-6}.

Autosomal Recessive Disorders

In autosomal recessive inheritance the disorder is only manifest clinically when the patient has a double dose of the abnormal gene, i.e. in the homozygous state. The patient has no normal allele at the particular locus involved, having inherited one abnormal gene from each parent. Usually both parents are heterozygous for the gene in question, and are clinically normal, the action of their normal allele at the locus being sufficient to compensate. Rarely one or even both parents are themselves affected homozygotes. In the usual situation, where both parents are heterozygous, a child has a 1 in 4 chance of being an affected homozygote, there is a 2 in 4 chance of being a heterozygote like the parents and a 1 in 4 chance of being normal.

In Britain the overall incidence of autosomal recessive disorders is about 2.5 per 1000 live births, and the commonest is *cystic fibrosis*. About 1 in 2000 are affected and about 1 in 22 people are heterozygotes, or carriers of the gene. The exact biochemical defect in cystic fibrosis is unknown, but there is a generalised alteration in mucus, with blocked pancreatic ducts leading to digestive problems, and blockage in the bronchial tree causing recurrent chest infections. A great number of autosomal recessive disorders are caused by an absent or inactive enzyme, preventing a step in a critical metabolic pathway—the so-called 'inborn error of metabolism' first elucidated by Garrod in the early years of this century. One fairly common example is a form of *adrenal hyperplasia* (*adrenogenital syndrome*). The deficient enzyme is 21 hydroxylase, the gene for which happens to be situated on chromosome 6 (Fig. 1.1). The resultant metabolic block causes increased activity in an alternative pathway leading to the excess production of androgens. These result in 'virilisation' of the female fetus with enlargement of the clitoris. More importantly the 21 hydroxylase deficiency interferes with the production of important cortical steroids. The clinical features of many inborn errors of metabolism are the result both of the accumulation of substances before and a deficiency of substances beyond the enzyme block.

The heterozygous state can be detected by biochemical tests in many autosomal recessive disorders and this can play an important part in genetic counselling. This fact also raises the question of whether a condition is truly recessive, if the gene produces a detectable effect in the heterozygous state. In practice the heterozygote is generally healthy and there is such a vast difference between the clinical manifestation in the heterozygous and the abnormal homozygous state that the use of additional categories such as intermediate or co-dominant disorders is

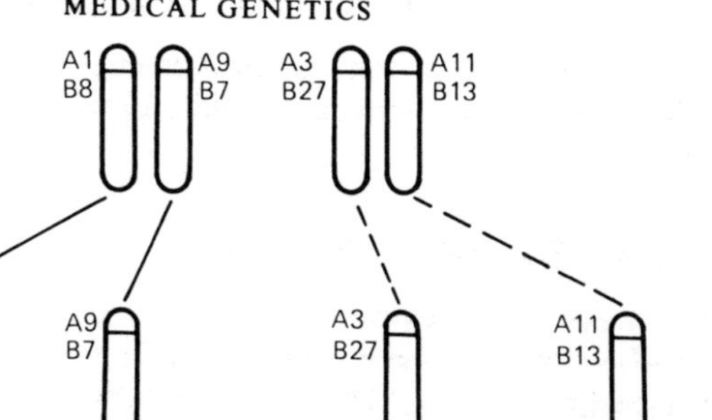

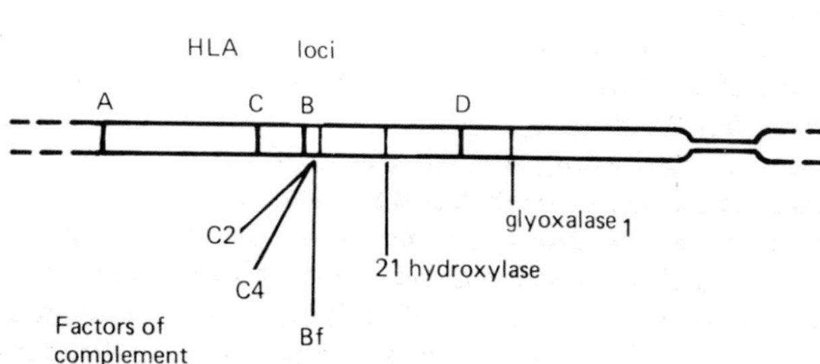

Fig. 1.1 A chromosome diagram showing the usual segregation of HLA haplotypes with no crossing over between Loci **A** and **B**. Below, a genetic map of part of chromosome 6.

unhelpful. *Sickle-cell anaemia* and *β-thalassaemia major* (*Cooley's anaemia*) can be regarded as autosomal recessive disorders even though the heterozygote or sickle-cell trait may have some *in vivo* sickling of their red cells with extreme anoxia, and people with β-thalassaemia trait may be slightly anaemic.

The incidence at birth of a recessive disorder in a population depends primarily on the incidence of the heterozygous state. Obviously early death will modify the frequency with which it is encountered in an older population, and a changing rate of cousin marriage can also have an effect. The extent to which new mutations maintain the frequency of heterozygotes for different recessive disorders is difficult to estimate, but natural selection has played the predominant role in sickle-cell disease and the thalassaemias. The sickle-cell trait affords some protection against malaria and analysis of DNA around the sickle-gene locus indicates that about 80% of West Africans with the sickle-cell trait inherited the gene from a common ancestor.

First cousins share one eighth of their genes in common and therefore they have a slightly increased chance of having children with recessive disorders compared to unrelated parents in the same population. Comparison between populations is not valid because a high cousin marriage rate over many generations tends to reduce the frequency of harmful recessive genes by natural selection.

X-linked Recessive Disorders

X-linked recessive inheritance produces a characteristic family pedigree, where males are affected and the gene is passed on by unaffected females. Using simple diagrams of the X and Y chromosome it is easy to satisfy oneself that an abnormal gene carried on one of the X chromosomes in a female will be passed on to half her daughters, who would be heterozygous like herself, and to half her sons who would manifest the disease because they have no compensating X. An affected male would produce only heterozygous daughters, but cannot pass the gene on to his sons, who only receive his Y chromosome. In a population where the X-linked red-cell enzyme defect *glucose-6-phosphate dehydrogenase (G6PD) deficiency* is common, an affected man may have an affected son, but only because his wife is also a heterozygote. Such a mating results in half the girls being affected homozygotes.

In some X-linked disorders a proportion of female heterozygotes are mildly affected, and this is the case with G6PD deficiency. Cytochemical staining of the red cells shows that about half are G6PD deficient and half are normal. The explanation (the Lyon hypothesis) lies in the fact that only one of the X chromosome pair is active in any one cell. The random inactivation of one or other X chromosome occurs in each cell early in embryonic development, and thereafter the descendants of a particular cell have the same inactive X. By chance some women heterozygous for G6PD deficiency have the normal X chromosome inactivated in 80–90% of their cells, and can therefore develop haemolysis, like the affected hemizygous males, when exposed to certain drugs such as sulphonamides and antimalarials.

In Britain the incidence of X-linked disorders is about 0.6 per 1000 total live births. *Duchenne muscular dystrophy* is the commonest with a birth incidence of about 1 in 4000 males. As we saw earlier, when there is an isolated affected male in the family, one of the clinical problems is to establish the probability of his disease being due to a new mutation. One can take the number of healthy males on the mother's side of the family into account, as well as the mother's plasma creatine kinase level. The enzyme leaks out of dystrophic muscle fibres and very high levels are found in the plasma of affected boys. The creatine kinase level tends to be increased in women heterozygous for the muscular dystrophy gene, but the distribution of values overlaps with the distribution of values from normal women, so only rarely can one be certain about the carrier status of the mother of an isolated case. Similar problems arise when counselling families with *haemophilia* (two distinct genes: one causing Factor VIII, the other Factor IX deficiency), which is another fairly common X-linked recessive disorder. Advances in assessing which female relative is a carrier for these X-linked conditions are coming from the development of Factor VIII and Factor IX gene-specific DNA probes, and with the use of chromosome region-specific DNA probes linked to the gene locus for Duchenne muscular dystrophy.

The term *X-linked dominant* has been used for the very few rare conditions where the heterozygous female is regularly affected. However, the hemizygous male is always more severely affected and in some instances, such as the X-linked form of *oral–facial–digital syndrome*, affected males rarely survive gestation to be born, so only female patients are encountered in clinical practice.

Reference is made to the X-linked form of the oral–facial–digital syndrome, because an almost identical syndrome can be caused by an autosomal recessive gene. There are quite a number of disorders that are virtually indistinguishable on ordinary clinical examination, but are caused by different genes, often with different patterns of inheritance.

GENETIC LINKAGE AND DISEASE ASSOCIATIONS

At meiosis homologous chromosomes pair up, and there is often exchange of a length of chromosome between the pair—so-called crossing over. Thus the single set of chromosomes that ends up in an ovum or sperm carries an assortment of the genes from both sets of chromosomes in the parent. If crossing over did not occur, all the genes on a particular chromosome would always be inherited *en bloc*, the characteristics they determine segregating together generation after generation in the family. Crossing over results in some genes that are carried on the same chromosome segregating independently, but obviously the closer two genes are situated on a chromosome, the less likely they are to be separated by crossing over and the more likely they are to be inherited together. Two such genes loci are said to be linked, and the genetic linkage could be demonstrated in a family, if it happens that different alleles are present at each of the two loci. In other words, one needs a tag on the four bits of chromosome one is interested in, to know what is going on.

The genes involved in the HLA system of tissue types illustrate some of these points. There is a large number of different histocompatibility antigens, which amongst other things are involved in rejection of foreign-tissue grafts. At present it seems there are four different HLA loci named HLA A, B, C and D. There are about 18 alleles at locus A, 34 for B, 8 for C and at least 12 for locus D. It will be recalled, however, that an individual can only have 2 alleles at each locus as illustrated in Fig. 1.1, which for simplicity just gives the HLA A and B specificities.

The particular combination of alleles (and the specific antigens they determine) on a single chromosome is called a haplotype, and because the HLA A and B loci are closely linked, the parental haplotypes are generally passed on unchanged. However, during meiosis about one time in a hundred a cross over between the two number 6 chromosomes occurs at a site between loci A and B, and the ovum or sperm will then carry a recombinant haplotype. A particular haplotype is not 'fixed' for evermore, even if it is transmitted unchanged for many generations. Given enough time and random mating, every combination of alleles at loci A and B should arise; and in theory the frequency of the combinations, or haplotypes, should be a reflection (actually the product) of the frequencies of the individual alleles. Where this is the case the alleles are said to be in linkage equilibrium.

When two alleles occur together more frequently, or less frequently than expected from the individual frequencies, they are said to be in linkage disequilibrium. Linkage disequilibrium can arise in a variety of ways. One allele may have arisen by mutation relatively recently (on the evolutionary time scale) and not yet achieved equilibrium, still reflecting the original combination. A particular combination may have a selective advantage or disadvantage and achieve disequilibrium by natural selection. The same principles of equilibrium and disequilibrium can apply to alleles of any two linked gene loci. The haplotype A1B8 occurs more frequently than the individual frequencies would predict, and therefore these two alleles show linkage disequilibrium.

A mild dominant disorder, the *nail patella syndrome*, shows genetic linkage with the blood group ABO locus, both the ABO and the disease gene locus being situated on chromosome 9. If the nail patella syndrome gene happens to be on a chromosome 9 that carries the allele for group A, then the disease and the blood group A will tend to be inherited together. However, because of eventual crossing over, or independent mutations leading to different affected families, the nail patella syndrome may be linked with blood group O in another family or group B in a third family. Thus there is genetic linkage, but no association with a particular blood group. Genetic linkage is a phenomenon demonstrable within families. By contrast association is a phenomenon demonstrated by comparing a population of affected individuals with a control population. People with blood group A are more likely to get cancer of the stomach than people of blood group O. This is an association between the group A allele and the cancer, but this does not necessarily mean that a cancer susceptibility gene is situated on chromosome 9 close to the ABO gene locus.

Confusion between genetic linkage and the disease associations arises because in cases of an association between a particular HLA antigen and a disease, one of the explanations for the association is genetic linkage between the HLA loci and a disease susceptibility gene *plus* linkage disequilibrium involving the particular allele at an HLA locus. Linkage disequilibrium is an essential part of this explanation, for as we have already seen with the nail patella syndrome and the ABO blood groups, genetic linkage alone does not result in a general association.

It should be realised that transplantation is not the only reason for the clinical importance of the HLA genes. There is increasing suspicion that genes concerned with the immune response are located in the HLA region, and therefore in close genetic linkage with the HLA loci. It is reasonable to guess that some common chronic diseases may be due, at least in part, to an abnormal immune response to certain infectious agents. It is these ideas that have given added significance to the associations that have been observed between certain HLA specificities and some diseases. By far the best example, and the strongest association, is between *idiopathic ankylosing spondylitis* and *HLA B 27*. Over 90% of Europeans with ankylosing spondylitis have HLA B 27, compared with only about 9% of the general population. HLA B 27 alone is not sufficient to the cause the disease, for if it were, the disease would show an autosomal dominant pattern of inheritance which it does not. Environmental factors are obviously also important.

MULTIFACTORIAL INHERITANCE

The correlation between the height of parents and their children's eventual height is clear for all to see. The inheritance of quantitative characters, like height, has been the subject of careful study for over a century, and it can be shown that the correlation between various relatives can be explained on the basis of many genes each of small effect segregating in a normal Mendelian fashion, i.e. obeying the same rules described so far in this chapter.

There is a significant genetic contribution to the cause of some common congenital malformations like *spina bifida, cleft lip ±palate,* or *congenital heart disease*, and it appears that this is on the basis of many genes each having a small positive or negative effect on the susceptibility of the foetus to the malformation. First-degree relatives (brothers and sisters or children) of an affected person have a considerable risk of being affected, but this increased risk diminishes rapidly when one moves to second-degree relatives (nephews, nieces and grandchildren) and is almost back to the general-population incidence for third-degree relatives (cousins). This general point about multifactorial inheritance is illustrated by cleft lip ± palate which has incidence of about 1 per 1000 live births in Britain. In first-degree relatives of an affected case the incidence is about 40 per 1000, but falls to 7 per 1000 for second-degree relatives and 2–3 per 1000 for third-degree relatives. When a couple has had two affected children, the risk to a further child is higher, about 14 %. In reality, of course, the risk has been the same for each pregnancy; what has increased is our information about how susceptible the children of this couple are to the malformation. It must be emphasised that largely unknown environmental factors also play an important part in the cause of these common malformations, and 'preventative measures' around the time of conception and in early pregnancy might be possible in the future. There is increasing evidence that maternal multivitamin and folic acid supplementation is associated with a reduction in the recurrence risk for spina bifida and anencephaly.

Many common disorders of adult life, such as *diabetes mellitus, arterial hypertension, epilepsy* or *schizophrenia* have a significant genetic component with close relatives having an increased risk of developing the disease. However, it is becoming clear that there are probably several causes of these conditions, some largely environmental, some genetic, whilst others are multifactorial, involving both the action of several genes and environmental factors.

Type I or insulin-dependent diabetes mellitus appears to be usually the result of virus-triggered autoimmune destruction of the β-islet cells in genetically susceptible individuals. The main susceptibility gene(s) are located on chromosome 6 within or close to the HLA gene complex, although they are probably not any of the HLA alleles themselves. Overall a sibling of an index case has a risk of about 5–6 % of developing diabetes mellitus by the age of 16 years. However if the sibling has inherited the same two number 6 chromosomes as the index case, that is they are HLA identical, the risk is much higher, perhaps 30 % by the age of 30; and it is correspondingly very low if the sibling has no chromosome 6 in common with the index case.

Type II or maturity-onset diabetes shows close to 100 % concordance in monozygotic twins (compared to just under 60 % concordance in monozygotic twins where one has Type I diabetes) indicating almost complete genetic determination. Obesity clearly contributes in some way; and if the index case with Type II diabetes mellitus is obese, the risk to a non-obese sibling is about 5 %, whilst with a non-obese index case the risk to an obese sibling is about 25 %. This brief account is obviously an oversimplification, for there is almost certainly further heterogeneity within the general description diabetes mellitus.

CHROMOSOME ABNORMALITIES

Chromosome abnormalities fall into two broad categories; disorders of chromosome number and rearrangements or changes in chromosome structure. The overall incidence in live births is about 5–6 per 1000 and it is estimated that about 50% of early spontaneous abortions are chromosomally abnormal, and of 1000 recognised pregnancies there are about 75 foetal or neonatal deaths due to chromosome abnormalities, the great majority arising as new mutations in the ovum, sperm or early zygote.

Simple monogenic disorders are not associated with any chromosomal change using routine karyotype analysis. However an X-linked form of mental handicap affecting 1 in 3–5000 boys and associated with large testes after puberty, features an unstainable gap or 'fragile site' at the end of the long arm of the X, when lymphocytes are cultured in folic acid deficient medium.

Disorders of Chromosome Number

During meiosis, the reduction division that leads to the ovum and sperm having a single, haploid, set of chromosomes, homologous chromosomes pair up before moving apart to the opposite poles of the dividing cell. Failure of the pair to associate in the first place, or failure to dissociate, can lead to an ovum or sperm with an extra chromosome, or one missing. The term non-disjunction, which assumes the latter mechanism, is often used for this error of chromosome segregation. The causes of non-disjunction are largely unknown, but the chance of it having occurred in the ovum increases with age. The resulting foetus will either have three copies of a particular chromosome (*trisomy*) or only one (*monosomy*). In practice the trisomies are the most important, monosomies in general being non-viable.

In some individuals the non-disjunction occurs after zygote formation, and in this case there are two cell lines each with a different chromosome complement. Such cases, which when they do occur often involve the sex chromosomes, are called *mosaics*, and overall they tend to manifest fewer abnormalities of development than the full trisomy, although this is not necessarily so in any one individual.

Anomalies of Sex Chromosome Number

Trisomies involving the X or Y chromosome are relatively common and lead to surprisingly minor physical abnormalities considering the size of the X chromosome (Fig. 1.2) and the many genes it carries. The explanation resides in the phenomenon of X chromosome inactivation described earlier. Only one X chromosome remains active in any one cell beyond an early stage of development and the inactive X chromosome becomes the X chromatin body (formerly known as the Barr body) which is visible close to the nuclear membrane in a proportion of cell nuclei in females. XXX females have two X-chromatin bodies in their cell nuclei, and the much rarer XXXX females have three X-chromatin bodies.

About 1 in 700 newborn males has the chromosome complement 47XXY, is X-chromatin positive, and has the clinical picture of

Klinefelter's syndrome. Those affected are outwardly nearly normal males, but the testes are always small after puberty with complete, or almost complete, azoospermia. There is often enlargement of the breasts, termed gynaecomastia, and concern about this, or infertility, are common ways for these patients to present. Some have moderate mental handicap, the distribution of IQ values being shifted down by 10 points compared to normal.

About 1 in 1000 newborn females has the chromosome complement 47XXX. Although disturbances of menstruation and fertility are common, many are essentially normal fertile females. Theoretically a proportion of their ova would carry two X chromosomes, leading to XXX or XXY offspring. This event has been observed, but there is probably selection against the abnormal ova.

With the relatively high incidence of 47XXY and 47XXX newborns, one would expect the complementary product of the non-disjunction, the 45X individual, to be common. It probably is at the time of conception, but about 98 % are lost as early abortions and only about 1 in 10 000 female births has the 45X chromosome complement with the associated clinical picture of *Turner's syndrome*. Affected females are short and fail to menstruate, their ovaries being replaced by streaks of connective tissue. There are often associated physical abnormalities, such as neck webbing and coarctation of the aorta, but intelligence is usually normal.

The XYY complement is found in about 1 in 700 newborn males. These individuals tend to be taller than average. Early surveys over-emphasised the association with aggressive, antisocial behaviour, and the majority are undiagnosed and lead a normal life.

Down's Syndrome Due to Primary Trisomy 21

Down's syndrome (mongolism), always due to an extra chromosome 21, is the commonest viable autosomal trisomy, presumably because of the small size of the chromosome involved. Overall about 96 % are due to a primary non-disjunction, and about 80 %, involve errors in the formation of the ovum rather than the sperm. In the other 4 % the extra chromosome 21 is attached to another chromosome and will be discussed in the next section. The incidence of Down's syndrome increases from about 1 in 1200 in mothers under 30 years to about 1 in 100 at the age of 40 years, and at present accounts for about a third of all cases of severe mental handicap of school age.

Chromosomal Translocations and Other Structural Abnormalities

With the introduction of banding of chromosomes, a special staining technique, individual chromosomes and parts of chromosomes can be identified (Fig. 1.2). This has allowed the accurate description of translocations and structural changes like small deletions.

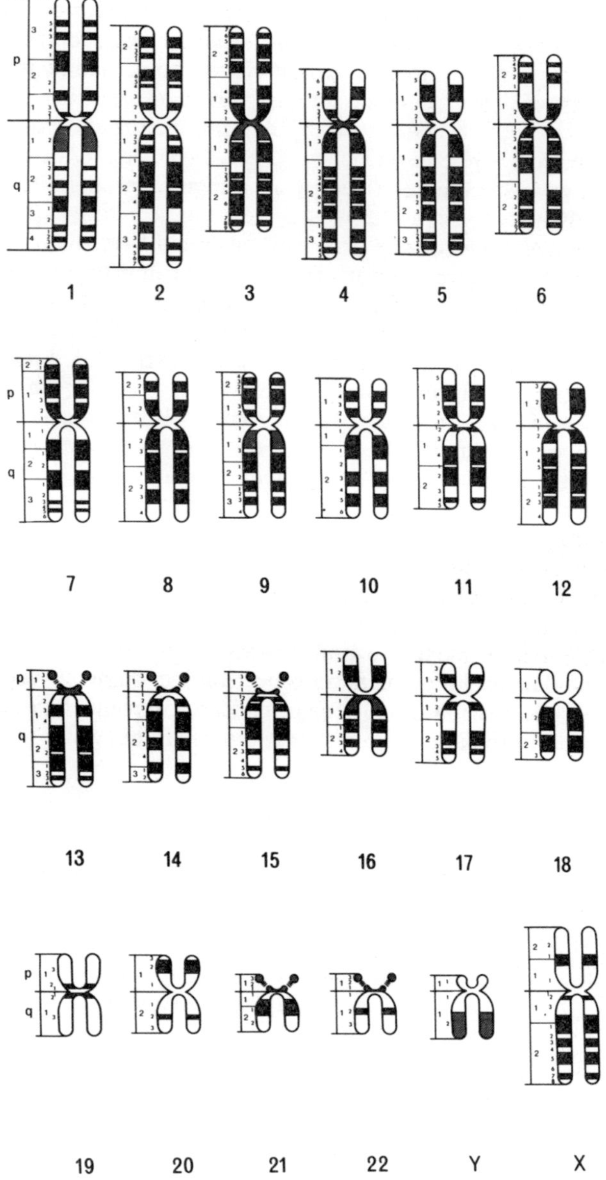

Fig. 1.2 Ideogram of the human chromosomes showing the banding pattern that allows each one to be identified. Chromosomes are analysed during division and each chromosome is shown divided into two daughter chromatids but attached at the centromere.

An internationally agreed shorthand is as follows: 'p' indicates the short arm, 'q' the long arm, and 't' a translocation. The total chromosome count is written first followed by the sex chromosome complement. A gain or loss of a whole chromosome is indicated by '+' or '−' before the number of the chromosome involved, e.g. 47XX+21 = Female Downs. A balanced reciprocal translocation between 1 and 3 would be written 46XXt(1; 3)(q32; q25), the position of the break points being described by arm, region and band for 1 and 3 respectively.

A *reciprocal translocation* occurs when two different chromosomes break simultaneously and a portion of one joins up with a portion of the other, and vice versa. Such a person has 46 chromosomes but part of two chromosomes, say a number 1 and a number 3, have been rearranged. There is no loss of genetic material and the carrier of this balanced reciprocal translocation is healthy. However, trouble can occur at meiosis, for normally just one of each homologous pair is passed on by the ovum or sperm. If the normal chromosome 1 and the normal chromosome 3 are passed on, a child with a normal chromosome complement will result. If the chromosome 1 carrying a bit of 3 and the chromosome 3 carrying a bit of 1 are passed on, a healthy child with a balanced translocation, like the parent, will result. However, if either of the other two combinations are passed on the child will have an unbalanced translocation and development can be severely disturbed. Risks vary with the particular translocation involved. A male or female carrier of a balanced reciprocal translocation ascertained because of an abnormal child has about a 20% chance of a subsequent child having an unbalanced translocation. The risk is about 5% if the carrier was picked up in some other way.

The effect of certain small constitutional deletions within a chromosome are now being delineated. Deletion of the band 11p 13 is associated with *aniridia* and *Wilms' tumour*; 13q 14 with retinoblastoma; and 15q 12 with the *Prader–Willi* syndrome.

Translocation Down's Syndrome

We have seen that primary non-disjunction is the main cause of Down's syndrome and increases with maternal age. However in about 8 to 10% of the subjects with Down's syndrome born to mothers under 30 years the extra 21 chromosome is attached by its short arm to the short arm of another acrocentric chromosome (13–15 or 21–22), usually chromosome 14. This type of fusion of two acrocentric chromosomes is termed a *Robertsonian translocation*. Thus the Down's syndrome child has 46 chromosomes, but one in fact is a composite chromosome 14^{21}.

In about a third of cases one or other parent carries the 14^{21} Robertsonian translocation. However they have only 45 chromosomes, including a normal 14, a normal 21 and the composite 14^{21}, and since they have the right amount of chromosome material they are healthy. Again the problems arise at meiosis, when the 14, the 21 and the 14^{21} chromosomes have to associate together and then segregate. Normal ova or sperm can be formed leading to normal offspring. The ova or sperm may carry the composite 14^{21} without the other 21 or 14, and produce healthy offspring carrying the translocation. Finally both the composite 14^{21} and the other 21 may pass into the ovum or sperm and a child with Down's syndrome will result. There is selection against the unbalanced gametes and a woman carrying a 14^{21} translocation has a risk of about 1 in 8 of producing a child with Down's syndrome, whilst for a man the risk is about 1 in 50.

DIRECT ANALYSIS OF DNA

Until recently the letters DNA in a patient's notes meant 'Did not attend'; increasingly it will indicate a test involving direct analysis of some of the patient's genes! The impact of the so-called 'New genetics' on clinical medicine stems from three main components: (a) the ability to isolate or construct specific sequences of DNA and clone these by exploiting the rapid replication of bacteria; (b) the fundamental discoveries concerning the organisation of human chromosomal DNA, or genome, made possible by (a); and (c) the ability to analyse certain specific genes in any individual using DNA from any tissue.

The 46 chromosomes represent a 6 000 000 000 long string of the nucleotide bases guanine, cytosine, adenine and thymine; but probably only a mere three per cent or so represent coding sequences for the body proteins. A coding sequence is 'read' in base triplets, or codons. Codons exist for the 20 amino acids and also for initiation and termination of translation. Each coding sequence for a polypeptide chain is interrupted by non-coding regions (*introns* or *intervening sequences*) which range in number from 2 in many genes to about 50 in one of the collagen genes. The blocks of coding sequence are called *exons*. The exons and introns plus short sequences at either end of the gene are all transcribed into a single stranded nuclear RNA (ribonucleic acid) molecule. Next the introns have to be carefully spliced out before the definitive messenger RNA, now with a continuous coding sequence, can move into the cytoplasm (Fig. 1.3). The term 'gene' is usefully applied to the whole transcription unit (plus sequences necessary for the initiation of transcription) for mutations anywhere in this DNA can cause a deficiency or abnormality of the gene product. In sickle-cell anaemia there is a point mutation (single base change) in the β-globin gene with the codon corresponding to the sixth amino acid GAG (glutamic acid) changed to GTG (valine). β^0-thalassaemia (complete absence of β-globin) can be due to point mutations that result in premature termination of translation; a point mutation that prevents splicing out

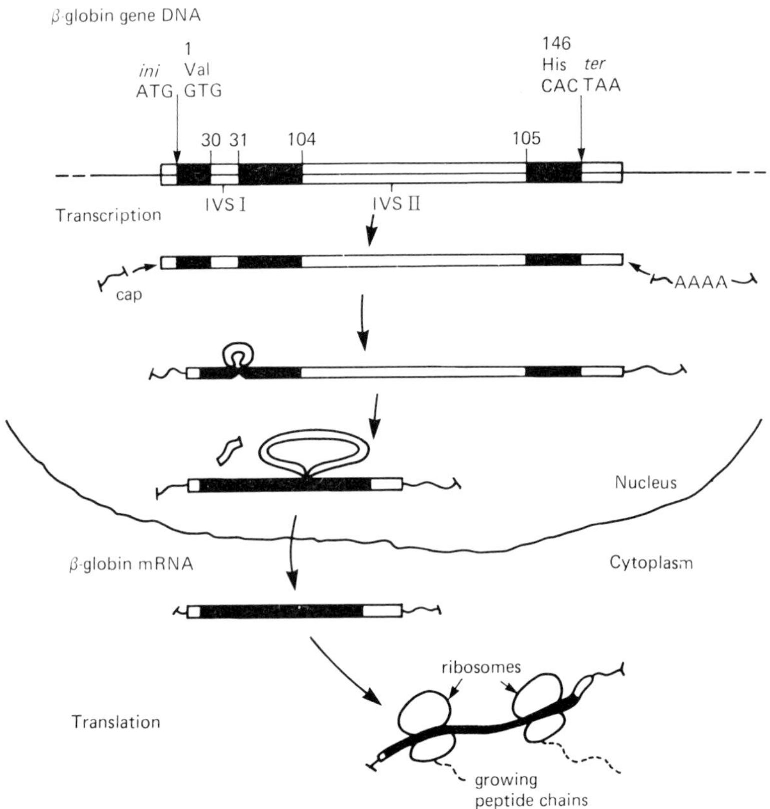

Fig. 1.3 Schematic representation of the β-globin gene and the way the gene sequence is transcribed into a nuclear RNA, which then has non-coding intervening sequences or introns (IVS I and IVS II) spliced out before passing into the cytoplasm as mRNA. The position of the initiation codon (ini), codon 1 (corresponding to the first amino acid of the β chain), codons 30, 31, 104, 105 and 146, and the terminator (ter) codon are indicated.

of the second intron; or a base deletion leading to a disasterous shift in the reading frame during translation, to name just some of the causes. β^+-thalassaemia, producing just a few normal β chains, can be due to a point mutation in the middle of the first intron that results in ambiguous splicing, with some mRNA molecules correctly assembled, but with the majority incorrectly spliced.

The discovery of this heterogeneity at the DNA level, which is likely to be even more marked in autosomal dominant and X-linked disorders, poses some problems for identification of genetic defects by direct analysis of the DNA. Elucidation of the exact point mutation or deletion in one family may tell one very little about the exact DNA defect in another family with the same clinical condition. A large deletion involving the gene, such as often occurs in α-thalassaemia, is the only type of mutation that can be simply detected; the others, in essence, require nucleotide sequencing.

Fortunately for the families with inherited disorders there are ways around the problems just mentioned. Rather than define the DNA defect within the gene, one tracks the inheritance of the particular region of chromosomal DNA that includes the gene locus. β-thalassaemia always involves the β-globin gene locus, which is situated on the short arm of chromosome 11. A homozygous affected child has inherited two number 11 chromosomes from his parents (each carrying some form of β-thalassaemia mutation); so if these two chromosomes can be distinguished from the parents' other two number 11 chromosomes, then transmission of the β-thalassaemia genes can be predicted in a future foetus. What are required are common genetic markers closely linked to the disease gene locus; in the same way that different HLA alleles can act as markers of that part of chromosome 6 that carries the 21-hydroxylase gene locus (Fig. 1.1).

One of the surprises in recent years has been the discovery that there is considerable variation in the DNA sequence between the two chromosomes of a pair. These differences are, of course, largely confined to the non-coding DNA, either the intergenic DNA between the genes, or the introns; but they can be exploited as markers for neighbouring gene loci by the use of *restriction enzymes* or *endonucleases*. There are many kinds of restriction enzyme and each cut double-stranded DNA at a specific site, a sequence of four or six nucleotides (Eco R1 cuts at the sequence GAATTC). If a DNA difference between two homologous chromosomes involves a restriction enzyme cutting site, then digestion of total DNA with that enzyme will lead to differences in the length of DNA fragments produced by the two chromosomes. These *restriction fragment length polymorphisms* can be used to track the inheritance of a disease gene in a family if each of the chromosome pair can be distinguished by its restriction fragment pattern on analysis and the disease gene is known to be closely linked to the sequence identified by the DNA probe. In this context, a DNA probe is a single stranded length of DNA labelled with ^{32}P that will hybridise with a unique complementary sequence from the human genome. The fragment with which it has hybridised can be revealed by autoradiography. A DNA probe can be either gene-specific (derived originally from mRNA for the gene product in question); or chromosome region-specific. There are already many gene-specific probes; those being introduced into clinical practice include β-globin (for β-thalassaemia and sickle-cell anaemia), α-globin (for α-thalassaemia), phenylalanine hydroxylase (for phenylketonuria), α1 antitrypsin, HPRT (for Lesch–Nyhan syndrome), and Factors VIII and IX (for Haemophilia A and B). Chromosome region-specific probes include RC8 and L1.28 that are linked to the gene locus for Duchenne muscular dystrophy.

Although the 'new genetics' is having an immediate impact as expected on the investigation of monogenic disorders, it would be wrong to imagine that its influence is limited to this group of disorders. There will be opportunities to define the main susceptibility genes in common multifactorial disease like *atherosclerosis* or *schizophrenia*, principally by asking the question—which bit of DNA is common to affected sibling pairs but not inherited by the unaffected siblings?

Another area where molecular genetics is making a dramatic contribution is in the field of cancer. The life cycle of RNA viruses includes a phase of integration into the DNA of the infected cell and it appears that, whilst roaming around the collective mammalian genome, certain viruses have picked up some cellular genes, that after various modifications, bestow the virus with tumorigenic properties. The viral DNA sequences necessary for transforming cells into a neoplastic state are called *oncogenes*. Thus with many oncogenes there are corresponding but somewhat different genes in the human genome presumably performing their regular function, although the gene products are for the most part still unknown. What are the differences between oncogenes and the human genomic equivalent (called proto-oncogenes) from which they were originally derived; and could the evolution from proto-oncogene to oncogene occur spontaneously in a human cell and thereby result in a neoplasm in the absence of a virus? In general the oncogene is characterised by a much greater rate of transcription than the proto-oncogene, and it is not difficult to see how an excess of a normal gene product might adversely influence cell behaviour. The protein encoded by a monkey sarcoma virus oncogene turns out to be closely related to platelet derived growth factor, which is important in normal healing in man. Although the relevance to human cancer is not yet established, clearly excess growth factor could be one step in the multistep path to neoplasia.

One way in which a proto-oncogene may be modified in the direction of the oncogene as it is found in tumour viruses, is by translocation to a different chromosomal location. Obvious places to start looking for support of this idea were malignancies associated with a characteristic chromosomal translocation. *Chronic myeloid leukaemia* is associated with the Philadelphia chromosome, which occurs as a result of an apparently balanced reciprocal translocation between chromosome 9 and 22. This translocation involves the human cellular equivalent (c-abl) of the transforming sequence of Abelson murine leukaemia virus. c-abl is normally situated on chromosome 9 but is moved to 22 with the translocation, and therefore may well be involved in the generation of chronic myeloid leukaemia.

It should be emphasised that viral infections per se have only been implicated in *Burkitt lymphoma* and a rare *T-cell lymphoma*. It is just that the various isolated viral oncogene sequences can act as probes to pick out the human genomic equivalents, and it is the study of these that may reveal more about the cause of human cancer. In a complete reversal of the traditional genetic approach, one starts with a bit of DNA which has been shown to be important and then aims to discover what protein it encodes and how this functions. A technological revolution that deserves the accolade 'the new genetics'.

GENETIC COUNSELLING AND PRENATAL DIAGNOSIS

The great majority of people seeking genetic counselling are couples who have had one child with an abnormality and want to know the risk to further children, and perhaps the risk to their affected child's offspring. Sometimes it is another relative, whose probability of being at risk has to be assessed from a combination of pedigree data and test results (often a complex calculation). The first responsibility is to give them as reliable an estimate of the risk as possible, and put it into perspective. In any random pregnancy the risk of any serious error of development is about 1 in 40 and this is a useful yardstick for the couple in assessing the degree of risk. Whether or not to go ahead with planning further children is clearly, in the end, the couple's own decision. The clinical geneticist should discuss the various options available including prenatal diagnosis followed by selective abortion of an affected foetus. There are some couples who will not entertain an abortion on any grounds, but there are many who see this as a way of having a healthy family. Most prenatal tests are specific, and for this reason it must be clear for what particular abnormality the foetus is at risk. In metabolic genetic disorders a precise biochemical diagnosis on the affected relative is essential before embarking on prenatal diagnosis.

Amniocentesis is done at about 16 weeks gestation, and ultrasound examination is an integral part of the process and is increasingly used to detect anatomical defects. Amniotic fluid contains cells of foetal origin and these can be cultured for chromosome or biochemical analysis. Sometimes the amniotic fluid can be used directly, for example, when measuring the α-foetoprotein level for the detection of open spina bifida.

Foetoscopy is playing an increasing role in prenatal diagnosis in the mid-trimester of pregnancy. It allows direct vision of the foetus, and facilitates sampling of blood from the foetal circulation, generally from the umbilical cord at its insertion into the placenta. Foetal blood samples allow the prenatal diagnosis of β-thalassaemia and haemophilia, although direct DNA analysis on tissue obtained by chorionic villi biopsy at 9 weeks gestation is likely to be the approach in the future. In common with all medical practice, the risk of the investigative procedure has to be taken into account and discussed fully with the patient.

In addition to prenatal diagnosis in specific families at risk, there are now two prenatal screening procedures that are available in many centres to women who wish to have them. Pregnant women of 38 years or over can be offered mid-trimester amniocentesis for chromosomal prenatal diagnosis, particularly for the exclusion of Down's syndrome. Spina bifida and anencephaly are relatively common congenital malformations in Britain, and a woman carrying an affected foetus tends to have a higher than normal serum α-foetoprotein level. Taken at 16–17 weeks gestation, the maternal serum α-foetoprotein level can be used to define an 'at risk' group, who can then be offered the definite prenatal diagnostic tests, measurement of amniotic α-foetoprotein, detection of a specific neural cholinesterase in amniotic fluid and careful ultrasound examination.

CHAPTER 2

PSYCHIATRY

INTRODUCTION

Psychiatry is concerned with difficult, distressing, or eccentric behaviour viewed from a medical aspect. The term 'behaviour' is broad, including everything people do, think, and say, and behaviour problems may arise in connection with any illness. There is no absolute division between those problems which count as 'psychiatric' and others dealt with within other branches of medicine, but psychiatrists tend to be asked to deal with the more spectacular or difficult behaviour problems. The separation of part of medicine with special interest in this field is an ancient practice which began when primitive medicine men tried to explain odd or eccentric behaviour as punishment inflicted by the Gods for misdeeds. In ancient Greece and Rome 'madness' was regarded as illness; but this idea was lost in the Middle Ages when insanity was attributed to demonic possession. By the nineteenth century humane views had revived and deluded and disturbed people were again seen as ill and in need of care.

During the past century knowledge of psychiatric disorder has increased enormously, being derived from several separate but complementary points of view. The description of clinical symptoms and signs, based on careful observation in the Hippocratic tradition, led to the identification of syndromes by Kraepelin, Bleuler and others which form the basis of current psychiatric classification. Psychological understanding was increased by the work of Freud, Jung and other psychoanalysts and latterly by contributions from social, behavioural and experimental psychologists. At the same time, developments in neurosciences have greatly increased knowledge of biological aspects of psychiatry and of drugs which may affect psychiatric illness. There has also been continuing interest in the ways in which a psychiatric patient may respond to his environment—for better or worse—both in hospital and in the community, where treatment efforts are increasingly directed.

PSYCHIATRIC ASSESSMENT

1. General

In psychiatry the task is to understand the patient and his problem, and to make sense of his behaviour. This is done by history taking and examination as elsewhere in medicine, except that in psychiatry examination is principally by observation during clinical interviewing. Clinical interviewing skills are therefore specially important in psychiatry.

Psychiatric *assessment* should be thought of as leading to *formulation*. A formulation summarises the patient's difficulties and their investigation and treatment. Formulation has five parts.

(a) *Descriptive Formulation*. This is a summary of the significant symptoms and signs (often called phenomena in psychiatry) noted on psychiatric examination. It comes first because description should precede explanation. It is not very sensible to try to explain something without clearly defining what it is that has to be explained. Thus a complaint of 'depression' for example should not just be taken at its face value, but explored in detail—it might refer, among other things, to tearfulness, worrying thoughts, indecisiveness, constipation, disturbing memories, etc. To put it another way, what the problem behaviour is should be clearly identified before attempts are made to account for it. Psychiatric examination is discussed in more detail later in this chapter.

(b) *Diagnostic Formulation*. This comes next because diagnosis in psychiatry is based upon the identification of syndromes according to agreed rules of thumb (set out in various official diagnostic manuals in general use). Syndromes are collections of phenomena, so that the psychiatric diagnosis represents a further summary of examination findings. Psychiatric diagnosis is important because it (i) is a communicable summary of examination findings, (ii) can indicate important things which the patient does *not* have, and (iii) can provide some (even though often limited) pointers towards treatment and prognosis. Diagnosis has sometimes been devalued in psychiatry by people who expect it to do what the problem formulation more appropriately does.

(c) *Problem Formulation*. One purpose of the psychiatric interview is to arrive at statements of the patient's problems which are useful in that they suggest and inform action. A similar principle underpins the problem-oriented approach developed in internal medicine by L. Weed in the USA in the early 1970s. In psychiatry the idea is to find the form of words which makes most sense of present problems to both patient and interviewer. The psychiatric interviewer should be able flexibly to approach the patient's problems in psychological, biological or social terms as seems most appropriate, and also to talk about problems in ordinary language intelligible to the patient. No single conceptual framework (brain chemistry, psychoanalysis, etc.) is appropriate in all psychiatric circumstances.

In a way, the problem formulation is like the descriptive one, in that each problem statement is a summary of observable 'things that happen'. 'Problems' are, however, broader than symptoms and signs, and although a descriptive diagnostic syndrome is sometimes also usefully called a problem (e.g. the problem of a depressive neurotic syndrome requiring treatment), many problems requiring clinical attention are not syndromes of illness. Thus a person with a depression problem may also have 'inadequate housing including poor washing facilities', 'problem of coping with educationally backward child', and 'problem of indecision about contraceptive preferences'.

(d) *Explanatory Formulation.* This is an attempt to account for the symptoms, signs, and problems which have been identified, indicating how they have arisen and how they may be linked together. This account again often needs to include psychological, biological and social aspects. The explanatory account should make sense to the interviewer and to the patient, with whom it should often be shared. For instance, the 'explanatory formulation' in a patient with a 'depression problem' might note long-standing inferiority feelings derived from childhood experience, a genetic predisposition to depression evidenced by a history of depression in a parent and grandparent, and several stressful recent events implicating the idea of loss, such as death of a pet dog, departure of a grown-up child from home, and theft of the family car.

(e) *Action Formulation.* This section summarises proposed action. It may be detailed, referring to one or more specific treatments (psychological, biological, and/or social), or general or provisional, perhaps only indicating the need for particular investigations or kinds of information still to be obtained. It is a key idea in the problem-oriented approach that problem statements should be based upon a specified data base; if the data base is incomplete then problems and action can usually only be specified generally and provisionally. If the action formulation is complete, then the data base has become sufficient.

2. History Taking

A psychiatric history is a careful account of the changes, problems, and symptoms that the patient has experienced or encountered; it is as simple as that. Sometimes students feel that psychiatric symptoms are less well defined than physical complaints, so that psychiatric history taking must be correspondingly more difficult; but this feeling can be overcome by attending sufficiently to the details of the symptoms—what they are, when and where they occur, what the experience is like, and so on—to make them well defined. It is important to remember that sometimes patients (i) are unaware of problems altogether; (ii) are unaware of the impact of their symptoms on others; (iii) minimise or even conceal symptoms; and (iv) have problems—impotence for example—which are manifest within a relationship rather than 'possessed' by an individual. For all these reasons a psychiatric history based on self-report may need to be supplemented by an account from one or more other informants—family member, spouse, friend, colleague, etc. Experience shows it is unfortunately only too easy to fail to see an informant. Time and again a clinical mystery is resolved by a meeting with a previously unseen relative.

Psychiatric symptoms involve highly personal aspects of life and often touch on experiences associated with pain, embarrassment, shame and guilt. The interviewer needs a tactful, accepting and understanding approach which allows the patient to tell his story in his own way while preventing him from straying too much from the point, and avoiding putting words into his mouth. Time is therefore required. It is simply not possible to make a detailed psychiatric assessment in a few minutes.

The history should be recorded in a formal way, but this does not mean that history *taking* should be a rigid procedure. It is usually best to allow the patient to talk as freely as possible at the start of the interview, leaving specific follow-up questions to later. The history should be set out under five headings.

(a) *Reason for Referral.* The reason for referral involves various questions:

What is the problem?

What are the symptoms that trouble the patient?

What led the patient to the doctor?

This should summarise both the presenting complaints and the means whereby the patient came to medical attention. For example, 'patient admitted to hospital after self-poisoning with aspirin, now complaining of persistent sadness, insomnia, and weight loss of three months' duration'.

(b) *History of Present Illness.* This account amplifies the presenting complaints. Special attention should be paid to details of the onset of symptoms as well as to their nature. The symptoms of psychiatric illness are often changes in degree from normal experience rather than qualitatively novel departures from it, and a degree of sadness, anxiety, etc. which may not appear excessive at interview may yet represent for the individual a change indicative of illness. Illnesses have onsets, and problems which do not have onsets—i.e. are very long-standing, more or less life-long—are usually best thought of as personality problems rather than as illnesses.

As well as inquiring about the onset, nature, and development of symptoms, the interviewer should note their temporal relations to possible precipitants. This is important because many psychiatric problems occur at least in part in response to stressful life events. Social changes—changes in interpersonal relationships, work efficiency, etc. should also be asked for and recorded, for many psychiatric disorders lead to problems of social role performance. One helpful tactic is to ask the patient to describe in detail a typical day in his life.

(c) *Family and Personal History.* The disorder must be set in its personal and social context. This involves inquiring into family background and personal biography. This inquiry naturally cannot and actually need not be prolonged and exhaustive in every case—commonsense and the time available affect the extent to which particular items should be pursued. For instance, a much briefer history is obtained during a single outpatient consultation than following a full inpatient assessment; and details of early childhood experience are usually of less immediate relevance with elderly patients than in adolescents. Nevertheless, at least some mention should be made under each heading in the following list:

(i) *Family*

1. Parents—ages, state of health, occupation;
2. Siblings—ditto;
3. Family relationships—parental discord, divorce, separation, overall evaluation of home, present status of relationships;
4. Family health—psychiatric disorder in blood relatives;
   Remember especially:
   - known inherited disorders
   - suicide
   - epilepsy
   - delinquency, including domestic violence
   - alcohol and drug abuse
   - mental handicap.

(ii) *Biography*

1. Origins—where born and brought up. Any known problems;
2. Education—age at which education stopped, academic and other attainments, general evaluation of schooldays, and psychological/behavioural problems;
3. Occupation—work record since leaving school: number of jobs, length of and reasons for periods of employment, reasons for leaving, personal evaluation of career (satisfied, bored, ambitious, etc.)

   Note: this is a most important section as much can be learned from performance in work roles and situations, and time is invariably well spent on it;
4. Health—medical and psychiatric problems and treatment. For women, also menstrual and obstetric history;
5. Relationships—friendships, psychosexual history, marital history, present domestic arrangements and current pattern of relationships within family.

(d) *Personality*. This term refers to 'the sort of person this is'. If the patient has experienced a novel set of symptoms amounting to an illness, then we are interested in what the person was like before the illness began—i.e., in the premorbid personality. However, sometimes patients do not complain of new experiences but rather seek help for longstanding aspects of themselves, i.e. for personality attributes which seem unsatisfactory in one way or another.

The assessment of personality should cover habitual patterns of personal and social behaviour, including sociability, gregariousness, and interests, and emotional responsiveness, stability, ability to cope with stressful events, general levels of drive and energy, ambitions, and moral standards. A person's self-description is often complemented usefully by the descriptions of others who know them well.

3. The Examination of Mental State

The assessment of mental state is based upon the patient's self-report and on the observations made by the interviewer of the patient's behaviour. The student will find it convenient to set out the mental state examination under five headings.

(a) *General Behaviour.* When this is extravagantly abnormal it is not hard to see that something is amiss! Often however behavioural changes are less obvious, or reported by relatives rather than by the patient personally (although sometimes subject and family all fail to notice very gradually developing abnormalities).

The observer should attend to the patient's dress, gestures, facial expression, and level of general activity, which may be increased as in states of excitement or agitation, or diminished or slowed, as in severe depression. Also, much may be learned by noting the appropriateness of the patient's behaviour to the interview situation—a patient may be flippant, aloof and unconcerned, or suspicious and on his guard. The examiner should note any failure to develop a customary sense of contact with the patient. While by no means pathognomonic, this may arise from the lack of human relating capacity found in schizophrenia, and therefore points to the possibility of this diagnosis. Schizophrenic patients sometimes display odd mannerisms (habitual expressive movements), grimace in unusual ways, or adopt odd postures.

(b) *Thought and Talk.* Notice how the patient talks, and his language. Is the talk fast or slow? Is the patient evasive or reluctant to talk? Is he circumstantial, does he drift off into irrelevancies or does he stick to the point? Is he over-talkative, or does his talk contain oddities such as puns or rhymes? Grossly abnormal speech amounting to incoherence is found in severe organic speech defects and in severe schizophrenia, where talk is sometimes fragmentary and disconnected or contains words invented by the patient (neologisms).

Disorders of thought have four aspects:

(i) *Stream.* The stream or flow of thought may be accelerated (as sometimes in states of agitation or anxiety) or slowed (e.g. in depression), or interrupted as in schizophrenic thought blocking where a train of thought stops and after a gap is replaced by a new one on a different topic (a superficially similar experience of thought stoppage occurs in normal people under stress—e.g. in oral examinations—and in anxiety states). Note that the flow of thought is usually accelerated in agitated depression and slowed in retarded depression. In severe psychomotor retardation the almost motionless patient may take 10–20 seconds plus to respond—correctly—to a simple question (though slowness of response to a question in depression may also be due to inattention, ignorance, suspicion, hostility, or preoccupation with hallucinations).

(ii) *Possession of Thought.* Some patients have disturbances of the control (or possession) of thought. Normally people feel their thoughts are their own, and are controllable; but schizophrenic patients may feel that their thoughts are inserted into their minds from without, or removed from them, or that their thoughts are known to others, or being broadcast (these symptoms of thought *insertion*, *withdrawal*, and *broadcasting* indicate that the individual is not experiencing the self as distinct from the outside world, as people normally do; the 'ego boundary' is impaired).

In contrast, the patient with *obsessional* thoughts knows the thoughts are his own, and does not feel they are inserted from outside. Obsessions include repeated, unwelcome, and subjectively resisted ideas, phrases, or acts which intrude in the patient's life in an unpleasant way (this usage of 'obsession' is distinct from the lay 'thinking a lot about' which usually refers to some welcome preoccupation).

(iii) *Form.* The form or structure of thought may be distorted. This can occur of course as a consequence of organic brain disease but among the 'functional' psychiatric disorders it is seen most characteristically in schizophrenia. A patient with this illness may lose the ability to use concepts clearly and consistently, particular difficulty occurring in the handling of abstract ideas. Trains of thought may merge imperceptibly into others, forming a sequence which leads nowhere. This is often accomplished using sentences of normal structure. A sequence of normally arranged words which convey little meaning and yet are delivered earnestly has a disconcerting effect on the listener.

(iv) *Content.* Things people think about a lot are called preoccupations. Sometimes people are preoccupied with something to an unusually intense extent, or with something which most people are unlikely to think much of; these are called overvalued ideas. They are not in themselves signs of mental illness, although psychiatric patients may have them. Overvalued ideas lack the qualities of delusions—although this is not always easily established. A delusion is a demonstrably false belief, held with absolute conviction, which is inappropriate to the person's sociocultural background. Delusions are *primary* when they arise spontaneously and cannot be understood empathically; primary delusions always suggest the diagnosis of schizophrenia, even though they may occur in some other illnesses. Sometimes delusions arise as a consequence of some other experience, most commonly a severe mood disturbance. These are *secondary* delusions. They can be understood empathically, given that the person has the prior emotional disorder. In severe depression the patient may believe he has no worth (worst person in the world, even); no bowels (body being eaten away by maggots, perhaps); and no hope (condemned to hell as a consequence of unforgivable sins, even); these are examples of *nihilistic* delusions. Persecutory and grandiose delusions of exalted status, etc., are referred to as *paranoid*. It is important to remember that paranoid delusions may occur in many illnesses, including organic disorders, affective illness, and schizophrenia; do not equate 'delusion' (or hallucination, come to that) with 'schizophrenia'.

(c) *Emotion.* Feelings are notoriously hard to describe; the range of words applicable to feeling is so great that it is rarely possible to sum up a patient's feelings in a single sentence. The most useful tactic is to gauge the prevailing emotional state of the patient. Many psychiatric syndromes are associated with extensive change of mood. Sadness, misery, dejection, pessimism and an overall feeling of unhappy wretchedness are commonplace in psychiatric disorders, particularly depression, but they are also found in other syndromes, e.g. in organic mental states.

It is important to assess whether the patient's emotional state is appropriate to the rest of his mental condition and whether it is constant or variable. Shallow emotional responses and lability of mood are other features to look out for—they can occur in organic mental states and in schizophrenia. Many patients are apathetic and say that they have lost all feeling. Others may be unnaturally elated, breezy or euphoric, whilst others may describe states of bliss or ecstasy. These latter exalted feelings are found in mania and in schizophrenia whilst episodic ecstatic states must raise the suspicion of temporal-lobe epilepsy.

It is helpful to think of feelings as having three components (see Fig. 2.1). When they speak about feelings, people sometimes refer to behaviour, sometimes to physiology, and sometimes to cognitive–subjective aspects. They may also refer simultaneously to any two components, or to all three. Hence 'depression' may mean sadness and hopelessness (subjective); immobility and gloomy expression (motor–behavioural); constipation, insomnia, and suicidal thoughts (physiological and subjective). In assessing mood the examiner should note which components of emotion are involved, and how they contribute to the clinical picture.

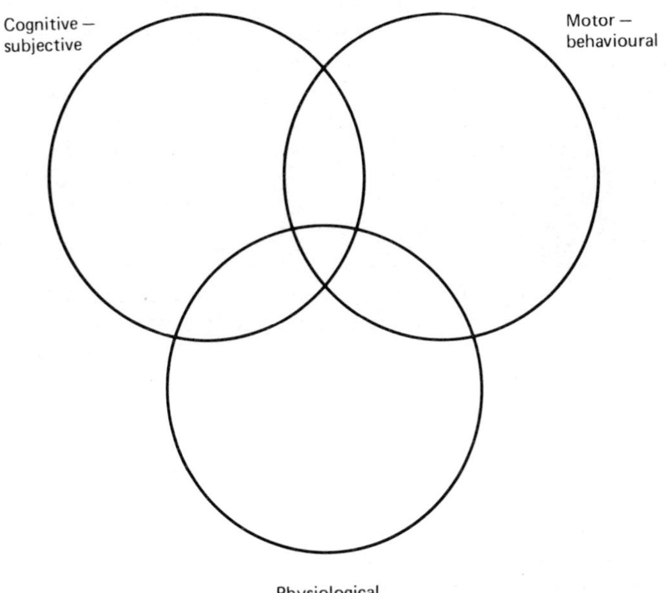

Fig. 2.1 Components of a feeling.

(d) *Perception.* The collection of sense data from all modalities—perception—is the basis of interaction with the environment. Perceptions may be heightened or dulled as in some toxic and delusional states or under the influence of hallucinogenic drugs. Illusions are distortions of environmental stimuli which can occur in states of fatigue and drug intoxication as well as in organic mental states and in schizophrenia. Hallucinations are perceptions which occur in the absence of an outside stimulus. Hallucinations do not always signify mental illness—they can for instance occur after prolonged sensory deprivation and while going to sleep (hypnogogic) and waking up (hypnopompic hallucination).

Hallucinations may arise in any sense modality but hallucinations of taste, smell, and touch are much less common than auditory and visual ones. Visual hallucinations suggest an organic mental disorder although they also occur in schizophrenia. Auditory hallucinations occur in many mental illnesses; but complex voices including third-person conversations about the subject, or commentaries on his actions, are uncommon except in schizophrenia.

(e) *Cognitive Functions.* Cognition is the means by which information is stored and retrieved. To test it involves giving simple formal tests of memory, general information, concentration and orientation for time and place. Cognitive function is always impaired in organic mental states. If there is disorientation and loss of recent memory, then the patient has some cerebral malfunction.

(i) *Orientation.* This includes orientation for time, for place, and for person. Test it by asking the patient to give the day, date, and time of day. Also make sure that he knows where he is. Remember that disorientation often fluctuates in organic states and may be marked at one assessment and absent a few hours later. Repeated observations are therefore very useful. In hospital cases, nurses' records are invaluable.

(ii) *Memory.* Give the patient a name and address. Ask him to repeat it and then ask him to reproduce it in five minutes. This is a simple but useful test of the ability to register, retain and reproduce recently learnt material. Ask about the activities of the day before.

(iii) *Concentration.* Ask the patient to subtract 7 from 100 and go on subtracting—again a simple but useful test.

(iv) *General Information.* Usually this can be assessed in interview, but if there is any doubt a good simple test is to ask the patient to name the capitals of six countries, the names of six large cities, the names of prominent public figures, etc.

(v) *Intelligence.* This can also usually be assessed in interview, and educational attainment is a pointer; or tests of intelligence may be informative.

(vi) *Insight.* Ask the patient if he feels that he is ill in any way. The object is to find out not only whether the patient is aware of his illness but also to find out whether he has a reasonable idea of its extent and implications. The importance of this heading is to draw attention to the way the patient's view of the problem(s) resembles or differs from that of the examiner.

Comment. Not every patient needs full cognitive assessment, but it is essential when there is any suspicion of physical illness. So of course are physical examination and whatever medical investigations may be indicated by it.

CLASSIFICATION

In the past there has been considerable disagreement about psychiatric diagnostic classifications. However the situation has been easier to understand since the 8th Edition of the *International Classification of Diseases* (published in the late 1960s) enshrined the principle that psychiatric disorders should be defined as syndromes (i.e. as collections of clinical phenomena). No classificatory system based on some other principle such as aetiology is justified in the present state of our knowledge. The current 9th Edition has evolved from the 8th which it resembles. Improved classificatory systems are being developed to accommodate psychiatric problems as they present in general practice; and the current system formed in the USA (DSM III, short for Diagnostic and Statistical Manual of Mental Disorder, 3rd Edition) differs somewhat from the ICD. The main diagnostic classes in psychiatry cover groups of recognisable disorders and the student should satisfy himself that he understands what each class includes. Following sections deal in order with affective disorders; schizophrenia; neuroses; personality disorders; and organic disorders.

AFFECTIVE DISORDERS

Affective disorders are all characterised by a primary disturbance of mood with symptoms in the areas of cognition, behaviour, and bodily functioning. There are polar extremes of affective disorder which range from intense excitement and elation (mania and hypomania) to severe depressive states. The term '*manic–depressive psychosis*' was originally given to these disorders, but is nowadays best restricted to cases in which episodes of elevation of mood (i.e. hypomania) and depression both occur. Another name for this is 'bipolar affective disorder', a term which emphasises the distinction from unipolar illnesses characterised by recurrent episodes of disturbance at one affective pole only. Unipolar illnesses are usually depressions—recurrent mania with no episodes of depression is extremely rare. The term 'psychosis' lingers, but is obsolete; the majority of depressives are not psychotic in the sense of being out of contact with reality. Nowadays 'psychotic' means little more than that a lay person might think the person was 'mad'. Likewise, the associated term 'neurotic' means little more than 'worrying' or 'upset'.

DEPRESSION

In depression a person becomes persistently sad and unhappy but the disturbance exceeds in intensity and duration the everyday shades of feeling and emotional response that colour human life. Abnormally depressed mood is disproportionate to any cause, real or fancied. The intensity or duration of the feeling may lead family and friends soon to recognise that something is wrong, perhaps before the patient does. Depression may come on suddenly or insidiously; and it may become chronic.

Depression occurs in three major kinds of illness—in bipolar affective disorder, in unipolar affective disorder, and as depressive neurosis. The diagnosis of bipolar illness cannot be made until and unless hypomanic and depressive episodes have both occurred. Patients with depression only may be classified as having either unipolar affective illness or depressive neurosis. These can be defined as distinct syndromes, but many patients are difficult to allocate to one or other category, and seem to have characteristics of both (the student may encounter the terms 'endogenous depression' and 'psychotic depression' and should regard these as synonyms for 'unipolar affective disorder').

Although neurotic depressives are often extremely distressed, most severely depressed (and never manic) patients tend to be classed as having unipolar affective disorder, because the marked biological and cognitive phenomena often thought to be characteristic of 'endogenous' depression are often simply a consequence of the severity of the mood disturbance. Some clinicians prefer a single diagnostic category, 'depressive illness'. However, the trouble with such a broadly defined class is that distinct depressive syndromes certainly occur. The writer's approach is to reserve 'unipolar' depression for patients in whom cognitive and biological features (see below) are marked, and to refer to other illnesses as neuroses, recognising that distinct syndromes may be recognisable within this class (also see below). (It is important to remember that the term 'reactive', which often enters this discussion, applies equally to manic-depressive, unipolar, and neurotic depressions, in the same sense that episodes of all of them may be precipitated by ('reactive' to) stressful life events.)

Aetiology. A genetic factor operates in unipolar affective psychosis (depressive or mania) and in bipolar affective psychoses (i.e. manic-depressive). These psychoses breed true, show a definite family incidence and a high concordance rate in monozygotic twins. Certain races, e.g. the Irish and Jewish people, are more prone to affective disorders than others. Also physical build is important: the endomorph with small hands and feet and large visceral cavities is more liable to affective illness. Brain biochemistry is important. Current theory stresses the importance of CNS transmitters—the catecholamines, dopamine and noradrenaline and the indoleamine, 5 hydroxytryptamine (5HT or serotonin)—as being involved in depression when their concentration in the hypothalamus and brainstem is decreased. Medication produces higher concentration and relief of depression, but the mechanism is not fully understood (see psychopharmacology).

Life events such as bereavement, moving house or losing a job, etc., can all contribute to depression. Also certain physical illnesses such as jaundice and virus infections can set off depression. The same is true of various drugs including reserpine, methyldopa, the sulphonamides, phenobarbitone and 'the pill'.

Social and family influences are hard to pinpoint, but there is at least more than a suggestion that loss of a parent in early childhood can lead to depression much later. An unduly strict and repressive family climate can mould children into depression-prone adults whose aggressive feelings cannot be expressed but can only be turned inwards.

Clinical Features.

Mood. Mood disturbance is usually prominent and may be described in terms of despair, pessimism, sadness, gloom, solemnity, apathy, hopeless self scrutiny and tearfulness—in short a range of feeling that cannot easily be summarised. Mood change may be constant or show diurnal variation and may have lost the responsiveness of normal moods to outside events.

Behaviour. This is often slow, faltering, and weary. Psychomotor retardation refers to a slowing of movement (and thought process) issuing from what amounts to inhibition of cerebral control processes. Retardation is shown by slowing of all movements and by delay in producing answers to all questions—the answers when they do come are to the point, if brief. Retardation is roughly opposite to agitation, wherein psychic and motor processes are accelerated, leading to restless pacing, continual wringing of hands, pressured distressed talk, and so on; psychomotor agitation amounts to half-organised worried over-activity. It is helpful to note the presence and predominance of retardation or agitation.

Thought Process. This is slow in retardation, and accelerated in agitation. Slowness is usually associated with poverty of thought—i.e. thinking few thoughts. In depression, concentration is poor because the patient is preoccupied. The memory performance may be poor, either because the patient feels too wretched to pay attention to what is going on, or because memory function has actually been impaired—presumably by some inhibitory process—as is particularly likely in elderly depressives, who often give the impression of being demented.

Thought Content. There is a cognitive triad in depression of helplessness, hopelessness and worthlessness, representing negative attitudes to one's capacity to act effectively on the environment, to the future and to self-evaluation. These negative attitudes should be sought whenever depression is in question, for they not only occur in response to disappointing, painful, or otherwise disturbing life events, but also tend to prevent the person from helping himself. The thought content of the depressive should be thought of as a long list of negatives—no help, no worth, no hope, no good, no health, no future, no interest, no energy, no God, no bowels, no enjoyment. Severely depressed patients may develop delusions, which may be hypochondriacal (delusions concerned with health matters), nihilistic ('nothing' ideas, as above, taken to a delusional degree), of guilt, or (less commonly) paranoid. Happily, the severest depressions in which these delusions arise are not often seen nowadays. Querulous and hypochondrial behaviour in depression may obscure the real diagnosis. It is the sense of badness about self and perhaps also others and the world which may lead to suicidal thoughts and intent in depression.

Perception. In depression a person sees the whole world in a dull light. Pleasant experience is no longer so, everything looks grey and lacklustre. In severe psychotic depression the patient can experience auditory hallucinations, usually voices that condemn him—the voice of the devil, etc. These symptoms are rare, since nowadays treatment starts early, but they occasionally occur in elderly people.

Insight. Is always impaired in depression. No depressed person is able to judge himself sensibly. He may appear to agree that he is ill, while knowing how bad it all is and that the doctor is wrong. This type of insightlessness can lead to suicide.

Other Symptoms. Depression can affect any aspect of personal functioning. Hence a wide range of symptoms can arise. Remember to inquire about:

(a) sleep disturbances—particularly early waking and lying awake;
(b) loss of energy, interest, volition—apathy and inertia;
(c) loss of appetite;
(d) hypochondriacal bodily complaints—especially involving bowels, abdominal churning, pains and headache;
(e) sexual dysfunctions and loss of sexual interest;
(f) irritability, anxiety and tension;
(g) indecision and self-doubt;
(h) deteriorating personal relationships and work performance;
(i) general malaise;
(j) self-neglect;
(k) suicidal thought, talk, and behaviour;
(l) recent abuse of alcohol or drugs.

These symptoms are easily overlooked. Many are non-specific in that they are found in physical illness, but when viewed as a whole they add up to the picture of depression. It is still the case that a patient can be extensively investigated while the diagnosis of depression is missed, because the one symptom is followed up and the patient is ignored.

Diagnosis. Apart from mood disturbance, the key symptoms to look for include general symptoms of lost function as outlined above. Depressive states are inevitably coloured by the individual's premorbid personality; the irritable person gets more irritable, the histrionic person becomes more demonstrative and unstable. The history should point out any precipitating events. Bereavement is a typical and important example. Mourning can merge into depression. Normal mourning is a healthy reaction to loss but is generally self-limiting in that people come to accept loss and adjust to normal living. However, if mourning extends for months it is more than likely to be abnormal. Space does not permit a full examination of normal and abnormal grief, but a good rule is that someone who is still grief-stricken after six months is depressed. In chronic and painful physical illness, true depression is hard to diagnose, since anyone in pain feels unhappy and lacks zest—a state of unhappy malaise that is sometimes called dysphoria.

Schizophrenia. Early mood change is always overtaken by basic schizophrenic symptoms: thought disorder, delusions, etc.

Organic Cerebral Disease. May cause diagnostic difficulty especially in middle-aged depressives who do not respond to treatment. Organic brain disease may then be suspected. Inevitably if organic brain disease is present it will cause memory and intellectual defect. It is wrong to diagnose organic brain disease without evidence.

Personality Disorders. Unstable people frequently are unhappy after personal crises, but their mood disturbance, though colourful, is labile.

Physical Illness. May mimic depression and vice versa. Important illnesses to look out for include myxoedema, Parkinson's disease, and pernicious anaemia.

Treatment.

Hospital treatment is most likely to be used for suicidal, elderly, and physically neglected patients. The most severely depressed patients require inpatient admission, but many depressives are better treated as day patients based at home but attending hospital during the day, so long as the domestic environment is supportive and supported by the staff. Most less severe depressives are treated as hospital outpatients or without hospital referral by general practitioners.

Psychological Measures. Sympathetic supportive acceptance of the depressive's painful predicament is essential. While depressed, people are often intensely sensitive to the feelings and attitudes of others. Breezy admonitions to 'pull yourself together' are unhelpful and usually interpreted by the depressive as lack of understanding and real concern.

Apart from this general psychological approach which is always important, specific psychological treatments are sometimes indicated. These are sometimes called cognitive therapies because they focus on ways of altering the depressive's negative ideas and attitudes. Also, marital or family therapy may be indicated where depression is intimately related to domestic or relationship problems. At present, all these specific therapies are applied to cases referred to specialist centres rather than to those treated in general practice.

Physical Treatment. The basic physical treatments of depression used nowadays are antidepressant drugs and of these the tricyclic series are the most widely used. Electroconvulsive therapy (ECT) is valuable in severe cases, and there is a definite but restricted place for monoamine oxidase inhibitors (MAOIs).

Prognosis. In general the prognosis is good. Acute onset favours speedy recovery and insidious onset suggests chronicity. Relapse is common and for this reason depressed patients often need long-term supervision.

General Comments. Depression is common, and is a disagreeable and wretched state to endure. There is no justification for waiting for spontaneous remission or letting the patient 'work through' depression. Once a patient begins to feel better with treatment he sees his problem in a more sensible light. The most important thing is to recognise depression and do something about it.

MANIA AND HYPOMANIA

Both of these are much rarer than depression.

Mania is a state of high elation and uncontrollable excitement. Psychomotor overactivity is excessive. The patient is noisy, bounds with energy and ebullient high spirits. Grandiose delusional ideas are common and the patient's clothing may be covered in fantastic decoration. Often there is a paranoid colouring and the breezy elation turns to rage. Talk is so fast and overloaded with content as to be disorganised, though connected by rhymes, puns and jokes, etc.

Hypomania is less severe than mania and more common. The onset may be sudden, or gradual and hard to date. The symptoms are sometimes an exaggeration of the patient's personality characteristics—he may always be more cheery and energetic than his fellows, gregarious, hardworking and the 'life and soul of the party'. In hypomania an acceptable level of energy, self-confidence, elation and wakefulness develop into restless overactivity, the patient perhaps becoming a talkative, importunate nuisance, doing too much, overspending, and being boastful and rude, scorning advice. Patients may need to be protected from the socially damaging consequences of hypomanic disinhibition which can lead to financial, sexual, or occupational indiscretions.

Diagnosis. The differential diagnosis of any state of excitement includes schizophrenia, affective psychosis, and organic states (including intoxication). In states of extreme excitement, peculiarly schizophrenic symptoms may be hard to elicit; time and medication usually clarify the picture.

The acute excitement of delirious states is distinguishable by the clouding of consciousness that is a characteristic feature. Manic episodes may herald neuropsychiatric disorders such as general paresis or encephalitis. Intoxication with alcohol, barbiturate, hallucinogens (LSD) and amphetamine can cause states of excitement resembling hypomania.

It should also be noted that overactive excited states also occur as stress reactions in some cultures in which vigorous physical activity is socially sanctioned. These acute disorders have been reported in some Asian cultures and in the West Indies, for instance, and immigrants in the UK sometimes present with acute noisy excited overactivity superficially resembling hypomania or schizophrenia when the diagnosis is really a culture-influenced stress reaction.

Treatment. Manic patients need admission to hospital because of their wild exhausted state. Compulsory admission may be needed (see Mental Health Act) because manic and hypomanic patients are often unwilling to accept help, at least until repeated episodes have taught greater insight and led to continuing contact with health services.

Physical treatments are vital. For the acute attack, the neuroleptics are the first line of treatment—usually the phenothiazines and haloperidol. For prophylaxis, continuous lithium therapy is vital. Lithium treatment needs proper medical monitoring.

Prognosis. The prognosis for manic and hypomanic episodes is good; episodes are usually short lived, but they are also recurrent. If lithium is tolerated and effective, episodes can be reduced in duration or intensity, or perhaps even prevented altogether.

SCHIZOPHRENIA

Schizophrenia is a syndrome of personality change and other symptoms, which tends to start in early adult life and which can lead to a severe disintegration of personality. Some symptoms are relatively specific, e.g. primary delusions, thought disorder, hallucinosis and social withdrawal. The illness always occurs in clear consciousness. The personality change is global and recovery, though often apparently complete, is rarely so. This makes diagnosis crucial since diagnosis implies a prognosis.

Aetiology. The notion of there being one cause for schizophrenia is now discarded in favour of a multifactorial aetiology which encompasses biological, psychological, family interaction and sociocultural factors as playing complementary roles in determining the probability of the illness occurring.

Biological Factors. The incidence in the general population is 0.85%. In Britain the admission rate for schizophrenia over the last 25 years has been around 15–20 first admissions per 100 000 psychiatric admissions per year. *Genetic inheritance* is important in that certain families do breed true, but 60% of schizophrenics have no family history. In the family of a schizophrenic the expected incidence may be as high as:

Parents	5–10%
Children	8–16%
Full siblings	10%

It was formerly said that concordance rates in monozygotic twins was as high as 90% but this has been refuted—the figure is probably 60 %. *Age* is important—most cases start early.

Biochemical and Metabolic Factors. Despite intensive searching for toxic, metabolic, serological and endocrine factors, there are really few hard data. Much contemporary research involves brain biochemistry.

One hypothesis is that in schizophrenia the brain produces an abnormal central transmitter in response to stress stimuli and that the build-up of the substance causes the symptoms in the same way that hallucinogenic drugs and amphetamines trigger off 'model' psychoses. *Temporal lobe epilepsy* is frequently associated with schizophrenic psychoses; this suggests a link between the TLE and the psychosis that is stronger than mere chance association.

Personality and Constitution. Many have commented on the asthenic body build of chronic schizophrenics and have described a premorbid personality—a schizoid personality characterised by aloofness, seclusiveness, shyness, emotional coolness and detachment. This is true but leaves unexplained the 50 per cent of schizophrenics who have a perfectly normal premorbid personality.

Psychological Factors. The original description of schizophrenia by Bleuler stressed the importance of 'loosening of thought processes', emotional incongruity and personality disintegration, but these were descriptions of the mental state rather than explanations of causality. Some psychological theories have postulated a basic perceptual disorder, and others have suggested a malfunction of learning processes.

Psychodynamic theories relate the development of schizophrenia to defects in the parent–child relationship in early life, causing faulty psychological maturation and hence psychosis in a specially vulnerable personality.

Life events have been shown to bear a significant relationship to onset and relapse (e.g. moving house, death of spouse, promotion, etc.).

Family Interaction and Social Factors. Sociologists and anthropologists have examined schizophrenic families and presented a number of theories. For example:

(a) Schizophrenic families use odd eccentric modes of communication which set up impossible conflicts in weaker family members who are victims of an ambiguous communication net.

(b) Schizophrenic parents use incomprehensible ways of relating to their children, e.g. the 'double-bind' situation where a child is ordered to obey a negative injunction and threatened with punishment whatever happens. This leads him to adopt immobile withdrawal as a form of self-preservation, which is then called 'psychosis'.

(c) The family may be a malign influence which edges the person into psychosis as an escape from a family which has selected one member for a psychotic role.

(d) Schizophrenia probably occurs more commonly in lower socio-economic groups than in higher, but in addition it is easier for a person in the lower end of the social scale to be diagnosed as schizophrenic.

(e) In certain countries schizophrenia is diagnosed casually, and the 'diagnosis' is used to 'treat' 'social deviants' and 'political extremists'.

Comment. Schizophrenia is likely to be a heterogenous mixture of syndromes with no unitary cause. The aetiologies so far mentioned are not mutually exclusive.

Clinical Features. Schizophrenia seems to be a useful label for syndromes with fairly definite symptoms and a poor prognosis. Schizophrenic symptoms can never be *understood* in the same way as depressive symptoms and they are never a logical reaction to a life experience. Specific symptoms include disturbances of form, content, and possession of thought; behavioural disorders; emotional disorders; and perceptual abnormalities. These phenomena are often accompanied by disabling changes in the way the person functions as a whole human being. The personality changes, giving the impression of fragmentation of mental faculties that, in health, function as a unity. Drive and impetus may be lost, and the person fails to initiate or complete sequences of goal-directed behaviour, so that purposeless social drifting ensues.

Delusion has already been defined. The true (or primary) delusion may arise out of the blue or be preceded by a premonitory feeling of unusual awareness or impending revelation or disaster. Once established, it is maintained with extraordinary conviction. Schizophrenic primary delusions may be grandiose, paranoid or hypochondriacal, and are sometimes bizarre. There maybe a conviction of being singled out in a special way. Schizophrenics may also have secondary delusions which are attempts to explain odd perceptions or feelings.

Form and possession of thought have also been discussed. Formal thought disorder refers to a basic flaw in conceptual thought which impairs reasoning. There may be thought blocking, knight's move thinking indicating abnormal connections between concepts, and the introduction of neologisms, new words invented by the patient. Thought disorder may be more evident in writing than in speech. Thought insertion, withdrawal and broadcasting are also important schizophrenic symptoms.

Behaviour Disorders. Many patients develop stiff awkward movements and strange symbolic movements which they repeat (stereotyped movement). They may become mute and stuporose—rare since physical treatment has been possible. Excitement and uncontrolled aggression can also occur—again rare nowadays. Rarely too a schizophrenic can get fixed in a weird posture with sluggish stiff limbs (waxy flexibility). Again some schizophrenics may behave impulsively and act in an inexplicable way without warning, e.g. shouting, violence or suicide. A common symptom is the feeling that the body is under outside influence or control—passivity feelings.

Emotional Disorder. Often in the early stages a patient feels unaccountably anxious and vaguely depressed. Others feel strangely blissful or ecstatic or feel that something is about to happen or be revealed. The most typical emotional abnormality is an incongruity between feeling and experience (e.g. laughing at bad news), but generally the incongruity is less extreme. Emotional responses are lowered and the patient becomes detached, cool, aloof, uninvolved and totally absorbed in his inner life. This comes across as a lack of empathy—like a pane of glass between him and others.

Perception. Perceptual disturbances occurring in schizophrenia include distortions and misinterpretations of sensory stimuli, and hallucinations. As previously noted, auditory hallucinations are the most common (though schizophrenics may also have visual hallucinations, even though these should suggest the possibility of organic disorder). Auditory hallucinatory phenomena include whispers, whistles and murmurs as well as the more familiar voices. Voices may be instructive or abusive, but these are not specific and it is voiced thoughts (hearing one's own thoughts spoken aloud), voices commenting on one's actions, and voices referring to the self in the third person, which should particularly suggest schizophrenia.

Clinical Types. Traditionally, four types are described—simple, hebephrenic, paranoid, and catatonic. However, although some patients are constantly typical of one type, other patients show features of different types at different phases of a continuing illness.

Simple. This type starts early and insidiously. Florid symptoms are few; the usual picture is of a fall-off in activity, thought and feeling. The patient is unaware of symptoms; it is the family who complains that he has slipped into inert self-neglect. Talk is sparse, answers are scanty or abrupt and there is a general impression of poverty of thought and emotion. The prognosis is bad: the patient may end up as a long-term patient, or at best a rather dull, empty person doing simple jobs under careful supervision.

Hebephrenic. Onset is usually insidious in late adolescence. The clinical picture is dominated by severe thought disorder, emotional incongruity and auditory hallucinations. Personality disintegration is extensive. A typical end point is one where the patient is fatuous, euphoric, buffoonish and thought-disordered. The prognosis is bad.

Paranoid. Onset is usually late (30–45) with paranoid delusions often very complicated (systematised) in the forefront. The delusions are often persecutory, though grandiose and exalted ideas are also common. The personality is well preserved, so the patient is better able to survive in the community. Drive and energy may be high and encourage the patient to act on his delusions in a forceful way. Thought disorder is hard to detect and paranoid schizophrenics are skilful in concealing paranoid content. Survival in the community is less easy if the delusions become too forcefully expressed, leading to acute crises caused by psychotic outbursts. The prognosis is generally better than in other schizophrenias since the personality is relatively well preserved. Emotionally the paranoid schizophrenic is remote, even callous, but inevitably absorbed in his delusions to the exclusion of everyone and everything else.

Catatonic. This type is comparatively rare nowadays. Onset is usually acute with either excitement or a quickly developing state of stupor. Early symptoms include odd gestures, stiff movements and weird postures. Catatonic excitement is severe to the extent of disorganised restlessness which may be aggressive or self-destructive. Bizarre acts and postures, and also echo reactions (mechanical repetition of the words or actions of the examiner) can occur as well as fixed rigid postures leading to stupor. This state requires total nursing care—feeding, washing, etc.—though ECT and neuroleptic drugs have made stupor and violent excitement short-lived and rare events.

Note on Social 'Symptoms'. Traditional descriptions of schizophrenia emphasised clinical mental state abnormalities found in hospital patients. More recently it has become clear that the 'clinical' state of the schizophrenic is in part a response to the social environment. Schizophrenics are prone to demoralisation, social withdrawal and careless personal care as a response to a dehumanised environment as can exist in a large institution such as a hospital or prison. Patients are also prone to acute symptomatic outbursts in response to socially overstimulating situations, as can arise with relatives with whom they are in serious conflict. Also a demoralised institutionalised state can persist in schizophrenics who are not in any institution but at large in communities in which they find they cannot fit. Much of the continuing distress of schizophrenics and their relatives derives not from 'mad' experiences—which may be private, or in abeyance—but from social difficulties. Assessment of a schizophrenic must include evaluating functioning (1) at work, and (2) at home; in relationships with (3) family, (4) colleagues, and (5) friends; and in relation (6) to accepted norms of good manners (self-care).

Diagnosis. The diagnosis of schizophrenia need not be difficult. The first step is to see if characteristically schizophrenic experiences have occurred. These 'first-rank' symptoms include ego-boundary disturbances (thought withdrawal, etc.); passivity experiences; ideas of influence; and certain kinds of auditory hallucinations, as already noted.

If first-rank symptoms are present, then the patient has probably either an organic schizophrenia-like psychosis, or schizophrenia. Many organic illnesses can occasionally cause a schizophrenia-like state, but amphetamine intoxication and temporal lobe epilepsy are specially important. These physical disorders are investigated in the usual way.

If first-rank symptoms are absent, then the patient may still have schizophrenia. First-rank symptoms are positive, active, experiences; many schizophrenics have positive symptoms only episodically or transiently, the chronic clinical picture being dominated by negative phenomena such as loss of emotional responsiveness, apathy, and social withdrawal. When a patient has negative symptoms, consideration of the course of the illness as a whole may clearly indicate the diagnosis.

Affective illnesses may resemble schizophrenic pictures, but are recognised by the primary mood disorder, and delusions can be understood as secondary to this; the form of thought is not disordered. Acute psychotic episodes in people with personality disorders and in people from different cultures may also resemble schizophrenia. Emphasis is again on the understandability of the relationship between moods and symptoms, and between symptoms and environmental difficulties (life events). In old age, paranoid symptoms are common and may be caused by organic illnesses or depression rather than by paranoid schizophrenia. This last illness is often very indolent and chronic in elderly people and sometimes called late paraphrenia. At any age, the occurrence of paranoid symptoms as the main mental problem should first suggest an organic psychiatric state rather than a schizophrenic illness.

Treatment. The aims of treatment include relief of distressing symptoms and the preservation of contact with reality, so as to return the patient as speedily as possible to normal social function. Aetiology is unclear, so causes cannot be treated, on the other hand aggravating factors can be modified, e.g. in family relationships, at work, etc.

Physical treatment. This consists mainly of the use of neuroleptic drugs which calm agitation, block hallucinosis and help the person to think more clearly and feel more at ease (see psychopharmacology). ECT is used mainly to shorten periods of excitement or if there is associated depression. For maintenance treatment, long-acting depot injections of phenothiazines (e.g. fluphenazine enanthate) are of value but require careful supervision.

Psychosocial treatment. A long stay in hospital can be harmful, encouraging institutionalism. Physical treatments make for earlier return to the community, where treatment has to be energetic, particularly in psychological and social aspects. The recovering patient may find the world and his family strange and unfamiliar, and the pace of life overstimulating and difficult to cope with; and relatives may find the patient odd, withdrawn, unpredictable, or frightening. Hence patient and relatives need understanding support and opportunities to discuss their questions, aspirations and worries. Social rehabilitation means enabling the patient to make best use of his residual capacities and assets, and a rehabilitation program will be needed based on an assessment of capacities and disabilities. Some patients for instance find post-illness slowness a major work disability; others are greatly disabled by unrealistic aspirations to achieve goals which are no longer open to them. The maintenance in the community requires coordinated hospital and community-based services and a high level of multiprofessional team work, often involving social worker, occupational therapist, community psychiatric nurse, clinical psychologist, and doctor. It is important to remember that schizophrenic patients require time for counselling and advice—it is a mistake to think that the schizophrenic requires nothing but medication. Patients and their relatives may need much thoughtful supportive counselling and some schizophrenic symptoms respond to specific psychological treatments. At the same time intensive deep psychotherapy is rarely helpful and may make schizophrenics worse.

Outcome. Hebephrenic and simple schizophrenia have the worst prognosis. Acute onset and onset following some obvious precipitant are good points. Insidious onset and low IQ are bad points. Approximately 50% of first admissions have no relapse; of the remainder, half do relatively well and the rest do badly. But all of the 'relapsers' show permanent personality change.

THE NEUROSES

Neuroses are very common. In a practice with 3000 patients, a general practitioner can expect about 30 new cases of depression in a year, and will probably have about 6 schizophrenics in the practice population. But he can expect roughly 10–20% of all his consultations to be about neurotic disorders. These are often accompanied by social and family problems. Neuroses can be extremely unpleasant and severe neurotic illnesses are among the most disabling afflictions to which man is heir. However, most neuroses are mild. Neurotic symptoms are part of everyone's experience, and the phenomena of neurotic illnesses are not qualitatively abnormal. What is meant by neurotic *illnesses* is that unpleasant experiences are more intense or more long lasting than they are ordinarily. So neurotic illness feelings differ from normal ones in intensity and/or duration. However, figures for neuroses in general practice sometimes include not only patients with neurotic illness as just defined, but also patients with less intense or less prolonged (but still disagreeable) feelings who attend doctors because they cannot (or feel they cannot) cope. Patients often lack the sort of family and neighbourhood network which sustains most people in times of stress. Sometimes their personality seems less than averagely resistant to adversity.

Of the various theories that have been advanced to account for neurosis, two are specially important. The first explains neurotic behaviour as maladaptive reaction to faulty upbringing and arrested emotional development based on early childhood experience. This would broadly summarise the psychodynamic theory. The other theoretical model is that neuroses are learned maladaptive responses—symptoms of faulty learning that have no unconscious dynamic significance. Others have suggested an existentialist basis for neurosis—the fear of 'non-being'. No theory is entirely satisfactory; the clinician may find an eclectic view most helpful.

Some symptoms are common in all neuroses. These include low energy, a feeling of malaise, worries about coping, insomnia, aches and pains, concern about relationships with others, and feelings of anxiety and tension. Naturally, these common symptoms do not distinguish one neurosis from another. Each neurosis is a syndrome defined by the phenomena which dominate the clinical picture. The most important syndromes are anxiety and phobic neuroses; depressive neurosis; obsessional neurosis; and hysteria. There are also hypochondriacal, depersonalisation and neuroasthenic neurotic syndromes, but these are less important and are not considered further here.

ANXIETY AND PHOBIAS

Anxiety is an unpleasant experience like fear or dread related to the possibility, but not the certainty, of something happening. The behavioural features of anxiety include motor changes varying from tremulous restlessness to 'fight or flight' or being 'paralysed with fear'. Physiological accompaniments issue from autonomic activity and accordingly may include dry mouth, nausea and vomiting, or diarrhoea; tremor, muscular tension, numbness, dizziness; tachycardia, palpitations and chest discomfort; sensations of a lump in the throat, or of butterflies in the stomach; and anorexia, insomnia, frequency of micturation, and erectile impotence.

Anxiety is in itself normal, serving to mobilise the person's resources in response to some threat. Morbid anxiety is abnormal (1) when it is a disproportionately intense or prolonged response to stress; (2) when it has no discernible relationship to stressful stimuli; or (3) when it occurs in response to something which is objectively not at all threatening or dangerous. (1) and (2) are varieties of 'anxiety neurosis'; (3) is 'phobic neurosis'. Anxiety not associated with an object is 'free floating' or 'non-situational'. A phobia is an irrational (i.e. unnecessary) fear.

Normal and abnormal anxiety can be linked together and with performance in the so-called Yerkes–Dodson law (see Fig. 2.2). If anxiety is too low or too high, performance suffers.

Anxiety Neurosis

Anxiety neurosis may be acute, disproportionately intense or prolonged in response to a stress, or without apparent relationship to stress; or chronic, when the major manifestations are often in the physiological domain.

Anxiolytic drugs play a part in the treatment of acute anxiety, but should be avoided in chronic cases, in which psychological treatments, especially behavioural psychotherapies, are extremely valuable. Supportive and intensive psychodynamic psychotherapy may also be useful.

Phobias

Mild phobias are very common, and normal, especially in children and in females. When severe they can be extremely disabling. Phobias

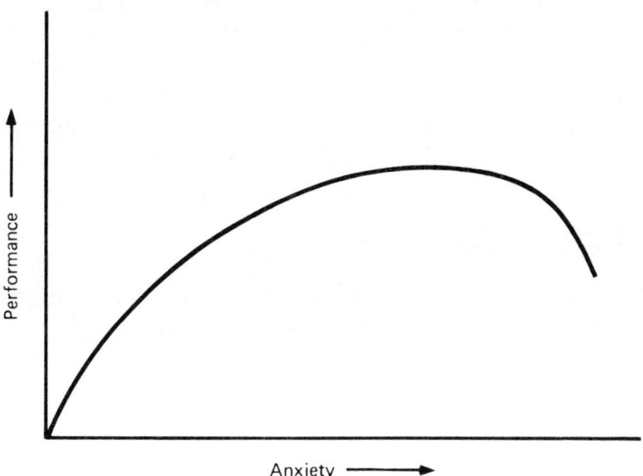

Fig. 2.2 Yerkes-Dodson law.

occur in three clinical groups: specific phobias; social phobias; and agoraphobia. Specific phobias include fears of spiders, cats, mice, birds, snakes and dogs; specific phobics are usually women whose fear dates from early childhood, have no other significant psychological problems, and respond extremely well to behavioural psychotherapy. Social phobias include fears of vomiting, speaking, eating, being seen, urinating, or drinking in public. Severe 'stage fright' is a social phobia. Social phobias are as common in men as women and are often closely linked with personality difficulties. Various psychological treatments may help.

Agoraphobia is the commonest severe phobic disorder. It occurs most often in young women (aged 18–35). Its core symptoms are of anxiety in, and consequent avoidance of, situations which mean being away from home and safety. The typical agoraphobic is anxious about travelling by car, bus, or train, or even on foot; about shopping or being in crowds; and perhaps about being trapped in enclosed places as well as exposed in open ones. Anxiety is usually reduced when the patient is accompanied by a trusted relative, friend or even by a pet or talisman. In addition to phobic anxiety, agoraphobics often also suffer 'free-floating anxiety', depression and unexpected non-situational peaks of anxiety termed panic attacks.

Treatment of agoraphobia includes drugs—tricyclic or MAOI antidepressants may be helpful, and anxiolytics may aid behavioural progress, although they should not otherwise be given regularly (lest they lead to dependence). Psychological treatment is essential—behavioural, supportive, and family treatments may all play their part. Day hospital attendance can be helpful. Agoraphobics often respond well to an enthusiastic 'total push' regime, and complete recovery is possible, even after years of disability.

Depressive Neurosis

Within depressive neurosis, several sub-syndromes can be distinguished. Important ones are (1) anxious depression; (2) hostile depression; and (3) depression with personality disorder. Anxious depression seems related to agoraphobia, except that phobic foci are less evident. MAOIs may be helpful. Hostile and personality-disorder-related depressions are often more difficult to manage than other depressions because the hostility and personality characteristics are difficult for staff to cope with. Often, these depressions are usefully viewed as needing marital or family therapy for the domestic problems which generated them, or as reflecting social difficulties requiring social remedies, rather than as illnesses requiring medical treatment.

Obsessional Neurosis

Obsessions include words, ideas, phrases and actions which a person feels compelled to repeat against a feeling of inner resistance. Obsessions are always unpleasant for the sufferer and may cause anxiety and severe depression. Obsessions have a quality that is very like the common childhood experience of 'having to' avoid cracks between paving stones or like some everyday superstitions that people observe in an embarrassed way. Obsessional neurosis starts early in life and persists with remissions well into middle and later years. Recent studies suggest that long-term prognosis is not as bad as had been suspected. Long periods of relative remission do occur and the end point is likely to be a compromise with symptoms. Depression is a common complication as is a relentless state of shame and tension perpetuated by the obsessions and rituals.

Treatment. Obsessions are regularly helped by (1) treatment of concurrent depression, and (2) admission to hospital (the obsessional benefits because hospital routine organises his time for him, reducing his freedom to behave obsessionally). Also, behavioural psychotherapy often helps, at least in less severe cases. Intensive psychotherapy aimed at analysing the symbolism of obsessions is of little value. Support is, however, invaluable. In severe intractable cases, especially those in whom tension is considerable, psychosurgical intervention may be helpful.

HYSTERIA

Hysteria is a difficult word because it is used inconsistently and can mislead. Laymen use it to describe uncontrolled behaviour, in which context it is not medically useful. It is also applied to a personality type, the hysterical personality, which many feel is better described as the histrionic personality. Its chief psychiatric use is to describe disorders in which there is *loss of function* in the central nervous system but no structural damage. These disorders are said to be caused by a dissociation of consciousness—a splitting off from consciousness of a function ordinarily under conscious awareness. Thus hysterical disorders include sensory and motor dysfunction as well as amnesia, trance-like states and fugues.

The general theory of hysteria is that these states of *conversion hysteria* are the result of unacceptable conflict which causes intolerable stress which can only be dealt with by unconsciously simulating illness. The most extreme examples of this follow severe ordeals, as in wartime and disaster, but the theory hardly accounts for long-term follow-up of people diagnosed as suffering from 'hysteria', many of whom show a disturbingly high incidence of unrecognised organic disease, suicide and mental illness. Hysterical disorders are rarer than they used to be; this is possibly because a patient no longer has to complain of physical symptoms in order to receive help. On the other hand many physically ill people develop hysterical exaggeration of symptoms, and also organic brain disease can trigger off a hysterical reaction when higher control is impaired.

Diagnosis. Bizarre mental states that mimic psychosis can be hysteria, and usually occur in highly stressed situations. The same is true of amnesia and fugues. Paresis is much harder to evaluate, particularly when it is chronic. The diagnosis should not be made because no physical signs can be found. There should be some definite conflict situation which can be shown to present the patient with a gainful solution of an impossible problem.

Treatment. The acute hysterical reaction can usually be treated by heavy sedation followed by powerful suggestion and reassurance. Chronic hysteria tends to be propagated by diagnostic uncertainty. In general, vigorous and positive support and rehabilitation with the careful use of medication are the mainstays of treatment. The chronic hysteric will need careful and skilled psychotherapy to deal with conflict and encourage the return of lost function.

ORGANIC SYNDROMES

Organic cerebral syndromes are caused by dysfunction at cellular level, whether resulting from ischaemia, toxins, inflammation, tumour or trauma. The damage may be transient, permanent or progressive. Organic brain disease causes symptoms of:

1. Intellectual impairment.
2. Memory defect.

3. Personality change.
4. Focal signs and symptoms.

Of these, the first three contribute to recognisable syndromes of organic brain disease, which present as psychiatric disturbance, whilst the focal symptoms usually present as neurological defect.

There are four basic types of organic cerebral syndrome. They may present in pure culture or they may overlap. They include:

1. Delirium.
2. Subacute delirium (confusional state). } 'clouded states'
3. The dysmnesic syndrome.
4. Dementia.

1. Delirium

Consciousness is badly clouded, concentration and attention are fleeting and narrow. The patient is disoriented, cannot grasp what is happening and the environment appears strange and frightening. In a sleepy state the patient misinterprets what is going on and may develop fragmentary delusions. The emotional state is usually fearful and terrified. Hallucinations often occur as well as illusions (perceptual errors). This general state of frightened uncertainty leads to excited overactivity and attempts to leave the ward. Onset of delirium is usually acute and the clouding of consciousness is worst at night when visual cues are less clear. Quiet calm nurses and doctors will do much to allay the frightened delirious patient.

2. Subacute Delirium (Confusional State)

This is marked by clouded consciousness, disorientation, perplexity and incoherence of thinking, feeling and activity. The onset is usually slow and the course prolonged—sometimes passing unrecognised for days or weeks. Subacute delirium is common in medical and surgical wards, and may not be spotted until the patient slips into frank delirium. Often the patient seems to be 'difficult and uncooperative', but when examined carefully he is muddled and vague or flat and querulous—all based on his perplexity.

3. Dysmnesic Syndrome

Severe loss of memory for immediate past events is the main symptom. This is associated with a total failure to retain immediate impressions and inability to recall them. Also there is disorientation for time and place and, most striking of all, a tendency to invent answers to make up for the memory defect (confabulation).

The emotional state is flat and mildly euphoric. The classic dysmnesic syndrome is Korsakov's psychosis where the dysmnesic syndrome and peripheral neuropathy occur in chronic alcoholism and thiamine deficiency. The lesion affects the dorsal thalamic nuclei. A Korsakov-like picture can be caused by injury, ischaemic disease and various toxins.

4. Dementia

This syndrome is the consequence of overall failure of brain function, with which focal signs may be associated. The symptoms are chiefly in the areas of (1) cognition, (2) emotion and (3) personality.

Cognition. There is failure to retain and remember recently acquired information—a reflection of the brain's ability to store and retrieve new material—though past information remains untouched until the process is so extensive as to be terminal. At first the patient cannot remember to keep appointments, etc., but can get by with a notebook. But this worsens to the point where he gets lost while out shopping or is so forgetful that everyone but he is concerned about it. Concentration falls off and thought is slow and muddled. Talk becomes sparse and repetitive. It is hard to shift from one topic to another; answers become non-committal. Flexibility of thought goes. As the process goes on disorientation in time and space, and personal disorientation become more pronounced.

Emotion. Affective symptoms may come on, especially when the patient is aware of failing mental powers. Usually, however, the emotional change is caused by lack of higher cerebral control. Mood change is labile—tears and laughter may come easily but have little depth. A shallow affective state prevails and the person remains unmoved by sad family events. Irritability, distress and rage are sparked off by trivia. The emotions are infantile and egocentric. Later 'emotional incontinence' occurs, i.e. there is no control over feelings which are displayed noisily and without substance.

Personality. Personality change is probably related to frontal lobe damage. There is loss of control of behaviour which at first seems merely exaggeration of the normal self but soon tends to coarsening of behaviour—tactlessness and rudeness go beyond eccentricity and lead to social disgrace, e.g. sexual acts with children, shoplifting. Jokes are lewd and uttered in an insightless way. The end-point is fragmentation of the personality and babbling shadowy incoherence.

Note. Some symptoms in organic states express the acuteness of the cerebral malfunction, while others express the extent or site of it. Thus clouding of consciousness occurs in acute states, while loss of recent memory and disorientation express general cerebral disturbance, acute or chronic. Organic syndromes indicate that the brain is malfunctioning, but not why this is so.

Note on Diagnosis. Organic states are identified by clinical observation, with special reference to disorientation, loss of recent memory, and clouding of consciousness. Depression may resemble dementia especially in old people, where slowness, forgetfulness and apathy can look like dementia ('pseudodementia'). Since depression is treatable, a confident diagnosis of dementia should always have excluded depression. Schizophrenia, particularly late onset and paranoid states, may appear to be organic states, but apparent clouding in schizophrenia is fleeting and there are no memory or intellectual defects. Personality disorders also sometimes give rise to diagnostic difficulty.

The identification of an organic syndrome is followed by investigation of its cause(s). Meanwhile, symptomatic treatment may be needed—tranquillising and neuroleptic drugs may be required to calm agitated and distressed behaviour. For a dementing patient for whom 'care' rather than 'cure' is required, admission to hospital is often in response to family and social needs.

Investigations. These follow careful mental state assessment.

A. Routine (1) Physical examination—may reveal systemic causes—e.g. congestive cardiac failure causing subacute delirium, chest infection, etc.

(2) Blood and serological tests—may indicate macrocytic anaemia, systemic lupus, lead poisoning, neurosyphilis, etc.

(3) Urine—Barbiturates, bromides; porphyria.

B. Psychological Testing. This is invaluable in establishing the extent of impairment. A baseline is useful because later retesting can indicate rate of cerebral deterioration.

C. Special Tests. Previous editions of this chapter have mentioned an encephalogram, ventriculogram, and carotid angiography as possible investigations of organic states. Recent development of brain scan techniques have, however, greatly reduced the need for invasive cerebral investigations. Electroencephalography and lumbar puncture remain useful, indicated on neurological rather than psychiatric grounds.

Notes on the Causes of Organic Psychiatric Syndromes

1. General

Since organic states are caused by the malfunction or destruction of brain cells, they may be caused by any process which can so affect the brain. So, for instance, the causes of dementia include the causes of progressive brain-cell death—degenerative disease, chronic inflammation, tumour, and untreated metabolic disorder such as hypothyroidism. At the same time a tumour or cerebral infarct may be surrounded by partially damaged, recoverable cells, so that acute or subacute delirium may overlay dementia.

2. Drugs

A wide range of drugs, but especially alcohol, barbiturates, bromides and steroids, may all cause clouded states.

(a) *Alcohol* in heavy doses causing chronic intoxication can produce a severe withdrawal syndrome of delirium tremens, i.e. tremors, hallucinosis and delirium; onset is usually acute. Treatment includes chlormethiazole which is a safe anticonvulsant and sedative plus vitamin saturation and treatment of any associated infection. Tranquillisers such as diazepam are useful. Food, fluids, good nursing are mandatory.

(b) *Barbiturates* in doses over 900 mg per 24 h cause chronic intoxication (dysarthria, nystagmus, ataxia) and withdrawal fits. Acute withdrawal causes fits and a delirium which may be indistinguishable from delirium tremens. Treatment consists of reintoxication with pentobarbitone to a state of slightly slurred speech and reducing the pentobarbitone by 100 mg daily.

(c) *Bromide* intoxication is rare nowadays, but presents a picture of rashes and subacute delirium with psychotic excitement and hallucinosis. Treatment consists of nursing, phenothiazines and the use of sodium chloride to hasten excretion.

(d) *Corticosteroids* can cause a wide range of psychiatric disturbance, though clouded states, excitement and labile mood disorder are the most common.

3. Infections

(a) *Acute* infections produce delirium in high fevers, but these disappear when the infection is controlled.

(b) *Chronic* infections such as neurosyphilis may present with a clouded state, the classic picture of GPI—Argyll Robertson pupils, tremor of lips, face and tongue are late signs. Early GPI often starts with headache, insomnia, irritability, fits and odd behaviour. Serology and CSF findings clinch the diagnosis. Treatment with antibiotics arrests the disease.

4. Metabolic Disorders

(a) *Renal failure* causes subacute delirium and coma—barbiturates are after all urea derivatives.

(b) *Hepatic failure* causes subacute delirium and coma as part of the syndrome of portal systemic encephalopathy; 'flapping tremor' and incoordination are well-known signs. The subacute delirious state may mimic irritable depression. Parietal dysfunction is common and for this reason a progress chart should always include the patient's writing and simple drawings.

(c) *Endocrine disorders* are frequently—if not invariably—associated with psychiatric symptoms. *Hypothyroidism* is often accompanied by depression, which may fail to respond to antidepressive treatment if the diagnosis is missed, and may also cause a paranoid psychosis (myxoedema madness). *Hyperthyroid* patients often have very high levels of anxiety; less often there is here, too, a paranoid state. In *Cushing's Syndrome*, as with exogenously administered steroids, affective syndromes (including anxiety, depression, and elation), delirious states and paranoid psychotic illness may all occur. In *Addison's Disease* a neurotic picture may delay diagnosis or there may be a subacute delirious state; the psychiatric symptoms respond to steroid replacement therapy.

(d) *Electrolyte disturbances* usually cause clouded states and are most commonly seen after gastrointestinal surgery. Fluid and electrolyte replacement always correct the disorder.

(e) *Porphyria* is a rare inherited metabolic disorder (Mendelian dominant). Symptoms include peripheral neuropathy and mental symptoms whose real significance is overlooked. Abdominal pain, skin changes, and fits are common, but the psychiatric symptoms may mimic neurosis or depression, though clouded states are common. Attacks are set off by drugs such as the barbiturates, ergot, alcohol, sulphonamides and chloroquine. Urinary findings clinch the diagnosis. Phenothiazines are useful in the acute attack.

5. Deficiency Diseases

(a) *Pellagra* is rare in England but is occasionally seen in alcoholics. The triad of 'diarrhoea, dermatitis and dementia' is classical but psychiatric symptoms can mask everything by presenting as neurosis, depression or 'personality disorder'. Untreated cases pass through clouded states to dementia, coma and death. Treatment consists of replacing the deficient substance nicotinic acid.

(b) *Pernicious Anaemia.* Anaemia and neurological signs usually present first but some patients develop an organic mental state with a normal peripheral blood picture.

(c) *Folate deficiency* may lead to a wide range of psychiatric symptoms. It is always to be remembered in patients on barbiturates or anticonvulsants.

6. Intoxications

These are rare but should not be forgotten: e.g. lead, encephalopathy and dementia; manganese, extrapyramidal signs and dementia; mercury, tremor and dementia; carbon monoxide, extrapyramidal signs and dementia.

7. Tumour

There is no simple rule that when applied to an organic cerebral syndrome will identify it as being caused by cerebral tumour. Obviously if there are focal signs, or if there are signs of raised intracranial pressure such as fits, vertigo, headache, nausea and papilloedema, then the diagnosis will be simpler, but in fact 30% of brain tumours start in 'silent' areas and 60% start with psychiatric symptoms. There is no special 'tumour' syndrome, a fact which has always to be considered when assessing any organic cerebral syndrome. Fits are usually early symptoms and often the earliest sign is personality change and memory defect; later more clear-cut organic changes appear. Two examples may illustrate the difficulty. A nineteen-year-old man was said to be 'work shy' and idle after gastroenteritis. He gave a history of nausea and vomiting in the morning. He had early papilloedema but no focal signs. Investigation showed an extensive fronto-temporal glioma. A thirty-five-year-old housewife was treated for anxiety and depression for three years. All her symptoms went when a meningioma was removed.

8. Trauma

After open or closed head injury the immediate sequel is often delirium, and depending on the extent of brain damage the outcome may be permanent organic impairment. Progressive encephalopathy is found in boxers who have had repeated knock-outs (punch drunk). Subdural haematoma should not be overlooked as a cause of dementia, especially in elderly patients, alcoholics and anyone with a history of repeated head injury.

9. Cerebrovascular and Degenerative Disorders

(a) *Subarachnoid Haemorrhage.* This may be followed by depression, intellectual impairment, or personality change, especially if the frontal lobes have been affected.

(b) *Cerebral Infarction.* Some degree of emotional, intellectual, and personality impairment is frequent following strokes, especially when a large part of the brain has been damaged. Cerebrovascular disease may cause profound dementia without initial focal neurological signs—hypertension may cause this, and be more severe in younger patients.

(c) *Arteriosclerotic Dementia* —now better called *multi-infarct* dementia, indicating the pathology—is a common disorder which may be hard to distinguish from senile dementia, although it tends to start at a slightly younger age (60s rather than 70s and 80s). In multi-infarct dementia onset may be insidious, or marked by an apparently recovered focal 'stroke', or by a delirious state. The course is typically progressively downhill though marked by episodic worsenings ('little strokes') with partial recovery. Mental symptoms may include marked anxiety, hypochondriacal complaints, and paranoid, querulous ideas, though all accompanied by the signs of organicity—recent memory failure, disorientation, etc. Survival with established multi-infarct dementia is rarely beyond two years.

(d) *Senile Dementia.* This is one of the major public health problems in Western societies. It is not uncommon in the 60s, frequent in the 70s, and very common indeed after 80 years. As women tend to outlive men, most very elderly patients with senile dementia are women. In some ways, the underlying process resembles accelerated normal ageing. The brain shows plaques of cell damage. The onset is usually insidious and the course steadily progressive; but downhill progress may be slow and many patients survive beyond two years.

(e) *Presenile Dementia.* This term refers to dementia occurring before 65 years. Possible causes are legion—all the kinds of illness already discussed in this section. In addition, there are some special presenile dementias, all rare.

Pick's and *Alzheimer's* diseases are clinically similar, though the pathology is different. In Pick's disease frontal lobe signs are predominant, and the illness is probably inherited. In Alzheimer's disease the process affects the whole brain and there is a higher incidence of fits and extrapyramidal signs.

Huntington's chorea is a rare hereditary dementia (dominant). The onset is usually in the 40s or 50s. Early symptoms include involuntary and choreiform movements. Neurotic or depressive symptoms are inevitably followed by dementia. Survival is rarely for longer than 10–15 years after diagnosis and the end is total helplessness and global mental deterioration. *Jakob – Creutzfeldt* disease is rare but of interest because it was recently shown to be due to a slow virus. *Normal pressure hydrocephalus* is another rare cause of presenile dementia, but important because potentially curable.

Psychiatric Aspects of Epilepsy

Psychiatric problems are particularly associated with temporal lobe epilepsy. Temporal lobe fits often start in early life following birth injury and may adversely affect psychosocial development, leading to personality disorder. Also, episodic aggression, ecstasy, or excitement may indicate temporal lobe epileptic activity. Also, fugue states (wanderings, losses of memory) may follow temporal lobe fits. Finally, a psychosis closely resembling paranoid schizophrenia occurs in a proportion of chronic temporal lobe epileptics.

PERSONALITY DISORDER

As already noted, personality characteristics are relatively longlasting and unchanging, and are what people mean when they say 'what sort of a person is this?' It is helpful to think of personality as a coin with two sides—one is the individual's view of himself, the other is other people's view of him. The concept of abnormal personality is important in psychiatry, since it provides a way of explaining and understanding persistent modes of behaviour and emotional experience that puzzle society and distress the patient and his family. Some people behave in an odd way from childhood, and their oddities may cause problems, either for themselves by causing conflict and distress, or for others or society at large, especially if they offend moral codes or break the law in a relentless way that is unaffected by punishment or 'treatment'. Indeed, a popular definition of the term 'psychopath' is Schneider's . . . 'a psychopathic personality causes suffering to the person, to society, or both'. However in Britain 'psychopath' sometimes refers to people who show persistently antisocial conduct; but the original use of the term related it more widely to personality disorder.

The important point for the clinician is that personality abnormalities start early and persist, unlike illness which has an onset and is clearly a change in experience or behaviour. It is useful to identify syndromes of personality disorder which, when present in marked degree, represent extremes of variation from normal. People with severe personality disorders are unusual and often very eccentric and therefore often find it difficult to fit into society. Extreme degrees of personality disorder are relatively uncommon and most patients with personality problems have only mildly anomalous or unusual personalities.

SYNDROMES OF PERSONALITY DISORDER

1. Schizoid Personality

The schizoid personality has been likened to an abortive form of schizophrenia; this is offset by the fact that only 50 % of schizophrenics have a premorbid personality that could be fairly described as schizoid. Schizoid people are inward looking and tend to be shy, quiet, self-absorbed and withdrawn. They usually have been 'model' children, being quiet, obedient and bookish. They cannot relate easily with others and this reinforces a tendency to be seclusive and aloof. A schizoid person is emotionally cool and detached and makes a poor and unloving spouse. On the other hand their dreamy detached intellectualism may be advantageous and many go through life unscathed. If schizoid traits are marked with fanatical zeal the patient may get into difficulty if he neglects himself or adopts a crankish diet or takes hallucinogenic drugs in a search for cosmic revelation. If he becomes depressed, the schizoid person may have rather atypical symptoms.

2. Obsessional Personality

Obsessional people are excessively perfectionistic and over-conscientious. Obviously to be conscientious is a valuable social trait but the obsessional personality tends to possess these traits to a degree that imposes handicap, since his exalted standards of perfection can never be attained. A moderate degree of obsessionality is useful in any professional or skilled person but when excessive it becomes a hindrance. Obsessionals make good subordinates but bad leaders. They tend to be indecisive and glum and over-concerned by bureaucratic trivia. They are often rigid in a wearisome and amusing way but are unimaginative and moralising and have little sense of fun. Their humour is dry and laboured and they suffer from guilt and self-doubt. Conscientiousness may be carried to absurd lengths; everything is listed and checked in a stultifying way. They are prone to depression and hypochondriasis, are easily upset by changes in routine and are usually loyal, diligent but rather dreary people. Their talk is larded with qualifying phrases and apology. They usually come from families where one parent has shown similar traits and where the family climate is strict with undue emphasis on self-control and keeping feelings out of sight.

3. Paranoid Personality

The paranoid personality is unrealistic often to the extent of being near deluded. He is suspicious, touchy and oversensitive, and overreacts to criticism, real or fancied. Criticism is borne hardly, something that his family or friends may sum up as a 'chip on the shoulder'. This makes it hard for him to settle in a job or relate with other people. Paranoid personalities often channel their basic sense of injustice into the support of a 'cause' but can prove to be an embarrassment to their associates by becoming fanatical. The paranoid tendency to overvalue ideas and resent criticism can build up into bitter, even violent feeling. In their most extreme forms certain paranoid personalities have influenced world history in a disastrous way.

4. Hysterical Personality

The criteria of maturity include stability, the ability to adjust to change and the ability to handle relationships in a sensible undemanding way without having to manipulate others to meet some pathological need. Mature people can accept success, failure, frustration and disappointment with relative equanimity. Immaturity is a state of emotional childishness. Children react stormily to frustration and the failure to achieve gratification of immediate needs. Growing up and maturation modify this response and encourage a state of independent self-reliance. Some never grow out of this infantile response pattern and become egocentric immature adults. Applied to personality, the term 'hysterical' means 'histrionic' rather than 'excessively prone to conversion hysteria', which it isn't. Histrionic people are usually emotionally labile—sudden bouts of desperate gloom pass quickly and are replaced by some capricious infatuation or enthusiasm which is dropped as quickly as it is taken up. Behaviour tends to be dramatic and the person is importunate and cannot tolerate frustration. The emotions are shallow—effuse demonstrations of feeling mean nothing and relationships with others are never stable. Sexual behaviour is often flirtatious with a façade of empty provocative eroticism.

5. Antisocial Personality (Psychopathic Personality)

The antisocial personality presents society with many problems, mainly because of repeatedly antisocial behaviour. The psychopath seems unable to control his impulses, learn from mistakes or show any foresight about the consequences of his actions. The impulsiveness of the psychopath is like that of a child who flies into a rage when an immediate wish is not granted. The failure to learn from experience suggests arrested emotional development—a failure in social learning. Many have commented on the youthful appearance of certain psychopaths and on the presence of immature patterns in the EEG. This does not apply to all psychopaths, but suggests that at least some of them are people who have a constitutional abnormality. Some psychopaths have emotional shallowness which can extend to callous brutality.

In general the antisocial psychopath is unreliable and untruthful, with little regard for any consideration beyond his own needs. Hence he disregards laws and moral codes with a nonchalance that society may find inexplicable. The psychiatrist may help sometimes by making problem behaviour more understandable (not excusable). This should not be confused with the idea that the psychopath should be treated as if his personality were an illness, which is a mistake which can seriously damage further the psychopath's precarious sense of responsibility for his acts.

Antisocial psychopaths are sometimes called sociopaths in the USA. Family studies of these individuals suggest an interplay of genetic and environmental factors. There is an increased incidence of parental alcoholism, psychosis, criminality and neglect in such families. Truancy, early institutionalisation and early delinquent behaviour all add up to a background that breeds psychopathy.

6. Inadequate Personality

This applies to people who cannot cope with life at any level. They are usually passive and submissive with a history of repeated failure at school, in work and in relationships. They drift from one job to another, are easily led and deceived. Often they are vaguely but persistently hypochondriacal and attend their doctor very frequently. They are usually feckless and may drift into minor criminality or the abuse of alcohol or drugs. Their lives are a catalogue of repeated mistakes and well-intentioned failure. They fill the ranks of recidivist offenders and often find a haven in institutional life, be it hospital or prison. Mood disturbance is labile.

7. Treatment

The antisocial psychopath presents the biggest problem because of his effect on society. There is good evidence to suggest that even severe psychopathic offenders improve as they grow older. Group therapy in prison or in hospital may help the patient to some awareness of the impact of his acts on others. Also regular supervision by probation officers can provide a stabilising influence. Other personality disorders can be helped by simple psychotherapy and guidance through periods of crisis.

Summary

Personality and its disorders are of considerable clinical importance because:

(1) personality disorders cause much personal, family, and social suffering;

(2) personality disorders tend to make psychiatric diagnosis more difficult;

(3) a person's personality characteristics affect the content of any psychiatric illness he may have, and also how well he copes with the illness and complies with treatment;

(4) psychiatric illness may occur in response to (i.e. be precipitated by) personality problems; and

(5) personality disorder predisposes to (i.e. increases the likelihood of) psychiatric illness and behaviour difficulties.

Personality problems predispose to two kinds of behaviour difficulty of especial medical and public concern—alcohol and drug abuse, and sexual deviations. These are therefore discussed next.

ALCOHOL AND DRUG DEPENDENCE

Human beings have an enormous capacity for damaging themselves in the pursuit of pleasure, whether through alcohol, drugs, riding fast motor cycles or smoking heavily. In the case of alcohol and drug abuse and dependence the doctor is presented with a condoned toxin (alcohol) and a proscribed or restricted group of toxins, namely 'drugs'. Drug misuse does not necessarily offend society, and much of it is at least partly caused by medical prescribing habits (e.g. iatrogenic analgesic or hypnotic dependence).

ALCOHOL

Alcohol is condoned by society and is potentially very dangerous, but at the same time provides revenue as well as profit. Chronic alcoholism is a state in which a person is unable to control the amount he drinks and so develops physical, psychiatric and social handicaps in consequence.

(a) *Physical Complications.* These can affect all body systems. They include hepatic cirrhosis, pancreatitis, gastritis, and increased susceptibility to peptic ulceration; cardiomyopathy; peripheral neuropathy, Wernicke's encephalopathy, liability to head injury and subdural haematoma; cerebral atrophy, and dementia; and increased susceptibility to chest infection, including tuberculosis.

Withdrawal symptoms occur when alcohol intake ceases in someone who is physically dependent. Withdrawal symptoms include tremor ('the shakes'); memory lapses ('blackouts'); delirium tremens ('the horrors'); epileptic fits; auditory hallucinosis; and the Wernicke–Korsakoff syndrome can be precipitated by withdrawal.

It is vital to obtain a full psychiatric, family and social history in anyone suffering from an alcohol-related illness. This is easy to miss out.

(b) *Psychiatric Problems.* Alcoholics are liable to depressive illness, suicide, and paranoid reactions of which delusions of the marriage partner's infidelity ('morbid jealousy') are particularly important. Delirium tremens, dementia, and hallucinosis have already been noted.

(c) *Social Problems.* These are of course closely linked with (b). Domestic problems are only too frequent in the families of alcoholics, in all areas of family life—money, child-rearing, job problems, sexual relations. Marital violence is unhappily common, and the prognosis for the marriage of alcoholics is bad.

Severe alcoholism is not really hard to diagnose, but doctors still sometimes have a blind spot for someone whose drinking is getting out of control, especially someone reasonably high in the social scale, such as another doctor. The signs of developing alcohol dependence include telling lies about alcohol intake that is steadily creeping up, avoiding the topic of drink, becoming preoccupied with having enough drink readily available at home or elsewhere; the drinker who is losing control starts drinking earlier in the day, has an excuse for a drink. Binges leading to total drunkenness may be frequent, although many alcoholics space their drinking throughout the day and never get insensibly drunk. The relationship between the amount of alcohol consumed and the development of alcohol problems is complex, but a useful guide is to assume a problem in a male who consumes an average of 10 units daily or a woman who habitually takes half this amount. (One unit equals one half pint of beer, one single measure of spirit, or one ordinary sized glass of wine.) Physical dependence is indicated by the development of withdrawal symptoms (see above) of which morning shakes usually develop first. It is temporarily relieved by alcohol so the history is of 'liveners' to get going in the morning. Tolerance for alcohol varies, so there are individual differences in dose resistance, although anyone will become dependent if he takes enough for long enough. Some alcoholics find they can tolerate less alcohol once they become dependent on it.

DRUGS—NON-MEDICAL USES

Non-medical use is a term which distinguishes casual drug abuse and dependence from therapeutic drug abuse and dependence. The former is related to the use of drugs for pleasure or to relieve distress while the latter is related to the 'accidental' discovery by a patient that a drug makes him 'high'. Drug abuse means taking a drug in a way that exceeds its proper medical use. Dependence means the development of a state in which a person has to go on taking a drug (or alcohol—itself a drug!) because he needs to get high on it or because he becomes sick if he stops. There is no need to distinguish too severely between physical and psychological dependence, except in two instances that are clinically important. The first is in the case of opiate drugs, where physical dependence usually is severe, though it presents no hazard to life. The second is in the case of alcohol/barbiturate dependence, where chronic dependence produces a state of intoxication in which acute withdrawal can cause fits which can be fatal, e.g. if vomit is inhaled.

Types of Drug Dependence

These are often classified according to the type of drug involved. This is currently unhelpful, since the last ten years have shown that multiple-drug use is likely to be the rule. A simple way of classifying the problem is to classify it as shown in the table:

	Physical dependence	*Psychological dependence*
Central stimulant dependence	nil	severe
Opiate dependence	severe	severe
Alcohol/barbiturate dependence	dose-related—severe	usually severe
Hallucinogenic	nil	may be severe

Assessment

As noted, the assessment of individuals with alcohol and drug-related problems requires adequate physical, psychiatric and social evaluation. Often, this is particularly difficult because the person is secretive, not easily trusting of others, defensive, and at best ambivalent about giving up his habit. It is best to be cautious about accepting too readily what the patient says about his alcohol (or drug) consumption. It is very important though often difficult to see the patient's close relatives, both to obtain further information and to enlist cooperation and perhaps participation in treatment plans.

Also as noted previously, the personality is particularly important in cases of alcoholism and drug dependence. These habits often develop as attempts to cope with life problems or stressful environmental events. If the personality has few weaknesses or vulnerabilities, then it will take more external pressure (plus social opportunity) to push the person into alcoholism or drug dependence. People with personality disorder are more vulnerable and liable to respond maladaptively to correspondingly (objectively) less stressful pressures. The stronger the personality, and the greater the environmental contribution to the alcohol or drug dependence, the better the prognosis.

Treatment of Alcoholism and Drug Dependence

In both cases the objectives are the same, namely abstinence and normal social functioning. In alcoholism, withdrawal is relatively easy and abstention is encouraged by social pressures and by the use of drugs such as disulfiram which cause severe symptoms if alcohol is taken. Patients should be encouraged to join AA (Alcoholics Anonymous), which promotes abstinence through self-help and the recognition that alcohol has defeated the individual. In the case of drugs, the principles are the same except that in the case of opiate dependence physical dependence is often so bad that maintenance prescription of the drug is necessary as a social measure aimed at limiting illicit drug traffic. This is done in the UK in special drug-dependency clinics. With barbiturate and central stimulants such as amphetamines and cocaine, prescribing the drug is useless and should not be practised. Withdrawal from drugs may require admission to hospital, though the patient's motivation is the key to success and people can be encouraged to stop drugs as part of an outpatient treatment programme. Continuing abstention can be encouraged by involvement in educational and readjustment groups, often run by ex drug-users and including a residential component. Some of these programmes are hospital based, while others have little to do with medical treatment. The aim is to help adjustment to a more realistic life style, and to the acceptance that a useful and satisfactory life can be lived without resorting to mind-altering drugs as a barrier between oneself and reality.

SEXUAL DEVIATIONS

'Sexual deviation' is a statistical term. That is, sexual deviations represent erotic preferences differing from those of the majority who prefer sexual activity with adults of opposite sex. In this sense *only* can homosexuality be regarded as a deviation. Recent estimates suggest that in current western societies perhaps 10% males have almost exclusively homosexual erotic preferences, while a much larger number (maybe 50–70%) are capable of homosexual and heterosexual responses, while usually preferring the latter.

Other variants from the majority pattern include *paedophilia* (sexual interest in children) and *bestiality* (interest in animals). These are naturally not socially acceptable forms of sexual expression.

Some sexual deviations are like part of the normal love-making process taken out of context and made ends in themselves. Dominating or submitting to a sexual partner become *sadism* or *masochism* when inflicting or enduring pain or cruelty become the means of attaining sexual gratification. Interest in possessions or representations of a loved one becomes *fetishism* when the boots, handkerchief or whatever become the vehicles for orgasm independently of the person. *Transvestism* implies wearing clothing of members of the opposite sex, again as a means to sexual gratification.

Sometimes transvestism is fetishistic—i.e. the clothing represents a preferred sexual partner in some way. It is not usually associated with any doubt in the mind of the transvestite that he (most transvestites are male) is male. Therein transvestism differs from *transexualism* in which condition there is a clear conviction of being psychologically of the gender opposite to one's external genital sex. Transexuals usually request, often with great earnestness, surgical treatment to make the body more appropriate to someone of the experienced gender. Operations such as penectomy and vaginoplasty may play a helpful part in the complex treatment programme required for someone seeking gender re-assignment.

Serious sexual deviations often require specialist advice or treatment. However, it may not be easy to decide whether or not any treatment is needed. A useful criterion for determining this is if the person is complaining about it or if the person's sexual partner finds it intolerable. Sometimes agents of society (courts, etc.) complain about behaviour which the individual has no wish to change—in such instances the chances of behavioural change are remote.

Doctors may be called upon to advise people suffering uncertainty, anxiety, or distress about their sexual orientation or about relations between sexual and other characteristics of the personality (e.g. inferiority feelings and low self-esteem associated with sexual failure and sexual guilt). General counselling principles apply (see later).

'PSYCHOSOMATIC' DISORDER

It is easy to pay lip service to the notion of 'whole-person' medicine, but difficult to practise it, since medical training correctly emphasises the importance of recognising and treating lethal physical illness. For this reason the psychosocial aspects of medicine tend to be studied as an afterthought. However, emotion colours all illness and emotion affects all doctors whether they care to admit it or not. Some illnesses seem to have an ill-comprehended emotional aspect and are called psychosomatic—which is misleading if it implies that any illness not so defined has no psychological aspects. Often the illnesses that have been labelled psychosomatic appear to have received the label on the rather dubious grounds that chronicity and recurrence must imply psychological causality. These illnesses have included rheumatoid arthritis, peptic ulcer, asthma, ulcerative colitis and hypertension. No one would deny that all of these are affected by feelings, but it is taking an unjustifiable step to assign prime importance to emotional causes. Much of medical practice is concerned with minor and self-limiting illnesses and emotional disturbances, and the effects on health of social disadvantage such as poverty, bad housing and poor education. The general population could improve their health overnight by stopping smoking, eating less, drinking less alcohol and taking more exercise. At the same time the doctor has to look out for early signs of serious illness in his patients. The conflict set up by this confusing role makes many doctors frustrated since they feel that the illnesses that were emphasised at Medical School have greater prestige than common minor illness. A sharper educational emphasis on the psychosocial aspects of medicine will no doubt help to ease this situation.

The stresses and strains of dealing with serious illness and of trying to apply complex technology to patients sometimes lead students and doctors to forget that illness affects family as well as patient and that patient and relatives may need to share questions and anxieties with staff. Nowadays a sensible view of psychosomatic medicine includes:

(1) *remembering to assess psychological and social factors in every clinical situation* (*for they may be relevant to any disease whatsoever*);

(2) *being able to examine a patient's mental state as necessary in any clinical setting; and*

(3) *seeing patient's relatives as often as is necessary*. In addition, the student should be aware that an important growing point is the application of psychological principles of behaviour analysis and modification beyond psychiatry elsewhere in medicine (e.g. eating behaviour problems including obesity, the modification of headaches, insomnia, blood pressure, etc.).

The idea of abnormal illness behaviour aids understanding of why some patients keep attending hospital departments with physical complaints but no physical cause and yet no definite psychiatric illness either. Such people have learned to express difficulties with life's stresses indirectly with medical complaints which produce caring responses from doctors. These responses are gratifying even though they do not affect the stress itself. Abnormal illness behaviour is less likely if social and psychological factors are assessed and if necessary tackled before the patient is referred for specialist medical tests.

It has recently been realised that hospital psychiatry only deals with a small proportion, say 10%, of the psychosocial problems with which people consult their family doctors. The commonest symptom patterns seen in primary care psychiatry are mild or moderate anxiety and/or depression, often with physical symptoms, often not really severe enough to be called 'illness', often due to stressful life events, and often relieved in a few weeks with simple counselling. The interplay between physical, psychological, family and social factors in illness is seen clearly in general practice but easily ignored when the patient is separated from the family in hospital.

ASPECTS OF PSYCHIATRY IN MEDICINE

ANOREXIA NERVOSA

This was first described by Sir William Gull in the late nineteenth century. It is a syndrome characterised by food refusal, weight loss, and amenorrhoea. Most patients are girls, only about 10 % being males. It is important to stress the term 'food refusal' because usually the anorexic patient has a normal appetite, it is merely that he or she refuses to eat and adopts numerous devices to avoid it. These range from the obvious such as hiding food or throwing it away to the less obvious such as self-induced vomiting and the use of excessive purgation. Weight loss can be severe and extremely rapid leading in extreme cases to severe electrolyte depletion with dehydration and dangerously low potassium levels. Some patients indulge in episodic bingeing and may therefore have had experience of being distinctly overweight. Amenorrhoea is often simply a consequence of starvation but is an early symptom in a proportion of cases and may precede significant weight loss. Anorexic patients may show significant depression of mood and also be much distressed by obsessional symptoms.

Aetiology. Food refusal is often based on a fear of being fat. The anorexic sees herself (her 'self-image') as being fatter than she really is. The fear is partly determined by social pressures, including advertising which extols the virtues of slimness—social factors probably account for the recent increased incidence of anorexia nervosa. It is in a vulnerable individual that conventional slimming gets out of control and becomes clinical anorexia nervosa. This vulnerability often includes maturational problems—i.e. changing from a child to an adult who is independent of parents, sexually mature, and socially competent. In a high percentage of cases disturbed family relations complicate the problem. By the time the patient is in hospital the whole topic of the patient's food refusal has become a matter of anxiety and concern within the family so that the parents will have over-reacted to an admittedly dangerous situation. Sir William Gull's original advice that the patient should be separated from the parents during treatment remains sound.

Management. Severe anorexia nervosa requires treatment in hospital, even though the patient may need much staff time and discussion before agreeing to it. The main object is to overcome the patient's food refusal and get her back to a reasonable weight which she can tolerate. In severe cases the patient may require intravenous fluid and electrolyte replacement particularly when potassium levels are low. Also in severe cases feeding via a narrow nasogastric tube may be life saving, though skilled nursing makes this very rarely necessary nowadays. The mainstay of treatment is supervised feeding with good support and encouragement from nursing staff. The patient learns to eat in order to achieve specific goals agreed beforehand in discussion with staff. These goals include events and activities which have rewarding properties for the individual (being allowed out of bed, having visits from friends, etc.). It is usually necessary to involve the family in treatment at some stage. Sometimes, psychotropic drugs such as chlorpromazine reduce tension and appear to facilitate weight gain, but drugs are of minor importance in this illness.

Prognosis. Anorexia nervosa has a mortality of about 4% and many patients require frequent re-admission after speedy relapses. Some patients maintain a chronic anorexic state for years. Others recover to normal weight and mature both biologically and psychologically (i.e. periods return, sexual activity occurs, etc.).

PSYCHIATRIC EMERGENCIES

(a) Acute Excitement

This means excessive motor activity, often largely purposeless, and excessive noise, associated with much anxiety in subject and observers. It is a clinical situation which may occur in home or hospital. The main causes are:

(1) organic brain syndromes;
(2) schizophrenia;
(3) mania; and
(4) disturbed behaviour of a psychopath usually intoxicated with alcohol or drugs.

Usually time does not permit detailed mental state examination, but it is important to try and find out whether consciousness is clouded or not, for this would suggest an organic state. Treatment of the basic illness follows calming of the acute excited state. The patient should be approached in a calm and quiet manner and medication used effectively. Sedatives such as the barbiturates should not be used as they disinhibit the patient and make matters worse. The best medications to use are the neuroleptics such as chlorpromazine and thioradazine given by mouth or by injection. These are effective in all excited states. It is also possible to start with a tranquilliser such as diazepam by injection; this calms the patient and the neuroleptics can be given thereafter. In cases of delirium, chlormethiazole is especially valuable and is the treatment of choice in alcoholic or barbiturate delirium. Feeding and fluids plus good nursing complete the management.

(b) Suicide and Attempted Suicide

The correlates of completed ('successful') suicide include being male; age over 50; social isolation (living alone, being widowed, divorced, or separated); recent loss of personal significance (bereavement, retirement); presence of serious—especially painful—physical illness; history of depressive illness and perhaps also recent treatment for depression; and presence of alcoholism (and less commonly schizophrenia or Huntington's chorea).

There is partial overlap between the 'suicide' and 'attempted suicide' populations, for many patients who complete suicide have a history of unsuccessful attempts, and some attempters will later complete suicide. Nevertheless, the statistical associations of attempted suicide (which in the majority of instances means self-poisoning) differ from those of suicide. Suicide attempts correlate with being female; age under 30; current interpersonal difficulties (e.g. arguments with parents or boyfriend, or unwanted pregnancy) and social unsettlement (no steady job or stable living arrangements); and personality disorder rather than psychiatric illness. Only a minority of attempted suicides have depressive illness, alcoholism or schizophrenia. Most attempted suicides are best understood as maladaptive responses to stressful life events.

Admission after self-poisoning is the commonest medical emergency under age 30. Each patient requires psychiatric assessment—which should be a collaborative affair between medical and psychiatric teams. Intensive treatment is likely to be needed for patients who, after self-poisoning, (1) articulate suicidal intentions; (2) are found to be alcoholic, significantly depressed, or possibly psychotic; (3) are judged to have significant problems of social adjustment (unsatisfactory home circumstances and work situation, and inadequate or absent network of supportive personal relationships); and (4) disclose serious unresolved life crises (e.g. unwanted pregnancy, impending court appearance). (3) and (4) are highly correlated with personality disorder and with the tendency to repeat self-poisoning. The social assessment is more important than the clinical one in many of these patients.

Some self-poisoning patients need only sensible counselling and advice. Others need little active help—beyond admission and assessment which are appropriate in all cases.

(c) Puerperal Psychosis

These are not specific psychoses but psychoses which happen to start after childbirth, and are either affective or schizophrenic. They usually respond very well to neuroleptics and ECT.

(d) Postoperative Psychosis

These may be organic delirious states, and if so, respond well to treatment as already outlined. Occasionally an acute affective or schizophrenic psychosis can be triggered off by surgery.

(e) Termination of Pregnancy

The 1967 Abortion Act ensured that unwanted pregnancy is rarely a psychiatric emergency but more a matter of psychosocial urgency. Psychiatric opinion is divided: some psychiatrists believe that there are no psychiatric grounds for terminating pregnancy and that the patient should get better with treatment and be supported through pregnancy. This is a minority view. The majority view is that termination is a reasonable way of dealing with the distress of unwanted pregnancy, particularly when there is severe mood disorder or psychosis.

PROBLEMS OF OLD AGE

People do not usually look forward to old age. The physical aspects, loss of elasticity, muscular weakness and stiffening joints are hard enough to bear. The increased risk of poor health or serious illness when for the average person good health is taken for granted is another burden of old age. In addition to this there are psychological changes in old age which do not make for a happy life. As people grow older they tend to become more rigid in outlook, tend to lose the range of emotions and drives that formerly had kept them going, and this tends to produce an impatient and intolerant reaction amongst younger people so that it is easy for the elderly person to feel progressively more lonely and rejected. Medical advances have not benefited the old as much as the young beyond the dubious advantage of prolonging life without improving its quality. In addition to this the older person is forced into senescence by having to quit work at a time when he may well be able to go on. Add to this the loss of a spouse and the departure of children, etc., and there are all the ingredients for emotional disturbance based on real loss of role and function plus relative poverty for most.

Important points to remember include the following:

(i) *Organic cerebral syndromes* in the elderly, whether caused by arteriosclerosis or senile dementia, may present as a subacute delirious state.

(ii) *Affective disorder* is common and may be misdiagnosed as dementia, especially where the picture is one of apathy and slowness. Elderly depressives respond very well to antidepressant treatment, either ECT or drugs.

(iii) *Paranoid states* are fairly common. These may be due to late-onset schizophrenia (paraphrenia), affective disorders with paranoid colouring, or they may be paranoid reactions in a life-long eccentric. The response to phenothiazines and antidepressants is very good.

(iv) *Neuroses* in the elderly are often overlooked. This group of patients too easily misses out on sympathy and understanding let alone psychiatric treatment.

MARITAL PROBLEMS AND SEXUAL DYSFUNCTIONS

The effect of medical practice reaches beyond the diagnosis and recognition of various obviously physical or psychological disorders. Increasingly doctors are expected, and rightly, to be able to offer advice, comfort and counselling to people whose lives have become troubled and unhappy through disharmony in their relationships within the family. Relationship problems contribute not only to psychiatric illness but to many other kinds of health problem, which are more prevalent in tense, stressed households than in calm, peaceful ones. Doctors should be aware of the common problems in marriage that may affect physical and psychological health.

Marital breakdown in the UK is on the increase, as it is elsewhere in the western world. Divorce rates are of course partly an expression of the rigour or otherwise of divorce laws; but divorce is but a sign that marital breakdown has already occurred, and where divorce is difficult to obtain, many broken marriages remain marriages only in name.

Factors contributing to marital disharmony and difficulty are many. Early age at marriage (age under 20) is highly correlated with divorce; often the partners in early marriage go on maturing from adolescence to adulthood after they are married and this leads them to grow apart.

Many marriages finally crumble after many years, in middle life. Sometimes this is associated for the husband with an excessive preoccupation and involvement with his work, leading him to neglect wife and family or even use his work as a way of avoiding a wife for whom he has grown to have little regard. On the other hand a wife may have perhaps over-identified with the rearing of children and diverted less time and affection to her husband. Commonly, however, the wife is suffering from plain overwork and exhaustion from raising a family and performing all the tasks traditionally expected of the housewife even in a more liberated age. A possible decline in sexual life, perhaps developing from sexual problems that have existed previously, adds to the factors potentially contributing to marital breakdown in the middle years. Alcohol problems, too, are frequent at this time of life—alcoholism is a most potent wrecker of a marriage.

A doctor consulted about marital disharmony needs to have a full and frank discussion with both partners if possible and find out exactly what is going on. Unhappily, however, one partner may be unwilling to participate in such a discussion. Sometimes it may be difficult to realise that a marital problem is present, for patients often present somatic complaints such as headaches, pains or tiredness instead of relationship difficulties about which they feel embarrassed or ashamed.

Once a marriage problem has been identified, and the willingness of both partners to be involved has been assessed, the doctor will need to decide whether he needs to refer for specialist guidance beyond his own counselling skills. Some general practitioners have marriage guidance counsellors working with them in their practices. Some psychiatric departments are able to provide marriage therapy; otherwise the various marriage guidance councils are the most likely source of aid.

Sexual Dysfunctions

Sexual dysfunctions are those problems which make sexual intercourse difficult or impossible. In the male they include:

(1) erectile impotence (failure to achieve or sustain an erection sufficient for coitus);
(2) premature ejaculation (ejaculatory control being impaired so that ejaculation occurs before it is desired); and
(3) retarded ejaculation (ejaculation simply fails to occur—this is a rare dysfunction).

Female dysfunctions include:

(1) failure to respond early on the sexual arousal cycle, leading to dryness, pain (if coitus is attempted), and difficulty in going on to orgasm;
(2) anorgasmia, when arousal begins but does not lead on to orgasm; and
(3) vaginismus.

Many established dysfunctions become accompanied by loss of sexual interest and inclination as the sexual difficulty leads to accumulated argument, anxiety, guilt and failure.

Sexual dysfunctions can be caused by structural or functional interference with local nervous or vascular pathways. Possible causes here are legion—diabetic autonomic neuropathy, antihypertensive and antidepressant drugs, and spinal-cord tumour are but three examples. Hypogonadism is a rare hormonal cause. In about 90% of cases of sexual dysfunction, no significant organic factor is present, even though they should be sought in all instances. The most important factors are usually *anxiety*, especially fear of sexual failure and anxiety about sexual performance; and *marital disharmony*—few couples continue active sexual lives when their general relationship is bad. Of course, general and sexual aspects of the relationship tend to feed each other, both for better and for worse.

Treatment of marital sexual problems is best based on the methods which evolved from the pioneering work of Masters and Johnson. The key features of this approach are:

(1) that both partners are involved;
(2) it is time-limited, involving
(3) 'homework' exercises for the couple to do at home designed to achieve specified treatment goals, and
(4) the results are assessed at the end of treatment.

Results are often very good, provided both partners are involved and genuinely seek progress.

Sexual dysfunctions have obvious links with many branches of medicine, and many disciplines can contribute to sexual dysfunction treatment. The person treating sexual disorders may need access to physician, urologist, gynaecologist, family-planning expert, venereologist, clergyman, social worker, psychologist, marriage guidance counsellor, or psychiatrist. Provided such links are readily available, the ability to treat the majority of sexual dysfunctions is readily gained by students or general practitioners as well as members of all these disciplines.

PSYCHIATRY: FORENSIC ASPECTS

Law and psychiatry interrelate in many ways. Laws are made to regulate society, to control criminality and to guarantee equity and justice for all citizens. Psychiatric aspects of the law that students should know about include civil and criminal responsibility, the Mental Health Act and testamentary capacity.

Responsibility

In law it is assumed that a man is sane and responsible for his actions—he intends their result and must bear responsibility for their consequences. This is true for both criminal and civil matters. In criminal acts the law bases responsibility on *actus reus* (the guilty act) and *mens rea* (the guilty mind). Responsibility implies liability to punishment. The prosecutor has to prove the guilty act and the defence has to prove that there is no intent, i.e. no *mens rea*. Age is important—a person may be too young to form intent. Or intent may be said to be absent by reason of mental disorder. This used to be governed by the M'Naghten rules. M'Naghten was a schizophrenic who killed Sir Robert Peel's secretary, thinking he was Sir Robert, whom he believed was persecuting him. The rules said insanity was a defence if the accused was 'labouring under such a defect of reason from disease of the mind as not to know the nature and quality of the act; or if he did know it, that he did not know that what he was doing was wrong'. The rules were hard to apply and led to the legal concept of Diminished Responsibility for Homicide stated in the Homicide Act 1957, whereby a person is not convicted of murder if he 'was suffering from such abnormality of mind . . . as substantially to impair his mental responsibility'. Such a plea, if accepted, reduces the charge to manslaughter.

Civil Responsibility. Sanity and responsibility are assumed—an anomaly here is that a drunk man can make a valid will, sign a valid contract or get married as long as he is not so drunk that he does not know what he is doing.

Absolute Liability. For some offences liability is determined by scientific tests, e.g. a blood alcohol over 80 mg % means unfitness to drive and loss of licence.

THE MENTAL HEALTH ACTS 1959 AND 1983

The 1959 Act was a model law which defined mental illness, subnormality and psychopathy and provided safeguards for the mentally ill against illegal detention and also guarded their rights and property. Compulsory treatment was provided for in a fair and humane way. This Act has been amended and brought up to date in the 1983 Mental Health Act which came into effect at the end of September 1983. The principle is still to encourage informal admission as the ideal with compulsion as something only to be used as a last resort, and the 1983 Act elaborates and extends the rights of those patients compulsorily detained and treated. The term *mental subnormality* has been replaced by *mental impairment*, which does not come under the Act unless it is accompanied with 'abnormally aggressive or seriously irresponsible conduct'. Consequently the Mental Health Act no longer applies to the majority of *mentally handicapped* people.

The student should be familiar with the sections dealt with in the 1983 Act (see Table 2.1).

Testamentary Capacity

Any one can make a valid will as long as he is of 'sound disposing mind'. Incapacity may be in question in cases of mental illness, especially organic states. The criteria for capacity are that the person should know the implications of the act of making a will, and know the extent of the estate and the likely beneficiaries. His judgement should not be impaired. Severe mental illness such as schizophrenia or dementia does not automatically make someone incapable, since there are often large islands of lucidity. Doctors should never witness a will made by a patient, over and above the obvious bar to witnessing a will of which the doctor is a beneficiary.

Table 2.1 The Mental Health Act 1983

Section	*Purpose*	*Application made by*	*Medical recommendation*	*Comment*
2	Admission for assessment	Nearest relative or approved social worker	Two doctors, one recognised as having special experience under Section 12 of the Act	Lasts 28 days, patient may apply to Mental Health Review Tribunal within 14 days of admission
3	Admission for treatment	As above	As above	Initially for 6 months. Patient may apply to Mental Health Review Tribunal in each 6 month period
4	Admission in an emergency	As above	Any doctor	Lasts for 72 hours
5	To detain a patient already in hospital	—	The doctor in charge of the case or nominated deputy	Lasts for 72 hours
5(4)	To detain a patient already in hospital where doctor in charge or deputy need to be contacted	—	A nurse of the prescribed class (registered mental nurse including registered nurses for mental handicap)	Lasts for 6 hours or until arrival of doctor, whichever is the shorter
37	Provides for compulsory treatment for offenders	—	Two doctors, usually prison MO and hospital consultant	Order is made by the Court. Hospital doctor has right to discharge. Crown Court may recommend restriction of discharge under Section 41
136	Provides facility for a police officer to remove to a place of safety persons in public places who appear to suffer from mental disorder	—	'Place of safety' may include examination by an approved social worker and doctor	Lasts 72 hours

PSYCHIATRIC TREATMENT

Psychological Effects

Psychological influences are operative whenever patient and clinician meet. Hence doctors have psychological effects on patients in every clinical setting. So do nurses, social workers, psychologists, and occupational therapists who also interact with patients. These psychological influences accompany pharmacological, surgical, nursing and other medical procedures, and are neither negligible nor unimportant. They affect patients' compliance with technical procedures and physical treatments, and also often affect responsiveness to physical treatment (e.g. relieving preoperative anxiety tends to reduce postoperative pain intensity and analgesic intake, increase benefit from postoperative physiotherapy, and reduce length of stay in hospital).

Treatments

A psychological treatment is a procedure whose aim is to achieve therapeutic goals by psychological means in prescribed treatment activities. Psychological treatments thus have their own structure—of meetings, sessions, etc. In this they contrast with 'psychological effects' which are informal and accompany other (non-psychological) procedures.

(1) **Types of Treatment.** One easy way of distinguishing different sorts of psychological treatment (synonym 'psychotherapy') is in terms of the personnel involved. Thus we can speak of three main varieties of psychotherapy:

(a) *Individual* —the therapist treats one patient.

(b) *'Natural group'* treatment—this means treating the patient as part of some group of which he or she is a member in ordinary life. This includes marriage therapies where treatment is of marriage partners and family therapy involving the whole domestic unit (usually parents and children, sometimes also in-laws, grandparents, etc.). In natural group treatments the couple or the family become the unit of treatment, even if one person was originally the referred patient.

(c) *Group therapy*—treatment involves a therapist (sometimes two therapists) and several patients. Small-group therapy includes 4–10 patients; large groups are less popular but can involve 30–50 patients or even more. Therapeutic groups can be usefully set up for outpatients, on wards for inpatients, or in day-hospital settings.

(2) **Length of Treatment.** Psychological treatments may be brief or prolonged, and time-limited or indefinite. (Individual segments of treatment ('sessions') may also vary in length, from a few minutes to 1–1½ hours, with about 50 minutes being most popular for formal individual treatment sessions, groups usually lasting 1–1½ hours.

Brief procedures require up to 10–15 meetings. Time-limited treatments take about 3–6 months. Treatments requiring not more than 10 sessions over 3 months are particularly important in busy Health Service settings where time and therapist personnel are scarce resources.

(3) **Therapists.** Doctors can readily gain psychological treatment skills. So can members of other health professions, and the doctor interested in psychotherapy learns to work in a multidisciplinary team of which the doctor may not always be the leader.

(4) **Aims and Approaches.** The goals of psychological treatment (and 'psychological effects' (see above) are relief, and/or behavioural change.

(a) *Relief.* The aim is the relief of unpleasant feelings, or the cessation of other disagreeable experiences—to 'feel better'. The general approach is to encourage the patient to talk about his problems and express distressing feelings, the therapist being attentive, accepting and ready to articulate his understanding of what the patient is communicating. That ventilation and communication bring relief is a cardinal principle of counselling both by professionals and by ordinary people seeking to aid their fellows in distress.

Naturally, such relief of distress occurs informally (as 'psychological effects'). But treatment whose goal is relief is frequently indicated as a formal procedure, usually brief and time-limited.

(b) *Behavioural Change.* This heading includes three treatment categories of differing conceptual and procedural complexity. There is a general shared aim of facilitating the occurrence of new behaviour of some sort.

(i) *Simple Measures.* These are often derived from common-sense notions of what the patient should do, or represent professional opinion of effects of illness on personal life. Thus simple measures designed to evoke behavioural change include giving advice about the effects of illness or operation; providing health-related information (e.g. sex education or publicising the dangers of cigarette smoking); and helping a patient to resolve indecision or conflict about marriage, abortion, or child rearing.

(ii) *More Complex Measures.* This heading includes most formal psychological treatments. They are all derived with varying degrees of cogency from one or other of the available theories applicable to behaviour. At the present time most treatments are either (1) psychodynamic—based on psychoanalytic theory or its derivatives; or (2) behavioural—based on learning theories; although there is an increasing tendency for treatments to be derived from other psychological approaches—personal construct theory, Gestalt psychology, a range of cognitive theories, and client-centred approaches, for instance.

(iii) *Personality Change.* This is sometimes the declared aim of intensive, indefinite treatments, especially psychoanalytic ones. These procedures are too costly of time and people, and their results too uncertain, to be of any great Health Service relevance. However, 'personality change' means 'extensive behaviour changes which persist and affect the subject's view of self and others and the world'; in this sense measures aimed at 'more complex' behaviour changes sometimes produce personality change.

(5) **Indications and Applications**. In general the aim is to fit the treatment to the individual patient's needs—not to think of particular treatment techniques for particular illnesses. It is however possible to suggest guidelines for aiding choice of psychological treatment.

(a) A 'relief' procedure should be thought of when (i) distress is intense, (ii) feelings are unexpressed, (iii) the patient is unable to think coherently about specific life problems and more specifically, (iv) when the patient has not worked through bereavement or other personally significant loss (loss of job, limb, pet, for instance, may cause grief-like states in people particularly sensitive to loss).

(b) Simple behaviour-change measures are always potentially relevant in medicine. Provision of information, advice and education should always be considered.

(c) Behaviourally based treatments programmes should always be considered with phobias, obsessions and sexual dysfunctions. They are often useful for patients with other disorders too, and the question the clinician has to ask himself is 'what might a behavioural approach have to offer in this case?'.

(d) Treatment programmes for interpersonal relationship problems, and for conflicts indicating difficulty in becoming mature usually require some psychodynamic basis. This applies whether the treatment is brief or more prolonged, and individual, or group.

(e) Brief, time-limited, treatments focusing on specific goals are preferable whenever possible.

(f) Family treatment not infrequently leads to improvement when more traditional treatments have failed. Family therapy should not, however, be considered only as a last resort; it should be considered as a possible initial treatment of choice when problems are closely involved with what is happening at home (e.g. many middle-aged women with depression, patients with anorexia nervosa and adolescent patients with severe psychiatric (and behavioural) problems).

Also a family meeting is often of great diagnostic help. While family *therapy* may be inappropriate, there are *no* contraindications to a diagnostic family meeting.

(g) Couple treatment (included above under 'natural groups') is the approach of choice for marital problems, including sexual problems in married people.

(h) A group approach is often helpful for people with interpersonal difficulties, for whom a group may offer greater opportunities for interpersonal learning than an individual approach. Groups are also helpful for patients who intend to become overly dependent in one-to-one situations.

Note. It should be remembered that relief, provision of information and advice, and behavioural change procedures can all be set up as individual, natural group, and group procedures. There is currently considerable interest in the therapeutic potential of information-giving groups—really amounting to educational classes—in medical settings.

Further Note. Every doctor should be prepared whenever necessary to use his counselling and psychological treatment skills to relieve distress and promote adaptive behavioural change. He may also wish to develop specific psychological treatment skills, according to inclination and the kind of work he does. Many skills within behavioural, group, and individual therapies are easily within the grasp of the doctor who can attain the fairly modest training required.

Social Methods

The relevance of social factors for illness is increasingly appreciated. Recognition of the harmful effects which may be brought about in susceptible patients by prolonged exposure to an unstimulating institutional environment has led to the current emphasis on community-based care for psychiatric patients. For patients with chronic illnesses this becomes essentially a matter of team-work. To manage a chronic schizophrenic patient at home, for instance, may require regular home visits from a community psychiatric nurse, regular meetings between a social worker and the patients' relatives, attempts to improve behavioural skills by a clinical psychologist, occupational retraining by rehabilitation therapists, and medical supervision of the whole package. The team approach applies in principle to all sorts of psychiatric disorder. The key to it is recognition of the considerable skills which can be brought to a clinical problem by members of all the professions which are relevant; the doctor must not perpetuate the fiction that only he has expertise in the field of psychiatric disorder.

PSYCHOPHARMACOLOGY

Psychopharmacology is a relatively new science which is concerned with the structure and mode of action of drugs that alter the mental state. These drugs can be broadly classified as psychotropic drugs in that they alter feeling, behaviour and perception without any significant change in consciousness, unlike sedatives and hypnotics which produce an altered mental state by dulling consciousness. The study of psychopharmacology has opened up many questions about the relationship between brain biochemical activity and behaviour. For instance, much interest has focused on the cerebral amine theory of depression. Central transmitting substances in the brain appear to play a definite role in affective disorder. The substances concerned are the cerebral amines, noradrenaline, 5-hydroxytryptamine (5HT or serotonin) and dopamine. These amines are found in high concentration in the hypothalamus and brain stem and are also stored in central neurone endings. The theory is that amine depletion causes depression and excess causes mania. Tricyclic antidepressant drugs probably act by blocking the reabsorption of free amines while monoamine oxidase inhibitors (MAOIs) probably act by preventing oxidative deamination, thus increasing amine concentrations.

Psychotropic drugs include three main groups, and lithium. A fifth category—psychedelic (hallucinogenic) drugs—is of no practical importance now but has stimulated research into the nature of the psychoses.

(a) **Neuroleptics.** These are antipsychotic drugs. Interest dates from 1952 when the antipsychotic action of chlorpromazine was demonstrated. In general the neuroleptics slow psychomotor overactivity, damp down feeling and block hallucinosis. This is probably related to their ability to diminish CNS arousal via the reticular activating system. There is little or no alternation in consciousness, and for these reasons the neuroleptics are most valuable antipsychotic drugs. There are many drugs in the neuroleptic group. Mention is made here of the two most important groups.

(i) *Phenothiazines*

Chlorpromazine—daily dose 75–400 mg. Most widely used.
Thioridazine—30–600 mg daily. Has some antidepressant effect.
Trifluoperazine—3–40 mg daily. Has some alerting effect.
Fluphenazine—see below.

Fluphenazine is most frequently used as the decanoate ('Modecate') given as a long-acting intramuscular injection, very useful in the maintenance treatment of chronic schizophrenia. Flupenthixol, though not strictly a phenothiazine, has a similar action and can also be given as a long-acting injection.

All phenothiazines have the capacity to cause extrapyramidal side-effects which range from acute Parkinsonian symptoms (treatable by anti-Parkinsonian drugs such as procyclidine) to chronic syndromes, of which tardive dyskinesia is disabling and difficult to treat. As its name suggests, tardive dyskinesia is slow to develop; it includes complex involuntary movements involving face, tongue, and/or limbs. Phenothiazines may also cause other side-effects, such as hypotension, jaundice ('chlorpromazine jaundice'), rashes, and blood dyscrasias.

(ii) *Butyrophenones.* Haloperidol is the most widely used drug in this group. It is quickly absorbed and slowly excreted so that a twice daily dose is effective (up to 15 mg daily). Extrapyramidal side-effects are common. It is mainly used to calm acute excitement in hypomania and schizophrenia, for which purpose it is often given by injection.

(b) **Tranquillo-sedatives.** These are the anxiolytic or minor tranquilliser drugs. This group is very widely prescribed. Most popular are the benzodiazepines, e.g.:

Chlordiazepoxide—daily dose 15–100 mg
Diazepam—daily dose 6–30 mg.

These drugs calm anxiety effectively, but should be used cautiously because of the risk of dependence—and because they may cause disinhibition and hence contribute to outbursts of aggressive behaviour. It is advisable to restrict the use of anxiolytic drugs to acute anxiety situations.

Benzodiazepines are believed to act on the limbic system. They cause little drowsiness and have valuable anticonvulsant effects. Excessive doses cause drowsiness, ataxia and dysarthria, and fits can occur in abrupt withdrawal. Intravenous diazepam is a treatment of choice in status epilepticus and in any state of wild uncontrolled behaviour.

We may also note that beta-blocking drugs such as propranolol can control some of the somatic concomitants of anxiety.

(c) **Antidepressants.** The availability of antidepressant drugs has greatly reduced the need for ECT. These drugs are of two main groups:

(i) *Tricyclic Antidepressants.* Over 30 tricyclics (as well as other compounds in more or less closely related categories) are available for prescription. The student should be familiar with the two which are of most proven value—imipramine, and amitriptyline. Both are given in a dose of up to 150 mg daily. Amitriptyline is more sedative and may be preferred in more agitated patients; most of the daily dose may be given at night and will then aid sleep. All tricyclics take up to three weeks to act, and a tricyclic should not be rated 'ineffective' until the patient has had it in reasonable dosage for a month. With all tricyclics, atropine-like side-effects are common; they include dry mouth, constipation, delayed micturition and erectile difficulties. They should be used cautiously in the elderly and in patients with glaucoma or prostatism. They may affect cardiac function, and one of the newer compounds such as mianserin is to be preferred in depressed patients with heart disease. Tricyclics should not ordinarily be combined with MAOIs and may interact adversely with drugs that lower blood pressure.

(ii) *Monoamine Oxidase Inhibitors (MAOIs).* These were the first antidepressants. There are several monoamine oxidases, which contribute to the uncertainty of action of these drugs. MAOIs may be very useful in phobic anxiety and in depressive neurosis. However, usual practice in treating these disorders is to begin with a tricyclic because patients on MAOIs must observe dietary restrictions which many find tiresome. The problem is that, if monoamine oxidases are inhibited, serious hypertensive crises may arise if the patient eats tyramine-containing foods—the resulting flood of noradrenaline may cause headache, collapse and intracerebral haemorrhage. Foods which must be restricted include cheese, yeast and beef extracts, broad bean pods and some red wines. MAOIs also potentiate sedatives, alcohol, narcotics and anaesthetics.

Popular MAOIs include phenelzine (30–45 mg daily), isocarboxazid (20–30 mg daily), and tranylcypromine (20–30 mg daily).

(d) **Lithium** has mood-stabilising effects and is a most important part of the treatment of manic–depressive disorders. It is somewhat toxic, and therefore requires specialist supervision. In excess it may cause hypothyroidism and renal damage. Serial blood lithium measures help to monitor therapy.

General Remarks on Psychotropic Drugs

(a) All psychotropic drugs are powerful. Dosage levels should always be kept at the minimal effective dose.
(b) Interaction with alcohol is common—patients should be warned of this.
(c) A good rule is to use one drug at a time, rarely two and never three.
(d) Patients on MAOIs should carry a card with the drug dose and a list of food and drugs to avoid.
(e) Weight gain on tricyclics can be very heavy—this puts people off taking them.

Other Physical Methods

Electroconvulsive Treatment or ECT consists of inducing a fit by passing a 100 V potential a.c. current across the head. This is done using thiopentone anaesthesia and muscle relaxants to avoid muscle or bone damage. It is used in affective disorders, where it can be life saving, and to a limited extent in schizophrenia.

Psychosurgery involving operation, e.g. to divide connections between the frontal lobes and the thalamus, tends to be used in cases where patients are in states of chronic tension either through chronic depression or obsessional disorder.

FURTHER READING

Bloch, S., (ed.), *Introduction to the Psychotherapies*, Oxford University Press, Oxford, 1979.

Curran, D., Partridge, M. and Storey, P., *Psychological Medicine. Introduction to Psychiatry*, 9th edition, Churchill Livingstone, London and Edinburgh, 1980.

Granville-Grossman, K., *Recent Advances in Psychiatry*, Churchill Livingstone, London and Edinburgh, Vol. I, 1971; Vol. II, 1976; Vol. III, 1979; Vol. IV, 1982.

Lishman, W. A., *Organic Psychiatry. The Psychological Consequences of Cerebral Disorder*, Blackwell, Oxford, 1980.

Taylor, F. Kraupl, *Psychopathology. Its Causes and Symptoms*, 2nd edition, Butterworth, London, 1979.

CHAPTER 3

THE ALIMENTARY SYSTEM

SYMPTOMS OF ALIMENTARY DISORDERS

Pain

There is still no general agreement either about the mechanism of abdominal pain or its classification. Following the observations of Kellgren, who showed that human volunteers could distinguish only two types of pain, a superficial variety elicited by stimulation of the skin and subcutaneous tissues and a deep variety felt when any structure deep to the subcutaneous tissues was stimulated, doubt has been cast on the validity of the traditional classification of abdominal pain into visceral and somatic types. Furthermore, the description of pain given by patients with visceral and somatic lesions, such as carcinoma of the stomach and retroperitoneal sarcoma, often fails to provide any distinguishing clue.

Nevertheless, certain types of pain are sufficiently characteristic to be of great value in diagnosis. *Colic*, originally pain arising in the colon, is a term now applied to painful spasm in any hollow muscular viscus, usually due to partial or complete obstruction of its lumen. Intestinal colic is a spasmodic pain, coming in a succession of waves which rise to a peak of intensity and then subside; renal and biliary colic, however, may persist at a steady and very severe level for an hour or more. The patient doubles up or writhes about when it is at its height and warmth applied to the abdomen helps to relieve it. There may be associated vomiting. Colic is usually poorly localised, but small intestine spasm is felt mainly in the centre of the abdomen, large intestine colic in the lower abdomen, renal colic in the loin radiating to the groin and testicle on the same side, bilary colic in the right upper quadrant or epigastrium sometimes radiating through to the back, and uterine colic in the lower abdomen.

Pain due to inflammation of the parietal peritoneum, on the other hand, is a sharp steady severe pain accurately localised over the site of the inflammation. Pressure on the area causes tenderness and reflex spasm in the overlying muscles (guarding or rigidity) and since the pain is aggravated by movement the patient usually lies quite still.

Patients with acute appendicitis provide a good illustration of these two types of pain. In the early stages when there is obstruction and consequent spasm in the appendix the patient has colicky pain vaguely referred to the area around the umbilicus, and he frequently vomits at the outset; but in a few hours, when inflammation has developed in the appendix and spread to involve the parietal peritoneum, the pain becomes sharper and shifts to the right iliac fossa directly over the site of the lesion.

Pain and tenderness occur in the liver only when its capsule is acutely stretched by sudden distension of the organ, as in congestive cardiac failure; and in the spleen when there is inflammation in its peritoneal covering, as by an infarct extending to the surface. The mechanism of pain in peptic ulcer is considered on p. 89.

Vomiting

Vomiting is produced by compression of the stomach between the muscles of the abdominal wall and the diaphragm, with simultaneous relaxation of the cardiac sphincter and reverse peristalsis in the stomach and oesophagus. The causes are very numerous, but fall into a few main groups:

(a) When due to *intra-abdominal disease* it is usually preceded by nausea. In pyloric obstruction the vomiting may be projectile, the gastric contents being ejected from the patient's mouth with great force, and frequently very large quantities of vomit are produced containing recognisable food taken many hours previously. In intestinal obstruction the reverse peristalsis throughout the gut may eventually cause faeculent vomiting.

(b) *Cerebral vomiting* occurs in patients with raised intracranial pressure and there is often no preceding nausea. Labyrinthine disturbances are also common causes of vomiting, as in patients with acute vertigo or travel sickness.

(c) *Psychological vomiting* is also common. Some people vomit from sudden fear or horror, as for example if they see an accident in the street; others do so for less obvious and more deep-seated psychological reasons. Repeated persistent vomiting without loss of weight is nearly always of this type.

Heartburn

A burning pain behind the sternum is a symptom common in many alimentary disorders and is therefore not very helpful in diagnosis. It is perhaps most commonly found in patients with peptic oesophagitis due to gastro-oesophageal regurgitation; these patients may also have *acid regurgitation*, complaining that from time to time a bitter-tasting fluid rises up into the throat.

Waterbrash

Waterbrash is filling of the mouth with a tasteless fluid (saliva) and nearly always indicates the presence of a duodenal ulcer.

Diarrhoea

(a) *Acute diarrhoea* is usually due to dietetic indiscretion, food poisoning, infections such as bacillary dysentery, or an exacerbation in one of the causes of chronic diarrhoea.

(b) *Chronic diarrnoea* occurs:

(i) after operations such as gastrectomy and vagotomy,
(ii) from lesions of the small intestine such as regional ileitis (Crohn's disease) and the malabsorption syndromes,
(iii) in diseases of the colon, such as carcinoma, diverticulitis, amoebiasis and ulcerative colitis.

Apart from alimentary disorders such as the above, chronic diarrhoea may be due to general causes, such as thyrotoxicosis or anxiety neurosis.

Constipation

Many men and nearly all women when asked about their bowels reply that they have always tended to be rather constipated. They mean that instead of having a daily bowel action, which the patent medicine advertisements have taught them is essential for normal health, their bowels move only once every two or three days. They have therefore fallen into the habit of taking a purgative every day or once or twice a week, and they believe that continuing with this ritual is essential to their well-being. In fact, however, variations in the normal rhythm of the colon are quite wide, and to evacuate the bowel twice a week is not constipation; it may be just as normal and healthy as to evacuate it twice a day. On the other hand, the taking of regular evacuants seldom does any actual harm and when a patient with a lifelong dependence on one of them comes into hospital with an organic complaint, undoubtedly the most sensible plan is to continue prescribing his usual laxative. The time is not appropriate to attempt re-education of bowel function, which in any case would be most unlikely to succeed.

Normal regular movement of the bowels is not to be expected in febrile dehydrated patients who are taking little or no solid food and a dose of cascara or senna or a simple enema every few days is all that is needed. Greater care must be taken to ensure a regular evacuation in weak, elderly patients, in whom impaction of a mass of faeces in the rectum tends to occur.

Dyschezia is constipation due to functional sluggishness of the bowel, due mainly to persistent failure to answer the call to stool. It is treated by patient retraining of a regular bowel habit, helped in the early stages by a mild aperient such as senna or by glycerine suppositories.

THE MOUTH AND THROAT

Inspection of the mouth and throat in a good light is an essential part of every medical examination for, apart from purely local conditions which will not be discussed here, it occasionally reveals evidence of some general disorder.

Furring of the tongue is too common to be of much help in diagnosis and is often seen in smokers who are in good health. The 'black hairy tongue' due to alteration in the normal flora of the mouth is mainly seen in patients who have been treated with broad spectrum antibiotics. The thickly coated tongue and uriniferous breath of the uraemic patient contrast sharply with the clean dry tongue and sweetish ketotic breath of the severe diabetic.

Atrophy of the filiform papillae of the tongue, making the normal velvety surface smooth and shiny, is seen in *iron deficiency*, when it appears first round the edge of the tongue; in *Vitamin B_{12} deficiency*, when it is usually first seen on the dorsum; in *riboflavin and nicotinic acid deficiency*, in this country usually the result of some intestinal disorder and sometimes associated with cracking at the angles of the mouth. It also occurs after oral administration of *broad spectrum antibiotics* where it may be caused by *Candida albicans* and responds to oral nystatin.

Brown pigmentation on the lips and on the buccal mucosa lining the cheeks is an important sign of Addison's disease, but it is also seen in normal people of mixed racial origin.

Sloughing ulceration of the mouth and throat is an important sign of agranulocytosis and acute leukaemia and in the monocytic variety of the latter disease there may also be swelling and infiltration of the gums and occasionally of the tongue.

THE OESOPHAGUS

PEPTIC OESOPHAGITIS

The squamous epithelium of the oesophagus is not designed to resist the digestive action of acid gastric juice and it frequently becomes inflamed and eroded in patients with gastro-oesophageal reflux. Such reflux occurs particularly, but not exclusively, in association with hiatus hernia. It should be noted too that other patients with hiatus hernia, with or without radiologically demonstrable reflux, suffer no ill-effects whatever.

Two important *symptoms* may arise from peptic oesophagitis. The commoner is *substernal pain*, similar in quality and distribution to angina pectoris; it is brought on, however, not by effort but by positions which encourage gastro-oesophageal reflux, mainly lying flat and stooping after a meal. The second symptom is *bleeding*, rarely presenting as haematemesis but sometimes causing severe and at first obscure anaemia.

Diagnosis. *Barium meal* examination in the Trendelenburg position demonstrates the gastro-oesophageal reflux and usually an associated hiatus hernia and the inflammation and erosion of the oesophageal mucosa can be confirmed by *oesophagoscopy*. Reproduction of the pain by introducing 0.1 N hydrochloric acid into the lower oesophagus (*Bernstein's test*) or even by drinking a hot cup of tea is useful confirmatory evidence.

Treatment. (1) *Medical.* Most patients can be treated successfully by a simple regime designed to minimise gastro-oesophageal reflux and to neutralise any gastric acid which finds its way into the gullet. These ends are achieved by sleeping in a 'head up' position, either well propped up on pillows or with the head of the bed blocked, by avoiding stooping, and by taking small frequent meals. A tablet of Gaviscon chewed and washed down with water after meals and at bedtime helps by forming a mechanical barrier to reflux at the cardia. Cimetidine given as for peptic ulceration reduces acid reflux and helps to control symptoms. Weight reduction if necessary and stopping smoking are important.

(2) *Surgical* repair of the oesophageal hiatus in the diaphragm usually gives excellent results in those patients in whom severe symptoms persist in spite of a reasonable trial on the above regime.

ACHALASIA OF THE CARDIA

Achalasia of the cardia is due to a disorder of motor function of the oesophagus. Essentially there is an absence of peristalsis through the lower two-thirds of the oesophagus and a failure of the cardia to relax. Normal peristalsis may be replaced by slow ring-like contractions. The oesophagus becomes dilated and its muscle wall is hypertrophied. Because it cannot empty properly the oesophagus may contain food residue. In severe cases these residues may spill over into the lungs to produce recurrent attacks of pneumonia.

Achalasia of the cardia is due to degeneration of the cells of Auerbach's plexus. This is most marked in the dilated portion of the oesophagus and results in denervation of the oesophageal muscle. At the cardia some innervation appears to persist, but it seems likely that the nerves which cause relaxation of the cardia have disappeared.

Clinical Features. Achalasia of the cardia may occur at any age, but is more common in middle age and in women. The chief symptoms are *dysphagia* and *regurgitation*. They may be gradual in onset or may start suddenly, sometimes following an emotional upset. The dysphagia is often worse when the patient is emotionally upset or worried. In the early stages of the disease radiographic examination with a barium swallow will show delay at the cardia and often considerable oesophageal activity in the form of spasm and ring contraction, but no proper peristalsis. Some patients complain of discomfort behind the sternum when the oesophagus becomes distended with food. X-ray of the oesophagus in advanced cases shows it to be grossly dilated and filled with food residue; when the level of barium in the oesophagus reaches a certain level the cardia opens momentarily to let a little through into the stomach. It is at this stage that spill-over into the lungs occurs and the patient develops recurrent attacks of pneumonia which may finally lead to severe lung damage. Other complications include the development of carcinoma of the oesophagus and of multiple arthritis. In the early stages of achalasia of the cardia the patient's general health remains remarkably good and there is no weight loss. When the condition becomes more severe weight loss may occur.

Treatment. Inhalation of octyl nitrite relaxes the cardia, but this effect lasts for only one or two minutes and treatment giving more permanent relief is always needed. Dilatation with an instrument such as the Starke dilator, which causes forcible rupture of muscle fibres at the cardia, is often very effective. If this fails, or if the gullet is obviously dilated, cardiomyotomy (Heller's operation) should be performed. Results are excellent except in patients with gross dilatation and tortuosity of the gullet who require more extensive surgical procedures.

Oesophageal Spasm

In this condition there are spontaneous contractions of the lower oesophagus which sometimes produce quite severe pain. Unlike achalasia, dysphagia is not a prominent symptom. The disorder may arise de novo and continue intermittently for years or may complicate carcinoma of the oesophagus or gastro-oesophageal reflux. A radiograph of the oesophagus shows the typical corkscrew appearance due to muscle spasm. There is no specific cure but treatment of the reflux, if present, will help.

Systemic Sclerosis (see p. 424)

The oesophagus may be involved with the disease process resulting in infiltration by collagen and muscle atrophy. Peristalsis decreases and the cardia becomes incompetent with resulting acid reflux. The main symptoms, due to reflux, are acid oesophagitis and dysphagia.

Treatment is with antacids and cimetidine.

CARCINOMA OF THE OESOPHAGUS

This condition, which is much commoner in men than in women, should be suspected in any patient of middle age or beyond who develops dysphagia. The growth may occur in any part of the oesophagus and usually, though not invariably, the patient can indicate fairly accurately the level at which his food appears to stick. The dysphagia is steadily progressive, so that whereas at first there is difficulty only in swallowing solid food such as meat, within a month or two semi-solids and eventually fluids are affected also. The other striking symptom is rapid loss of weight.

Diagnosis. Barium swallow shows an area of narrowing which is rigid and may be irregular. Oesophagoscopy enables a biopsy to be taken for histological confirmation of the diagnosis.

Treatment. In general the prognosis is extremely bad, but carcinoma at the lower end of the oesophagus can occasionally be successfully resected. Alternatively, a Mousseau-Barbin tube, inserted at operation, may delay complete obstruction in swallowing for a month or two. Radiotherapy is usually ineffective, but occasional palliation of symptoms occurs after use of the supervoltage techniques available with the linear accelerator or cobalt unit.

THE STOMACH AND DUODENUM

Acute Gastritis

Acute gastritis is due to an irritant such as excessive alcohol or food poisoning, or occasionally to an acute specific infection such as influenza. The symptoms are loss of appetite, nausea, vomiting and abdominal discomfort; diarrhoea often occurs too, due to an associated enteritis. The vomited material is occasionally blood-stained. The symptoms subside spontaneously within a few days and usually all that is needed in the way of treatment is to keep the patient warm and comfortable and avoid any further irritation of his stomach. Occasionally, however, severe haematemesis necessitating transfusion occurs from acute superficial gastric erosions; sometimes these follow the taking of aspirin, of which even the soluble forms are common causes of minor gastric bleeding, but more often the aetiology is unknown.

Chronic Gastritis

Although chronic gastritis is a diagnostic label frequently attached to middle-aged and elderly patients with dyspeptic symptoms, it has no clear-cut pathology or clinical picture. The best-known variety is that due to chronic alcoholism. The patient complains of loss of appetite and nausea, particularly in the early morning, and frequently vomits mucus which has collected in the oesophagus and stomach during the night. He does not feel well until he has had another drink or two and so the vicious circle goes on. The only treatment of any value is complete and permanent abstention from alcohol.

PEPTIC ULCER

Peptic ulcers may be acute or chronic. They occur in the lower oesophagus, stomach or duodenum, or occasionally in the upper jejunum or at a gastro-enterostomy stoma.

Acute ulcers cause little in the way of symptoms and are seldom diagnosed unless they cause serious bleeding or perforation. They usually heal rapidly but often recur. Aspirin is a gastric irritant and may cause superficial gastric erosions which bleed.

Chronic peptic ulcers nearly all occur in the stomach or duodenum; when they co-exist the gastric ulcer usually develops second. A hereditary factor in gastric and duodenal ulcer has long been suspected from their frequent occurrence in several members of a family; furthermore, both types of ulcer have a higher incidence in persons of blood group O and are also more common in those who are unable to secrete their blood group substances in the saliva and gastric juice. This is a genetically determined factor; non-secretors number about 20% of the general population and 30–35% of the ulcer population.

Patients with duodenal ulcer as a group have twice as many parietal cells in their gastric mucosa as healthy people or patients with gastric ulcer and in general the further an ulcer is from the cardia the more hydrochloric acid is secreted by the stomach. Patients with duodenal ulcer also secrete more pepsin and have a tendency to nocturnal hypersecretion of acid. Gastric ulcers on the other hand tend to be associated with a low or normal acid secretion and with a gastric mucosa affected histologically by chronic gastritis; whether the latter is cause or effect is not known.

Chronic peptic ulcers occur at any age but are particularly common in middle life; gastric ulcers tend to arise in rather older people than duodenal ulcers. The sex incidence of gastric ulcers is almost equal; duodenal ulcers are 3–4 times more common in men than in women. In Western countries gastric and duodenal ulcers now seem to be significantly more common in poor people. There is no firm evidence to show that psychological factors, physique or personality are important in the cause of ulcer, but anxiety, overwork and stress of various kinds often lead to exacerbation of symptoms.

The increased incidence of duodenal ulcer in patients on renal dialysis is probably due to defective removal of circulating gastrin, and in patients with hyperparathyroidism to increased gastrin release induced by hypercalcaemia.

Oesophageal peptic ulcers arise in patients with hiatus hernia and gastro-oesophageal reflux. **Stomal ulcers** are particularly common in patients with gastroenterostomy in whom no procedure to reduce acid secretion, such as vagotomy, has been performed. **Upper jejunal ulcers,** usually at the duodeno-jejunal flexure, are associated with gross hypersecretion of gastric juice, which is produced continually at a maximal rate. This is the Zollinger–Ellison syndrome (p. 97).

Clinical Features. The principal and often the only symptom is *pain*, which is usually accurately localised to the centre of the epigastrium. It has two very characteristic features. The first is its *time-relation to food*: duodenal ulcer typically causes a hunger pain, which comes on when the stomach is empty and is relieved by the taking of food; in gastric ulcer the timing is often less regular, but the pain tends to come on about half to one hour after meals. The pain of duodenal ulcer often wakes the patient up at about 2 a.m., but curiously there is seldom pain before breakfast. Though typically localised to the epigastrium, the pain is occasionally referred to the lower abdomen, to the chest or to the back. The second very characteristic feature is the *periodicity*. Apart from treatment the history invariably tells of remissions, with complete freedom from symptoms for weeks or months, and subsequent relapses which are particularly liable during the winter months.

Mechanism of the Pain. For many years there has been debate between those who believe that the pain is due to spasm and those who ascribe it to irritation of the ulcer by acid, but neither of these theories is entirely satisfactory. It has been shown that pain is dependent on the presence of acid in the stomach, but it is also dependent on inflammation in the ulcer. From time to time a chronic peptic ulcer becomes inflamed and sensitive and at these times the action of acid, and other stimuli, cause pain; at other times they do not, even though the ulcer is still demonstrable by X-ray or gastroscope. The cause and mechanism of these episodes of inflammation constitute one of the basic unsolved problems of the disease. It is clear, however, that the state of tone in the stomach and duodenum and the acidity of their contents are largely incidental in the production of pain and that the administration of antispasmodics and antacids at times when the ulcer is in a quiescent phase is unlikely to serve any useful purpose.

Other symptoms including vomiting, a common event in patients with severe pain, when it is followed by relief, and in those with pyloric obstruction from either spasm or cicatricial stenosis; and waterbrash, or the filling of the mouth with tasteless watery saliva.

Physical signs are of minor importance. The ‘pointing sign’ is probably the most helpful: the patient when asked where his pain is places his finger tip on the centre of the epigastrium. There may also be some epigastric tenderness.

Diagnosis depends on *barium meal* screening of the patient by an experienced radiologist. The great majority of gastric ulcers occur in the middle third of the lesser curvature and are quite easily demonstrated in profile as a niche projecting from this aspect of the stomach. Ulcers occur only in the first part of the duodenum, referred to by the radiologist as the duodenal bulb or cap, and are much more difficult to demonstrate, being identified with certainty in little more than half the cases. They are more often seen '*en face*' than in profile, appearing as a round pool of barium a millimetre or two in diameter surrounded by a clear halo, and sometimes mucosal rugae can be seen radiating from this area. Frequently, however, the only signs are irregularity, irritability and tenderness of the duodenal cap.

Endoscopy. With a modern instrument employing fibre-optics, ulcers (or other lesions) in the stomach or duodenum can be directly seen, and if necessary a biopsy may be taken. This is a very helpful examination when the diagnosis remains in doubt and should be performed on all patients with a gastric ulcer to exclude malignancy.

Tests for occult blood in the stools are usually positive in patients with active peptic ulcer.

Complications

(1) **Haemorrhage.** Slight bleeding always takes place from the raw surface, but if the ulcer is a deep one it may erode into an artery in the wall of the stomach or duodenum and lead to massive haemorrhage. The patient may vomit a large quantity of blood (this is a *haematemesis*) and it is obvious at once that serious bleeding is in progress, but if the blood goes the other way down through the intestines the diagnosis must be made first on the signs of internal haemorrhage and later on the appearance of a large amount of altered blood in the stools making them black and tarry. The latter event is a *melaena.* Internal haemorrhage should be suspected in any patient who complains of sudden faintness and is found on examination to be pale and sweating, with a fast thready pulse and a low blood pressure.

(2) **Perforation** is the most dangerous complication and is almost confined to men. The discharge of acid gastric or duodenal contents into the peritoneal cavity causes severe generalised abdominal pain and board-like rigidity of the abdominal muscles. The patient lies quite still, because any movement aggravates his pain, and he shows signs of shock (pallor, sweating, fast pulse and low blood pressure). The diagnosis is usually easily made from this striking clinical picture and emergency operation to close the perforation should be done without delay.

(3) **Pyloric stenosis** is a complication of ulcer in the duodenum or rarely in the pyloric canal itself and results from contraction of scar tissue laid down in the base of the ulcer. In many patients, however, the syndrome of pyloric obstruction is due mainly to spasm in association with an active ulcer and clears up as the ulcer heals. Obstruction at the pylorus leads to distension of the stomach, which is evacuated from time to time by vomiting, which is often copious and projectile; and if the vomit contains recognisable articles of food, such as tomato skins, known to have been eaten many hours previously, this provides clear evidence of delay in gastric emptying. Patients with pyloric stenosis lose weight and become dehydrated and the alkalosis resulting from loss of

hydrochloric acid may lead to tetany, either overt (carpopedal spasm) or latent (positive Chvostek and Trousseau's signs). The only satisfactory treatment for pyloric stenosis is gastroenterostomy.

(4) **Hour-glass stomach** is the result of scarring from a chronic lesser curve ulcer and is usually simply an incidental X-ray finding. It is nearly always seen in women and is now rare.

Treatment of Peptic Ulcer

(1) **Medical Treatment.** The treatment of peptic ulcer has been revolutionised by the introduction of the H_2 receptor antagonist drugs *cimetidine* (Tagamet) and *ranitidine* (Zantac). Cimetidine is given in doses of 400 mg twice daily; or ranitidine 150 mg twice daily. The usual course lasts 6 weeks by which time the great majority of ulcers have healed, but the bedtime dose is often continued on a long-term basis to prevent relapse. Initial suspicions about the safety of prolonged administration have not been confirmed. These drugs suppress both basal and stimulated gastric acid secretion and also reduce the secretion of pepsin. They have very largely replaced the anticholinergic drugs such as poldine, previously given to limit gastric acidity.

Antacids such as aluminium hydroxide and magnesium trisilicate give symptomatic relief and when given in large doses one and three hours after meals have been shown to promote healing of duodenal but not gastric ulcers. Sodium bicarbonate and sodium hydroxide relieve pain quickly, but prolonged use may cause alkalosis.

Carbenoxolone has been shown to accelerate the healing of gastric ulcers. It is given in doses of 100 mg three times daily. Since it causes fluid and salt retention the patients, particularly if elderly, must have their blood pressure and weight checked weekly. An increase in weight of 2 kg or more is an indication for adding a thiazide diuretic and Slow K to the regime. A preparation of deglycyrrhizinated liquorice (Ulcedal or Caved S) may be given to elderly people instead of carbenoxolone since it is substantially free from side-effects.

Prolonged rest is seldom necessary today but when symptoms are severe a few days in bed at the onset of treatment may be very helpful. Special ulcer diets are no longer employed but patients should have regular meals and avoid items known to upset them. Milky drinks may be taken between meals and at night to relieve pain. Smoking should be avoided.

The healing of gastric ulcers should always be checked endoscopically as a precaution against missing early gastric carcinoma.

The Treatment of Massive Bleeding. A patient who has had a large haematemesis or melaena is always an anxious and difficult problem in treatment. In the hope that the bleeding will stop spontaneously he must be kept as quiet as possible; an injection of morphine 15–20 mg is therefore given on admission and repeated in a few hours if restlessness returns. Blood is taken for grouping and for haemoglobin estimation and an hourly pulse and blood pressure chart is started. The haemoglobin level does not reflect the severity of the bleeding until several hours later, so that the pulse and blood pressure give a better immediate indication. *Transfusion* may not be necessary if the patient is young and the haemorrhage relatively slight, but an elderly patient who has bled severely must be given at least two pints of blood without delay. For a patient whose bleeding is thought to have stopped transfusion at the rate of one pint in four hours is satisfactory, but the blood must be run in much more quickly if the bleeding is continuing. In addition to the obvious immediate risk to life, two serious hazards of failing to replace lost blood may be mentioned: in the elderly, severe anaemia may lead to cardiac failure by inducing an increase in cardiac output; and very occasionally recurrence of bleeding in a severely anaemic patient leads to permanent blindness. A good rule to follow is: 'When in doubt, transfuse.' At one time these patients were given only ice to suck, in the mistaken idea that this would rest the stomach. An empty stomach is in fact much more active than a full one and it is wiser to give the patient a *diet* corresponding to the first stage of the usual ulcer regime as soon as he can take it. *Cimetidine* 200 mg IV 6-hourly may be given and a change made to oral administration when possible. However, its usefulness in treating haematemesis is still debated. Emergency *operation* may be needed if the bleeding continues or recurs, but carries a high mortality in these severely ill patients; the decision whether to operate, and when, calls for a high degree of clinical judgment on behalf of both physician and surgeon and cannot be made according to any hard and fast rules.

(2) **Surgical Treatment.** The **indications for surgery** are:

(a) Failure of the symptoms of a duodenal ulcer to remit, or failure of a gastric ulcer to show radiological or endoscopic evidence of healing, after an adequate period of efficient medical treatment.
(b) Pyloric obstruction.
(c) Severe bleeding, particularly if it has recurred and the patient is above middle age.
(d) Doubt whether a gastric ulcer may be malignant. Duodenal ulcers are never malignant.
(e) Perforation.

For benign chronic gastric ulcer the operation of choice is *subtotal gastrectomy* (Billroth 1) and gastroduodenal anastomosis.

For chronic duodenal ulcer the popular operations today are (1) *truncal vagotomy and pyloroplasty* and (2) denervation of the parietal cell mass without drainage (*proximal gastric vagotomy*). The incidence of postoperative syndromes has declined since these procedures largely replaced the Billroth 2 operation (distal three-quarters gastrectomy with closure of the gastric stump and gastrojejunostomy) but the recurrent ulcer rate is slightly higher.

Postoperative Syndromes

(1) *Gastro-oesophageal reflux* is sometimes troublesome after either vagotomy or gastrectomy. Symptoms can usually be controlled by raising the head of the bed and giving metoclopramide (Maxolon) 10 mg four times daily.

(2) *Diarrhoea* is common after truncal vagotomy (up to 25 %) but quite rare after proximal gastric vagotomy. Spontaneous improvement usually occurs. Small frequent meals and codeine phosphate 30 mg up to three times daily help to control the symptom.

(3) *Dumping syndrome* occurs in about 20 % of patients after gastrectomy and is occasionally seen after vagotomy. Symptoms start either during a meal or within half an hour with abdominal fullness and sensations of 'rolling' or 'churning', nausea, palpitations, dizziness and faintness. Soon afterwards the patient usually complains of weakness, fatigue or exhaustion which may persist for up to 3 hours. Severe attacks may be precipitated by large meals or less often by sweet foods or drinks. The symptoms are probably the result of excessive jejunal stimulation: they can be reproduced by various abnormal jejunal stimuli such as entry of iced water, hypertonic solutions or distension by a balloon. Barium meal shows precipitate gastric emptying, the meal leaving the stomach within ten minutes. Inadequate handling of a glucose load, with a lag type of glucose tolerance test and a reduction in plasma volume have been demonstrated and tolbutamide 0.25–1.0 g ten to thirty minutes before meals may help to prevent attacks. Dry meals rich in protein and poor in carbohydrate and lying down after eating are other helpful measures.

(4) *Late hypoglycaemic attacks* occur $1\frac{1}{2}$–3 hours after meals and are due to functional post-prandial hyperinsulinism. Symptoms are dizziness, faintness, sweating and palpitations. The patients are frequently rather nervous unstable people who have been subject to similar but milder attacks before the operation. They require treatment by reassurance, correction of malnutrition if necessary, and should take small frequent meals with a low carbohydrate content.

CARCINOMA OF THE STOMACH

Carcinoma of the stomach is the third commonest cancer in the UK (after breast and bronchus) and occurs twice as often in men as in women.

Clinical Features. Early diagnosis is of the utmost importance if the patient is to have any chance of radical cure, and to this end the possibility of malignant disease of the stomach should be borne in mind when a patient of early middle age or beyond develops for the first time dyspeptic symptoms which persist for more than two or three weeks. The symptoms are very variable, but the most common are anorexia and epigastric pain which usually does not show the clear-cut relation to food seen in patients with peptic ulcer. Within a few months most patients show obvious loss of weight and anaemia, though occasional very slowly growing gastric cancers may cause only very vague symptoms for as long as two years. Frequently a good deal of bleeding occurs from the surface of the carcinoma, and the vomiting of altered blood which looks like coffee grounds is a characteristic feature. On the other hand, negative tests for occult blood in the stools do not exclude this diagnosis, for the infiltrating type of growth (causing the 'leather-bottle stomach') may extend widely in the wall of the stomach without causing surface ulceration. Some patients develop symptoms and signs of pyloric obstruction; less often a fundal tumour obstructs the cardia and the patient complains that his food appears to stick at the lower end of the gullet. In some unfortunate patients the earliest symptoms are those due to metastases in the liver or elsewhere.

Physical signs are usually present only in patients whose disease has advanced beyond the reach of curative surgery. Common findings at this stage are a hard fixed mass in the epigastrium and evidence of secondary deposits; important among the latter are an enlarged irregular liver, a hard lymph-node above the clavicle (described by Virchow), deep-vein thrombosis in the leg (Trousseau's sign), or on rectal examination bilateral Krukenberg tumours in the ovaries or a hard mass in the rectal pouch from transcoelomic spread. The only sign sometimes found in early cases is slight epigastric tenderness.

Diagnosis depends mainly on the *barium meal* examination, which classically shows a filling defect and failure of peristaltic movements over the affected part of the stomach. It is now thought that not more than about 1 % of peptic ulcers of the stomach undergo malignant change; in this group a very large ulcer and a suggestion of filling defect at one end of its are signs arousing suspicion of carcinoma. A leather-bottle stomach is small, indistensible and inactive and the barium runs straight through it into the duodenum. Biopsy of the lesion by *endoscopy* leads to histological confirmation of the diagnosis. There is usually a *hypochromic anaemia* and a raised *sedimentation rate* but both of these may also be found in patients with simple gastric ulcer.

Treatment. Radical surgery provides the only opportunity for cure, but the prognosis is among the worst for all forms of carcinoma and five-year survivals are below 10 %. Even in advanced cases the primary growth should be resected whenever possible, for apart from possible prolongation of life symptomatic relief makes the procedure worth while.

DISORDERS OF THE INTESTINES

THE MALABSORPTION SYNDROMES

These disorders are characterised by failure of absorption of essential food factors by the small intestine, with consequent chronic diarrhoea and malnutrition. All somewhat rare, the more common members are coeliac disease in children, idiopathic steatorrhoea, and tropical sprue. Similar effects may result from resection of part of the small gut, especially when a blind loop has been formed, from Crohn's disease, from pancreatitis, from drugs such as neomycin or phenindione and from the very rare Whipple's disease (intestinal lipodystrophy).

Tropical Sprue (p. 710)

Sprue is endemic in certain countries in the Far East, notably India, Sri Lanka, Indo-China, and the East Indies. It occurs also in the West Indies but is apparently rare in Africa. It particularly affects Europeans living temporarily in an endemic area, though usually not until after many years' residence. The gut shows abnormal or atrophic villi but the cause of the disease is obscure; at present the most popular theory for the failure of intestinal function is an alteration of the normal bacterial flora following recurrent dysenteric infection.

GLUTEN ENTEROPATHY (Idiopathic Steatorrhoea)

This is the adult counterpart of coeliac disease (which will not be described here) and sometimes the symptoms can be traced through a series of remissions and exacerbations back to childhood. It was noted in Holland after the second world war that children with coeliac disease who had been making good progress under conditions of near starvation during the German occupation began to deteriorate when wheat and rye were introduced into the diet. Further investigation soon confirmed that there was an intolerance to gluten, the protein part of the wheat, rye or barley germ, but curiously enough not to the glutens in other cereals. It is probable that intolerance to wheat and rye glutens is also the cause of idiopathic steatorrhoea. The cause of this intolerance is either deficiency of the enzyme which normally hydrolyses the toxic peptide part of the gluten or damage to the intestinal mucosa from an abnormal immunological reaction.

The disease is familial: siblings are about 100 times more likely to suffer from it than members of unaffected families. There is a high incidence of tissue antigen HLA-B8.

Clinical Features. There is usually an insidious onset of looseness of the stools, general weakness, and loss of weight. The diarrhoea is persistent, though most patients have exacerbations from time to time followed by remissions in which the stools become temporarily almost normal. During exacerbations the stools typically are pale, bulky, frothy, and greasy; but they may be fluid and not obviously fatty, though analysis will usually reveal an excess of fat. Flatulence is usually severe and the distension of the abdomen contrasts with the progressive emaciation of the rest of the body. Clubbing of the fingers occasionally develops. Other symptoms and signs result from failure of absorption of essential food factors:

Factor Deficient	*Clinical Effect*
Iron	Hypochromic anaemia } (The anaemia is usually of mixed type)
Vitamin B_{12}, Folic acid	Macrocytic anaemia } (The anaemia is usually of mixed type)
Vitamin B complex	
aneurine (thiamine)	Peripheral neuritis (rare)
riboflavin, Nicotinic acid	Glossitis, Stomatitis
Vitamin D, Calcium	Tetany, Osteomalacia
Vitamin K	Haemorrhagic tendency
Potassium	Weakness, apathy, and mental disturbance

Diagnosis. A number of screening tests have been used, of which the xylose absorption test and the serum folate level are probably the best, but if the disease is suspected clinically peroral jejunal biopsy (using a special capsule) must be performed on two occasions. The first demonstrates the typical mucosal lesion; the second shows the response to gluten withdrawal.

Treatment of Gluten Enteropathy. Although most patients respond completely to a strict gluten-free diet within a few weeks, some require supplements of iron, Vitamin B_{12}, folic acid, calcium or Vitamin D. A few continue to have diarrhoea or relapse, usually from failing to keep to the diet; it should be made clear from the onset, therefore, that wheat gluten will probably have to be avoided for life. In the UK gluten-free foods are prescribable under the NHS (on EC 10), and patients derive help and moral support in keeping strictly to their diet by joining the Coeliac Society. If the patient is severely ill prednisolone may be given in addition to a gluten-free diet and usually causes improvement in the general condition and in the mucosal lesion.

Complications. There is a high incidence of lymphoma of the small bowel in these patients, most often reticulum-cell sarcoma of the jejunum. They are also more prone to carcinoma of the gastrointestinal tract and even in other parts of the body.

About 60% of patients with dermatitis herpetiformis have a gluten enteropathy. The reason for this association is not known.

Treatment of Sprue. Europeans who develop sprue in the tropics usually recover spontaneously when they return to a temperate climate. Sometimes a course of tetracycline, 250–500 mg 6-hourly for five days, is of benefit, probably by altering the bacterial flora of the gut. It is usual to give a diet rich in protein and vitamins and low in fat and roughage. Vitamin B_{12} is given intramuscularly, starting with 100 μg on alternate days and gradually increasing the interval between injections during recovery. Folic acid 10–20 mg three times daily is given by mouth. Other vitamin and mineral deficiencies are corrected as necessary.

Other Causes of Malabsorption

Obstructive jaundice impairs the digestion of fats and in long-standing cases the resulting steatorrhoea may lead eventually to osteomalacia. In *chronic pancreatitis* lack of pancreatic digestive enzymes impairs the digestion of fat and protein and leads to steatorrhoea and heavy loss of nitrogen in the stools; absorption of glucose, iron, folic acid, and vitamin B_{12} is usually normal.

Extensive resection of the small gut may be followed by malnutrition, but in organic disease of the small intestine malabsorption results not from loss of absorbing surface but from bacterial activity. The normally sterile small gut may be invaded by coliform organisms, as a result of stasis, either above a *stricture* (as in Crohn's disease) or in a *blind loop* formed by a fistulous communication or surgical bypass, or as a result of direct access through a *gastrocolic fistula*. In the very rare *Zollinger–Ellison syndrome*, probably as a result of gastrin secretion by the pancreatic tumour always present, there is heavy and continuous outpouring of gastric juice and the usual clinical presentation is severe and intractable peptic ulceration, but sometimes the contents of the small intestine are rendered acid and steatorrhoea results from inactivation of the pancreatic enzymes. Another very rare cause of steatorrhoea and progressive wasting is *Whipple's disease* or intestinal lipodystrophy; the cause is unknown and the diagnosis can be made with certainty only by biopsy of the small intestine to show large foamy macrophages, filled with an unidentified glycoprotein, in the tunica propria, and lipogranulomatosis in the mesenteric lymph-nodes. The disease is progressive, but temporary remission of symptoms may be induced by corticosteroid therapy.

Disaccharide Intolerance

Digestion of disaccharides such as lactose, sucrose and maltose takes place within the mucosal cells. If one of the enzymes lactase, sucrase or maltase is lacking the corresponding disaccharide accumulates and may cause diarrhoea and malabsorption. Patients with *lactase deficiency* may give a history of diarrhoea after drinking milk; the diagnosis is supported by demonstrating a flat blood sugar curve after a loading dose of lactose. The deficiency may be an inborn error or the result of various diseases affecting the small intestine. Symptoms are relieved by a milk-free diet.

CROHN'S DISEASE

In this disease of unknown aetiology there are single or multiple sharply demarcated areas of intestine, mainly in the lower ileum and in the colon, which become grossly thickened by lymphoid hyperplasia, ulceration, oedema, and secondary infection. Complications include cicatricial stenosis of the bowel, localised perforation, abscess, and the formation of fistulae. The sex incidence is approximately equal and symptoms usually begin in the twenties or thirties.

Clinical Features. Symptoms usually develop very gradually and there are often long natural remissions so that the history commonly extends over several years by the time the diagnosis is made. Most patients present with attacks of colicky pain round the umbilicus or in the right iliac fossa, with associated mild diarrhoea and general weakness. Loss of weight is usual and there is often low fever. The most helpful and important *physical sign* is a tender fixed mass, usually in the right iliac fossa, and the *barium 'follow through'* examination demonstrates gross filling defects and narrowing of the lumen of the affected segments of intestine. The blood count shows anaemia and some leucocytosis and a high sedimentation rate. Fistulous *complications* may lead to peri-anal abscess and fistula-in-ano, dysuria and passage of wind *per urethram* from ileovesical fistula or abscess in the abdominal wall. An associated granular proctitis is common.

Systemic Complications. Transient arthritis, usually confined to one large joint, is common; about 5% of patients have ankylosing spondylitis; and about 20% have symptomless sacro-iliitis, revealed by X-ray. Erythema nodosum is commonly seen, particularly in women; more serious is pyoderma gangrenosum, a term applied to deep ulcers with a sloughing base seen mainly on the legs, but sometimes on the face, thought to be a result of vasculitis. Iritis, episcleritis and conjunctivitis are important ocular complications. There is a high incidence of both gallstones and kidney stones. Cirrhosis of the liver is a rare association.

Treatment. The patient should be confined to bed during febrile exacerbations and should be advised at all times to avoid exhaustion from either physical or mental overstrain. Improvement does sometimes seem to follow the resolution of emotional problems and worries, but in the individual patient it is seldom that any useful action can be taken in this connection. Sulphasalazine is given as for ulcerative colitis (q.v.) to reduce the incidence of relapses and exacerbations. Rapid relief of symptoms often follows treatment with steroids, but the improvement is not always maintained and it is probably wise to reserve steroid therapy for the control of exacerbations. A suitable course would be prednisolone 40–60 mg daily for a few days until the fever and other symptoms have subsided, then a maintenance dose of about 20 mg daily for two or three weeks, after which the dosage should be gradually tailed off. Azathioprine is sometimes useful when other forms of medical treatment have failed. The usual dose is 2.0 mg/kg/day and regular blood counts are necessary as there is a risk of bone marrow depression. Operation should be avoided if possible during the stage of active ulceration but about three quarters of the patients will ultimately require surgery for the relief of complications such as perforation, cicatricial obstruction or fistulae. Resection of the affected segment of bowel is the treatment of choice.

Prognosis. Although most patients with Crohn's disease are able to lead a reasonable life, their survival rate is below that of a control population. About half the patients who have a surgical resection will relapse within ten years and some will require further surgery.

ULCERATIVE COLITIS

This is a serious and chronic disease of the colon and although temporary remission of symptoms is common, relapse nearly always follows after a variable interval of months or years and complete recovery is very rare. The cause of ulcerative colitis is unknown. Its acute stage is very similar to bacillary dysentery, which suggests that an infection might be responsible, but no specific organism has ever been isolated. Some authorities have been very struck by the characteristic personality of many of these patients, who are said to be fussy, tidy, meticulous people, emotionally immature and showing an abnormal dependence on one or other parent, and by the fact that the onset of the illness or exacerbations in its severity quite often appears to be precipated by an emotional crisis associated with marriage, childbirth, or the death of a parent or near relative. It has therefore been suggested that the changes in the bowel are secondary to some psychological disturbance. Controlled psychiatric studies on small groups of patients have not supported this theory.

Clinical Features. It usually starts in early adult life and is slightly more common in women than in men. The principal symptom is *diarrhoea*, which continues in some degree throughout the whole course of the illness. During acute relapses the stools are greatly increased in number and contain *blood and mucus*, abdominal pain is often severe, the temperature is raised and the patient becomes very weak, anaemic and emaciated; in remissions the general health becomes more or less restored, but there is nearly always some persistent looseness of the stools. The severity of the disease varies greatly in different patients. There is an acute fulminating variety which renders the patient gravely ill, even moribund, within a few weeks; at the other end of the scale is a mild type which causes only relatively trivial inconvenience; and between these extremes the majority of patients require admission to hospital from time to time over many years and are always more or less severely disabled by their disease.

Physical signs are few, though there is usually some tenderness over the affected part of the colon. The blood count reveals *anaemia* which is sometimes severe and usually a *leucocytosis*. The *sedimentation rate* is very high during relapses and seldom falls completely to normal even during remissions. *Sigmoidoscopy* shows a very red, granular, bleeding, and superficially ulcerated mucosa. The *barium enema* in moderately severe or advanced cases shows the affected bowel to be shorter and narrower than normal and to have a rather fuzzy outline devoid of the normal haustral markings; these appearances are particularly helpful in assessing how much of the colon is involved. The double-contrast technique involves insufflation of air into the bowel after most of the barium has been removed and provides better definition of mucosal lesions.

Complications. Stricture of the bowel, peri-anal abscess, toxic dilatation of the colon, perforation leading to abscess or peritonitis, severe haemorrhage and the development of carcinoma in the diseased colon are complications particularly to be feared in the younger patients with severe ulcerative colitis. Opinions differ about the frequency of malignant change, but it certainly occurs sufficiently often in patients who have had a severe form of the disease for ten years or more to be a powerful argument in favour of treatment by colectomy. Increasing dilatation of the colon is a serious complication seen in very ill patients and is an indication for immediate operation.

The various *systemic complications* of Crohn's disease (p. 98) are also seen in patients with ulcerative colitis.

Treatment. There is no specific therapy and during the acute stages undoubtedly the most important measure is a period of complete *rest* in bed. The *diet* should be high in protein and in total calories; a milk-free diet may be worth trying in patients with persistent mild symptoms. Vitamin supplements should be given. For the relief of anaemia fresh *blood transfusion* is the most effective treatment and in addition often seems to be of benefit to the patient's general condition. *Iron* is indicated too and should be given parenterally (see p. 611 for details) if oral preparations appear to aggravate the diarrhoea. To control the diarrhoea tab. codeine phosphate 30–60 mg three or four times daily or diphenoxylate (Lomotil) 2 tablets three or four times daily are the most useful preparations and propantheline 15–30 mg three or four times daily may help to relieve colic.

It is now usual to give oral *sulphasalazine*, which has been shown to reduce the incidence of relapses. The initial dose is 2.0 g daily in divided doses. Side-effects include nausea, headaches, blood dyscrasias and rashes. For long-term maintenance the dose can be reduced. This treatment must be continued over many months or years.

In the acute stage the most effective drug to induce a remission is prednisolone. It should be given locally (a daily Predsol enema) and systemically (prednisolone 5.0 mg four times daily). After the acute attack has subsided it should be gradually withdrawn as prolonged treatment with this drug will lead to steroid toxicity. The immunosuppressive drug azathioprine may be tried in patients failing to respond to the above regime, but careful supervision with regular blood counts to detect early bone-marrow suppression is essential; the dose is 2.0 mg/kg daily.

Many patients need surgery but there is no general agreement about the *indications for operation.* The procedure employed is total colectomy, and although it is occasionally possible to join the ileum to the rectal stump, most patients are left with a permanent ileostomy. With modern techniques, however, patients with this disability are able to lead almost normal lives. The present tendency therefore is not to regard surgery as the final desperate gamble for an almost moribund patient, but to advise operation after a reasonable trial of medical treatment. The improvement in health is usually well worth the price of the ileostomy and, as mentioned above, the risk of malignant change and other complications is a further incentive to relatively early surgery.

Intestinal Ischaemia

Ischaemia of the gut is rare because of the good collateral blood supply. It is seldom seen in patients under 60. *Acute ischaemia* causes sudden severe abdominal pain, often with diarrhoea and rectal bleeding, and with signs of intestinal ileus. It is an acute surgical emergency. *Chronic ischaemia* causes abdominal pain which starts soon after a meal and persists for an hour or two. Distension, diarrhoea and loss of weight are other features. As time passes it may be noted that smaller meals bring on the pain and do so more quickly. There are no characteristic physical signs and *diagnosis* depends on coeliac, superior and inferior mesenteric angiography. Arterial grafting may relieve the symptoms.

Protein-losing Enteropathy

In some gastrointestinal diseases, notably ulcerative colitis, regional ileitis, idiopathic steatorrhoea and carcinoma of the stomach, exudation of plasma occurs into the lumen of the gut. The faecal nitrogen is not increased, since most of the plasma is digested and reabsorbed; but hypoproteinaemia and resulting oedema may develop in view of the liver's limited reserve capacity to synthesise albumin.

DIVERTICULAR DISEASE OF THE COLON

This expression is now preferred to the older terms diverticulosis and diverticulitis. Two varieties are recognised.

Diffuse diverticular disease becomes very common after middle age and is found in most elderly people. Diverticula with short necks and wide mouths occur throughout the colon and are probably the result of muscular atrophy without any increase in intraluminal pressure. Usually there are no symptoms, but occasionally a diverticulum perforates or leads to massive haemorrhage from the bowel; indeed, this is the commonest cause of the latter symptom.

Localised diverticular disease is most common in the sigmoid colon; it is thought that a rise in intraluminal pressure, due to irregular contraction of the hypertrophied muscle, forces diverticula through the thickened bowel wall so that their necks are often long and narrow. At first there may be obstructive symptoms such as distension, flatulence, and colicky pains, but later inflammatory changes may cause more persistent pain with fever and a tender mass may become palpable. A fistula between the colon and either the bladder or vagina should be suspected if the patient develops frequency of micturition or vaginal discharge.

Treatment. Diverticular disease does not occur in parts of the world where a high-residue diet is eaten, and the addition of miller's bran to a Western diet, a tablespoonful two or three times daily, is usually effective in relieving symptoms. Appropriate surgical treatment may be needed for inflammatory complications.

IRRITABLE BOWEL SYNDROME

This term is applied to many patients who complain of disordered action of the bowels, usually diarrhoea, often with abdominal pain, distension and flatulence, in whom thorough examination and investigation fail to reveal any evidence of organic disease. Formerly such patients were often said to have a 'spastic colon'. Symptoms usually start before the age of 30 and may date back to childhood; it is unwise to make this diagnosis in patients presenting after the age of 50.

Treatment. Increasing dietary fibre by giving miller's bran 1 tablespoonful three times daily, is often helpful; and dramatic improvement may follow the recognition and treatment of underlying anxiety or depression. Supportive follow-up is also beneficial.

ACUTE GASTROINTESTINAL BLEEDING

This is a common and serious medical emergency with a mortality rate of about 10%. The outlook is particularly bad in elderly patients with associated cardiac or pulmonary disabilities. It is useful to classify the patients as having upper or lower gastrointestinal bleeding according to whether the source of bleeding is above or below the duodeno-jejunal flexure.

UPPER GASTROINTESTINAL BLEEDING

This may be revealed by haematemesis and/or melaena, but frequently has to be inferred from signs of internal haemorrhage: these are sudden faintness or collapse with rapid pulse and low blood pressure and in the elderly the reduced perfusion of heart or brain may lead to myocardial infarction or stroke. In this situation routine rectal examination may be invaluable in revealing melaena stool.

The Cause of the Bleeding. Duodenal ulcer and the gastric ulcer are the commonest causes, in that order, and together account for about 50% of the cases. Acute gastric or duodenal erosions (up to 10%), oesophagitis (about 5%), oesophageal varices (about 3%) and Mallory–Weiss tears (up to 5%) are other important causes; rare ones include gastric carcinoma and bleeding disorders. However, full investigation including endoscopy fails to reveal the site of bleeding in at least 20% of cases. Acute 'stress' ulcers have long been recognised as complications of severe burns or neurological disease, but are now known to occur in patients critically ill from any cause.

Clinical Assessment. The Hb level is not a reliable index of acute blood loss since dilution of the blood takes some hours to develop; a low Hb at this stage suggests chronic blood loss previously. Frequent observations of pulse rate and blood pressure should be made, a low diastolic level being particularly significant. Sometimes a patient who has bled seriously may appear to have a satisfactory pulse rate and blood pressure while at rest in bed but become faint with tachycardia and hypotension on standing. Conversely the absence of these postural effects suggests that the patient has not had a major haemorrhage.

Differential Diagnosis. (a) *History.* A history of ulcer dyspepsia suggests (though its absence does not refute) that the bleeding is from a peptic ulcer. Ingestion of aspirin within 24 hours, particularly in association with alcohol, favours acute erosions in the stomach or duodenum. A history of alcohol abuse raises the possibility of bleeding oesophageal varices (though in many cirrhotics a peptic ulcer is found to be the source of the bleeding). A haematemesis coming after massive vomiting (often related to alcoholic excess) suggests a mucosal tear at the cardia (*Mallory–Weiss syndrome*).

(b) *Examination.* Epigastric tenderness favours peptic ulcer or oesophagitis; a palpable mass may indicate a gastric carcinoma; stigmata of liver disease suggest bleeding varices; haemorrhage from other sites or telangiectasia point to a bleeding diathesis.

(c) *Investigations.* Emergency barium meal and/or endoscopy may be necessary to establish the site and nature of the lesion.

Acute Lower Gastrointestinal Bleeding

Diverticular disease of the colon has long been recognised as a common cause of acute lower gastrointestinal bleeding, and Meckel's diverticulum a rare one; more recently a microvascular abnormality of unknown cause (angiodysplasia) has been identified as a common cause of acute haemorrhage, usually from the right half of the colon, in elderly patients. The diagnosis is often difficult and if barium follow-through, double-contrast barium enema and colonoscopy fail to reveal it, mesenteric angiography while the patient is still bleeding may demonstrate the source of the haemorrhage.

DISEASES OF THE LIVER

JAUNDICE

Definition. Jaundice is an increase in the amount of bilirubin in the blood resulting in yellow discoloration of the sclerotics of the eyes, the skin, mucosae, and certain body fluids.

Physiology of Bile (Fig. 3.1). After circulating in the blood for about 120 days red corpuscles are removed and broken up by cells of the reticuloendothelial system, mainly in the liver, spleen, and bone marrow. The haemoglobin is split into two fractions, an iron-containing part which is returned to the bone marrow for resynthesis into haemoglobin and an iron-free porphyrin fraction from which the pigment bilirubin is derived. When liberated into the blood for transport to the liver this bilirubin is insoluble in water and being protein-bound it is unable to pass into the urine. It is said to be *unconjugated.* The bilirubin is taken up by the liver cells, where it becomes conjugated through its carboxyl groups with glucuronic acid to form water-soluble bilirubin diglucuronide (*conjugated bilirubin*).

In this form bilirubin passes down the bile duct to the duodenum, where it is converted into stercobilinogen, the pigment responsible for most of the normal colour of faeces. Some of this is absorbed (as urobilinogen) from the small intestine into the portal bloodstream; and though nearly all of this fraction is removed again by the liver cells and returned to the biliary passages, traces of it usually escape through the liver into the general circulation and are excreted in the urine.

Bile salts are the end product of cholesterol metabolism and consist of cholic acid and chenodeoxycholic acid conjugated with glycine and taurine. They are excreted in the bile and play an important part in fat absorption. In the terminal ileum they are changed by bacterial action

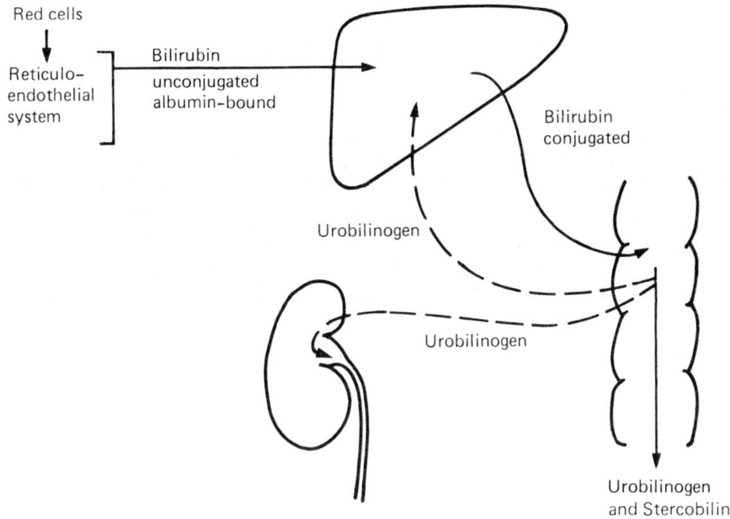

Fig. 3.1 Circulation and excretion of bile pigments.

into deoxycholic acid and lethocholic acid which are reabsorbed and excreted again, unchanged by the liver. About 20 g of bile salts are excreted each 24 hours and only 0.8 g are eventually lost in the faeces, so there is considerable recycling.

Types of Jaundice

It is obvious that jaundice may result either because too much bilirubin is liberated into the blood from excessive breakdown of red corpuscles (*haemolytic jaundice*) or because too little bilirubin is removed from the blood in its passage through the liver. The latter can occur in two ways. The function of the liver cells may be deranged so that they cannot excrete bilirubin into the bile; this is known as *hepatocellular* or *hepatic jaundice*. Obstruction to the biliary system will prevent the flow of bile and this is now known as *cholestatic jaundice*. If the obstruction is in the main ducts outside the liver it is said to be *extrahepatic* and if the defect is in the small bile ducts and canaliculi within the liver it is *intrahepatic*.

Haemolytic Jaundice. This is the least common of the three main types of jaundice and the yellow discoloration of the skin and other tissues is seldom more than slight. The *urine* contains no *bilirubin* since the bilirubin in the blood is highly protein bound. As more bile pigment than normal is being produced and consequently an excess of urobilinogen is formed in the duodenum more of this pigment is absorbed into the portal bloodstream than the liver cells can remove and an *excess of* *urobilinogen* passes through into the urine. The stools retain their normal colour and chemical analysis shows that they too contain an excess of urobilinogen (sometimes called stercobilinogen in this context). The causes of haemolytic jaundice are discussed under haemolytic anaemia (pp. 615).

Cholestatic (Obstructive) Jaundice. This can be due to interference with bile flow in the main bile ducts (extrahepatic) or in the small bile ducts (intrahepatic).

Table 3.1 The main causes of cholestatic jaundice

Extrahepatic	*Intrahepatic*
Gall stones	Viral hepatitis
Carcinoma of the pancreas, bile ducts or gall bladder	Drugs
	Recurrent jaundice of pregnancy
Secondary deposits	Primary biliary cirrhosis
Biliary stricture	Inflammatory bowel disease
Chronic pancreatitis	Recurrent idiopathic

In extrahepatic cholestasis there is mechanical obstruction to the bile ducts with dilation of the biliary system. In intrahepatic obstruction the mechanism is not known. The major bile ducts and gall bladder are empty and the disorders appear to be a defect in biliary secretion or biliary flow.

With both types of obstruction there is a rise in the plasma concentration of conjugated bilirubin and when this exceeds the renal threshold of 34 μmol/l bile passes freely into the urine, the conjugated form being water soluble. As little or no bile reaches the intestine, the stools are pale. No urobilinogen is formed and thus none is found in the urine. Bile salts are also retained by the liver and are believed to be responsible for the pruritis which is common in patients with this condition.

Prolonged obstruction of the biliary system causes damage to liver cells which leads to fibrosis with distortion of the normal liver pattern, and ultimately cirrhosis (secondary biliary cirrhosis). In addition, extrahepatic obstruction may be complicated by biliary tract infection (cholangitis).

In cholestatic jaundice the plasma alkaline phosphatase is raised roughly in parallel with the bilirubin and similar changes are found in the 5-nucleotidase. Unlike hepatocellular jaundice the serum aspartate aminotransaminase is usually only moderately raised but may be high if there is complicating cholangitis (see Table 3.2).

The distinction between intra- and extrahepatic obstruction may be easy on clinical grounds; however, this is not always so and biochemical tests may not help. Three useful investigations are:

Table 3.2 Laboratory investigation of jaundice

Test	*Normal range*	*Hepatocellular jaundice*	*Cholestatic jaundice*	*Haemolytic jaundice*
Serum bilirubin	Up to 23 μmol/l	Conjugated raised	Conjugated raised	Non-conjugated raised
Stools		Variable	Pale	Normal
Urine bilirubin	0	Usually present	Raised	0
Urobilinogen	0–trace	Increased in early stages	0	Raised
Serum aspartate-aminotransferase	Up to 43 μg/l	Raised	Normal or slightly raised	Normal
Alkaline phosphatase	20–90 μg/l	*Normal or a little raised	Raised	Normal
5-Nucleotidase	0–13 μg/l	Normal or a little raised	Raised	Normal
Albumin	30–46 g/l	Reduced	Normal	Normal
Globulin	20–38 g/l	May be raised	Normal	Normal
Gluteryl transpeptidase	< 40 μg/l	An index of enzyme induction. Raised in alcoholic liver disease and also in cholestatic jaundice.		
Cholesterol	3.6–8.0 mmol/l Varies with age	Normal or decreased	Raised	Normal

*Sometimes in viral hepatitis the alkaline phosphatase is high, suggesting a cholestatic element.

(a) ultrasound scanning, which will not only reveal gall stones but will show dilated bile ducts in about 90% of patients with extrahepatic obstruction;
(b) percutaneous transhepatic cholangiography (PTC) in which contrast medium injected into the bile ducts will show their outlines;
(c) endoscopic retrograde cholangiopancreatography (ERCP), in which contrast medium injected via the ampulla of Vater outlines the biliary tree and pancreatic ducts.

Hepatocellular Jaundice. In this group the jaundice is due primarily to difficulty in the transport of bilirubin through the hepatic cell, and possibly in its conjugation; but the pattern of bile pigments in the serum is in fact identical with that which follows occlusion of the bile duct, and the jaundice must be due partly to regurgitation from the bile canaliculi. In addition, diminished red cell survival is found in all patients with this condition, and adds a haemolytic component to the jaundice. There is usually a stage in the disease in which the stools are pale and the urine contains bilirubin but no urobilinogen, as in cholestatic jaundice; there may also be a misleading rise in the serum alkaline phosphatase. Elevation of enzymes, which is due to cell damage, is the characteristic biochemical finding. The total serum cholesterol is usually decreased.

Causes of hepatocellular jaundice include:

viral hepatitis	yellow fever
drugs	leptospiral jaundice
chemicals	

Familial Hyperbilirubinaemia

This condition, of which a number of varieties have been described in recent years, causes few if any symptoms and is usually detected on routine blood examination, so that in published cases there has been a high incidence in doctors and other hospital workers. The most common type is that described by Gilbert; there is a defect in the transport of bilirubin to its site of conjugation in the liver cell and non-conjugated (water-insoluble) bilirubin accumulates in the blood. Liver function tests are normal, needle biopsy shows normal hepatic structure, there are no complications and prognosis is excellent. The importance of the condition lies in distinguishing it from haemolytic jaundice and progressive hepatic disease. In the rarer *Dubin-Johnson* variety the hold-up occurs after conjugation and the clinical picture is that of cholestatic jaundice; liver biopsy reveals a dark brown pigment in the liver cells. Diagnosis is important so that these patients may be reassured that they are not suffering from serious liver disease.

INFECTIOUS HEPATITIS

There are two strains of virus causing acute hepatitis and differing mainly in their mode of transmission and incubation period. Virus A has an incubation period of about a month (20–40 days) and is present in the patient's stools, being transmitted by faecal contamination of food or water. Where hygienic standards are high only sporadic cases are seen, but where large groups of people live under relatively primitive conditions in a warm climate widespread epidemics may occur. Thus, during the war there were large outbreaks among troops in India and the Middle East. Under these conditions flies are important agents in the spread of the infection.

Virus B hepatitis is usually called serum hepatitis. It has an incubation period of about three months (60–160 days) and is found only in the patient's blood. Some healthy people harbour this virus in their blood for prolonged periods (perhaps indefinitely) and people found to be virus B positive should be excluded from service as blood donors. Transmission to susceptible individuals occurs through transfusions or injections containing plasma, or even from the use of inadequately sterilised syringes or needles. Patients presenting with infectious hepatitis should therefore always be asked if they have been given any injection during the preceding four months. Virus B hepatitis is a particular hazard in dialysis units treating patients with chronic renal failure; and as the virus may be present in body fluids such as saliva, vaginal secretions and seminal fluid, the infection may be acquired by close personal contact, particularly sexual intercourse.

A third type of hepatitis (non-A non-B hepatitis) is now the commonest post-transfusion hepatitis in some areas.

After recovery the patient usually has life-long immunity, but only to infection with the same strain of virus. Furthermore, there is some evidence that the virus of infective hepatitis causes only a mild gastroenteritis in young children and that those who acquire the more severe illness in adult life are those who have escaped childhood infection and consequent immunisation. This is known to apply to some other virus infections, such as poliomyelitis, which are more serious in adults than in children.

Clinical Features. The illness starts with fever, general malaise, aching in the back and limbs, nausea, and loss of appetite; arthralgia and urticaria are common prodromal symptoms of serum hepatitis not seen in infectious hepatitis. *Anorexia* is a very constant symptom and its occurrence for a few days before the appearance of icterus is one of the most important points distinguishing hepatitis from other causes of jaundice. Clinical jaundice usually becomes manifest within a week and about the same time the temperature settles and the patient starts to feel better. At this stage the liver is usually somewhat enlarged and tender and in about 20% of patients the spleen can be felt too. In the pre-icteric phase the *urine* usually contains an excess of urobilinogen; then when intrahepatic biliary obstruction occurs the urobilinogen disappears, bilirubin is found in the urine (which is consequently dark in colour) and the stools become pale; and finally during recovery after bilirubin has disappeared from the urine there may be a temporary return of urobilinogen in excess before the urine reverts to normal. The great majority of patients are jaundiced for only a week or two and then make a complete recovery. Very occasionally, however (less than 0.5%), fulminating infection may cause death even before the appearance of jaundice; or, equally rarely, recovery (from virus B or non-A non-B hepatitis but not virus A hepatitis) is incomplete and slowly progressive hepatic damage leads eventually to cirrhosis. Very mild cases never develop clinical jaundice (infective hepatitis sine ictero) and usually escape recognition except during epidemics. Raised serum transaminase levels are a sensitive index of hepatocellular damage; they are found even in anicteric patients (and are helpful in tracing the course of an epidemic) and may persist for several months in patients who are recovering normally.

A long convalescence is advisable after this illness, since depression and tiredness are often rather persistent and it may be some months before the patient recovers his full mental and physical vigour. Abstention from alcohol for about three months is also a wise precaution.

A small number of patients with chronic hepatitis have been found to carry the virus B antigen in the blood. These patients are clinically similar to those with chronic active hepatitis (see below) but do not usually have evidence of multisystem disease. This finding suggests that chronic liver damage can occur as a result of the persistence of virus B.

Treatment. There is no specific treatment for infective hepatitis. Prolonged bed rest used to be advocated, but it has been shown that the course of the illness and the incidence of complications are no different in patients permitted such activity as they feel inclined to undertake. Particular care should be taken in the disposal of excreta and the washing of hands after attending the patient. Diet should be regulated by the patient's appetite rather than the physician's fancy.

A short course of prednisone, starting with 40–50 mg daily and tailing the dosage off over about a week, may be tried in patients who continue to be deeply jaundiced after six weeks or more and sometimes appears to hasten recovery. If the patient is so ill that he cannot tolerate 1000 Calories by mouth the regime for acute hepatic failure (p. 116) should be instituted. Human gammaglobulin 0.06–0.12 ml per kg body weight, given not later than 6 days before the onset of symptoms of hepatitis A, modifies the disease and its administration may be considered for specially debilitated patients at risk.

CHRONIC HEPATITIS

This is defined as a chronic inflammatory reaction in the liver persisting without improvement for at least 6 months. It is subdivided into:

(a) **Chronic persistent hepatitis** in which the portal zones are expanded by mononuclear cells and some fibrosis but the limiting plate of liver cells between portal zones and liver cell columns is intact and the course is benign;

(b) **Chronic active hepatitis**, in which the portal areas are greatly expanded by inflammatory cells which extend into the liver lobule causing erosion of the limiting plate. The clinical course often, but not invariably, progresses to cirrhosis.

Both varieties may result from virus B or non-A non-B hepatitis, from alcohol abuse or as a reaction to certain drugs (isoniazid, methyldopa, paracetamol and cytotoxic agents). In addition, chronic persistent hepatitis may complicate long-standing inflammatory bowel disease such as ulcerative colitis and Crohn's disease.

'Lupoid' chronic active hepatitis is a variety seen mainly in women either at puberty or the menopause. The serum IgG is very high, smooth muscle antibodies are found in 60 % patients, antinuclear antibody may be found in high titre and LE cells can be demonstrated in 15 % patients. Liver biopsy reveals very florid chronic active hepatitis, usually with cirrhosis.

Treatment. 'Lupoid' hepatitis responds to steroids which should be continued until the liver function tests return to normal and liver biopsy shows no activity. The usual dose of prednisolone is 30 mg daily reducing to a maintenance dose of about 10 mg daily. If steroids fail, immunosuppression with azathioprine should be tried.

In hepatitis complicating viral infection the response to steroids is less satisfactory and there is no preferred treatment at present.

CIRRHOSIS OF THE LIVER

The word cirrhosis means tawny and was introduced by Laënnec because of the slightly icteric tinge sometimes seen in the livers of patients who have died of this disease. Later it became realised that a much more characteristic feature than the tawny colour is the presence of a great deal of fibrous tissue and cirrhosis has come to mean diffuse hepatic fibrosis. This may be the result of a number of different pathological processes, so that cirrhosis should be regarded as analogous with pulmonary fibrosis rather than as a disease entity.

Clinical Features. *Laënnec's cirrhosis* occurs most often in the forties and fifties and the alcoholic variety is commoner in men than in women. The disease is usually brought to light by the discovery of splenomegaly, hepatomegaly, jaundice, gastrointestinal bleeding, or ascites. In alcoholics there is usually a history of epigastric discomfort, loss of appetite—particularly for breakfast—and morning sickness with vomiting of mucus, symptoms attributable to alcoholic gastritis; but patients with idiopathic cirrhosis have frequently had no symptoms up to the time of diagnosis. Furthermore, in about one third of cases seen at autopsy the disease has been unsuspected in life.

The clinical features arise from two main causes, hepatocellular failure and portal hypertension:

Hepatocellular failure may have many different effects. *Low-grade fever* often with leucocytosis is seen in about half the patients. More common is the development of *vascular spiders*, each consisting of a central dilated arteriole from which a number of tiny vessels radiate; these appear on the face, neck, upper half of the trunk and upper limbs. Their cause is not known; it is probably not the high blood oestrogen level, as once thought. Erythema of the thenar and hypothenar eminences and of the pads of the fingers ('*liver palms*') is also common. Mental and physical *fatigue*, *loss of weight* and vague *indigestion* are the rule. *Foetor hepaticus*, which can be detected in the breath and urine, is a common sign; it is presumably due to a substance from the gut which is normally detoxicated by the liver. It is a sweetish somewhat faeculent smell which is usually likened to that of a freshly opened corpse. It is a grave sign, often quickly followed by hepatic coma, in patients with severe hepatocellular failure, though in patients with extensive portacaval venous anastomoses it may be present intermittently for quite long periods and does not necessarily imply such a bad prognosis.

Hepatic coma is probably related to failure of the liver to convert ammonia to urea and the blood ammonia level is raised. It is more common in patients with portacaval connections and may be precipitated by a high protein diet, by the taking of nitrogenous compounds, or by gastrointestinal haemorrhage, intercurrent infection or the rapid removal of ascitic fluid. Coma is preceded by a stage of lethargy with mental confusion, irrational behaviour and a typical 'flapping' tremor of the outstretched hands.

Jaundice in cirrhosis, due to failure of the liver cells to excrete bilirubin, is not very common and usually slight; when present it implies a bad prognosis.

Portal hypertension in cirrhosis is due to the combined effect of diminution in the portal vascular bed, the result of both fibrosis and the pressure of regenerating nodules of liver tissue against small portal venous radicles, and of the increased transmission of hepatic arterial pressure to the portal venous system. It leads to congestive *splenomegaly* and to the opening up of portacaval anastomoses. The two situations in which these distended veins are of clinical importance are:

(a) The abdominal wall, since here they are readily seen and are helpful in diagnosis. Portal blood passes to the umbilicus through the para-umbilical veins to reach collaterals of the caval system. There are usually only one or two distended veins, the classical 'caput medusae' being rare, but it can be demonstrated that the flow of blood is radially away from the umbilicus. This helps in the distinction from inferior vena caval obstruction in which the blood in the distended abdominal veins always flows from below upwards.

(b) Varicose veins in the *oesophagus and fundus of the stomach* are the most dangerous effect of portal hypertension, since bleeding from this source is always serious and often fatal. They may be demonstrated by barium swallow, using a thin emulsion to delineate the delicate mucosal pattern, though negative findings on X-rays do not exclude their presence. The spleen is almost invariably palpable in patients with portal hypertension and, as in any condition associated with splenomegaly, *pancytopenia* is frequently found in the peripheral blood (see hypersplenism, p. 624).

Ascites develops in cirrhosis from the combined effect of portal hypertension and the reduced plasma osmotic pressure which follows hepatocellular failure and diminished albumin synthesis. Accumulation of fluid in the peritoneal cavity reduces the effective body fluid volume and compensatory mechanisms to retain fluid in the body come into operation and lead in turn to increase in the ascites; they include increased secretion of antidiuretic hormone from the neurohypophysis and of aldosterone from the adrenal cortex.

Clinical features of obscure origin, sometimes seen in cirrhosis, include *clubbing of the fingers*, *gynaecomastia*, and *scanty or absent body hair*. In acute hepatocellular failure the circulation is overactive, as shown by a rapid collapsing pulse, high pulse pressure, warm extremities and increased jugular venous pressure. The *diagnosis* of cirrhosis is difficult to establish in the early stages. The first biochemical test to show abnormal results is usually the bromosulphthalein (BSP) retention test; later the serum albumin is reduced, the globulin raised and the serum transaminase levels elevated. Sometimes the serum bilirubin level is slightly raised. In early cases the diagnosis can be made with certainty by needle biopsy, but the indications for this procedure must be carefully assessed for each patient as it incurs a slight risk of haemorrhage which is occasionally serious.

Assessment of Liver Damage in Cirrhosis

In patients with jaundice the severity of liver cell damage is indicated by the height of the serum bilirubin level, the degree of reduction in the serum albumin and of rise in the serum globulin levels, and elevation of the serum asparate aminotransferase level (normal < 35 u/l).

In patients without jaundice the bromosulphthalein (BSP) retention test is an accurate index of the severity of liver damage. 1 ml of a 5 % solution per 10 kg body weight is injected intravenously and 30 minutes later a sample of venous blood is taken from the other arm; normally the serum at half an hour contains only 0–10 % of the injected dose. This test can also be used as an accurate index of recovery after infective hepatitis; it cannot be used, however, when the serum bilirubin is above 35 μmol/l.

Treatment. Whatever the aetiology of the cirrhosis the patient must abstain completely from alcohol for the rest of his life. An adequate mixed diet is important, but there is no advantage in giving protein supplements. Special indications are as follows:

(a) For **oedema and ascites** give a diet containing no added salt, frusemide 40 mg daily and spironolactone 100 mg four times daily with potassium supplements to reduce the danger of inducing hepatic coma. Paracentesis should be avoided if possible.

(b) **Haematemesis and/or Melaena.** Bleeding may be due to either oesophageal varices or to peptic ulceration. In patients with liver failure cimetidine 200 mg 6-hourly by injection will usually prevent bleeding from ulceration or if haemorrhage occurs it will be more easily controlled. Bleeding from varices is usually better controlled by intravenous pitressin than by the inflatable balloons of a Sengstaken tube. If bleeding continues emergency operation (portacaval anastomosis, or Tanner's operation if the portal vein is not patent) may be considered unless there is hepatocellular failure or gross ascites.

(c) **Coma** from **Acute Hepatic Failure.** Neuropsychiatric symptoms of incipient coma are an indication for reducing the protein content of the diet to 20 g daily. In established coma enough calories must be given as intravenous glucose, if necessary by intracaval catheter, to minimise endogenous protein catabolism; ammonium absorption from the gut is reduced by giving oral neomycin 1 g four times daily and lactulose syrup 40 ml three times daily will help to empty the bowel; paracentesis, thiazide diuretics and sedative drugs must be avoided; and it may be necessary to give potassium if the serum level is reduced due to secondary aldosteronism.

(d) **Renal Failure in Cirrhosis.** A majority of patients with advanced cirrhosis of the liver have impaired renal function and often renal failure. This is rarely due to structural renal disease but much more commonly to what is termed functional renal failure, the most obvious aspect of which is renal vasoconstriction. The cause is not clear and has been variously attributed to endotoxins or to pooling of blood in the splanchnic vascular bed. The use of diuretics is an additional factor.

In the early stages the features are those of renal hypoperfusion with oliguria and a hyperosmolar urine; later the symptoms of established acute renal failure develop.

Any precipitating factors should be corrected and diuretics must be stopped. Otherwise the treatment is as for acute renal failure (see p. 471).

Special Types of Cirrhosis

(1) **Obstructive Biliary Cirrhosis.** Some patients with chronic ex-

trahepatic cholestasis, usually due to stone in the common duct, carcinoma of the head of the pancreas, compression from peri-biliary lymph nodes or surgical injury to the common duct, eventually develop diffuse hepatic fibrosis which in turn may lead to portal hypertension and hepatocellular failure. This sequence of events occurs particularly in patients with long-standing partial or recurrent obstruction complicated by cholangitis and the clinical course is often punctuated by bouts of rigors and pyrexia (Charcot's 'biliary remittent fever'). The only effective treatment is surgical relief of the obstruction.

(2) **Primary Biliary Cirrhosis.** In this rare disease the primary disorder appears to be diffuse intrahepatic biliary cholestasis of unknown cause. Most of the patients are middle-aged women. Insidious onset of itching of the skin is slowly followed by the appearance of jaundice of cholestatic type without fever or abdominal pain. The spleen is palpable at an early stage and later the liver becomes greatly enlarged; eventually signs of portal hypertension and hepatocellular failure develop. Pigmentation and skin xanthomata are quite often seen. Bone pain and thinning are common and are due to Vitamin D deficiency. The prognosis is better than in Laënnec's cirrhosis; some patients recover and others run a very prolonged downhill course. A remission sometimes follows treatment with penicillamine, the usual dose being 600 mg daily, and it should be given a trial in patients who are doing badly. Steroids are contraindicated as they are of no benefit and may make the bone condition worse. Cholestyramine helps to control the irritation and Vitamin D will arrest the osteomalacia.

(3) **Haemochromatosis.** The primary lesion is probably an inborn metabolic defect which results in the absorption of a slight excess of iron. There is no mechanism by which this extra iron can be eliminated from the body and it is laid down in various tissues and organs, where eventually functional and structural changes may be induced. Symptoms rarely appear before early middle age. The disease is extremely rare in women (5–10 per cent of cases) and in them appears at a later age than in men, probably because the loss of iron in menstruation and pregnancy delays or prevents the clinical expression of the disease. Cirrhosis is a constant feature and the diagnosis should be considered in patients found to have a very enlarged firm liver and greyish pigmentation of the skin, notably over exposed parts. Impotence and general weakness are early symptoms and testicular atrophy with absent or scanty body hair are found much more commonly than in other forms of cirrhosis. Diabetes develops in about two-thirds of the patients. Death usually results from hepatocellular failure or heart failure, the result of impregnation with haemosiderin of the liver cells or the myocardium. The *diagnosis* may be confirmed by serum iron studies; the combination of a raised serum iron level with complete or almost complete saturation of the serum iron-binding capacity is almost pathognomonic. If any doubt remains needle biopsy of the liver will

settle the matter. *Treatment* is by regular bloodletting; in most patients a pint a week can be taken for many months before early signs of iron deficiency appear in the blood picture. Thereafter a pint should be removed every month or two to prevent reaccumulation of iron in the tissues.

(4) **Syphilitic cirrhosis** (hepar lobatum) is now extremely rare but may be suspected in patients with hepatomegaly and gummata elsewhere in the body. Serological tests for syphilis are positive and the diagnosis is confirmed by the favourable response to antisyphilitic treatment.

(5) **Cardiac Cirrhosis** (see p. 124).

(6) **Hepatolenticular Degeneration** (Wilson's disease; see p. 556).

ACUTE HEPATIC FAILURE

In addition to complicating cirrhosis, acute hepatocellular failure can result from several other causes. It may be due to drugs including isoniazid and overdosage with paracetamol or may occur during the course of a severe viral hepatitis.

Clinical Features. The onset of symptoms is rapid. Jaundice is usual and encephalopathy, starting with impairment of mental function and proceeding to coma in severe cases, is common. Several factors are probably responsible for the encephalopathy, retained toxins absorbed from the gut and electrolytic disturbances playing a major role. The unwise use of drugs will exacerbate symptoms and the chief offenders are central depressants (particularly opiates) and potassium-losing diuretics which increase hypokalaemia. There is reduced production of clotting factors by the liver and gastrointestinal bleeding may occur, although oesophageal varices are rare. Salt and water retention with oedema and ascites are due to a low plasma albumin and to disturbances of renal function (see p. 113).

Treatment. The general treatment of hepatocellular failure is considered under cirrhosis on p. 114. When liver failure is due to causes other than cirrhosis, there is a reasonable chance that the liver can regain normal function if the patient can survive the initial damage. A number of support systems have been tried to tide the patient over the acute stage of the disease including the temporary perfusion of a pig's liver and haemodialysis, but no satisfactory system has yet been available. The survival rate of severe failure is about 20–30%.

Drug Induced Liver Damage

There are a variety of drugs which may produce liver damage.

(1) **Hepatocellular.** Certain substances including the *chlorinated hydrocarbons (carbon tetrachloride) and benzene derivatives (trinitrotolu-*

ene, dinitrophenol) are liver poisons and will produce necrosis of liver cells. This is probably due to direct action of the toxic agent on the liver. Industrial workers exposed to such hepatic poisons should be examined regularly for enlargement or tenderness of the liver and the urine should be tested weekly for bilirubin or urobilinogen.

Other substances only occasionally produce liver necrosis, which when it occurs however may be severe and fatal. This group includes some of the monoamine oxidase inhibitors and *paracetamol* overdose, *halothane, isoniazid* and *methyldopa.*

(2) **Chronic Active Hepatitis.** Isoniazid causes liver damage in older patients, particularly if combined with rifampicin. Other drugs which rarely cause hepatitis are methyldopa and paracetamol.

(3) **Cholestasis.** Certain drugs may occasionally produce the clinical picture of intrahepatic cholestasis. The mechanisms involved are not known. On withdrawal of the drug recovery is the rule. This type of dysfunction may occur with:

Chlorpromazine and some other phenothiazines
Methyl testosterone
Thiouracil
Mestranol
Ethinyloestradiol
Chlorpropamide
Nitrofurantoin
PAS
Phenytoin

Thrombosis of the Portal Vein

Cirrhosis accounts for about half the cases of portal vein thrombosis but it is a rare complication seen in only about 1% of cirrhotics. Other causes are malignant disease, portal phlebitis secondary to cholangitis, pancreatitis, or appendicitis, and increase in blood platelets (thrombocytosis) such as occurs in polycythaemia vera and after splenectomy. The clinical features are abdominal pain, splenomegaly, haematemesis, and ascites and distinction from intrahepatic portal obstruction is difficult. Absence of hepatomegaly and signs of hepatic failure are sometimes helpful but the diagnosis can be established with certainty only by splenic venography (which can be performed by percutaneous injection of the dye). The only practical importance in recognising the condition is that it precludes portacaval anastomosis.

Hepatic Vein Thrombosis (Budd–Chiari syndrome)

This very rare condition is usually a complication of renal or hepatic carcinoma, thrombophlebitis migrans or polycythaemia. It causes sudden vomiting, enlargement of the liver, slight jaundice and ascites which is very resistant to treatment. Anticoagulant therapy should be instituted, but it is difficult to be sufficiently sure of the diagnosis for this to be done. The prognosis is very bad.

Bone Disorders and Chronic Liver Disease

Osteomalacia and osteoporosis are now recognised as complications of various types of chronic liver disease including primary biliary cirrhosis, multilobular cirrhosis and various types of cholestasis.

Osteomalacia appears to be due to a lack of Vitamin D rather than to inability to hydroxylate Vitamin D to 25 hydroxycholecalciferol. The reason for the deficiency is not clear but a number of factors are probably involved. The cause of osteoporosis is unknown. Osteomalacia will respond to 1-α-hydroxycholecalciferol 1.0 μg daily.

TUMOURS OF THE LIVER

Adenomas

There has been an increase in the incidence of adenomas of the liver and this has been linked, though not conclusively, to the use of oral contraceptives.

Clinical Features. Adenomas which may be single or multiple may cause no symptoms, occasionally there may be pain over the liver and rarely a tumour may rupture into the peritoneal cavity with severe bleeding.

Treatment is by resection if possible.

Hepatomas

These primary malignant tumours of the liver are particularly common in China, Japan and south-east Asia. Aetiological factors include cirrhosis of the liver and possibly previous viral infection and carcinogens in the diet.

Clinical Features. A hepatoma may arise during the course of cirrhosis or symptoms may develop de novo. Commonly there is weight loss, weakness and anorexia. The patient may complain of pain in the upper right quadrant of the abdomen and on examination the liver will be found to be enlarged and frequently tender.

A useful diagnostic test is for the elevation of the plasma *α-foetoprotein* level which occurs in about 50% of the patients. The tumour may be localised by isotope or CAT scanning and the diagnosis confirmed by biopsy.

Treatment. Occasionally it is possible to remove the tumour surgically. Adriamycin given as a single dose of 60–75 mg/m^2 IV every 3–4 weeks has some palliative effect. The prognosis is poor.

Secondary Tumours

These are very common and rarely respond to any form of treatment.

DISEASES OF THE PANCREAS

ACUTE PANCREATITIS

The cause of this relatively common disease is not known, but about half the patients also have disease of the biliary tract and many of them are alcoholics or morphine addicts. An acute attack may occur during or soon after an alcoholic bout. It is thought that the characteristic lesions are produced by pancreatic enzymes which have escaped from their normal channels. They include necrosis and haemorrhagic oedema of the gland and plaques of fat necrosis on the mesentery and peritoneum as well as on the pancreas.

Clinical Features. The main symptom is extremely severe and persistent pain in the epigastrium or left upper quadrant of the abdomen passing through to the back, with vomiting and sometimes profound shock. There is deep epigastric tenderness and frequently some abdominal distension. A serum amylase level of 900 u/l or higher (normal range 70–300 u/l) is practically pathognomonic of the disease, though smaller increases in the level may be the result of spasm of the sphincter of Oddi induced by morphine and are occasionally found in other intra-abdominal diseases.

Treatment. Unless there is doubt about the diagnosis laparotomy should be avoided as it incurs a high mortality. If pethidine 100 mg intramuscularly every few hours fails to relieve the pain, morphine 15–20 mg may need to be given in spite of its tendency to cause spasm of the sphincter of Oddi. Shock must be combated by restoration of normal fluid and electrolyte balance, antibiotics such as penicillin 500 000 units with streptomycin 0.5 g twice daily are given to prevent secondary infection of the damaged pancreas, and pancreatic secretion is minimised by giving nothing by mouth and administering a vagal blocking agent such as atropine sulphate 0.6 mg IM every 3 or 4 hours. Aprotinin (Trasylol) is said to inhibit trypsin and may be of value if given in the first 24 hours. A million units are given IV followed by 100 000 units hourly for 3–4 hours.

CHRONIC PANCREATITIS

Chronic pancreatitis is the term applied to the extensive fibrosis and atrophy of the acinar and islet tissue which may follow repeated attacks of acute or subacute pancreatitis and which may lead eventually to pancreatic insufficiency and diabetes mellitus. The condition is usually seen in middle-aged men and the most common associated conditions are cholelithiasis and alcoholism. The *clinical history* starts with recurrent episodes of upper abdominal pain as described above; a stage may then be reached in which attacks recur every week or two or pain may become almost continuous and extremely demoralising; and finally diabetes mellitus and/or pancreatic insufficiency may develop. Occasionally the final stage may be reached without any history of severe pain. Pancreatic insufficiency is characterised by loss of weight and the passage of bulky fatty stools. Calcification of the pancreas seen on X-ray strongly favours chronic pancreatitis. More precise diagnosis can be made by radiological demonstration of the pancreatic ducts (ERCP), abdominal ultrasound and analysis of the pancreatic juice obtained after a secretion test. Estimation of the serum amylase level is less helpful than in the acute disease, though it is usually somewhat raised.

Treatment. The diet should be started containing 50 g of fat and increased until steatorrhoea appears and enough protein and carbohydrate should be given to ensure adequate calorie intake and nutrition. Strong pancreatin powder BNF 0.25–2 g should be given with each meal together with cimetidine to reduce gastric acid. Alcohol should be forbidden. In patients with severe intractable pain sphincterotomy or even partial or complete resection of the pancreas may have to be performed, but no operation gives consistently good results and the mortality is high. Diabetes if present is controlled in the usual way.

FURTHER READING

Bouchier, I. A. D., *Gastroenterology*, 3rd edition, Baillière, London, 1982.

Sherlock, S., *Diseases of the Liver and Biliary System*, 6th edition, Blackwell, Oxford, 1981.

CHAPTER 4

THE CARDIOVASCULAR SYSTEM

INTRODUCTION

Diseases of the cardiovascular system are the commonest cause of death. With an ageing population it seems likely that there will be further increases in the incidence of those varieties of cardiovascular disease which occur in both middle and advanced age, namely coronary artery disease and hypertension.

THE EXAMINATION OF THE CARDIOVASCULAR SYSTEM

Cyanosis

The colour of a part in terms of its redness or pallor depends on the amount of blood in the capillaries of that part and the thickness of the overlying tissues—where that issue is thin, e.g. lips and conjunctivae, the colour may be very deep. The colour of blood depends on its haemoglobin and therefore the state and amount of the haemoglobin also influence the colour of the part.

When the capillary blood contains an excess of reduced haemoglobin, it looks blue and produces a blue shade in the skin and mucosae. This is cyanosis. Five grams of reduced haemoglobin per 100 ml are required to produce detectable cyanosis.

Cyanosis may be of two kinds:

(a) *Peripheral cyanosis*, which is due to stagnation of blood in the capillaries, is best seen in the extremities and the lips and is often associated with coldness of the part. It may be abolished by warming the part. It is not seen in the tongue or mouth. It may occur in heart failure or be due to local causes such as poor circulation in the hands or feet. Normal people who are 'blue with cold' have this type of cyanosis.

(b) *Central cyanosis* is due either to inadequate uptake of oxygen in the lungs secondary to pulmonary disease or to a right-to-left cardiac shunt which results in deoxygenated blood bypassing the lungs and passing directly to the systemic circulation. It is characterised by cyanosis which affects the mouth and tongue as well as the extremities, which are warm.

Temperature of the Extremities

Coldness of the extremities is due to vasoconstriction or obstruction of the superficial blood vessels so that the blood supply to the skin is reduced. In heart disease it is often due to the peripheral vasoconstriction which follows a fall in cardiac output. Conversely, in conditions with a high cardiac output the peripheral vessels are dilated and the skin is very warm.

Clubbing of the Fingers

Clubbing of the fingers may occur in cardiac disease. In congenital cyanotic heart disease it is related to the degree of cyanosis and is often very marked, the fingers having a drumstick-like appearance. It is also seen in patients with cor pulmonale and in infective endocarditis. The possibility of other causes, including chronic lung suppuration, carcinoma of the bronchus, ulcerative colitis, the malabsorption syndrome, and cirrhosis of the liver, must not be forgotten.

The Arterial Pulse

The pulse rate and rhythm as usually determined by feeling the radial pulse.

(a) *Rate.* During the first year of life the normal pulse rate is about 100–110/min. As the child grows up the pulse becomes slower and by puberty it has slowed to the adult rate, which is usually between 65–85/min. Athletes, however, may have a resting rate of 50/min or less. Increase in pulse rate is called *tachycardia* and may be due to emotion, exertion, fever, thyrotoxicosis, bleeding, intrinsic heart disease, paroxysmal tachycardia, atrial flutter or atrial fibrillation. Sleep eliminates emotion and exertion and therefore the sleeping pulse rate may be a valuable observation.

Undue slowing of the pulse is called *bradycardia* and is much less common; it may be due to sinus bradycardia as in hypothyroidism, obstructive jaundice or raised intracranial pressure and is quite commonly found in young fit people; it may also be due to disorders of the pacemaker or conducting system of the heart. It may also result from overdosage of digitalis or β blockers.

(b) *Rhythm.* Abnormalities of rhythm are considered on page 148.

(c) *Tension.* Measurement of the systolic blood pressure by digital compression of the pulse is misleading. It can only be accurately measured by the use of a sphygmomanometer.

(d) *Amplitude.* The amplitude of the pulse is dependent on the pulse pressure and is often better appreciated at the carotid artery than at the wrist.

A small amplitude pulse means a small stroke volume or obstruction to the outflow from the left ventricle together with a high peripheral resistance. It is found in severe heart failure, shock and mitral stenosis. In aortic stenosis the pulse wave may be of low amplitude but it is also slow rising and prolonged. It is called a *plateau pulse.*

A large pulse amplitude is associated with a wide pulse pressure and a low peripheral resistance as in persistent ductus arteriosus, thyrotoxicosis or an arteriovenous fistula, or it may be due to the large stroke volume of extreme bradycardia (complete heart block). It may also be found with the rigid aorta of old age. In aortic incompetence there may be a very wide pulse pressure producing a *collapsing (water hammer) pulse*. This is best appreciated by lifting the patient's arm and grasping the wrist with the whole hand when the pulse can be felt as an abrupt but forcible tap.

(e) *Pulse Wave*. There are a number of variations in the pulse wave which may be helpful in diagnosis. They are best appreciated by feeling a large artery, for example the carotid rather than the radial.

(i) *Pulsus Bisferiens*. Pulsus bisferiens is a double pulse wave and is found in patients with combined aortic stenosis and regurgitation or in pure aortic regurgitation.

(ii) *Pulsus Alternans*. Pulsus alternans consists of alternate weak and strong pulse waves. It may be appreciated on palpation of the pulse, but is more easily shown with the sphygmomanometer. It is found in left ventricular failure.

(iii) *Pulsus Paradoxus*. Pulsus paradoxus is found in constrictive pericarditis and pericardial effusions. Normally inspiration sucks blood into the right ventricle with a corresponding rise in right ventricular output to fill the expanded pulmonary vascular bed. If the right ventricle cannot expand due to rigidity or a surrounding effusion, this compensating rise in right ventricular filling cannot occur and cardiac output falls. It can also occasionally occur in asthma where there is a sharp fall in intrathoracic pressure on inspiration, which increases the capacity of the vascular bed of the lung and thus temporarily reduces the flow of blood.

The Venous Pulse

The neck veins should be examined in the recumbent patient with the head and shoulders raised 30° from the horizontal. At this angle the column of blood in the jugular system should reach the level of the clavicle. The normal jugular venous pressure is measured with reference to the sternal angle and is usually recorded in cm of blood. In normal individuals the range is between +3 and −6 cm with the subject horizontal. Where precise measurement is required a catheter may be introduced into the right atrium for continuous monitoring of pressure which is then sometimes called *central venous pressure*, but which really indicates right atrial pressure. An elevation of jugular venous pressure is found in *heart failure* and in certain conditions associated with a high cardiac output. It is also raised in superior vena caval obstruction when pulsation is absent. Finally minor degrees of elevated venous pressure may occur in conditions with increased intra-abdominal pressure such as pregnancy. The external jugular veins may be compressed as they pass through the cervical fascia; it is therefore best to observe the right internal jugular vein.

With the normal jugular *venous pulse* it is possible to observe 'a' and 'v' waves. The 'a' wave is caused by contraction of the right atrium and coincides with the first heart sound. It is followed by the 'x' descent due to relaxation of the right atrium. Pressure recordings in addition show a notch on the 'x' descent which is called the 'c' wave and is probably due to transmitted carotid pulsation. Following the 'x' descent the 'v' wave represents the rise in pressure which occurs when the right atrium fills with the tricuspid valve closed; it coincides with the second heart sound. Finally the tricuspid valve opens in ventricular diastole causing a fall in atrial pressure which is seen in the venous pulse as the 'y' descent.

Large 'a' waves are seen in tricuspid stenosis or when there is increased rigidity of the right ventricle due to hypertrophy such as occurs in pulmonary stenosis or with pulmonary hypertension. Very large 'a' waves or *cannon waves* are seen when the right atrium contracts against a closed tricuspid valve due to atrial and ventricular contractions being nearly synchronous. This occurs regularly in nodal rhythm and nodal tachycardia, and irregularly in complete heart block and rarely with ventricular ectopic beats. The 'v' wave is increased in right ventricular failure.

Large waves corresponding to ventricular systole occur in tricuspid incompetence due to the systolic pulse being transmitted to the right atrium.

A deep and abrupt 'y' descent is found in constrictive pericarditis and is due to the ventricular walls being sprung apart early in ventricular diastole. It may also occur in right ventricular failure due to rapid ventricular filling early in diastole.

The Liver

With a rise in venous pressure such as occurs in congestive cardiac failure the liver becomes congested and enlarged. It may be painful and tender on palpation if the enlargement is rapid. Expansile pulsation in the liver is found in tricuspid incompetence. Chronic congestion may lead to some interference with liver function and result in slight jaundice and even *cardiac cirrhosis*.

Hepatojugular Reflux

Continuous pressure over the liver or abdomen increases the filling of the right atrium and ventricle; in the normal heart this can be accommodated without raising jugular venous pressure but in right ventricular failure the neck veins become distended.

Dyspnoea, orthopnoea, and *oedema* are discussed on p. 138.

THE BLOOD PRESSURE

Introduction. The intermittent rise and fall of pressure within the arteries depends on the ejection of blood from the left ventricle. The peak pressure developed is called the systolic pressure and the lowest pressure the diastolic pressure. The difference between systolic and diastolic pressures is called the pulse pressure.

The height of the blood pressure depends predominantly on the cardiac output and the peripheral resistance to blood flow. An increase in cardiac output causes a rise in mean blood pressure, the systolic pressure being more affected than the diastolic pressure. A rise in resistance to flow or a rise in pulse rate causes a rise in mean blood pressure, the diastolic being more affected than the systolic pressure.

The rise in blood pressure which occurs on exercise or with emotion is predominantly due to a rise in cardiac output and this may often be associated with a fall in peripheral resistance. In uncomplicated essential hypertension, however, the cardiac output is normal and the elevated blood pressure is due to increased resistance to blood flow.

Another factor which modifies the blood pressure is the elasticity of the arteries. In youth when the arteries are elastic the pulse pressure tends to be low, even in the face of a high peripheral resistance. With increasing age the arteries become less elastic and the pulse pressure increases and may result in the development of so-called benign systolic hypertension of the aged, with a blood pressure in the region of 200/90 mmHg. This type of raised blood pressure may be of less significance than that due to an increased peripheral resistance.

Finally, increases in blood volume and in blood viscosity will raise the blood pressure.

Measurement of Blood Pressure. When measuring the blood pressure the subject must be at rest both physically and mentally as both recent exercise and anxiety may cause a transient rise. It is customary to take the blood pressure in the right arm, although, except where there is obstruction to the arterial supply to one limb, there is not usually more than a few millimetres of pressure difference between the two arms. It is important to ensure that the sphygmomanometer cuff is firmly and evenly applied. The cuff is fully inflated and then deflated and the pressure at which the brachial pulse returns is determined by palpation. This gives a rough guide to the systolic pressure. The cuff is then reinflated and the stethoscope applied over the brachial artery. The *systolic blood pressure* is the pressure at which sounds appear. In the UK the *diastolic blood pressure* is taken as the pressure at which there is a change from loud clear sounds to muffled sounds (phase 4). The complete disappearance of sounds (phase 5) is usually 5–10 mmHg lower and is taken as the diastolic pressure in the USA.

As the sphygmomanometer cuff is deflated, there is sometimes a pressure range between the systolic and diastolic pressure when no sound is heard. This is called the 'silent gap' and if the blood pressure is being measured by the auscultatory method, the return of sounds at the end of the silent gap may be mistaken for the true systolic pressure. This mistake is avoided if the systolic pressure is first determined by palpation.

THE HEART

Inspection. The apex beat may be visible and its position should be noted. A search should be made for other pulsations. A characteristic 'lift' can sometimes be seen between the apex and the left sternal border in patients with right ventricular hypertrophy, and if the pulmonary arteries are dilated this may extend up to the second or third left intercostal spaces. Aneurysm of the first part of the aorta produces pulsation in the second right intercostal space.

Palpation. The position of the *apex beat* should be confirmed; if it is difficult to locate, palpation should be carried out with the patient sitting forward and expiring fully. Normally the apex beat is in the 5th intercostal space just internal to the midclavicular line. It may be displaced either by shift of the mediastinum or by cardiac enlargement. In *left ventricular hypertrophy* the apex beat is displaced downwards and to the left and is of a characteristically localised and thrusting nature. Sometimes in left ventricular failure a double impulse starting in late diastole can be felt at the apex. This is due to forceful atrial contraction followed by left ventricular contraction (see Heart Sounds, below). If hypertrophy is combined with dilatation the apex beat feels more diffuse. With *right ventricular hypertrophy* a forceful impulse can be felt just to the left of the lower end of the sternum; if hypertrophy is minimal but there is a large flow through the right ventricle as in atrial septal defect the impulse has a tapping character.

Careful examination must be made for *thrills*. These are vibrations which may be appreciated by the hand and are really palpable murmurs. Systolic thrills can be felt in the appropriate areas in both aortic and pulmonary stenosis and in mitral incompetence. A systolic thrill can also be felt over ventricular septal defects and aortic aneurysms. A diastolic thrill may be felt in mitral stenosis. The presence of a definite thrill is always abnormal, and must be distinguished from the slight vibrations which may be felt over a forcibly beating heart.

Occasionally it may be possible to feel valve closures. For instance, the loud first sound in mitral stenosis due to forcible closure of the mitral valve may be actually palpable and it is sometimes possible to feel the second heart sound in the pulmonary area in pulmonary hypertension.

Percussion. It is doubtful whether percussion affords any more information than can usually be found on palpation, but it is customary to percuss out the left and right borders of the heart. By this means the cardiac area can be roughly outlined and percussion may occasionally be useful in the diagnosis of a pericardial effusion or of an aneurysm of the ascending aorta.

Auscultation. Auscultation must be carried out over the whole praecordium and not merely in the classical mitral, aortic, pulmonary, and tricuspid areas.

Heart Sounds (Fig. 4.1)

There are four groups of heart sounds.

(1) Sounds produced by valve closure—namely the first sound, caused by closure of the tricuspid and mitral valves, and the second sound from closure of the aortic and pulmonary valves.
(2) Sound produced by valves opening—namely the opening snap of the mitral valve.
(3) Sound produced by rapid ventricular filling.
(4) Extracardiac sounds.

Some of the sounds may be heard in both normal and abnormal hearts; others only occur in the diseased heart.

(1) *Sounds of Valve Closure.* The *first heart sound* is produced by the closure of the mitral and tricuspid valves. In health it is either single or closely split. In right, and left, bundle branch block the splitting may be quite wide due to the asynchronous closure of the mitral and tricuspid valves.

The *loudness* of the first heart sound depends on the position of the A-V valves at the beginning of ventricular systole. If they have been forced well down into the ventricular cavity by the flow of blood from the atria they have a long way to snap back when systole begins and the first sound is therefore loud. This occurs particularly with a short P-R interval, and in mitral stenosis. In the latter condition it is probable that

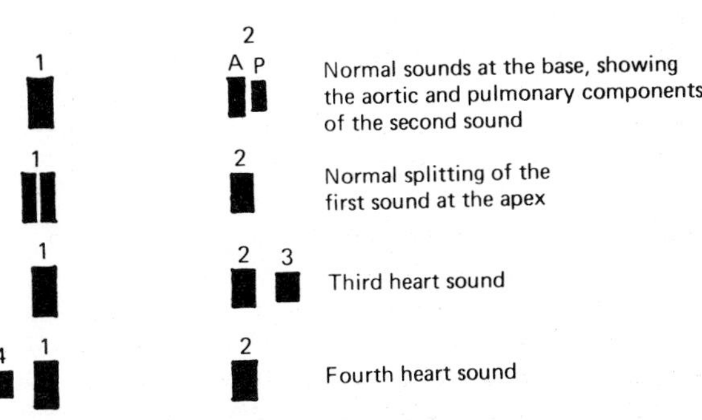

Fig. 4.1 Heart sounds.

the rather prolonged blood flow through the stenosed mitral valve together with shortening of the chordae tendineae keeps the valve deep in the ventricle until systole starts. Loud first heart sounds are also heard in nervous people with tachycardia, in thyrotoxicosis and in anaemia and are due to the rapid ventricular contraction forcibly closing the A-V valves.

The *second heart sound* at the base of the heart is composed of the closure of the aortic and pulmonary valves. In most children and in many adults the second sound in this area can be heard to be closely split, the first element of the split being due to aortic valve closure and the second element to pulmonary valve closure. Normally this split increases with inspiration, probably due to a momentary increase in the stroke volume of the right ventricle with a prolongation of systole. In *right bundle branch block* the split is wide and widens on inspiration, in *atrial septal defect* the split is wide and fixed.

In *left bundle branch block* the splitting of the second sound may be reversed so that the aortic component follows the pulmonary component. In this case the sound come closer together on inspiration.

(2) *Sounds Produced by Valves Opening.* The most important of these sounds is the *opening snap of the mitral valve*. It is best heard between the apex beat and the lower sternum. It is a sharp, high-pitched snap and occurs in early diastole. It is almost, but not quite, diagnostic of mitral stenosis and suggests that the valve is mobile. It is rarely heard in mitral incompetence.

Ejection clicks are high-pitched sounds occurring in early systole; they are found in valvar aortic or pulmonary stenosis and are due to sudden distension of the stenosed valve at the start of systole. Occasionally a click may be heard in midsystole, often associated with a late systolic murmur (see p. 184).

(3) *Sounds Produced by Rapid Ventricular Filling (Triple Rhythm).* These extra sounds are probably produced by rapid distension of the hypertrophied and rigid ventricles. They are low-pitched and can thus be readily distinguished from the high pitched sounds of valve opening and closure.

The *third heart sound* is produced by rapid ventricular filling with sudden tensing of the ventricular walls and mitral valve in early diastole. It is a soft low frequency sound and is often heard at the apex in normal young adults, but in people over the age of 40 it is associated with increased rigidity of the ventricular muscle. It is heard best at the left sternal edge in right ventricular failure, and at the apex in left ventricular failure.

The *fourth heart sound* is produced by rapid filling of the ventricles associated with forceful atrial contraction and occurs just before the first heart sound in late diastole. It is a low-pitched sound and is best heard a little way inside the apex beat and is found particularly in hypertension and aortic valve disease. It does not necessarily mean that there is left ventricular failure but indicates left ventricular overload. It cannot be present if there is atrial fibrillation and may disappear if the overload is removed (i.e. if hypertension is treated). If the heart is beating rapidly the three sounds may assume the cadence of a horse's hooves when galloping. This is called *gallop rhythm.*

Sometimes both third and fourth heart sounds may be present and if the heart rate is rapid these additional sounds may blend to produce what is sometimes called a *summation gallop* or *canter rhythm.* It is always of serious significance and suggests gross failure of ventricular function.

(4) *Extracardiac Sounds.* These sounds are usually heard in the latter half of systole. They are of a scratchy or crunchy nature and often sound rather superficial. They alter in intensity with respiration and position. They have a variety of causes and are usually innocent.

A special type of extracardiac sound is the *pericardial friction rub.* It may be heard at the base or apex of the heart and may be systolic or diastolic in timing or sometimes both. It is a scratchy or crunchy sound. There is usually other clinical evidence to suggest pericarditis.

Heart Murmurs

Heart murmurs are caused by eddies set up in blood as it passes from a narrow to a wider channel. They may be caused by pathological narrowing of valves, by their incompetence, or by undue distension of channels. Eddies may also be produced by the unduly rapid passage of blood through the heart as in thyrotoxicosis. When describing murmurs the following points should be noted:

(1) Site and radiation.
(2) Timing.
(3) Loudness. This is usually graded 1–6 for systolic and 1–4 for diastolic murmurs, grade 1 being very soft and grade 6 very loud.
(4) The pitch of the murmur.
(5) The presence or absence of a thrill.

Murmurs can be classified:
(1) Systolic murmurs.
(2) Diastolic murmurs.
(3) Continuous murmurs.

(1) *Systolic Murmurs* (Fig. 4.2). Note that these are usually high-pitched.

(*a*) *Ejection murmurs* are caused by the ventricles forcing blood through a narrowed orifice usually a stenosed aortic or pulmonary valve, or through a normal orifice into a dilated vessel such as an aortic

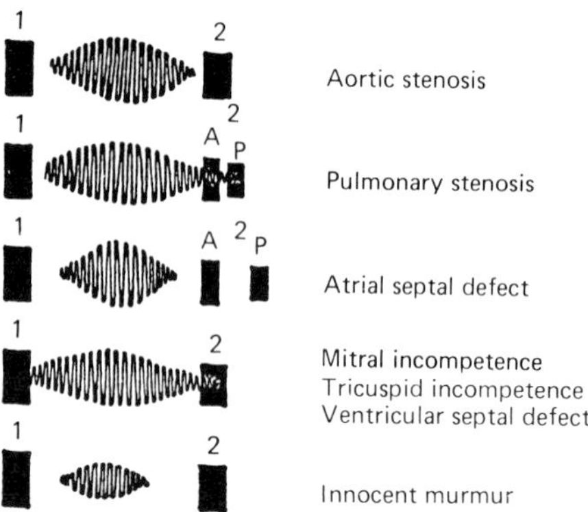

Fig. 4.2 Systolic murmurs.

aneurysm or a dilated pulmonary artery as in atrial septal defects. They can also be produced by rapid flow through a normal valve (see below).

Characteristically this type of murmur commences after the first sound, rises to a crescendo in midsystole and dies away before the second sound.

(*b*) *Pansystolic murmurs* are due to incompetence of the mitral or tricuspid valves or to a ventricular septal defect. They last throughout systole up to the second sound, they are more or less constant in intensity with sometimes a late systolic crescendo.

(*c*) *Late systolic murmurs* are found in coarctation of the aorta. Apparently normal subjects may occasionally have a *midsystolic click* followed by a *late systolic murmur*. This is believed to be associated with various congenital abnormalities of the mitral valve, including elongated chordae or voluminous valves. Occasionally late systolic murmurs are found in hypertrophic obstructive cardiomyopathy (see p. 193) and are due to a combination of obstruction to the outflow from the left ventricle and to mitral incompetence.

Innocent Systolic Murmurs. A great many systolic murmurs are not due to organic disease. The cause of such murmurs is not fully understood but many of them may be associated with a high velocity of blood flow and can be considered to be attenuated ejection murmurs. They are particularly liable to occur with pregnancy, anaemia, or fevers. They are commonly heard along the left sternal border or at the apex and they are rarely very loud. Their timing varies but they are usually of short duration. They nearly always begin in early systole and finish by midsystole. Their differentiation from organic systolic murmurs will depend partially on the character of the murmur and partially on the presence or absence of other evidence of cardiac disease.

(2) *Diastolic Murmurs* (Fig. 4.3).

(*a*) *Ventricular Filling Murmurs.* These murmurs are due to the flow of blood through stenosed mitral or tricuspid valves. They are separated from the second heart sound by a short gap of variable duration. In patients in sinus rhythm the murmur rises to a crescendo just before the first heart sound due to the contracting atria causing a momentarily increased rate of flow through the narrowed A-V valve. These murmurs are always low-pitched and rumbling.

The murmur of mitral stenosis is heard best with the patient lying on the left side. In mitral incompetence and ventricular septal defect there is increased blood flow through the mitral valve in diastole and although the valves are normal they may produce a low pitched diastolic murmur.

(*b*) The *Austin Flint Murmur*. This is an apical diastolic murmur heard in aortic regurgitation and is due to vibration of the anterior cusp of the mitral valve between the regurgitation flow from the aorta and the flow from the left atrium.

(*c*) *Regurgitant Diastolic Murmurs.* They are soft and high-pitched and are due to regurgitation of blood through the aortic or pulmonary valves. They are heard best with the patient sitting forward and in full expiration. They start immediately after the second heart sound, are loudest at their onset and die away before the end of diastole.

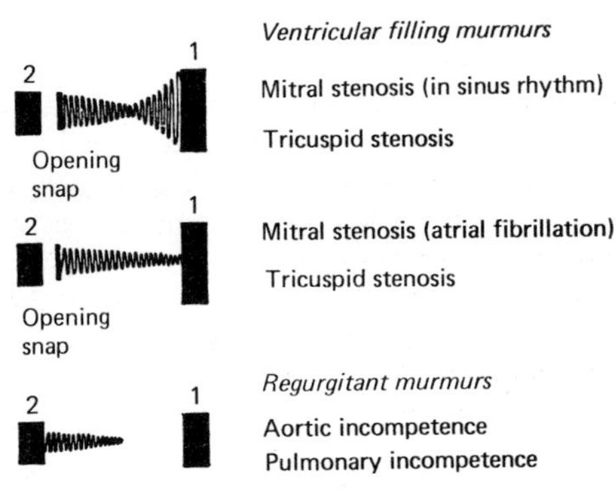

Fig. 4.3 Diastolic murmurs.

(3) *Continuous Murmurs* (Fig. 4.4). Certain murmurs continue throughout systole and diastole. They are found when there is blood flow between high and low pressure vessels, most commonly when a persistent ductus connects the aorta with the pulmonary artery.

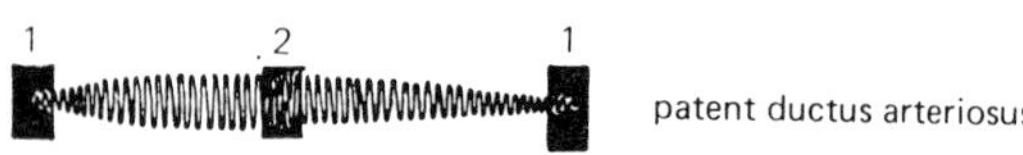

Fig. 4.4 Continuous murmurs.

THE ELECTROCARDIOGRAM (ECG)

The electrocardiogram records the electrical changes produced by the depolarisation and subsequent repolarisation of the heart muscle, associated respectively with systole and diastole. These changes are amplified and recorded on moving paper. The potential changes are recorded by electrodes attached in various combinations to the body. Each of these attachments is known as a 'lead'.

There are two main groups of leads, known as bipolar and unipolar. *Bipolar* leads record the potential changes between two points of the body surface, the leads in common use being:

Lead 1—which records the potential difference between the right and left arm.
Lead 2—between the right arm and left leg.
Lead 3—between the left arm and left leg.

Unipolar leads record potential change at one position on the body's surface. This is done by connecting the leads from both arms and the left leg, the potential change from these three leads being zero. A further electrode is then placed at various positions on the body's surface and the potential changes at these positions recorded. The most usual positions are the chest leads which are numbered V1-6 and the limb leads which are designated a VR (which is the right arm), a VL (left arm) and a VF (left foot).

Tracings from all parts of the body have certain common characteristics. The first wave, which is usually upright, but may be inverted, is called the P wave and represents atrial contraction. The next wave is a small downward deflection known as the Q wave and this is followed by an upright deflection, the R wave, and a further downward deflection, the S wave. This QRS complex represents ventricular contraction (Fig. 4.5).

The P-R interval, measured from the beginning of the P wave to the beginning of the R wave, represents the time taken by the wave of excitation to pass down the bundle of His and should not exceed 0.2 second in the normal subject. The duration of the QRS complex represents the time taken for the wave of excitation to spread through the ventricle and should not exceed 0.1 second in the normal subject. The QRS complex is followed by a short interval and then by a deflection which is usually upright. This is the T wave and represents the recession of the wave of excitation through the ventricle. Changes in the S-T

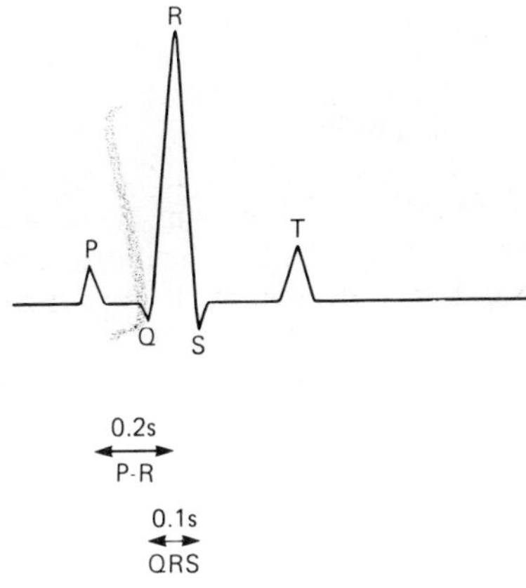

Fig. 4.5 The normal electrocardiogram.

segment and T wave area are of importance in the diagnosis of damage to the heart muscle.

In normal people the basic deflection in each lead is of one of three types. This depends on whether the electrode faces the right ventricle, the left ventricle, or the ventricular cavity. If the heart is in the normal position, leads aVF and Vs 1 and 2 have complexes arising from the right ventricle. Leads aVL and Vs 4, 5, and 6 have complexes arising from the left ventricle and lead aVR has complexes arising from the ventricular cavities. The *right ventricular lead* is characterised by a small R and large S waves and the absence of Q waves, *the left ventricular lead* by a small Q wave followed by a large R wave and small or absent S wave. In the *ventricular cavity lead* the P wave is inverted, the QRS complex consists of a negative deflection and the T wave is also inverted.

If the heart is in an abnormal position, then of course the distribution of these complexes is changed.

In reading an ECG the following points should be noted:

(1) Heart rate.
(2) Heart rhythm.
(3) Nature and direction of the P waves.
(4) The duration of the P-R interval.
(5) The direction of the main deflection and general shape of the QRS complex.
(6) The width of the QRS complex.
(7) The size of the complexes.
(8) Any depression or elevation of the S-T segment.
(9) The direction and character of the T waves.

ECHOCARDIOGRAPHY

This is a method of investigation which is becoming increasingly important. It is non-invasive and harmless and can be carried out in a short time. Essentially it consists of recording the echoes obtained from a sound source of 1000 pulses per second. This shows the pattern of movement obtained from the pericardium, the interventricular septum and posterior wall of the left ventricle, the mitral, triscuspid, aortic and pulmonary valves and the left atrium. It is particularly useful in the diagnosis of:

(1) *Left atrial myxoma* (see p. 194).
(2) *Mitral valve disease.*
(3) *Left ventricular function.* The movements of the left ventricular wall and septum can be measured during systole together with the rate of change. The thickness of the left ventricular septum can be measured and this can be useful in the diagnosis of *hypertrophic cardiomyopathy.*
(4) *Pericardial effusion.* Echocardiography shows two echoes, one from the moving posterior myocardium and one from the inert pericardium.

RADIOLOGY OF THE HEART

The heart can be examined by chest radiography, by fluorescent screening or by introducing radio-opaque substances into the heart or coronary arteries which is then X-rayed—this is known as angiocardiography.

In a plain radiograph of the heart, the right side of the cardiac silhouette is made up of the right atrium, the ascending aorta, and the superior vena cava. The left border is formed by the aortic arch, the pulmonary artery and the left ventricle. When the heart is examined by X-ray screening it should also be viewed in the left and right anterior oblique positions. If a little barium emulsion is swallowed the back of the heart is outlined and slight enlargement of the left atrium can easily be seen, especially in the right anterior oblique position.

Cardiac Enlargement. A general idea of the size of the heart can be obtained by measuring the maximum transverse diameter of the heart and the maximum transverse diameter of the chest; normally the heart diameter should not be more than half that of the chest.

Enlargement of individual heart chambers can also be demonstrated radiologically. *Left ventricular enlargement* causes rounding of the left lower border of the heart shadow on PA view, and in the LAO position the left ventricle can be seen bulging backwards and overlying the spine. *Right ventricular enlargement* causes increase in the transverse diameter

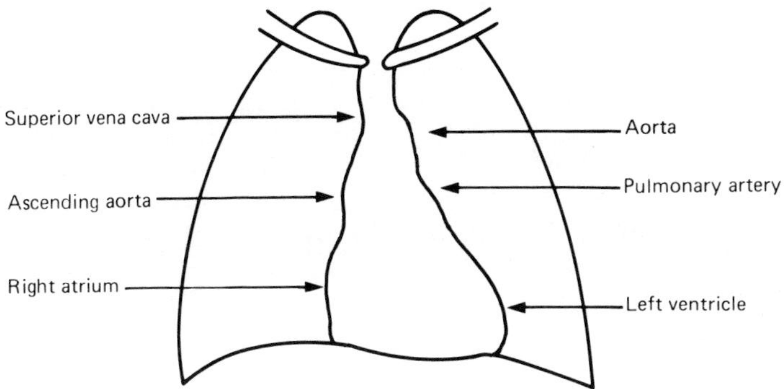

Fig. 4.6 A posterio-anterior view of the heart.

of the heart and there is often straightening of the left border of the heart caused by enlargement of the outflow tract of the right ventricle. *Left atrial enlargement* is best seen in the RAO position when it can be seen to indent the oesophagus following a barium swallow. In the PA view the enlarged left atrial appendage appears on the left border of the heart, below the pulmonary artery. *Right atrial enlargement* produces a bulge at the lowest part of the right cardiac border.

A *pericardial effusion* also produces an increase in the cardiac shadow which is usually pear-shaped with clear-cut margins and the lung fields frequently appear clear. It is not always easy to differentiate between enlargement of the heart and a pericardial effusion so that aspiration or echocardiography may be necessary to settle the diagnosis.

By radiological methods it is also possible to assess the great vessels leaving the heart and to demonstrate calcification of the heart valves.

The Lungs. The lungs may show changes which are secondary to cardiac disease, the most important being:

(a) *Congestion.* There is a haziness of the lung fields extending out from the hilar region. Oedema of the interlobular septa produces the horizontal lines usually in the lower lobes and known as Kerley B lines. In the early stages dilation of the veins draining the upper lobes may be the only sign.
(b) *Pulmonary Plethora.* Increased pulmonary blood flow occurs when there is a left to right shunt and therefore a large volume of blood passing through the lungs. There is a general increase in lung vascular markings and the large vessels become dilated.
(c) *Pulmonary Oligaemia.* Decreased pulmonary blood flow occurs in pulmonary stenosis and Fallot's tetralogy. There is a decrease in the pulmonary vascular markings.
(d) *Pulmonary Hypertension.* The pulmonary arteries are dilated but the vascular markings in the peripheral fields are reduced.

CIRCULATORY FAILURE

Failure of the circulation occurs when the heart is unable to maintain an adequate output. It can be of both acute and chronic forms which produce differing clinical pictures.

ACUTE CIRCULATORY FAILURE

In this condition there is a sudden fall in cardiac output and blood pressure which is due to two causes:

(1) *Hypovolaemia*—where there is inadequate venous return to the heart and thus a failure of output. This is commonly secondary to *haemorrhage, sodium deficiency* and *trauma.*
(2) *Pump failure*—where the myocardium cannot maintain an adequate output of blood. It occurs commonly after *cardiac infarction* or *pulmonary embolism.*

Septicaemia. Circulatory failure may also complicate septicaemia particularly by Gram-negative organisms. The mechanisms here are complicated.

The clinical distinction between pump failure and hypovolaemia may be clear from the history and physical signs. In cases of doubt and to monitor progress the measurement of various haemodynamic parameters can be useful:

(a) Central venous pressure. This is the easiest and least invasive measurement but does not give any direct information about left ventricular function.
(b) The pulmonary artery and pulmonary artery wedge pressure (which reflects left atrial and thus, left ventricular filling pressure) can be measured by a Swan Ganz catheter.
(c) Arterial blood pressure.
(d) The cardiac output can be estimated by dye or thermal dilution methods.

In uncomplicated hypovolaemia both the central venous pressure and the pulmonary artery wedge pressure will be low, whereas in pump failure they will be raised. It must be remembered, however, that the situation may be more complicated and that hypovolaemia and pump failure may coexist.

Clinical Features. The picture is one of adrenergic overactivity with pallor and cold extremities due to vasoconstriction, sweating and tachycardia. The blood pressure is low. In severe cases perfusion of vital organs is impaired causing confusion, acute renal failure (see p. 469), and acidosis due to overproduction of lactic acid. *Shock lung*, in which there is increasing dyspnoea with hypoxia and bilateral shadows on

X-ray, can develop and will require artificial ventilation.

Treatment. This depends on the cause. If the inadequate circulation is due to pump failure treatment is difficult and various agents have been tried to encourage the failing myocardium. Dopamine by continuous intravenous infusion increases the cardiac output by an effect on the myocardium and also causes dilation of renal blood vessels in the lower dose range and thus to some degree guards against acute renal failure. The initial dose is 2–5 μg/kg/minute and this is increased as required. Dobutamine which acts largely on the heart is also used. Generally however, the prognosis is bad. In hypovolaemia, circulating volume should be restored by infusion of plasma expanders such as dextran (or blood if due to haemorrhage), using central venous pressure or pulmonary artery wedge pressure as an index of adequate replacement. Causative factors such as infection should be treated vigorously with antibiotics which may be combined with 500 mg hydrocortisone IV 6-hourly or methylprednisolone in doses of 0.5 mg/kg/day by intravenous infusion. With severe shock the dose may be increased up to 30 mg/kg for a short period.

CARDIAC FAILURE

Cardiac Function in Heart Failure

The essential defect in cardiac failure is the inability of the heart to maintain a sufficient output of blood for the needs of the body. In health the stroke volume and cardiac output are influenced by three factors:

The preload
The state of the myocardium
The afterload.

(a) *The Preload.* This is dependent on the volume of blood in the ventricles at the end of diastole which determines the endiastolic filling pressure of the ventricles and thus the stretch applied to the ventricular muscle fibres. In a healthy heart an increase in endiastolic pressure leads to a rise in stroke volume and cardiac output in accordance with the well known Frank–Starling curve (see Fig. 4.7). In cardiac failure the normal relationship between endiastolic filling pressure and cardiac output is disturbed so that a rise in venous pressure is not followed by a rise in stroke volume and output. This is partly due to changes in the myocardium produced by hypertrophy and partly due to the myocardium working at a disadvantage as a result of ventricular distension.

(b) *The State of the Myocardium.* It is self-evident that a healthy myocardium is essential to meet the ever-changing demands made on the heart. The myocardium may be rendered less efficient by disease, particularly coronary disease and cardiomyopathies. Hypertrophy in response to increased afterload (see below) may ultimately interfere with

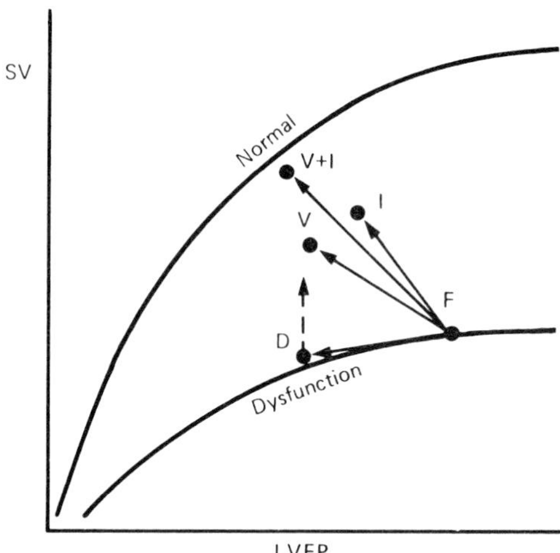

Fig. 4.7 Frank–Starling left-ventricular function curve relating left ventricular filling pressure (LVFP) to stroke volume (SV). Depressed curve of heart failure can be shifted toward normal by inotropic drugs (I) or vasodilator drugs (V), and these effects are complementary when the drugs are infused together (V + I). Note that diuretics (D) usually reduce filling pressure (F) without augmenting output. The dashed line suggests that stroke volume may later rise, perhaps by virtue of a gradual improvement in ventricular function. Reprinted by permission from the *New England J. Medicine* **297,** 27, 1977.

myocardial function by making the muscle stiffer and by upsetting the balance between coronary circulation and muscle.

(c) *The Afterload.* This is the impedance to the expulsion of blood from the ventricles, and in health it is determined by the pulmonary and systemic blood pressures. In diseased states the afterload may be increased by hypertension or by aortic or pulmonary stenosis. In addition cardiac failure can produce vasoconstriction and thus a further rise in peripheral resistance and afterload. The response to an increased afterload is hypertrophy of the ventricular muscle and for a time this will compensate for the extra work load but ultimately compensation is inadequate and cardiac failure develops.

In practice it is usual for more than one of these three factors to be involved in cardiac failure, and although one may predominate they are frequently interdependent.

Consequences of Cardiac Failure

(1) *Salt and Water Retention.* In heart failure there is a decrease in the blood flow to the kidneys resulting in retention of sodium and water.

Although the reason for this has not been fully elucidated it seems that the balance between glomerular filtration and tubular reabsorption is disturbed so that more of the filtered load of sodium is reabsorbed. Increased secretion of aldosterone may play a part in advanced heart failure but in the early stages this is not usually a factor.

In long-standing heart failure, particularly after vigorous treatment with diuretics, a further disorder of electrolyte and water balance may develop. The kidneys retain proportionally more water than sodium producing a *dilutional hyponatraemia*. This is often associated with considerable potassium depletion, partly due to the action of diuretics and possibly aldosterone and partly to the leakage of potassium from chronically hypoxic cells (sick cell syndrome).

Oedema. Salt and water retention leads to an increase in blood volume and the appearance of excess fluid in the tissue spaces, the distribution of this fluid being influenced by gravity so that it collects in the lower part of the legs, feet and ankles if the patient is ambulant or over the sacrum of those who are in bed. It is known as dependent or cardiac oedema and characteristically it pits on pressure. In severe heart failure ascites or pleural effusions may develop.

Another factor in the development of oedema is a rise in pressure at the venous end of the capillary (see below), which further increases the amount of tissue fluid.

(2) *Raised Venous Pressure*. This can be most easily appreciated in the external jugular veins, and the liver may be enlarged due to congestion. The rise in venous pressure is due to:

(a) Salt and water retention causing an increase in circulating blood volume.
(b) Failure of the heart to increase cardiac output in response to a rise in endiastolic venous pressure (preloading).

(3) *Heart Rate*. An increase in the heart rate produces a rise in cardiac output. Tachycardia due to increased adrenergic activity is a compensating mechanism in heart failure. If the adrenergic drive is removed by β adrenergic blocking agents, heart failure is made worse.

(4) *Dyspnoea*. This is caused by the effects of heart failure on the lungs. With the rise in left atrial pressure the lungs become congested and when the pressure in the left atrium and pulmonary veins reaches about 30 mmHg exudation of fluid from the pulmonary capillaries into the alveoli occurs. If this develops acutely it produces pulmonary oedema, if it develops more gradually it leads to thickening with fibrosis of the alveolar walls. Dyspnoea is due to:

(a) Oedema and fibrosis interfering with gas exchanges.
(b) Increased 'stiffness' of the lung with reduced compliance.
(c) Increased sensitivity of lung stretch reflexes.

In cardiac failure dyspnoea is usually first noticed on effort but may later occur at rest (see left ventricular failure). As it progresses patients become dyspnoeic on lying flat (orthopnoeic). This is believed to be due to increased pulmonary congestion which develops in the horizontal position. Changes in position also alter cardiac output but this plays only a small part in the genesis of orthopnoea.

(5) *Cyanosis* is of the peripheral type and is the result of slowing of the circulation with consequent venous and capillary stagnation of blood.

(6) *Tiredness and weakness* are common symptoms associated with a low cardiac output and are due to poor peripheral perfusion.

It is customary and useful to divide heart failure into left and right ventricular failure, for although in most cases of left ventricular failure the right ventricle will ultimately fail too, it often starts with failure of only one ventricle.

LEFT VENTRICULAR FAILURE

The chief causes of left ventricular failure are:

(1) Hypertension.
(2) Myocardial infarction.
(3) Aortic valvular disease.
(4) Cardiomyopathy.
(5) Mitral incompetence.
(6) Acute pulmonary oedema may also complicate mitral stenosis but is due to left atrial and not left ventricular failure.

The left ventricle may be called on to do increased work (afterloading), either because an obstruction to output causes a rise in pressure (hypertension or aortic stenosis) or because there is an increased volume of blood to be handled (mitral or aortic incompetence). The ventricle hypertrophies and for a time is able to maintain an adequate circulation, but eventually it is unable to do so. A similar situation arises if the myocardium is diseased, usually as a result of cardiac infarction. In both cases the pressure rises in the left atrium (preloading) and pulmonary veins, leading to increased pulmonary venous pressure and ultimately to pulmonary oedema.

Clinical Features. Left ventricular failure may develop gradually or suddenly. When it is of slow onset the patient usually complains first of dyspnoea on effort. In addition, his sleep is disturbed. At first he is restless when lying flat and is relieved by two or three pillows (*orthopnoea*); later sleep is broken by *paroxysmal nocturnal coughing*, relieved by sitting up and hanging the legs out of bed; later still, *paroxysmal nocturnal dyspnoea* or *cardiac asthma* appears. In some instances the patient experiences several short attacks of dyspnoea during the night. These are due to exaggerated bouts of Cheyne–Stokes respiration and are severe enough to rouse the patient from sleep. Left ventricular failure of *abrupt* onset, which is often due to myocardial infarction, may present with cardiac asthma without preceding symptoms. In the fully developed attack of paroxysmal nocturnal dyspnoea the patient goes to sleep and awakens an hour or two later in a state of great alarm, with a sense of suffocation and fighting for breath. He sits up and may throw open the windows. In severe attacks copiously frothy sputum is expectorated, which may be blood-stained and which is due to pulmonary oedema. After an hour or so the attack passes off and the patient sleeps until morning. Rarely does a first attack prove fatal.

It is not entirely clear why these attacks occur at night, but a number of factors, including the recumbent position, which increase the extent of the pulmonary venous congestion, are operative.

Examination at the time of the attack may show evidence of left ventricular hypertrophy; if however left ventricular failure complicates myocardial infarction this may be absent. *Tachycardia* is usual and on auscultation *a third or fourth heart sound* may be heard. *Late inspiratory crackles* from pulmonary oedema are heard at the lung bases, and there may be rhonchi from associated bronchospasm and bronchial oedema. If the attack is severe, there may be a fall in the systolic blood pressure. *Pulsus alternans* (p. 123) may be detected; when the difference in the systolic pressure exceeds 15–20 mmHg, and particularly when the alternation persists after the tachycardia has subsided, it is of grave prognostic significance.

The *electrocardiogram* nearly always shows some evidence of S-T or T wave changes over the left ventricle. A *chest radiograph* will show the hazy shadows of pulmonary oedema spreading out from each hilum into the lung fields.

Prognosis. It used to be said that the prognosis after an attack of cardiac asthma was poor, most patients dying within a year or two. With improved methods of treatment this is no longer true and some patients may do quite well, particularly if the underlying disease, such as hypertension, is amenable to treatment.

RIGHT VENTRICULAR AND CONGESTIVE FAILURE

The chief causes of right ventricular failure are:

(1) Following left ventricular failure.
(2) Mitral valvular disease.
(3) Tricuspid valve disease.
(4) Pulmonary heart disease.
(5) Certain types of congenital heart disease.
(6) Following pulmonary embolism.
(7) Thyrotoxicosis.
(8) Cardiomyopathy.

Tricuspid stenosis and constrictive pericarditis can also cause marked systemic venous congestion.

Clinical Features. Right ventricular failure is usually seen in patients who already suffer dyspnoea and orthopnoea from pulmonary congestion due to left ventricular failure or mitral valvular disease, and it is then often called *congestive cardiac failure.* When right ventricular failure occurs without pulmonary congestion or pulmonary disease, or when the lungs are spared congestion as in tricuspid stenosis, marked dyspnoea or orthopnoea is not usually a prominent feature although usually present to some degree. Other symptoms include tiredness, weakness, and loss of appetite.

The main signs of right ventricular failure are found in the systemic venous system. In a normal subject reclining at 30°, the neck veins are empty above the clavicles. In right ventricular failure, the *increased venous pressure* causes distension of the veins above this level. The pulsation in the distended veins can readily be distinguished from that of the carotids by the diffuse nature of the venous pulse, in which it is usually possible to distinguish at least two elements, and by the fact that the venous pulse can easily be obliterated by the finger. With severe right ventricular failure, there is stretching of the tricuspid ring leading to functional tricuspid incompetence and a consequent large systolic venous wave which can be seen in the neck and may be felt over the liver. It may disappear with treatment. Distension of the liver with blood, which follows right ventricular failure, may give rise to pain in the right hypochondrium. Palpation shows that the *liver is enlarged and tender*. If the congestion is of long duration the liver may be damaged, resulting in slight jaundice. Loss of appetite is common due to congestion of the stomach. Dependent *oedema*, for reasons already stated, occurs in right ventricular failure. If the oedema is severe it may be associated with ascites and pleural effusions. *Muscle wasting* is common but may be obscured by oedema. *Cyanosis* is common, partly due to poor oxygenation of the blood passing through the oedematous lungs and partly due to peripheral stagnation. In heart failure, the urine is usually diminished in volume, of high specific gravity, and may contain protein.

Treatment of Cardiac Failure

Treatment has two main aims:

(1) To improve cardiac function.
(2) To correct the underlying defect if possible.

A consideration of the factors involved in heart failure (p. 137) suggests that cardiac function could be improved in three ways (Fig. 4.7):

(a) By improving the inotrophic activity of the myocardium. This may be achieved with digitalis or other agents such as dopamine and dobutamine.

(b) By reducing preload (i.e. lowering venous pressure). This may be achieved by giving diuretics or by vasodilator drugs which pool blood in the peripheral vessels.

(c) By reducing afterload. This may be effected by vasodilator drugs which reduce peripheral resistance or by relieving valvular stenosis if present.

The effects of these different modes of treatment are shown in Fig. 4.7 and it will be noted that a combination of methods may produce a better result than a single type of treatment. The details of treatment which depend on the nature of the cardiac failure and the clinical situation, are considered below.

Acute Left Ventricular Failure

(1) The patient is kept upright supported by pillows; if possible the legs should be dependent to allow as much oedema fluid as possible to drain away from the lungs.

(2) *Morphine* 10–15 mg should be given intramuscularly. Its action in this condition is not fully understood, but its good effect is probably due largely to its sedative action which decreases anxiety and reduces hyperventilation. It is also a vasodilator and lowers venous pressure and thus preloading.

(3) Reduction in blood volume lowers venous pressure, relieves overfilling of the heart and leads to the disappearance of oedema. It is usually achieved by a diuretic, and *frusemide* 20–40 mg IV is effective.

(4) *Aminophylline* 250 mg slowly intravenously is useful particularly if there is associated bronchospasm.

(5) Pure oxygen should be given if available.

(6) Digitalisation is not required unless rapid atrial fibrillation is believed to have precipitated ventricular failure.

With these measures it is usually possible to relieve the patient of an acute attack. Thereafter he should be treated as for congestive failure with rest and diuretics (see below). If the underlying cause is amenable to treatment, this should be dealt with. For the next few nights, many patients have difficulty in sleeping and a hypnotic (temazepam 20 mg) is useful.

Right Ventricular and Congestive Failure

(1) *Rest* is important in the treatment of heart failure. The patient is nursed in bed and may find breathing easier if he leans forward resting his arms on a bed-table. This upright position allows the oedema fluid to drain away from the lungs and relieves dyspnoea. If an adjustable bed is available the patient will be able to sit with his legs lowered which, by

reducing the venous return to the heart, further relieves pulmonary congestion. An excellent alternative is a high-backed armchair; many patients find this very comfortable and so rest and sleep more easily. If at all possible he should be allowed up to use a commode. Complete rest should not be continued for more than a few days except for the seriously ill as it may be complicated by venous thrombosis. Thereafter, a gradual return to modest activity should be started.

(2) *Diet* should be light and easily digestible. There is no reason for severe salt restriction but in the early stages no salt should be added to the food at meal times. Fluid intake need not be reduced unless dilutional hyponatraemia develops.

(3) With prolonged rest prophylactic anticoagulation with heparin 5000 units twice daily by subcutaneous injection may be used.

(4) *Digitalis* was the standard treatment for cardiac failure although with the introduction of effective diuretics it lost much of its importance. There is no doubt that it is highly effective in controlling heart rate and improving failure in rapid atrial fibrillation. Its place in cardiac failure associated with sinus rhythm is less clear for although it can be shown to produce a positive inotrophic effect at the start of treatment there is no evidence that it persists after the initial stages of treatment. There is however good evidence that in patients with sinus rhythm who have been receiving the drug for long periods, it can be withdrawn without deterioration in their condition. There are several preparations of digitalis in use. They are all similar in their pharmacological action, but differ in the speed of onset and duration of effect and in the proportion of the oral dose which is absorbed. The most commonly used preparations are shown in Table 4.1. After absorption, digitoxin is largely protein bound and is metabolised by the liver, so that accumulation does not occur in renal failure. Digoxin is excreted fairly rapidly by the kidneys, and retention occurs with impaired renal function.

Table 4.1 Common preparations of digitalis

Preparation	*Route of administration*	*Maximum effect*	*Duration of half life*	*Percentage absorbed by oral route*	*Elimination*
Digoxin	IV	2 hours	40 hours		Largely renal
	oral	6 hours		70%	
Digitoxin	IV	6 hours	5 days		
	oral	12 hours		95%	Hepatic

Actions of Digitalis on the Heart

In therapeutic doses digitalis has no effect on the normal heart but in heart failure the following occur:

(a) Depression of conduction in the bundle of His so that in atrial fibrillation less impulses pass from the atria to the ventricles and the ventricular rate is slowed. This is the most important therapeutic action.
(b) Increased force of contraction of the ventricular muscle.
(c) Slowing of the heart by an effect on the sino-atrial node, partly mediated by the vagus and partly by direct action.
(d) In addition, digitalis produces depression of the S-T segment in the ECG.

These result in a rise in cardiac output and a fall in venous pressure. The increased renal blood flow causes a diuresis. Although digitalis has been used for all types of cardiac failure its main use is in controlling rapid atrial fibrillation. It is of little use in the treatment of heart failure associated with anaemia, acute myocarditis or beri-beri.

Dosage. There are many schemes of dosage of digitalis. They all aim at giving a loading dose fully to saturate the heart muscle with the drug followed by maintenance doses to replace the daily loss of the drug.

Two schemes of dosage are given below.

(a) *Routine Digitalisation.* The initial dose is 0.5 mg twice or three times daily depending on the size of the patient. Thereafter the dosage is adjusted to keep the ventricular rate between 70 and 80 per minute. The maintenance dose usually lies between 0.25 and 0.5 mg daily.

Digoxin is excreted largely via the kidneys and for this reason patients with impaired renal function and especially the elderly are liable to accumulate the drug and develop signs of overdosage. Digoxin tablets containing 0.0625 mg of the drug are available and may be useful in such cases where the correct dose usually lies between 0.0625 and 0.125 mg daily.

Equivalent amounts of digitoxin can be used (tablets of digitoxin 0.1 mg = digoxin 0.25 mg).

(b) *Emergency Digitalisation.* This is rarely required and is not without risk. Digoxin 0.5 mg is given *slowly* intravenously and is followed by digoxin 0.5 mg orally after four hours and then digoxin 0.25 mg t.d.s. until a satisfactory response is obtained. ECG monitoring is desirable. Intravenous digoxin should not be given to a patient who has received digitalis within the last two months. Nearly as rapid a result can be obtained if the initial dose of digoxin is given orally.

Digitalis Blood Levels. It is possible to measure the concentration of *digoxin* in the blood. The therapeutic levels lie between 1.0 and 2.0 ng/ml. Toxicity usually occurs at levels over 2.0 ng/ml. There is, however, considerable variation with overlap between therapeutic and toxic levels and digoxin assays are not often necessary in controlling treatment. They are however useful in checking compliance and possible toxicity.

Signs of Overdosage. The most important signs of overdosage are:

(a) *Coupled beats.* This is due to increased excitability of the ventricles leading to ventricular premature systoles which occur after every normal beat. If overdosage is allowed to continue ventricular tachycardia or fibrillation may occur.

(b) *Undue slowing of the pulse*—a resting pulse below 65/min suggests too much digitalis is being given.

(c) *Atrial tachycardia* with atrio-ventricular block may sometimes occur.

(d) *Nausea, vomiting,* and *diarrhoea.* Overdosage with digitalis can cause central vomiting—but it should be remembered that vomiting is sometimes a feature of heart failure itself.

(e) *Xanthopsia.*

It is usually sufficient to omit the drug for a day or two to abolish these effects but serious ventricular arrhythmias should be treated with lignocaine or phenytoin (see p. 153) and the plasma potassium level should be restored to normal if necessary.

Potassium and Digitalis. The presence of potassium ions decreases the toxicity of digitalis and vice versa. This means that overdosage of digitalis can be temporarily reversed by giving potassium salts. It will also be found that patients who are losing potassium ions (for instance, due to treatment with a thiazide diuretic or frusemide) may become more sensitive to digitalis and develop evidence of overdosage.

(5) *Diuretics* are extremely useful in patients with heart failure for they lead to decrease in extracellular fluid volume and lower venous pressure.

(a) *The Thiazides.* This group of diuretics prevent the reabsorption of sodium, potassium and water by the renal tubule. They are given orally. There are several drugs in this group with similar actions but differing in dosage.

Chlorothiazide	0.5–2.0 g
Hydrochlorothiazide	50–200 mg
Hydroflumethiazide	50–200 mg
Bendrofluazide	5.0–10 mg
Cyclopenthiazide	0.25–1.5 mg

Their diuretic action lasts about twelve hours. They are given usually orally each morning on a regular basis. Chlorthalidone in doses of 50–200 mg is similar, but its action lasts up to 48 hours.

In the upper dose ranges these diuretics will produce some potassium depletion. This is important as it potentiates the effects of digitalis and may lead to signs of digitalis overdosage. Patients on diuretics should therefore receive potassium supplements (see below). The benzothiadiazines also have some blood pressure lowering action and therefore increase the effect of hypotensive drugs.

Side-effects are not common, but benzothiadiazines cause some uric acid retention and may precipitate an acute attack of gout. Rarely they produce diabetes mellitus, which however usually recovers when the drug is withdrawn.

(b) *Loop Diuretics.* These diuretics act predominantly on the ascending limb of the loop of Henle. They act rather more quickly than the thiazides and are more powerful, they also cause potassium depletion.

Frusemide is given orally in doses of 40–200 mg daily and produces a diuresis lasting about 6 hours. It is also very effective intravenously (see left ventricular failure) in doses of 10–40 mg, causing an intense diuresis which lasts about 2 hours. *Bumetanide* is very similar to frusemide, the oral dose usually lies between 1–4 mg daily and the IV dose is 1–2 mg.

Care must be taken when using these powerful diuretics as they can produce acute sodium and water depletion with hypotension and collapse.

(c) In addition *spironolactone*, which antagonises the action of aldosterone, has been used in patients with obstinate oedema. It acts on a different site in the renal tubules to the usual diuretics and can be useful. The dose is 100 mg one to four times daily and it must be combined with another diuretic.

(d) *Triamterene* increases the excretion of sodium and water but reduces that of potassium. It is most effective when combined with one of the benzothiadiazines, the dose being 200 mg daily. *Amiloride* is similar to triamterene but is rather more powerful. The dose is 10–20 mg.

Amiloride, spironolactone and triamterene can cause potassium retention and for this reason must be used with great care in renal failure.

(e) *Potassium supplements* will be required by patients on thiazides or loop diuretics. Potassium chloride can cause ulceration of the gut, and Slow K (a slow-release preparation containing 8.0 mmol K) in doses of 3–6 tablets daily is satisfactory. As an alternative, a thiazide or a loop diuretic may be combined with a potassium sparing diuretic such as amiloride. This reduces potassium loss and is considered by some to be a more effective method of conserving potassium.

(6) *Peripheral Vasodilators.* Drugs which cause arterial vasodilation lower peripheral resistance (i.e. afterload) and thus allow the myocardium to work more efficiently. Likewise, drugs which dilate veins lower venous and thus endiastolic pressure (i.e. preload) and improve cardiac function. Several drugs have been used for this purpose both in chronic cardiac failure which is resistant to other forms of treatment and in the more acute and sometimes intractable failure which follows cardiac infarction.

Sodium Nitroprusside is a short acting drug which relaxes both arterial and venous smooth muscle. It is given by IV infusion and the initial dose is 1.0 mcg/kg/min and increased every ten minutes as required. *Prazosin* is an arterial and venous dilator. The initial dose is 0.5 mg by mouth three times daily, and this is increased cautiously until improvement occurs. *Hydralazine* is an arterial vasodilator, the initial dose is 25 mg twice daily. It is liable to cause tachycardia.

It must be stressed that when starting treatment with vasodilator drugs the blood pressure must be watched carefully. When there is a fixed resistance to blood flow as occurs in valvular stenosis vasodilators are not likely to be effective and should not be used.

(7) *Sedation* is important in these patients as they are often restless and anxious. Temazepam 10–20 mg is usually satisfactory but occasionally, for an ill patient, a *small* dose of an opiate is very useful.

(8) *Oxygen* may be required in patients with severe heart failure and may be given either by a Ventimask or by an oxygen tent. The indications are cyanosis or distress.

(9) If the oedema is very severe, or if there are collections of fluid in the chest or abdomen, recourse must be made to tapping the chest or abdomen (*paracentesis*).

(10) Rarely it may be necessary to remove excess fluid by peritoneal dialysis.

After recovering from cardiac failure the patient should make a steady return to activity. At this stage it may be necessary to consider any measures required to relieve the underlying cause of his heart failure (i.e. valvular disease, etc.). His ultimate mode of life will be conditioned by the limits imposed by his disease.

ABNORMALITIES OF RHYTHM

EXTRASYSTOLES (Ectopic Beats)

Extrasystoles, or more accurately premature systoles, are due to the cardiac impulse arising in an ectopic focus which may be in the atria, the atrioventricular node, or in the ventricles. As the contraction is premature the ventricles are only partially filled so that the resulting pulse wave is diminished or even impalpable at the wrist. The subsequent normal pulse falls in the refractory period so that no contraction occurs. During the pause more blood enters the ventricles than normal and the next beat is unusually forceful.

Extrasystoles are extremely common and most people have them at some time in their lives. Their incidence increases with age; they may occur only occasionally or may be as frequent as every alternate beat, this rhythm being known as pulsus bigeminus or coupled beats. They are often noticed when the patient is lying in bed at night, and though they disappear during exercise they may appear after exertion. They are often more frequent when the patient is tired or worried or during a feverish illness. In some people they may also be related to over-indulgence in tobacco, coffee, or alcohol. Extrasystoles may also occur in heart disease.

Many patients fail to notice their own extrasystoles. Others complain of a thump in the chest which is due to the powerful contraction after the compensatory pause. Sometimes patients notice the compensatory pause and complain of a 'dropped beat'.

Extrasystoles can usually be diagnosed by the pulse, when a premature beat followed by a pause is felt. Multiple extrasystoles can be confused with atrial fibrillation; the former will, however, disappear on exercise, whereas atrial fibrillation will become more marked. Some confusion may also result if the extrasystoles cannot be detected at the wrist. They can, however, always be heard on careful auscultation of the heart.

Electrocardiogram. In supraventricular ectopics the ECG (Fig. 4.8)

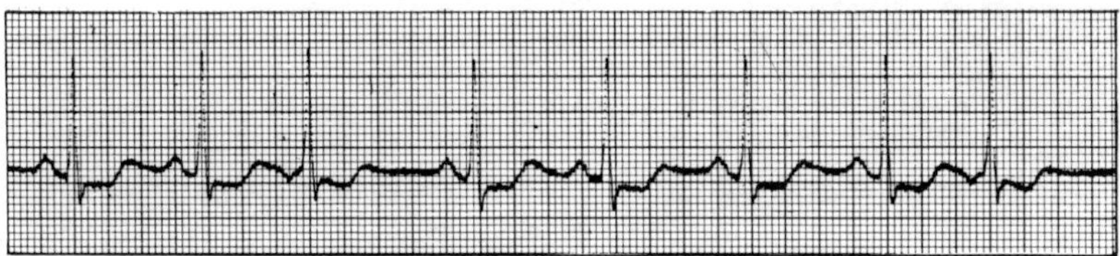

Fig. 4.8 Electrocardiogram showing supraventricular ectopics.

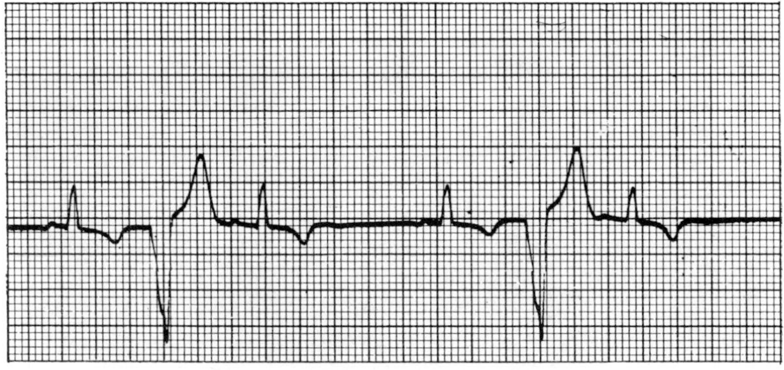

Fig. 4.9 Electrocardiogram showing ventricular ectopics.

will show a premature P wave followed by a normal QRS complex. In ventricular ectopics the ECG (Fig. 4.9) shows a premature and abnormally wide QRS complex.

Prognosis and Treatment. Extrasystoles by themselves are of no significance. Their presence calls for a careful examination and if no abnormality is found reassurance should be vigorous. If extrasystoles are found at a routine examination in an otherwise normal heart it is usually best not to tell the patient.

Occasionally in subjects with heart disease multiple extrasystoles may herald the onset of a more serious arrhythmia; e.g. the occurrence of ventricular extrasystoles after a coronary thrombosis is sometimes followed by ventricular fibrillation (see p. 160). In those taking too much digitalis ventricular extrasystoles cause coupled beats (pulsus bigeminus) and indicate that the drug should be discontinued for a day or two.

Drug treatment is rarely required for extrasystoles; reassurance and the avoidance of obvious precipitating factors are usually sufficient, and if the extrasystoles are very frequent and distressing, quinidine in doses of 200 mg three times daily or propranolol 20 mg three times daily will sometimes abolish them within a few days.

TACHYCARDIAS

Sinus tachycardia results from an increased rate of discharge from the S-A node.

Paroxysmal tachycardias are due to rapid discharge from an ectopic focus or may arise from re-entry phenomena. They are classified according to their site of origin:

supraventricular
ventricular

Supraventricular Tachycardia. This type of tachycardia may be due to an ectopic focus in the atria or A-V node but is more often due to a re-entry phenomenon in which the A-V node is reactivated via an accessory pathway so that a rapid circus movement is initiated. These accessory pathways may be purely functional or may, as in the Wolff–Parkinson–White syndrome (p. 163), have an anatomical basis and be associated with pre-excitation of the ventricles and a short P–R interval on the ECG.

Attacks of atrial tachycardia are not usually associated with cardiac disease but may complicate thyrotoxicosis and excess of digitalis, alcohol or caffeine. They often start in youth and tend to recur.

The ECG (Fig. 4.10) shows a regular rhythm, with a rate of 150–240 per minute and the QRS complexes appear normal. There is usually 1:1 conduction between atria and ventricles but at higher rates a 2:1 block may develop. Sometimes intraventricular block occurs with wide QRS

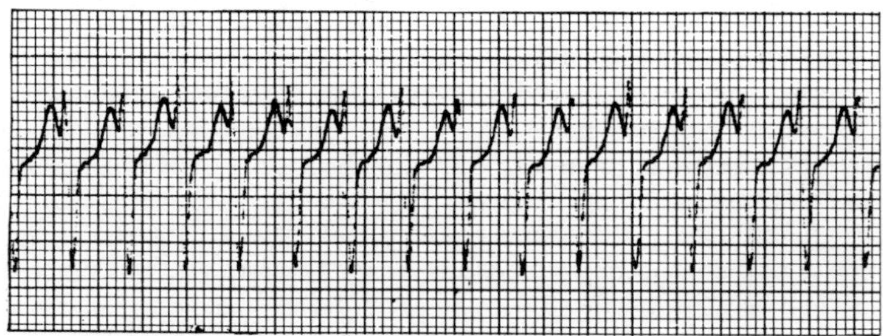

Fig. 4.10 Electrocardiogram showing atrial tachycardia.

complexes and this may be difficult to distinguish from a ventricular tachycardia. The P waves are abnormal and frequently inverted in Lead I. They may be difficult to identify and although they may precede or follow the QRS complex they often coincide with it.

Ventricular Tachycardia. This type of tachycardia usually occurs in patients with myocardial disease and is a common and potentially dangerous feature immediately following cardiac infarction. Recurrent attacks may complicate ischaemic heart disease, cardiomyopathies, thyrotoxicosis and digitalis overdosage, and are more likely to occur in conditions with hypokalaemia.

They arise from an ectopic focus in the ventricles and may be preceded by ventricular extrasystoles. The ECG (Fig. 4.11) shows wide and abnormal QRS complexes at the rate of about 120–160 per minute. There is dissociation between the P waves and the QRS complexes.

Clinical Features. An attack of paroxysmal tachycardia starts suddenly. The patient may remember the moment when his heart began to beat rapidly. The tachycardia may be described as palpitations or as a

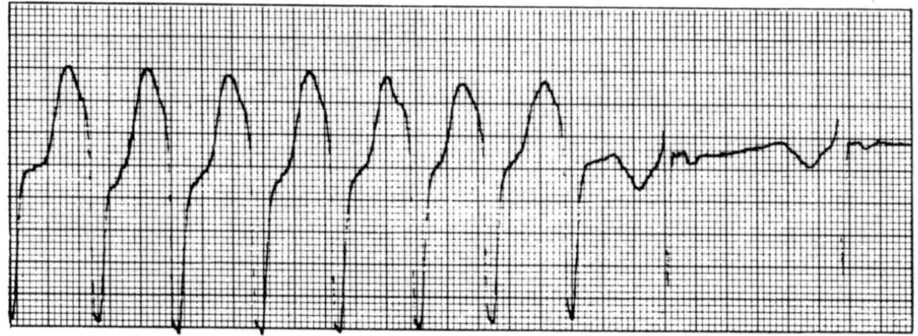

Fig. 4.11 Electrocardiogram showing the onset of ventricular tachycardia.

fluttering in the chest. It is always quite regular. Sometimes the attacks may start without warning and on other occasions they may be precipitated by a sudden movement or emotion. The attacks last any time from a few seconds to a day or two, then stop quite suddenly and normal rhythm is resumed; sometimes they are followed by extrasystoles. They may recur every few hours or only once or twice in a lifetime.

The degree of constitutional upset varies. Some patients are not disturbed by the attacks whereas others are anxious, feel faint or may complain of discomfort or even an anginal type of pain across the chest. Rarely patients may develop signs of heart failure during the attack, particularly if it lasts more than a day or so and more particularly if there is underlying heart disease.

Prognosis and Treatment. The prognosis in paroxysmal tachycardia, both of the acute attack and of subsequent events, depends on the presence or absence of underlying heart disease. If the heart is healthy the outlook is extremely good, though the paroxysms may cause a good deal of worry and distress.

In treating an attack of paroxysmal tachycardia it is important to know whether it arises from a supraventricular or from a ventricular focus. This is best determined by an electrocardiogram. Occasionally physical signs help. Rapid venous 'cannon waves' (p. 124) caused by the atria contracting against a closed atrioventricular valve, suggest a supraventricular tachycardia. Sudden slowing produced by carotid sinus stimulation suggest supraventricular origin.

Treatment

Supraventricular Tachycardia. The object is to terminate the attack by interrupting the circus movement when re-entry is the underlying mechanism or by suppressing the ectopic focus when present.

(1) *Carotid Sinus Massage.* Stimulation of a carotid sinus increases vagal tone and may thus break the re-entry circuit and stop the arrhythmia. It may also slow the ventricular rate in supraventricular arrhythmias by producing second-degree heart block and this manoeuvre is thus of some use in distinguishing between supraventricular and ventricular tachycardias.

(2) *Drugs.* If carotid sinus stimulation fails, then verapamil 5.0 mg given intravenously over five minutes is often successful. It slows conduction and thus interrupts the re-entry circuit. Verampamil may be repeated at five-minute intervals to a total of 15 mg. If this fails the following should be considered:

(a) When there is no hurry the patient can be given digitalis which may stop the attack.
(b) Amiodarone 5.0 mg/kg infused over 1–2 hours may be given.
(c) If it is felt that the heart is under undue strain as a result of the tachycardia, electrocardioversion should be used.

Remember the following contraindications:

(i) Verapamil should not be combined with a β blocker for although practolol can be used to treat a supraventricular tachycardia the combination has a powerful negative inotrophic effect.
(ii) Disopyramide can also be used but may rarely provoke a rapid ventricular rate.
(iii) Digoxin should not be used in tachycardias associated with the Wolff–Parkinson–White syndrome as it will facilitate conduction in the accessory bundle and may cause ventricular fibrillation.

To prevent a relapse digoxin and/or a β blocker is effective. If this fails amiodarone or disopyramide can be used.

Ventricular Tachycardia. The management of ventricular ectopic beats or tachycardia following myocardial infarction is considered on p. 214.

The drug of choice in treating an established attack is intravenous lignocaine. If this fails, or if the patient is seriously ill, the situation is best managed by DC cardioversion. As an ancillary measure the plasma potassium should be kept around 5.0 mmol/l and hypoxia (if present) should be corrected.

Drugs which are used to prevent recurrence include oral amiodarone and disopyramide. Medical treatment is, however, not always successful in preventing recurrence and a variety of surgical and electronic methods are being tried in resistant cases.

ATRIAL FLUTTER

Atrial flutter is less common. It is nearly always associated with heart disease, commonly rheumatic, hypertensive, or coronary disease. The mechanism of flutter is not entirely settled. Until recently it was thought to be due to a wave of contraction circling round the atria, but more recently it has been suggested that it is due to an excitable focus in the atria, discharging at a high rate, usually between 210–300/min. The ventricles are unable to respond at this rate so that there is usually some degree of partial atrioventricular block, the ventricles responding only to every second, third, or perhaps fourth atrial contraction (Fig. 4.12).

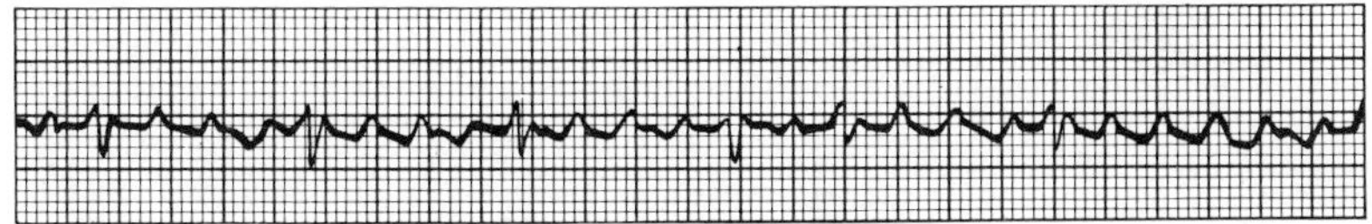

Fig. 4.12 Electrocardiogram showing atrial flutter with variable block.

Table 4.2 Drugs used to reduce cardiac excitability

Drug	*Action*	*Use*	*Administration*	*Half-life*	*Therapeutic blood levels*	*Contraindications*
Lignocaine	Suppresses ectopic foci	Ventricular arrhythmias	IV bolus 50–100 mg followed by infusion of 4.0 mg/min for 30 min and thereafter 2.0 mg/min. In presence of liver congestion or failure of circulation, metabolism slowed and infusion no more than 1.0 mg/min	2 h with normal metabolism	2–5 μg/ml	Heart block or idioventricular pacemaker
Mexiletine	Similar to lignocaine	Similar to lignocaine	IV bolus 150 mg infusion 250 mg over 1 h followed by 250 mg over 2 h followed by 0.5–1.0 mg/min. Reduce dose with liver or circulatory failure. Oral 400 mg followed after 2 h by 200 mg 8-hourly	16–18 h	0.6–2.5 μg/ml	As for lignocaine
Procainamide	Similar to lignocaine. Hypotension if given IV. SLE with prolonged use.	Prevention of ventricular arrhythmias	Oral 250 mg four times daily	2.0–3.5 h	4–8 μg/ml	
Phenytoin	Reduces excitability. Little effect on conduction	Ventricular and atrial arrhythmias	IV bolus 125 mg over 5 min. Orally 300 mg daily	10–40 h (blood level may require monitoring)	12–18 μg/ml	

Quinidine	Suppresses ectopic foci. Slows conduction	Preventing relapse of atrial arrhythmias.	Oral 200 mg four times daily	8 h	2.5–5.0 μg/ml	Conduction defects
Disopyramide	Similar to quinidine Very negatively inotrophic	Atrial arrhythmias	IV bolus 50–100 mg. IV infusion 0.4 mg/kg/h. Oral 100–150 mg four times daily	6 h. Longer with renal failure	2–4 μg/ml	Conduction defects or heart failure. Marked anticholinergic action
Verapamil	Interferes with action of Ca on myocardium. Slows conduction	Atrial arthythmias	IV 5.0 mg over 5 min. Oral 80 mg 6-hourly	5 h	—	Cardiac failure. Do not combine with β blockers
β blockers	Suppress ectopic foci. Slow conduction	Atrial arrhythmias	Practolol 5.0 mg IV over 5 min Atenolol 100 mg orally daily. 2.5 mg slowly IV repeated to a maximum of 10 mg	Practolol 8 h Atenolol 8 h	Practolol 10 μg/ml	Cardiac failure or obstructive airways disease
Amiodarone	Prolongs the refractory period	Atrial and ventricular arrthythmias	600 mg daily for 10 days then 200 mg daily orally	—	—	Care with β-blockers, digoxin, and Ca antagonists as can produce bradycardia. Also can cause corneal deposits which are reversible. Causes disorders of thyroid function

The *symptoms* of atrial flutter are variable. The patient may complain only of symptoms due to the underlying heart disease and the flutter may be found on examination. Sometimes there may be a complaint of palpitations of sudden onset. Examination may show little, especially when there is a considerable degree of heart block so that the ventricular rate is perhaps only 80/min. Sudden change in the degree of heart block resulting in doubling or halving of the pulse rate is characteristic of flutter. Halving of the pulse rate can sometimes be induced by pressing on one carotid sinus. In some patients, continuous variation in the degree of A-V block leads to complete irregularity of the pulse, which feels similar to that of atrial fibrillation. The rather unstable rhythm in atrial flutter may be troublesome to the patient and in most cases an effort should be made to induce a more stable rhythm.

The ECG (Fig. 4.12) shows the typical saw-tooth flutter (F) waves at about 300/min which are seen most clearly in leads II and VI. There is usually a 2:1 or 3:1 A-V block.

Prognosis and Treatment. The prognosis of flutter depends largely upon the underlying heart disease and is, therefore, variable. Flutter is treated by giving full doses of digitalis; this usually converts the flutter to atrial fibrillation. If the digitalis is then stopped about 40 % of patients will revert to sinus rhythm. The remainder will either continue to fibrillate or return to flutter. The decision whether to continue digitalis indefinitely or to try to restore sinus rhythm (see below) depends on the underlying heart disease.

ATRIAL FIBRILLATION

Atrial fibrillation is a common and important cardiac arrhythmia. Groups of muscle fibres in the atria contract independently at a rate between 400–500/min. These contractions can be seen as the 'F' waves in the electrocardiogram. The result of this disordered atrial activity is that there is no coordinated atrial contraction and the ventricles are stimulated in an irregular and often rapid fashion. This in turn throws a greater strain on the ventricular myocardium and may precipitate failure in an already damaged heart.

Atrial fibrillation is usually associated with heart disease, classically with mitral stenosis or thyrotoxicosis; it is, however, also quite common in coronary artery disease, in cardiomyopathy, in hypertension and it occasionally occurs in acute fevers. It may also be seen in constrictive pericarditis and carcinoma of the bronchus involving the myocardium. Sometimes it follows alcoholic excess or very heavy smoking and it is frequent after thoracotomy. Occasionally it occurs without any apparent cause. It may be paroxysmal or permanent. Atrial fibrillation is rare in aortic valve disease and in most forms of congenital heart disease.

Clinical Features. The onset of atrial fibrillation may pass unnoticed by the patient. More commonly he will complain of palpitations and may notice the irregularity of the pulse. Occasionally the onset is more dramatic, with fainting and collapse, and followed perhaps by acute cardiac failure. The *diagnosis* can be confirmed by feeling the pulse, which is characteristically completely irregular in force and rhythm. Exercise makes the arrhythmia more obvious (cf. extrasystoles p. 148). Further examination will usually show evidence of underlying heart disease.

Paroxysmal Atrial Fibrillation and Lone Atrial Fibrillation. Although atrial fibrillation is usually associated with heart disease, it is sometimes found when the heart is otherwise normal. These patients may either have paroxysms of atrial fibrillation or permanent fibrillation. Follow-up studies of these patients indicate that their prognosis is excellent, except for a number who develop the arrhythmia later in life and who may subsequently show evidence of underlying heart disease.

The ECG is characterised by complete irregularity of the QRS complexes and the disappearance of P waves with their replacement by small rapid fibrillation waves.

Treatment. The majority of patients with established atrial fibrillation have heart disease, perhaps with associated heart failure, and are best treated with digitalis. Occasionally the combination of a β blocker with digitalis will make control easier, but it must be used with care in patients with cardiac failure. Patients with mitral stenosis and atrial fibrillation should be anticoagulated to minimise the very real risk of systemic emboli. Patients with lone fibrillation and a slow ventricular rate often need no drug treatment.

In a small group of patients with atrial fibrillation an attempt should be made to restore sinus rhythm. This applies when there is no underlying heart disease, when thyrotoxicosis has been relieved and following a successful mitral valvotomy. Cardiac failure, any degree of cardiac enlargement or other evidence of severe heart disease are all contraindications. The presence of atrial fibrillation for more than a few months is said to increase the risk of embolism when sinus rhythm is restored.

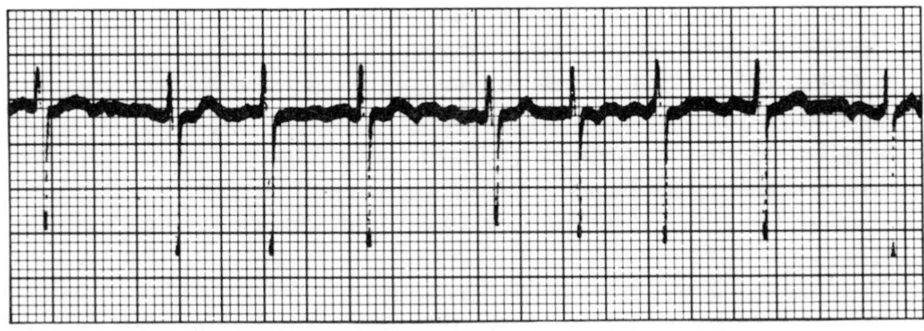

Fig. 4.13 Electrocardiogram showing atrial fibrillation.

The method of choice in restoring sinus rhythm is cardioversion by direct current shock. Drugs are now rarely used.

Electrical Cardioversion. This is a useful and safe way to restore sinus rhythm in supraventricular arrhythmias and in ventricular tachycardia. In the digitalised patient cardioversion may be delayed for 48 hours after the late dose, but if immediate cardioversion is deemed necessary, digitalisation is not a contraindication. Patients with mitral stenosis or a history of thromboemboli should first be anticoagulated to minimise the risk of systemic emboli.

Cardioversion is performed under short-duration anaesthesia and the shock is delivered synchronously with the down stroke of the R wave of the electrocardiogram. The initial shock should be 100 joules and if this fails it should be increased to 200 joules and if necessary to 400 joules. The shock depolarises the heart muscle and allows the sinu-atrial node to resume as the cardiac pacemaker.

Although cardioversion is successful in some 80% of patients with atrial fibrillation, about 60% of these relapse over the next year. Maintenance treatment with oral quinidine 200 mg four times daily or disopyramide 150 mg four times daily combined with digoxin may help but is not always effective.

HEART BLOCK

A block in the conducting system may occur either between the S-A node and the atrium (sinu-atrial block), or in the bundle of His, between the atria and the ventricles (atrioventricular block).

Sinu-atrial Disease

Sinus bradycardia is found in healthy athletes and as a complication of obstructive jaundice and raised intracranial pressure. It may also occur as a result of disease of the node itself and two syndromes can be recognised.

(a) *Sinus Arrest and Sinu-atrial Block*. This may be due to a progressive fibrosis of the node or may complicate cardiac infarction.

(b) *Bradycardia–Tachycardia Syndrome* (*Sick Sinus Syndrome*). In which bradycardia alternates with supraventricular tachycardia or atrial fibrillation.

Clinical Features. Attacks of dizziness or fainting occur with the bradycardia. The diagnosis may not be obvious as the ECG is often normal for much of the time, but 24-hour monitoring of the ECG is useful.

Treatment. When this disorder complicates cardiac infarction it can be relieved temporarily by atropine 0.3 mg IV. In chronic cases pacing will be required. The prognosis with pacing is good.

Partial Block

There are two degrees of partial heart block:

(a) Prolongation of the P-R interval (first-degree block).
(b) Dropped beats (second-degree block: partial block).

Interference with conduction may occur high in the conducting system in the region of the A-V node, in which case the His-bundle system is intact, or below the division of the bundle.

(1) *Prolongation of the P-R Interval.* The P-R interval exceeds 0.2 s. This is an electrocardiographic finding and produces no physical signs.

(2) *Dropped Beats.* There are two types of partial heart block with dropped beats:

(a) *Mobitz Type I.* The block is high in the conducting system. The P-R interval lengthens with successive cycles until a beat is dropped (*Wenckebach's periods*). With the next beat the P-R interval returns to normal and the process is repeated.
(b) *Mobitz Type II.* The block is below the division of the bundle of His. The P-R interval remains constant but there is a regular failure of A-V conduction with a dropped beat every second, third or more cycles.

Clinically, partial heart block can be diagnosed by noting regular dropped beats. It requires electrocardiographic confirmation. The elucidation of the underlying electrophysiology may also require electrocardiographic studies of the bundle of His.

Complete Heart Block

The atria and ventricles contract in complete dissociation, the stimulus to ventricular contraction arising in an ectopic focus which may be ventricular or nodal. If the ventricular pacemaker is high in the region of the A-V node the ventricular rate is about 50 beats per minute and the QRS complex is normal, indicating normal spread through the conducting system. If it arises low in the conducting system, it is usually slower (30–40 beats/minute) and the QRS complex is widened. The heart is usually slightly enlarged. The jugular pulse may show occasional 'cannon' waves when the atrium contracts against a closed tricuspid valve. With careful auscultation it is sometimes possible to hear the sound produced by the contracting atria and the first heart sound varies in intensity owing to the varying intervals between the atrial and ventricular contractions.

Causes of Heart Block. Heart block may be congenital (10% of cases), in which case it is usually high in the conducting system. It is most commonly due to a degeneration of the conducting system of unknown aetiology but which is related to age. It may complicate rheumatic fever, diphtheria and digitalis overdosage. Acute conduction defects may follow cardiac infarction (see p. 214).

Clinical Features. Disorders of conduction may produce a variety of symptoms, usually as a result of bradycardia or transient cardiac arrest. These include attacks of dizziness, fainting or fits. They are particularly liable to occur in elderly patients whose cerebral circulation may be impaired. When the diagnosis is in doubt, monitoring of the ECG for 24 hours may be very helpful.

Prognosis and Treatment. The prognosis of heart block depends upon the underlying causes. In congenital heart block the outlook is very good and it does not influence expectation of life. In patients developing A-V block with pre-existing heart disease the prognosis should be guarded. Patients with congenital heart block and those without symptoms in whom the block is high in the conducting system and the idioventricular rate is about 50 beats/minute do not usually require treatment. Those with a slower rate and particularly those with symptoms either due to transient asystole or to a low cardiac output due to bradycardia require pacing. Although treatment can be attempted with slow release isoprenaline (Saventrine) 30 mg 8-hourly, it is not often successful.

Stokes–Adams Attacks

These are attacks of unconsciousness from cerebral anoxia resulting from circulatory standstill. Fifty per cent are caused by cardiac arrest, 25% by ventricular tachycardia and 25% by ventricular fibrillation. All cause effective pumping by the heart to cease.

When due to cardiac arrest they are associated with acquired heart block, particularly when the rhythm is unstable and is fluctuating between partial and complete block; circulatory arrest is due to a delay in ventricular contraction when complete block develops suddenly. In the attack the patient falls suddenly to the ground, blue and pulseless and breathing increasingly deeply; if the asystole lasts more than a few seconds convulsions occur. With the commencement of the heart beat, the patient develops a characteristic flush and consciousness returns.

Attacks may occur with varying degrees of frequency and any one may prove fatal.

Treatment

The Acute Attack (*Circulatory Arrest*). The following treatment is used in patients with acute circulatory failure due to cardiac arrest or ventricular fibrillation. This may occur in patients with recurrent Stokes–Adams attacks, it is common in the period immediately after cardiac infarction, and occurs in those who are gravely ill from a variety of causes.

The immediate signs of ventricular asystole or ventricular fibrillation are:

(1) loss of consciousness;
(2) absent pulses, the carotid being the best artery to palpate;
(3) cessation of respiration;
(4) dilated pupils, which occur within thirty seconds.

Resuscitation must be started at once as irreversible damage to the cerebral cortex may occur in two minutes. The immediate treatment is aimed at maintaining circulation and ventilation.

(a) The patient must be laid supine on an unyielding surface and external cardiac massage applied by sharp compression of the lower end of the sternum about 60 times a minute.

(b) The airway must be cleared and the lungs inflated 10–12 times a minute. This can be done by either mouth-to-mouth respiration or better by an inflating bag (e.g. the Ambu bag) connected to air or oxygen.

(c) As soon as possible 100 ml of 8.4 % sodium bicarbonate should be given intravenously to reduce the rapidly developing acidosis, and repeated as required.

If at this time an ECG record is readily available, it is possible to decide whether circulatory arrest is due to asystole or to ventricular fibrillation, or whether normal rhythm has returned. But if further resuscitation is required it should not be delayed when no ECG is available. Electrodes are applied to the lower sternum and below the left axilla.

If the heart is in ventricular fibrillation DC defibrillation at 200 joules should be tried, if this fails a second attempt should be made at 400 joules as soon as possible. If the fibrillation continues after five shocks lignocaine 100 mg IV should be given and defibrillation repeated.

When the heart is in asystole, the shock may restart it, but if asystole persists ventricular fibrillation should be proved by giving 10 ml of 1:10 000 adrenaline and 10 ml of 10 % calcium chloride IV. Sinus rhythm may then be restored with the defibrillator. If spontaneous rhythm is unsatisfactory, pacing will be required. If normal rhythm has not returned after ten minutes of maintained circulation recovery is unlikely.

Preventative. Stokes–Adams attacks can sometimes be prevented by giving slow release isoprenaline (Saventrine) 30 mg 8-hourly by mouth.

Generally, however, the development of Stokes–Adams attacks is an absolute indication for a pacemaker, which is a much more reliable form of treatment.

The Pacemaker

A pacemaker is used to induce the cardiac cycle in various disorders of rhythm. Pacemaking may be *temporary* when the pulse generator is outside the body and the conducting wire is introduced via the subclavian vein or an arm vein and the tip is wedged into the apex of the right ventricle. The paced electrocardiogram should resemble a LBBB pattern. Temporary pacing is used for arrhythmias following myocardial infarction, for repeated Stokes–Adams attacks (permanent pacing will usually be required later), bradycardias and occasionally difficult tachycardias.

In *permanent* pacemaking the pulse generator is inserted subcutaneously and the electrode placed in the surface of the heart (epicardial). The main indication for permanent pacing is Stokes–Adams attacks and will include patients with sinu-atrial disease and second degree or complete A-V block. Occasionally cardiac function appears to be improved by pacing.

The pulse generator may produce a fixed rate pulse which is satisfactory provided the pacemaker stimulation does not coincide with the depolarisation period caused by spontaneous cardiac activity. If this is considered a risk, a demand pacemaker which is inhibited by spontaneous cardiac activity should be used. This is important when changes in conduction are likely to occur as after cardiac infarction or with varying block.

Bundle Branch Block

Until recently it was thought that the bundle of His divided into left and right branches which supplied the appropriate ventricles. It is now realised that the bundle divides into three branches, a left posterior division supplying the posterior part of the left ventricle, a left anterior division supplying the anterior and lateral aspects of the left ventricle and a right division. Each of these divisions can be damaged separately by disease processes.

Bundle branch block may occur acutely following cardiac infarction, it may be due to progressive disease of the conducting system of unknown aetiology and it is found with atrial septal defect. Right bundle branch block may also occur in normal hearts.

Clinical Features. Bundle branch block by itself produces no symptoms. Examination will show evidence of underlying heart disease if present and in addition, right bundle branch block causes a wide and fixed splitting of the second heart sound in the pulmonary area. Bundle branch block can only be diagnosed with certainty by an ECG.

Prognosis and Treatment. The prognosis depends on the underlying heart disease, often no treatment is required. The importance of recognising that the conducting system is trifascicular is that the ECG may show changes which suggest progressive damage to the system and give warning that complete block with its attendant risk of cardiac asystole is imminent. This is particularly important following cardiac infarction as asystole may be avoided by using a pacemaker.

The changes in the ECG which should be noted are:

(1) Right bundle branch block causes widening of the S wave in lead 1 and in the left ventricular surface leads and a wide R wave in lead 3.

(2) Complete left bundle branch block causes widening of the R wave in lead 1, a VL and over the left ventricle and a wide S wave in lead 3.
(3) Block of the anterior division of the left bundle leads to the development of left axis deviation of more than $-60°$.
(4) Block of the posterior division of the left bundle leads to the development of right axis deviation of more than $+120°$.

The combination of right bundle branch block with either anterior or posterior left bundle branch block following cardiac infarction is usually considered to be an indication for pacing although the prognosis is poor whatever is done.

Isolated left or right bundle branch blocks do not usually require pacing unless for associated reasons.

The Wolff–Parkinson–White Syndrome

This congenital disorder is due to an accessory pathway which connects atria to ventricles and bypasses the A-V node. The main features of the syndrome are an abnormal ECG and a tendency to atrial arrhythmias. The ECG shows a short P-R interval (less than 0.12s) and a broad QRS complex.

The arrhythmias are of three types:

(a) A supraventricular tachycardia due to re-entry via the accessory pathway.
(b) Attacks of atrial fibrillation which can be dangerous because conduction down the accessory pathway is not limited as in the bundle of His and very rapid ventricular rates may result. There is an increased incidence of sudden death in the WPW syndrome.
(c) Occasionally there are disorders of the function of the sinu-atrial node.

Treatment consists largely of managing arrhythmias as they arise. Supraventricular tachycardias, as long as the rate is not too high, respond to intravenous verapamil (see above). In atrial fibrillation however, the rate may be very high and it is better to block the accessory pathway which is responsible. This is achieved by electrical cardioversion or by giving disopyramide infused at the rate of 0.4 mg/kg/h.

Digoxin should not be used in treating supraventricular tachycardias associated with the WPW syndrome as it facilitates conduction in the accessory bundle and may provoke ventricular fibrillation.

HYPERTENSION

It is impossible to define normal blood pressure, for the term in this sense is without meaning. The average blood pressure for a group of apparently healthy people can be found and this average increases with age, being about 120/80 at the age of 20 and rising to about 160/90 at 60.

It has also been found that the higher the blood pressure is in youth, the greater is the rise with increasing age.

It can be seen therefore that within a group of apparently healthy people there is a wide range of blood pressures. For the purpose of life insurance and similar medical examinations 150/90 is usually taken as the upper limit of normal pressure.

Blood pressure also fluctuates throughout the day, being highest in the morning on waking and falling during sleep. In normal subjects the diurnal variation is about 30 mmHg systolic and 10 mmHg diastolic. Blood pressure is also raised by emotion, exercise and cold.

Patients whose blood pressure undergoes big swings so that sometimes it is 'normal' and sometimes raised may be said to have *labile hypertension*. It is usually assumed that sooner or later such patients will develop sustained hypertension although there is not much evidence that this actually occurs.

In terms of general management, it is best to assume that a proportion of subjects with labile hypertension will ultimately develop sustained hypertension, and their blood pressure should be checked at intervals, perhaps annually.

Causes of Hypertension. When a blood pressure which is above the usual level for the patient's age group is discovered the possible causes should be considered. They are the following:

(1) Essential hypertension (95 %).
(2) Hypertension associated with renal disease (4 %).
(3) Rare causes:
    (a) Hypertension associated with endocrine disease, i.e.:
        (i) Cushing's syndrome.
        (ii) Phaeochromocytoma.
        (iii) Primary Aldosteronism. (Conn's syndrome)
    (b) Coarctation of the aorta.
(4) A small proportion of women taking the contraceptive pill develop hypertension which is reversible when the pill is stopped although it may take six months or longer to return to normal.
(5) Toxaemia of pregnancy.
(6) Long-term treatment with steroids and chronic alcoholism can cause raised blood pressure.
(7) Elevation of plasma calcium is associated with a raised blood pressure and there is a high incidence of hypertension in hyperparathyroidism. The reason for this is not known.

Investigation of Hypertension. The discovery of a raised blood pressure calls for a careful case history which may give a clue to the cause, and a full clinical examination. Particular attention should be paid to the cardiovascular system, including the femoral pulses, the retinae and to examination of the urine. It is important to know whether the rise in blood pressure is a permanent feature or merely the result of anxiety due to visiting the doctor. If the blood pressure is found to be raised the reading should be repeated after five minutes' rest and if still elevated two further readings should be obtained on separate occasions. Hypertensive patients should have the following investigations:

(a) chest X-ray;
(b) electrocardiogram;
(c) blood urea or creatinine;
(d) serum electrolytes;
(e) plasma lipids.

More extensive investigations including pyelography, estimation of urinary VMA and other tests of endocrine function are needed only in the young hypertensive who has no family history or when there is a clinical suspicion of some underlying cause for the hypertension.

These tests should answer the two important questions which should be asked when hypertension is discovered:

(1) Is the diagnosis essential hypertension or is there some underlying cause?
(2) Is the raised blood pressure damaging the target organs, i.e. the heart, the vascular system or the kidneys?

ESSENTIAL HYPERTENSION

The cause of essential hypertension is unknown. There is at present a widespread opinion that patients with essential hypertension merely represent the extreme uppermost limit of normal variation in blood pressure in the population. There is little doubt that heredity plays a part and it is common to find evidence of hypertension in the patient's father or mother. Other factors which have been implicated are stress, salt intake, some derangement of sodium transport and sympathetic overactivity but evidence is incomplete. It is however clear that the immediate physiological abnormality is a raised peripheral resistance.

Clinical Features. The blood pressure may remain raised for many years without producing any symptoms or signs; in fact if a blood pressure of over 150/90 is considered abnormal, quite a large proportion of the older people of this country have essential hypertension which in the majority of cases causes them no harm for many years. Many such subjects die in old age of some other complaint.

The symptoms and signs of hypertension are really due to the effects of the raised blood pressure on the cardiovascular system and more rarely on the kidney. These complications are particularly liable to occur when the pressure is high and when hypertension develops at a relatively early age; they are more common in men than in women. Other risk factors are smoking and hyperlipidaemia. *It must be emphasised that many patients with mild or moderate hypertension show no abnormal physical signs except for the raised blood pressure.* The signs detailed below are evidence that the target organs have suffered damage.

(1) *The Heart.* The heart is the organ most frequently affected by hypertension. The left ventricle must work against an increased resistance and may in time fail. The *symptoms* are those of left ventricular failure: dyspnoea on effort and paroxysmal dyspnoea at night. *Examination* in a fully developed case shows a full pulse with some thickening of the wall of the radial artery. The heart is enlarged and the apex beat is of the left ventricular type. In some patients there is a triple rhythm with a presystolic (atrial) extra sound best heard at the apex. Although the triple rhythm is common in the more severe hypertensives, it does not necessarily imply a failing left ventricle and is not of great prognostic significance. The aortic component of the second sound is loud. A systolic murmur either at the apex or base is quite common; it is usually due to flow through the aortic valve and only rarely to aortic stenosis or a functional mitral incompetence. Eventually the left ventricular failure may progress to congestive failure with raised venous pressure and peripheral oedema.

(2) *The Blood Vessels.* The increased pressure within the blood vessels leads to thickening of the walls of the medium-sized arteries and this change may be palpable in the radial artery at the wrist. Hypertension also predisposes to atheroma with an increased incidence of coronary artery disease. High pressures lead to fibrinoid necrosis of arterioles which further raises peripheral resistance and in the kidney may lead to renal failure (see below).

Hypertensive Retinopathy. The arteries of the retina may show a series of changes which have been subdivided:

Grade I	Narrowing and increased tortuosity of the retinal arteries.
Grade II	Arterial changes more marked and nipping of the veins at the arteriovenous crossing due to the thickened arterial wall pressing on the vein.
Grade III	Grades I and II with the addition of haemorrhage and/or exudates.
Grade IV	Previous grades with papilloedema.

Cerebral Arteries. The cerebral arteries are affected in hypertension. Microaneurysms will develop which may ultimately rupture, causing cerebral haemorrhage. Headaches are no more common in hypertensives than in the normotensive population, but with severe hypertension morning headaches may be a problem. In severe hypertension attacks of cerebral oedema occur, producing the clinical syndrome of *hypertensive encephalopathy* with blinding headaches, fits, unconsciousness, and transient palsies.

(3) *The Kidney*. In the majority of patients with essential hypertension there is no evidence of serious interference with renal function and death from renal failure is rare. In the more severe cases the urine may contain a little protein and patients with impaired renal function frequently show some microscopic haematuria. In malignant hypertension (see below) there are marked changes in the blood vessels of the kidney, particularly fibrinoid necrosis of the afferent artery to the glomerulus, and in these cases there is a progressive decrease in renal function and death may occur from renal failure.

Malignant Hypertension (Accelerated Hypertension)

Malignant hypertension, which is relatively uncommon, may be regarded as the most severe grade of essential hypertension, although this view is not universally accepted. It is characterised by a high diastolic pressure (usually over 140 mmHg), by marked arterial changes in the retina with papilloedema, and by progressive renal failure. It arises most commonly in men of early middle age.

Renin and Hypertension

Renin is released from the juxtaglomerular apparatus of the kidney. It acts on a circulating a_2 globulin to release *angiotensin I*, which is subsequently converted to *angiotension II* in the lungs. This substance has two actions which raise the blood pressure.

(a) vasoconstriction;
(b) stimulates release of *aldosterone* by the adrenal cortex, which in turn causes sodium retention by the kidney and thus increased circulatory volume.

In essential hypertension the patients can be divided into low plasma renin (30 %), intermediate plasma renin (60 %) and high plasma renin (10 %) groups. The renin levels in essential hypertension are unrelated to total exchangeable body sodium or potassium and the clinical significance of these groups has not been resolved.

Drugs may alter the renin levels, and in particular diuretics increase levels and β blockers reduce them; however, these changes do not appear to be related to the patient's therapeutic response.

In *primary hyperaldosteronism (Conn's syndrome)* due to an adrenal adenoma, there are high plasma levels of aldosterone with low levels of renin caused by feedback suppression, the total body exchangeable sodium is increased and potassium decreased. In *secondary hyperaldosteronism*, which complicates accelerated hypertension and renal disease, plasma renin and plasma aldosterone levels are both raised.

Prognosis of Hypertension

The results of many studies now show that any elevation of blood pressure carries increased risks in terms of both morbidity and mortality. It is important to assess the prognosis as accurately as possible for this will largely determine the management of the patient.

Generally speaking the factors which influence prognosis are:

(1) Sex of the patient—women have a better prognosis than men.
(2) The height of the blood pressure. Both the systolic and diastolic pressures are important. A diastolic pressure of over 130 mmHg carries a bad prognosis.
(3) The degree of arterial change (particularly the retinal changes).
(4) The degree of hypertrophy of the left ventricle.
(5) Evidence of renal involvement.
(6) Plasma lipid levels.

It would seem that the majority of patients with mild or moderate essential hypertension, particularly middle-aged or elderly women, will live for 10 or 20 years or more, but even those with diastolic pressures of 100 will on an average have their life expectancy reduced by a few years. In those with high pressure and evidence of marked arterial or cardiac change the prognosis is considerably worse. Most patients with untreated malignant hypertension are dead within one year.

Treatment

General Measures. Most patients with hypertension require some *reassurance*. Their mode and tempo of life may require modification, but they should lead as normal a life as possible. There is no evidence that *diet* plays any part in the genesis of hypertension, but if the patient is overweight this should be corrected as loss of weight may cause some fall in blood pressure.

Because of the high incidence of coronary disease in these patients it is important to treat any associated hyperlipidaemia (p. 549) and the patient should stop smoking.

Sedation should be used in those patients who are unduly anxious. Diazepam 2.0 mg three times daily is usually satisfactory.

Drug Treatment. It is now widely accepted that in severe hypertension treatment will reduce morbidity and mortality. The incidence of strokes and heart failure is diminished. Until recently lowering blood pressure did not appear to influence the risk of cardiac infarction but the use of β blockers may achieve this effect. There is as yet no drug which is entirely satisfactory and free from side-effects. Drug treatment is therefore usually confined to those with a blood pressure of over 170/100, although many experts would also treat the milder grades of hypertension, particularly in younger male patients. In patients over 65 there is no evidence as yet available that lower blood pressure improves prognosis and side-effects from treatment can be troublesome. In the present state of knowledge therefore, it seems best to treat only older patients whose hypertension is either severe (diastolic > 115 mmHg) or is causing target organ damage. If the blood urea is over 15 mmol/l due to renal damage, lowering of the blood pressure may well precipitate acute renal failure.

The drugs available are:

(1) *β Blockers* (Table 4.3). β blockers reduce the cardiac output and lower blood pressure. The fall is not postural but may be associated with a decrease in peripheral blood flow. They will also exacerbate cardiac failure and bronchospasm. They can be divided into β_1 blockers (selective) which affect mainly the heart and $\beta_1 + \beta_2$ blockers (non-selective) which also affect the bronchi and arterioles. For lowering the blood pressure there is nothing to choose between these two groups but for patients with obstructive airways disease a selective blocker is to be preferred. β blockers should be avoided in asthmatic patients.

Table 4.3 β blockers

		Initial Dose
Non-selective	Propranolol (long acting)	160 mg daily
	Oxprenolol (slow release)	160 mg daily
	Sotalol	80 mg b.d.
Selective	Metoprolol	100 mg b.d.
	Atenolol	50 mg daily

The dose is increased gradually until a satisfactory control of blood pressure is obtained.

Labetalol is both an α and β blocker although its α effect is not marked. It may be useful in patients who are resistant to simple β blockade. The initial dose is 100 mg three times daily and this may be increased.

(2) *Centrally Acting Group*. *Methyldopa* lowers blood pressure by a central action. The initial dose is 250 mg three times daily. The full effect is not seen for about five days, so dosage is increased gradually until control is satisfactory. The usual dose is 1.0–1.5 g daily. Symptoms from postural hypotension are not common. Some patients complain of drowsiness early in treatment, also dry mouth and occasionally pyrexia. Water retention may occur but responds to diuretics.

Clonidine lowers blood pressure mainly by a central action. The initial dose is 50 μg three times daily and this is increased as required. It may cause depression in susceptible patients. *It should not be stopped suddenly as this may cause a dangerous rebound hypertension.*

(3) *Vasodilators*

(a) *Hydralazine* has a direct effect on the arteriole. It causes tachycardia and is therefore best combined with a β blocker. The initial dose is 25 mg b.d. High doses may lead to an SLE-like syndrome. It can also be used intravenously in a hypertensive crisis in a dose of 20 mg.

(b) *Prazosin* is probably an α blocker. The initial dose is 0.5 mg three times daily. The initial dose may cause collapse due to a sudden fall in blood pressure and the patient should be warned of this side-effect.

(c) *Minoxidil* is a powerful vasodilator which is used in resistant hypertension. The initial dose is 5.0 mg daily. Side-effects include salt and water retention (combine with a diuretic), hypertrichosis and, rarely, a pericardial effusion.

(d) *Captopril.* This drug inhibits angiotensin-converting enzymes and thus prevents the formation of angiotensin II. It can be used alone but if not effective it should be combined with a diuretic. The initial dose is 12.5 mg t.d.s. which can be increased to a maximum of 50 mg t.d.s. If this fails a thiazide diuretic should be added to the regime. Side-effects include proteinuria, myelosuppression and a metallic taste in the mouth.

(e) *Calcium Antagonists.* Nifedipine, by blocking calcium transport into the cells, interferes with muscle contraction in the arterial wall and acts as a vasodilator. The usual initial dose is 20 mg of the slow release preparation b.d. Side-effects include ankle oedema and, rarely, gastric disturbances and headaches.

(f) *Diazoxide* and *Sodium Nitroprusside* are given intravenously in treating a hypertensive crisis (see p. 171).

(4) *Diuretics.* The benzothiazide group (p. 146) is effective. Their mode of action is not clear. They produce a transient fall in blood volume but their hypotensive effect seems to depend on other factors. They are very effective when combined with hypotensive drugs, particularly captopril or β blockers, both of which may cause salt and water retention. Satisfactory diuretics are:

Bendrofluazide 2.5–5.0 mg daily;

Chlorthalidone 50 mg daily or on alternate days.

Frusemide is generally less effective than thiazides but is sometimes useful in patients with impaired renal function. Potassium supplements are not normally required provided the patient is on a full mixed diet.

Use of Hypotensive Drugs. Opinions differ as to the relative efficacy of these drugs in hypertension. In mild hypertension a β blocker alone is effective in about 50% of patients. If this fails to control the blood pressure a diuretic may be combined with a β blocker. In severe or resistant cases the combination of a β blocker, a diuretic and either hydralazine or prazosin is usually effective. The exact role of calcium antagonists and captopril is still being determined. The elderly present a special problem and side-effects are more common. A thiazide diuretic with or without a β blocker is probably best but there is a risk of developing diabetes or gout with long-term treatment with thiazides, and the problem of worsening cardiac failure and poor peripheral circulation with β blockers.

The more severe hypertensives will require admission to hospital for treatment, so that the blood pressure can be measured frequently while it is being brought under control. Mild hypertensives can usually be treated as outpatients.

In severe hypertension a reduction of blood pressure to about 160/100 is satisfactory, but in mild cases the aim should be to reduce it to 140/90 or lower. In *asthmatics* β blockers should be avoided and the most suitable drugs are thiazides, vasodilators and methyldopa. In *diabetics* selective β blockers can be used but the patient must be warned that the symptoms which usually accompany hypoglycaemia are suppressed.

Hypertension in Pregnancy. Pregnancy may exacerbate pre-existing hypertension or may induce it. At levels above 160/100 there is a risk of developing eclampsia. Blood pressure should therefore be carefully controlled. Methyldopa is usually used. Although there are theoretical reasons for avoiding β blockers, evidence is accumulating that they are effective and safe. Thiazides should be avoided. In addition to drugs rest is an important aspect of treatment.

Hypertensive Crisis and Hypertensive Encephalopathy

This usually occurs when there is a rapid rise in blood pressure. It is most common in malignant hypertension, acute nephritis and eclampsia. Symptoms are headaches, nausea, vomiting, clouding of consciousness and occasionally fits. The diastolic blood pressure is usually very high.

It is important to lower the blood pressure smoothly and not too rapidly as there is a risk of cerebral thrombosis and ischaemia. A number of drugs is available:

(a) Sodium nitroprusside 0.5–8 μg/kg/min by IV infusion, adjusted to keep the diastolic pressure about 100 mmHg.
(b) Hydralazine 20 mg slowly IV.
(c) Labetalol 50 mg slowly IV (not in cardiac failure or asthmatics).
(d) Nifedipine. A 10 mg capsule can be cut and the contents squeezed into the mouth. Absorption is rapid producing a fall in blood pressure within 20 minutes.

Thereafter the hypertension should be treated in the usual way.

RHEUMATIC HEART DISEASE

ACUTE RHEUMATIC FEVER

Acute rheumatic fever is a disease affecting connective tissue, particularly that of the heart and its valves and the joints.

Aetiology. It is a disease of childhood and adolescence, about 90 % of cases occurring between the ages of 8 and 15. It is common in temperate climates, as for example in the British Isles, and it affects the poorer classes, its incidence probably being increased by bad housing and overcrowding. The exact cause of the disease is unknown, but in many patients it follows about two or three weeks after a sore throat due to infection with haemolytic streptococcus (Lancefield Group A). It is possible that other organisms or viruses may play a part. There has been a sharp decline in the incidence of the disease in this country in the last 50 years, possibly related to an improvement in social conditions.

It seems probable that the heart and other organs and the streptococcus share a common antigen so that the antibody provoked by a streptococcal infection will have widespread effects.

Clinical Features. The attack of rheumatic fever nearly always follows seven to twenty days after a streptococcal throat infection. Typically but not invariably, the illness starts suddenly with fever, pain, stiffness, and sometimes swelling in one or more of the larger joints, namely the elbow, wrist, shoulder, hip, knee, or ankle. After a day or two the pain leaves the joint first affected and appears in another one; this *flitting from joint to joint* is unusual in other forms of arthritis and is a useful pointer to the diagnosis. Small joints are rarely affected. Skin rashes are sometimes seen in rheumatic fever; the most typical is *erythema marginatum* which consists of red rings of irregular size and shape which have slightly raised edges and normal centres. They tend to coalesce, and come and go rather quickly. In parts of the body where bones lie immediately under the skin, particularly shins, forearm, elbows, wrists, ankles, and scalp—*rheumatic nodules* may be felt. They are not tender, usually about the size of a pea and are not attached to the overlying skin.

In some children the rheumatic process takes a much milder and more insidious form which can easily be overlooked, though it is as likely as the more obvious type of rheumatic fever to be associated with active heart disease. Thus about half the patients who are later found to be suffering from chronic rheumatic heart disease give no history of rheumatic fever or chorea.

Evidence of Cardiac Involvement. The rheumatic process affects the endocardium, myocardium and the pericardium. In the endocardium the changes are mainly confined to the valves and consist of inflammation with deposition of fibrin and platelets along the margin of the valves. The myocardium shows the characteristic Aschoff bodies and the pericardium may be involved in a non-specific inflammatory process sometimes with an effusion. The following findings may be taken as evidence of cardiac involvement:

(1) *Tachycardia.* Patients with active rheumatic carditis nearly always have a raised sleeping pulse rate and awaking pulse dis-

proportionate to the degree of fever; that is more than 20 beats per minute rise per degree (C) of fever.

(2) *The Development of Cardiac Murmurs.* There are two types of cardiac murmur which indicate active rheumatic carditis. The *Carey Coombs murmur*, a short mid-diastolic murmur heard at the apex is the earliest indication of involvement of the mitral valve. When the rheumatic process resolves this murmur may disappear or if the valve is sufficiently damaged it may develop the typical presystolic accentuation of mitral stenosis. The typical rumbling murmur of mitral stenosis results from scarring of the valve, and takes two years at least to appear. The Carey Coombs murmur may be associated with a *pansystolic murmur* at the apex indicating mitral regurgitation.

Similarly the *soft early diastolic murmur* heard best down the left or right border of the sternum is typical of aortic incompetence and implies involvement of the aortic valve.

Isolated apical systolic murmurs are difficult to interpret in rheumatic fever because they are common in healthy children, but generally it can be said that the louder, rougher and more prolonged the murmur the more likely it is to indicate active carditis. It must however be emphasised that both systolic and mitral diastolic murmurs may disappear when healing of the rheumatic process occurs. The aortic diastolic murmur nearly always persists.

(3) *Cardiac Enlargement.* The development of cardiac enlargement indicates active carditis. It may be due to dilatation of the heart or to the presence of a pericardial effusion, or both.

(4) *Pericarditis.* The finding of a pericardial friction rub indicates active heart involvement.

(5) *Heart Failure.* The appearance of heart failure in acute rheumatic fever indicates a severe myocarditis. Rheumatic myocarditis may also be responsible for patients with established heart disease developing heart failure.

Laboratory Investigations. The blood shows a moderate leucocytosis with some anaemia and the ESR is almost invariably raised. The antistreptolysin titre in the blood is usually elevated. A figure above 200 Todd units is considered significant, though it must be realised that this merely indicates a recent streptococcal infection and is not diagnostic of rheumatic fever. The electrocardiogram shows no specific abnormality, but there may be various conduction defects.

Treatment. The seriousness of this disease lies in the risk of carditis occurring at some time in the illness and resulting in chronic rheumatic heart disease.

The most important principle in the treatment is *rest.* The patient should be semirecumbent on a firm mattress with two or three pillows. Sweating may be profuse. If the joints are very painful they may be supported by pillows and the pressure of bedclothes relieved by a cradle.

The specific drugs in the relief of rheumatic fever are the *salicylates* and high dosage is essential. Soluble aspirin should be given 4-hourly, the initial dose being 140 mg/kg body weight (max 10 g) daily for two days and thereafter 70 mg/kg body weight daily. (The daily dose should not exceed 5.0 g.) If side-effects such as tinnitus, nausea and vomiting are troublesome the dose should be reduced. If possible the blood salicylate level should be kept at 300–350 mg/l. With this treatment the fever and joint pains should be relieved in two to three days.

Prednisolone 40 mg daily is useful in the severely ill patient who is not responding to salicylates.

Although it is unlikely that salicylates alter the extent or severity of the valve damage, they do relieve the symptoms.

A course of *penicillin* should be given to eradicate any residual streptococcal infection, but it does not alter the course of an acute attack. It should also be used to prevent further streptococcal infections (see below).

Duration of Treatment. Complete rest must be enforced until all evidence of active disease has gone, which means the disappearance of all signs of infection and the return of the ESR to normal. It must be remembered that high blood salicylate levels cause acceleration of the ESR; conversely it is reduced if heart failure appears. Consequently the ESR must be interpreted in the light of the whole clinical picture. It rarely requires less than six weeks to return to normal and patients may have to be confined to bed for many months. Thereafter a graduated return is made to normal activity, a careful watch being kept for recrudescence of acute rheumatism.

After Care. On return to normal life the child should not be fussed over, but exposure to cold and dampness should be avoided as much as possible. Because of the danger of further damage to the heart from relapses, streptococcal throat infections should be prevented by giving sulphadimidine 0.5 g daily or phenoxymethylpenicillin 250 mg twice daily or benzathene penicillin 1.2 mega units monthly if compliance is poor. Prophylaxis should be continued until the age of 18 in childhood rheumatic fever or for five years if the disease starts after the age of 13. With prophylactic treatment it is possible to cut the relapse rate to around 4%.

Prognosis. Approximately half the children with acute rheumatic fever will have valve involvement and of these about half will be left with permanent valve damage. About 70% of those with a diastolic murmur will develop permanent valve damage but the prognosis with a systolic murmur is considerably better. The older the child at the time of the acute attack the less likely are the valves to be permanently affected. The incidence of permanent valve damage increases with increasing evidence of carditis and is more common after recurrent attacks.

RHEUMATIC CHOREA (Sydenham's Chorea)

Chorea may be considered as a manifestation of the rheumatic process in which the brain is affected. About 20% of patients with chorea develop chronic rheumatic heart disease identical with that found after rheumatic fever. In a certain number of cases there may also be other manifestations of the rheumatic process. Chorea commonly occurs in childhood and adolescence, but a particularly severe though rare type of chorea is associated with pregnancy. It is commoner in girls.

Clinical Features. The child developing chorea is first noticed to be very restless and fidgety and some time may elapse before it is appreciated that her jerkiness and clumsiness indicate illness rather than original sin. All four limbs are usually affected though occasionally the disorder may be confined to one arm or leg or one side of the body (*hemichorea*). When the disease is at its height the *involuntary movements* are the most prominent feature. The child is constantly grimacing and making sudden, jerky, and ever varying movements of the limbs; these movements cease in sleep. In doubtful cases it is a useful test to ask the child to grasp one's hand, as she is unable to maintain a steady pressure and the intensity of her grip will be found to be always waxing and waning. The *muscles are weak* and have a *poor tone*, so that the joints can be moved through an abnormally wide range, and typically the outstretched hands are held with the wrists slightly flexed and the fingers hyperextended at the metacarpophalangeal joints. These movements must be differentiated from nervous tics, the most important point being that unlike tics they are not purposive and never repetitive. *Emotional changes* are common, consisting of depression, weeping, uncontrolled laughter, and hysteria. Examination of the cardiovascular system may show evidence of cardiac involvement similar to that described under rheumatic fever. The ESR is usually normal unless the heart is involved.

The average *duration* of the disease is about two months, though occasionally chorea may last up to six months or longer. After apparent full recovery odd choreiform movements may persist and be particularly noticeable when the child is under stress. These movements are often considered hysterical, but recently it has been suggested that they represent residual brain damage.

Treatment. *Rest* is the most important part of the treatment of this disease, in order to prevent or limit permanent heart damage. To achieve complete rest in this type of patient is not easy. Some children are happier in a single room, others prefer the company of a general ward. The cot or bed should have sides to prevent the child falling out and there should be padding to prevent injury. One or two pillows are satisfactory and great care should be taken of the child's skin and cleanliness. Feeding may be difficult and great patience will be required by the nurse or mother.

There is no specific treatment for chorea. Soluble aspirin 300 mg t.d.s.

together with diazepam 0.8 mg/kg/day in divided doses or haloperidol 0.05 mg/kg/day in two or three divided doses can be used to control restlessness.

Following an attack of chorea prolonged convalescence is required with efforts to improve general health as far as possible. About one-third of patients with chorea will have a further attack. *Prophylaxis* similar to that for rheumatic fever is recommended.

CHRONIC RHEUMATIC HEART DISEASE

Following acute rheumatic fever, the heart may return to normal; but in about half the patients the valves are so severely damaged that ultimately they will become deformed and scarred and will be unable to function properly.

The incidence of involvement of the various valves is approximately:

mitral valve	80 % of cases
aortic valve	45 % of cases
tricuspid valve	10 % of cases
pulmonary valve	1 % of cases
mitral valve alone	50 % of cases
mitral and aortic valves together	20 % of cases

The natural history of the condition starts with the acute rheumatism, usually between the ages of 8 and 15. There may have been one or several attacks. There is then usually an asymptomatic period of 15–20 years until the patient begins to notice dyspnoea.

By about the age of 30 many patients have had their first attack of congestive cardiac failure, which is often precipitated by the onset of atrial fibrillation or perhaps some extra strain such as ill-advised pregnancy. The attacks of cardiac failure become less and less amenable to treatment and death usually occurs in the mid-thirties. It must be realised that the foregoing account is merely an average course of events. In some patients the course is even shorter, whereas others may live to middle or even old age without developing any symptoms from their heart lesion.

ACQUIRED LESIONS OF THE HEART VALVES

MITRAL STENOSIS

Mitral stenosis is the commonest valve lesion and is nearly always due to previous rheumatic infection, although only about half the patients give a clear history of rheumatic fever. It is possible that a few cases may follow a viral endocarditis and it is rarely due to congenital fusion of the valve commissures. It occurs more commonly in women than in men. It is probable that at the time of the acute rheumatic infection the mitral valves fuse at the point of insertion of the chordae tendineae. At first there may be little interference with the flow of blood from the left atrium to the left ventricle, but subsequently there is gradual contraction and narrowing of the mitral orifice and if the orifice is reduced below a size of about 1.0 cm^2 the passage of blood into the left ventricle is seriously obstructed. In addition there may be fibrosis and calcification of the valve cusps and thickening and shortening of the chordae.

There is thus a rise in pressure in the left atrium, which is transmitted back to the pulmonary veins, the pulmonary capillaries, and finally the pulmonary arteries, leading to pulmonary congestion. This passive rise in pressure is not very great, the pulmonary artery pressure being usually about 40 mmHg, but it would be sufficient to force fluid from the pulmonary capillaries into the alveoli and thus produce pulmonary oedema. This is prevented in two ways:

(1) There is a certain amount of thickening of the alveolar walls which becomes less susceptible to oedema.
(2) In about 20% of patients there is active vasoconstriction of the smaller branches of the pulmonary artery which 'protects' the pulmonary capillaries from the pressure developed by the right ventricle. The active pulmonary vasoconstriction, although lowering capillary pressure, causes a considerable rise in pulmonary artery pressure which is often about 80/40 mmHg.

Sometimes these protective mechanisms fail. This is liable to occur in the early stages of the disease when alveolar thickening has not developed and when the pulmonary artery vasoconstriction suddenly relaxes. Such patients develop attacks of *acute pulmonary oedema* which are always serious and may be fatal. In the majority of patients, however, the passive pulmonary congestion runs parallel with alveolar thickening. Such patients do not develop active pulmonary vasoconstriction or have attacks of pulmonary oedema. The *pulmonary congestion* does, however, lead to increased 'stiffness' of the lungs which plays a large part in causing dyspnoea which is a leading symptom of mitral stenosis. The changes in the walls of the alveoli also reduce oxygen uptake.

Finally the right ventricle fails and the fully developed picture of congestive cardiac failure emerges.

Clinical Features. *Dyspnoea* is the commonest presenting symptom of mitral stenosis and usually develops 10–20 years after the acute attack of rheumatic fever. It may be of two types:

(1) *Dyspnoea on effort* which becomes progressively more severe and is sooner or later accompanied by *orthopnoea*. This dyspnoea is due to increasing pulmonary congestion.
(2) A small proportion of patients with mitral stenosis present with attacks of *pulmonary oedema* similar symptomatically to those

found in acute left ventricular failure. The mechanism of the oedema is considered above. These attacks frequently follow some undue excitement such as a dance or other unusual exertion; they may also be precipitated by pregnancy or by the onset of atrial fibrillation.

Pulmonary congestion is also responsible for two other symptoms of mitral stenosis, *bronchitis* and *haemoptysis*. The former is usually more marked in the winter but may be troublesome throughout the year. Haemoptysis may be confined to mere blood streaking of the sputum but sometimes takes the form of a frank haemoptysis presumably due to rupture of a congested blood vessel.

The low cardiac output which is often found with mitral stenosis of any severity is probably responsible for the general symptoms of *weakness* and *tiredness* which are found in the developed condition.

Chest pain similar to angina occurs in a similar proportion of patients, the cause is not known.

Sooner or later most patients with mitral stenosis develop *congestive cardiac failure*. This may occur insidiously, but common precipitating factors are:

(1) the development of atrial fibrillation;
(2) intercurrent infection;
(3) further acute rheumatic carditis;
(4) infective endocarditis;
(5) pregnancy;
(6) pulmonary emboli;
(7) anaemia.

Complications. There are three complications of mitral stenosis which are not uncommon and which may seriously affect the patient's prognosis. *Thrombi* commonly form in the left atrium of patients with mitral stenosis, particularly in the older patient with atrial fibrillation. In about 20% of patients clots may break off from these thrombi and passing out into the systemic circulation obstruct arteries and produce a variety of symptoms and signs. Thrombi may also form in the deep veins of the legs leading to *pulmonary infarcts*; these are sometimes very intractable and precipitate cardiac failure which may be irreversible. Finally patients with mitral stenosis may develop *infective endocarditis*; this is, however, uncommon if atrial fibrillation is present.

Physical Signs. The patient with mitral stenosis occasionally has a slight cyanotic flush on the malar region of the cheeks (*mitral flush*), which is due to the low cardiac output. If heart failure has supervened the patient will be orthopnoeic and slightly cyanosed. The pulse will be small and may show atrial fibrillation. The blood pressure is usually on the low side with a narrow pulse pressure.

Examination of the neck veins may show evidence of heart failure and in addition a small group of patients who are in sinus rhythm will show a large 'a' wave indicating pulmonary hypertension or co-existing tricuspid stenosis.

The *apex beat is tapping* and the lift of the *enlarged right ventricle* can be felt between the apex and the left border of the sternum. In uncomplicated mitral stenosis the apex beat is rarely displaced. A *diastolic thrill* may be palpable at the apex.

If the mitral valve is still mobile the first heart sound is loud. This is due to the valve cusps being kept wide open by the prolonged flow of blood until the end of diastole. On ventricular contraction they close with a louder sound than normal valves, which are already half closed at this time. Careful auscultation at the lower end of sternum will also show a sharp, clear sound following the second heart sound; this is the *opening snap of the mitral valve.* The high left atrial pressure causes the mitral valve to open rapidly and the sound is due to the sudden check of the anterior cusp. It denotes a mobile valve. The pulmonary component of the second sound is loud and may even be palpable. As the mitral valve becomes progressively less mobile due to fibrosis and calcification the loud first heart sound and the opening snap will disappear.

The typical *murmur of mitral stenosis* is a low-pitched, rumbling diastolic murmur, localised to the apex (ventricular filling murmur). It is best heard with the patient lying on the left side and is accentuated after exercise. It is due to the blood rushing through the narrowed mitral valve and if the patient is in sinus rhythm there will be a presystolic accentuation due to the left atrium contracting and forcing the last portion of the blood even more rapidly through the mitral valve. The presystolic accentuation usually disappears with atrial fibrillation. In severe mitral stenosis the murmur extends from the opening snap to the first heart sound; in less severe stenosis it is shorter. If severe pulmonary hypertension develops the mitral diastolic murmur may become brief and insignificant due to the associated low cardiac output.

Very rarely there may be heard a pulmonary diastolic murmur down the left border of the sternum (*Graham Steell murmur*) due to pulmonary incompetence subsequent upon dilatation of the pulmonary artery; it must be stressed, however, that such a murmur is very much more commonly due to associated aortic incompetence.

An ECG may show large wide P waves of atrial fibrillation; there may also be right ventricular hypertrophy. A *radiograph of the heart* may show some cardiac enlargement. The dilated left atrium forms a double contour above the right atrium on the right border of the heart. The left atrial appendage can be seen just below the left pulmonary artery. Screening in the right oblique position with barium in the oesophagus will show left atrial enlargement. Calcification of the mitral valves may be seen but this can also occur in mitral incompetence. The pulmonary arteries are often dilated particularly if pulmonary hypertension is present. The lung fields will be congested if heart failure has supervened. *Echocardiography* is useful in confirming the diagnosis.

Normally the flow of blood through the lungs is higher in the lower than the upper lobes. In mitral stenosis there is constriction of the arteries to the lower lobe and thus a redistribution of the pulmonary circulation, so that pulmonary congestion affects both upper and lower lobes. As left atrial pressure rises fine horizontal lines appear in the costophrenic angles (*Kerley B lines*) which are due to oedema of the interlobular septa. With even higher atrial pressure the characteristic

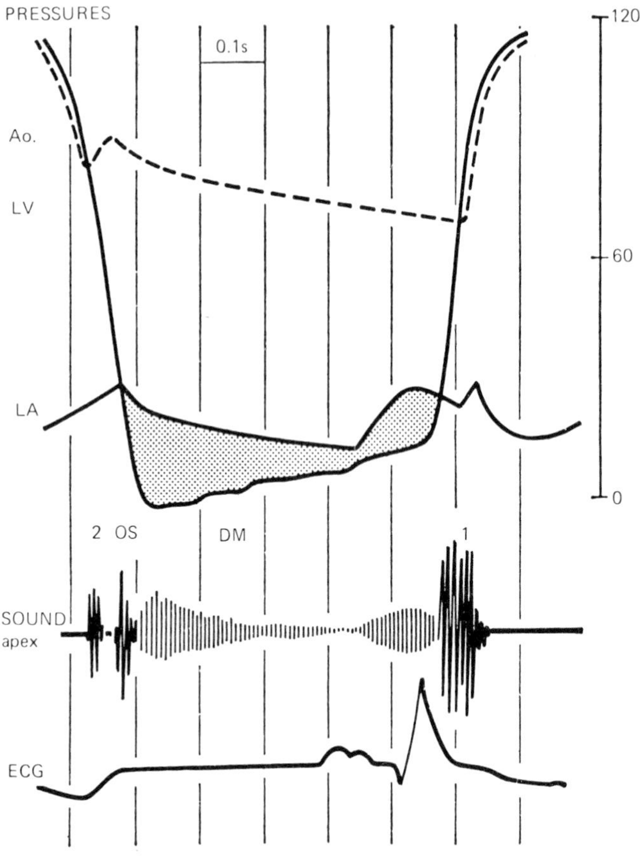

Fig. 4.14 The haemodynamics of the diastolic murmur of mitral stenosis with sinus rhythm. Mitral stenosis produces a persistent diastolic pressure gradient between the left atrium (LA) and left ventricle (LV). The gradient is represented by the shaded area in the figure. Note how, owing to the mitral obstruction, the gradient falls slowly in diastole and is sharply increased by atrial systole. The intensity of the diastolic murmur (DM) is related to the A-V pressure gradient, with a pre-systolic accentuation. The opening snap (OS) coincides with the opening of the mitral valve.

fine hilar haze of pulmonary oedema may develop. Echocardiography allows some assessment to be made of mitral valve movements.

Left heart catheterisation is useful in that it allows the left atrial pressure and the gradient across the mitral valve to be measured. Right heart catheterisation is rarely necessary but gives information as to the pulmonary artery pressure and the pulmonary wedge pressure (indirect left atrial pressure).

Treatment. Minor degrees of mitral stenosis, producing no symptoms and without evidence of cardiac enlargement, are no contraindication to leading a normal life, although extreme effort must be avoided.

Cardiac failure, with or without atrial fibrillation, should be treated as outlined previously (p. 143).

Operations and dental extractions should be covered by antibiotics to prevent infective endocarditis (see p. 221).

Anticoagulants are indicated after an embolism or in the older patient with atrial fibrillation.

The main indications for operation are:

(a) The onset of significant symptoms.
(b) Attacks of pulmonary oedema—this includes pulmonary oedema in pregnancy.
(c) Systemic emboli.

It is a mistake to wait until congestive cardiac failure has developed.

If the symptoms, signs and investigations suggest the patient has pure mitral stenosis with a mobile valve, the closed operation is satisfactory, with a mortality rate of less than 5 % and about 80 % of patients obtain a satisfactory result. With calcified valves or with a significant degree of mitral incompetence open operation will be necessary, the mortality is higher and the results less satisfactory.

Restenosis occurs at the rate of about 5 % of patients per year and depends on the state of the valve and the success of the previous valvotomy. Repeated emboli are best treated by valvotomy, but if this is impossible long-term anticoagulation may be required.

Lutembacher's Syndrome

In this disorder, mitral stenosis is combined with an atrial septal defect. This results in a marked left to right shunt through the septal defect and the development of right heart failure without concomitant pulmonary congestion.

MITRAL REGURGITATION

Mitral incompetence may be due to dilatation of the mitral ring which is caused by general dilatation of the left ventricle and found in such conditions as aortic valvular disease or hypertension.

This group accounts for the loud apical murmur which may be heard with gross dilatation of the left ventricle and which will sometimes disappear when the associated heart failure is successfully treated.

It may also be due to rheumatic affection of the mitral valve and can occur as a result of rupture of the chordae tendineae or damage to the papillary muscle as in infective endocarditis or myocardial ischaemia. It is often found in mitral valve prolapse and may be associated with cardiomyopathies and Marfan's syndrome.

RHEUMATIC MITRAL REGURGITATION

Rheumatic mitral regurgitation is slightly more common in men. The essential lesion is contraction and fibrosis of the chordae tendineae and thickening of the valve cusps so that the normal valve mechanism is unable to function. When the left ventricle contracts blood regurgitates into the left atrium so that the left ventricular stroke volume increases and the left ventricle dilates and hypertrophies. Left atrial pressure rises rapidly in ventricular systole but is not sustained and so pulmonary pressure is rarely as high as in mitral stenosis.

Clinical Features. Symptoms usually develop some years after the attack of rheumatic fever and generally a little later in life than in mitral stenosis. The presenting symptom is dyspnoea due to pulmonary congestion in which left ventricular failure will sooner or later play a part. The enlarged left ventricle may bulge into the right ventricle (*Bernheim effect*) producing some right ventricular obstruction and this may be partially responsible for producing the congestive failure which ultimately develops. The course is then usually rapidly downhill.

The pulse is frequently of small volume and atrial fibrillation is quite common. The apex beat is hyperdynamic and suggests left ventricular enlargement. A third heart sound is often present. The first sound at the apex is not accentuated, the typical harsh pansystolic murmur is heard best at the apex and spreads towards the axilla, it is loud and may be associated with a thrill.

A short mitral diastolic murmur is quite common in mitral regurgitation. It is due to a rapid flow of blood through the rigid mitral orifice and is brief because pressure equalisation between left atrium and ventricle occurs rapidly.

Radiography shows left ventricular enlargement and often considerable dilatation of the left atrium, perhaps with expansible pulsation in ventricular systole; the valve may be calcified.

Treatment. The treatment is that of heart failure when it supervenes; infective endocarditis should be avoided as for mitral stenosis.

Surgical treatment consisting of valve replacement or refashioning has so far not proved very successful.

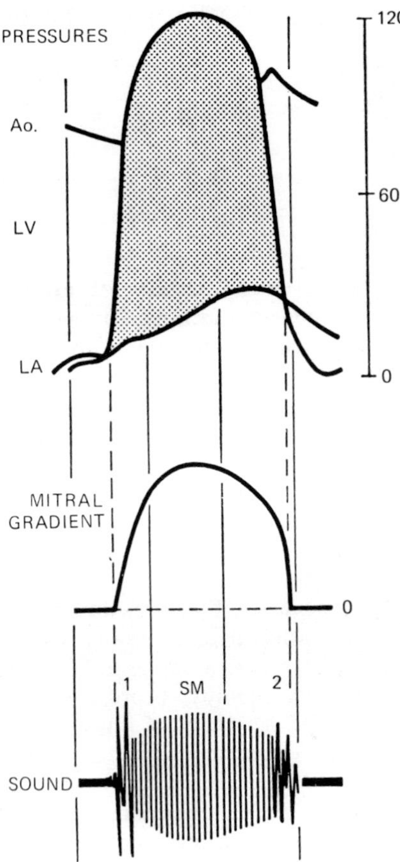

Fig. 4.15 The haemodynamics of the pansystolic murmur of mitral regurgitation. Aortic, left ventricular and left atrial curves, with phonocardiogram and pressure gradient across the mitral valve (not to scale). Note how the mitral pressure gradient and the regurgitant murmur last throughout systole.

Other Types of Mitral Regurgitation

Rupture of the chorda or papillary muscle. Chordal rupture is usually due to infective endocarditis. Rupture of the papillary muscle occurs after myocardial infarction or, more rarely, in cardiomyopathy. There is usually an acute onset of pulmonary oedema with severe dyspnoea together with the development of a regurgitant murmur.

MIXED MITRAL STENOSIS AND REGURGITATION

In many patients with rheumatic mitral disease there is a mixture of stenosis and regurgitation and the physical signs show features suggestive of both these lesions.

MITRAL VALVE PROLAPSE

This is due to myxomatous degeneration of the mitral valves. There are usually no specific symptoms, although a few patients complain of chest pain or dyspnoea on effort. On auscultation there is a midsystolic click followed by a late systolic murmur. Echocardiography is useful in confirming the diagnosis. Prognosis is good but occasionally the disorder is complicated by chordal rupture, infective endocarditis or ventricular arrhythmias.

INNOCENT APICAL SYSTOLIC MURMURS

It must be clearly understood that the majority of apical systolic murmurs are not due to mitral valvular disease. A small proportion are transmitted from other areas: for example, they may be aortic systolic murmurs which can quite commonly be heard at the apex. The majority are benign murmurs due to a variety of physiological causes. These benign murmurs are not associated with other evidence of cardiac disease, such as cardiac enlargement or thrills, they may disappear at various phases of respiration, they alter considerably in intensity with changes in posture and they are usually neither harsh nor loud. If a murmur shows these characteristics it can usually be disregarded.

TRICUSPID VALVE DISEASE

Tricuspid Regurgitation

Tricuspid regurgitation may be functional and due to dilatation of the tricuspid ring in association with right ventricular failure. It is common in the late stages of mitral stenosis and may occur in pulmonary heart disease and with various congenital lesions. Organic tricuspid regurgitation is usually rheumatic but may be part of the carcinoid syndrome (p. 554) when cardiac involvement occurs.

Clinical Features. The patient will nearly always have the symptoms and signs of congestive heart failure. In addition, the effects of the direct transmission of right ventricular systole to the veins is apparent. Marked pulsation of the cervical veins is seen, both superficial and deep, so that if the neck is viewed from the front in silhouette it widens perceptibly with each beat. The lobes of the ears are moved by this forceful deep pulsation. Expansile pulsation of the liver may be felt, and even superficial veins in the back of the hands can be seen to pulsate (sign of Levine). If tricuspid regurgitation is not rapidly relieved then *cardiac cirrhosis* of the liver results, and prolonged renal congestion may cause heavy *proteinuria*. The combination results in markedly reduced serum albumin levels, with generalised oedema. There is a systolic murmur lasting throughout systole and best heard over the lower end of the sternum. It becomes louder during inspiration.

Treatment is generally similar to that for congestive failure and in functional regurgitation this alone may banish the signs of valve incompetence. Organic changes in the tricuspid valves can be treated surgically.

Tricuspid Stenosis

Tricuspid stenosis is nearly always rheumatic and is associated with rheumatic lesions of other valves.

Clinical Features. It is characteristic that these patients do not complain of much dyspnoea or orthopnoea, because the stenosed tricuspid valve guards the lungs against congestion. The main symptoms as the disease advances are weakness due to the low cardiac output together with peripheral venous congestion with liver enlargement and oedema.

There is a raised pressure in the neck veins and if the heart is in sinus rhythm a large presystolic wave ('a' wave) is present due to the right atrium contracting against the narrowed tricuspid valve and resulting in a sharp rise in pressure in the atrium and great veins. On auscultation a diastolic murmur similar to that of mitral stenosis can be heard over the lower end of the sternum. It is sometimes more marked on inspiration.

Treatment is along the usual lines for congestive cardiac failure.

AORTIC VALVE DISEASE

AORTIC STENOSIS

Aortic stenosis can be divided into valvar and subvalvar. Valvar stenosis may be congenital, may follow rheumatic fever or be due to atheroma of the valve. Although the commonest cause of isolated aortic stenosis is probably congenital, the exact frequency with which these three causes operate is still debatable because the end result, whatever the initial lesion, is a scarred, deformed valve, with deposits of atheroma, so that identification of the original aetiology is very difficult.

If, however, aortic stenosis is combined with mitral stenosis it can be presumed to be rheumatic and if it is diagnosed in infancy it is obviously congenital in origin.

Subvalvar stenosis may be due to muscle hypertrophy (see Cardiomyopathies, p. 193), or to a fibrous ring.

When the aortic valve orifice is reduced to about one half its normal size the flow of blood is so restricted that the left ventricular pressure rises above the aortic pressure. This is followed by hypertrophy of the left ventricle and finally failure with pulmonary congestion.

Clinical Features. Aortic stenosis may produce no symptoms, but in the majority of cases sooner or later the strain on the left ventricle produces heart failure. This may present as *dyspnoea on effort*, often with attacks of acute left ventricular failure causing pulmonary congestion with *paroxysmal nocturnal dyspnoea*. Once heart failure develops the downhill course is progressive and death usually occurs within five years.

The narrowed aortic valve reduces the cardiac output, which cannot be increased to meet the demands of the body on exertion. *Exercise syncope* is an important symptom for it indicates severe stenosis and in general carries a poor prognosis. The high intraventricular pressure in diastole reduces coronary flow leading to *effort angina* although this can also be due to coincident coronary artery disease. Sudden death may occur probably due to ventricular fibrillation, although long survivals are recorded.

The *pulse* in aortic stenosis is typically small, with a slow rise and a low pulse pressure; it may, however, be normal. In a fully developed case the heart shows evidence of *left ventricular hypertrophy* with a heaving apex beat. There is a *systolic thrill in the aortic area*. A *harsh systolic murmur* which is maximal in midsystole (an ejection murmur) can be heard extending from the aortic area up into the neck and often also down to the apex. It is best heard in expiration. An ejection click may be noted between the first heart sound and the systolic murmur. This is due to tensing of the aortic valve. It is heard if the valve is pliable, and is not heard in subvalvar stenosis.

A short blowing early diastolic murmur may be heard down the left border of the sternum; it is due to minimal aortic regurgitation and is caused by the damaged valves failing to close completely. The second sound at the base is absent or greatly reduced.

Not all patients with aortic stenosis show all the signs enumerated above. Sometimes the diagnosis may be suspected on the grounds of a harsh systolic murmur transmitted to the neck, without obvious abnormalities of the pulse or the presence of a thrill, but it must be remembered that innocent systolic murmurs at the base of the heart are very common and a diagnosis of aortic stenosis should only be made if the murmur is loud and quite characteristic and does not disappear with changes of posture or during different phases of respiration.

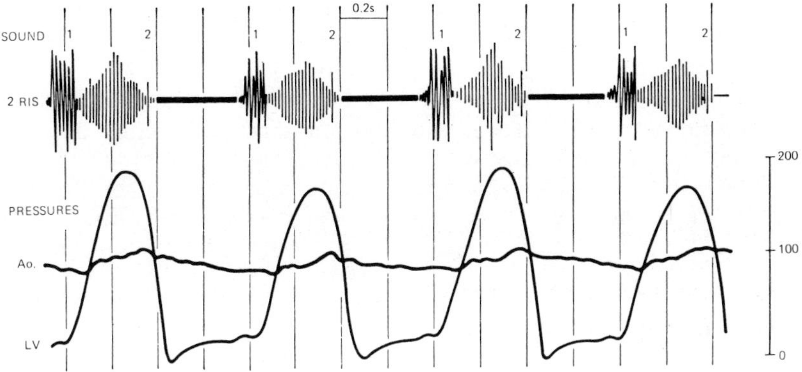

Fig. 4.16 Alternation of the intensity of the ejection murmur in aortic stenosis with left ventricular pulsus alternans. Note the left ventricular pressure rising above the aortic pressure and the short diamond-shaped murmur. There is also pulsus alternans due to left ventricular strain. Sound is taken from the second right intercostal space.

An ECG shows left ventricular hypertrophy usually with a vertical heart. *Radiography* of the heart confirms the left ventricular hypertrophy and careful screening may show *calcification of the aortic valves.* The aorta may show post-stenotic dilatation, particularly in valvar stenosis.

Left heart catheterisation shows a considerable gradient across the valve often in excess of 50 mmHg.

Treatment. Asymptomatic cases of aortic stenosis with no evidence of left ventricular hypertrophy require no treatment except for the avoidance of undue physical effort; they may otherwise lead a completely normal life. Operations and dental extractions require antibiotic cover to prevent infective endocarditis. When heart failure develops it should be treated along the usual lines (p. 142).

Several surgical procedures are now available to relieve aortic valve disease. The main indications for operation are related not only to the severity of the stenosis but also to the state of the myocardium and are:

(1) severe angina of effort;
(2) developing cardiac failure;
(3) syncopal attacks;
(4) ECG and catheter evidence of severe stenosis, particularly in children, may be an indication for open valvotomy even in the absence of symptoms.

In aortic stenosis it may be possible to perform a simple valvotomy, but for severely damaged or calcified valves, or if there is aortic regurgitation some form of valve replacement is required. This may be either a homograft aortic valve, or some form of prosthesis, of which the Starr–Edwards ball valve is probably the most satisfactory at the present time. In the best hands the operative mortality is down to about 5%. The principal postoperative complications are infection or thrombosis on the prosthesis, or residual valve leak with homografts.

AORTIC REGURGITATION

Aortic regurgitation may result from the following conditions:

(1) *Rheumatic valvular disease*, which commonly gives rise to a combination of regurgitation and stenosis.
(2) *Aneurysm of the ascending aorta* affecting the aortic valve ring, which becomes stretched and renders the valve incompetent.
(3) *Infective endocarditis.*
(4) *Rupture of an atheromatous aortic valve cusp.*
(5) A small proportion of patients with *severe hypertension*, especially those with coarctation of the aorta have some degree of aortic regurgitation.
(6) It may complicate *ankylosing spondylitis* and *Reiter's syndrome.*
(7) *Bicuspid aortic valves* may become incompetent when associated with infective endocarditis or with coarctation of the aorta.

If the aortic valve is incompetent blood flows back from the aorta to the left ventricle during diastole. This produces certain signs in the peripheral circulation and also imposes a strain on the left ventricle due to increased volume load. The freer the regurgitation the more striking are the peripheral signs and the greater the left ventricular strain with resulting dilation and hypertrophy. The rapid ventricular filling in diastole, due to the regurgitant flow, may cause premature closure of the mitral valves and thus limit ventricular filling from the atrium.

Clinical Features. The commonest presenting symptoms of aortic regurgitation are those of developing left ventricular failure, namely *dyspnoea on effort* and perhaps attacks of *cardiac asthma*; once heart failure develops the downhill course is usually rapid and death ensues within two or three years. Aortic regurgitation, particularly if due to rheumatic infection, can, however, exist for many years before heart failure develops.

Aortic regurgitation may be complicated by *angina of effort* because the low diastolic pressure found in this condition leads to poor filling of the coronary arteries. When angina occurs in aortic incompetence due to syphilitic aortitis an additional factor may be the involvement of the mouths of the coronary arteries by the gummatous process.

The *pulse in aortic regurgitation* is typically collapsing in nature, due to the rapid flow of blood forwards through the dilated peripheral arterioles and backwards into the left ventricle during diastole. It is best appreciated if the patient's wrist is grasped by the whole hand, when it can be felt as a distinct tap, which has been likened to a water-hammer. For similar reasons pulsation can sometimes be seen in the peripheral capillaries, particularly those of the nail bed, lips, and forehead. Marked pulsation can also be seen in the carotid arteries and the patient may complain of palpitation and throbbing in the head. There is a large pulse pressure, the systolic pressure being slightly raised and the diastolic very low. These peripheral signs are not present if there is only a slight leak back through the aortic valve.

The heart usually shows evidence of *left ventricular hypertrophy*, particularly if there is free regurgitation. The typical *aortic diastolic murmur* is soft and blowing and is not associated with a thrill. It is best heard with the patient sitting upright and with his breath held in expiration. It may be loudest down the left or right sides of the sternum or even at the apex. It is maximal immediately after the second sound and dies away through diastole (Fig. 4.17).

There may in addition be an aortic systolic murmur, which is not due to aortic stenosis but to the greatly increased blood flow through the aortic valve.

If there is gross enlargement of the left ventricle it may be possible to hear a rumbling diastolic murmur at the apex, similar to that found in mitral stenosis. This may be due to blood passing through normal mitral valves into the dilated left ventricle or to eddies produced by the regurgitant stream of blood around the medial cusp of the mitral valve. It is known as *Austin Flint murmur*.

ECG changes often occur quite late in the disease and consist of increased amplitude of the QRS complexes over the left ventricle and later, depression of the S-T segment. Radiography of the heart shows left ventricular enlargement.

The chief complications of aortic regurgitation are heart failure and infective endocarditis.

Treatment. Surgical treatment for aortic disease is considered on p. 187. Complications should be treated as they arise. If the incompetence is syphilitic in origin, the syphilis should be treated, but this will not cure the leaking valve. Generally speaking the physical activities of patients with aortic incompetence should be limited. Operations and dental extractions must be covered by antibiotics to prevent infective endocarditis.

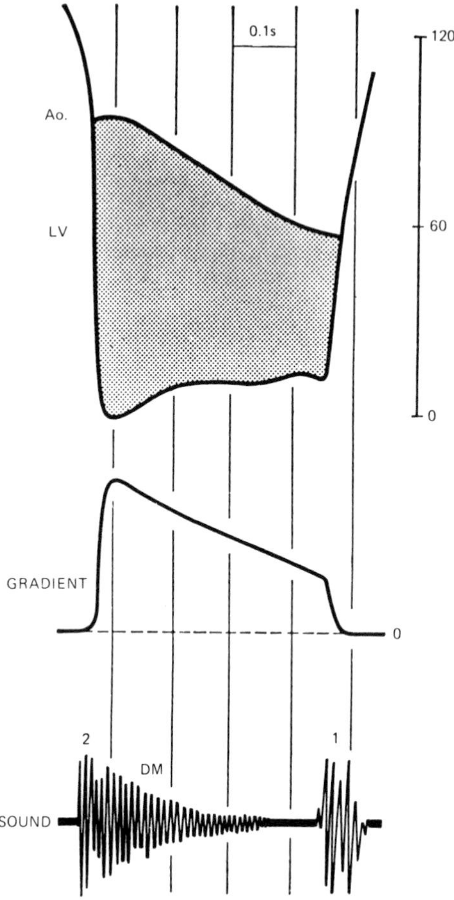

Fig. 4.17 The haemodynamics of the early diastolic murmur of aortic regurgitation. Simultaneous aortic and left ventricular pressure curves. The shaded area represents the gradient which is responsible for the regurgitant flow and murmur. The gradient is shown below (not to scale) and corresponds to the intensity of the murmur.

Aortic Regurgitation of Acute Onset

This may complicate infective endocarditis, or sometimes a valve damaged by rheumatism or atheroma may rupture spontaneously. There is a rapid fall in cardiac output and pulmonary congestion may develop. The patient may complain of sudden onset of dyspnoea or may develop a shock-like state. Examination usually reveals a loud sound in diastole. Heart failure may be difficult to control and surgical replacement of the valve is often necessary.

COMBINED AORTIC STENOSIS AND REGURGITATION

In rheumatic aortic disease it is common to get some degree of stenosis and regurgitation. This produces a combination of signs with both systolic and diastolic murmurs.

Treatment is the same as for single aortic lesions.

ANEURYSMS OF THE AORTA

Aneurysms of the aorta are usually due to atheroma sometimes complicated by a dissection (see below). Syphilitic aortitis which was a common cause is now rare in the UK.

Clinical Features. In many patients aneurysms cause no symptoms until they are discovered by chance on radiography. If there is concurrent aortic valve disease or coronary artery disease these can cause angina of effort or left ventricular failure. The classical symptoms and signs described below are rarely seen now that syphilitic aortitis has almost disappeared.

An aneurysm of the ascending aorta may erode the anterior chest wall, producing severe local pain and tenderness, and in addition may press on the superior vena cava causing obstruction.

It may be possible to percuss out the aneurysm to the right of the upper part of the sternum; and the aneurysm may finally appear on the surface as a pulsatile swelling which ultimately ruptures. It is common to find a harsh systolic murmur and thrill over the aneurysm. There may also be the typical murmur of aortic regurgitation.

An *aneurysm of the arch of the aorta* may compress the *trachea* and left bronchus causing a typical brassy cough and sometimes collapse of the lung, the *oesophagus* causing difficulty in swallowing, the *recurrent laryngeal nerve* causing paralysis of the left vocal cord and a hoarse voice, and the *sympathetic chain* causing Horner's syndrome (p. 333). When the aneurysm expands during systole it may push downwards on the trachea and left main bronchus causing a downward *tug on the trachea* and larynx which is best felt by standing behind the patient and palpating the cricoid cartilage. It may involve the origins of the great vessels and cause *inequality of the pulses.*

Aneurysms of the *descending aorta* rarely produce dramatic signs, but may cause *pain in the back and chest* wall by pressure and erosion of the spine and ribs. The fourth thoracic vertebra is most usually affected.

A radiograph will confirm the presence of aneurysmal dilatation arising from the aorta. Theoretically, on screening it should be easy to see expansile pulsation of the aneurysm, but this is not always so, partially because it may be confused with transmitted pulsation from the heart and partially because the sac of the aneurysm may be lined with blood clot which prevents pulsation. *Calcification* of the ascending aorta is suggestive of syphilitic aortitis.

Treatment. Aneurysms of the ascending aorta carry a poor prognosis and should be treated surgically if possible. In the descending aorta surgery should be confined to large aneurysms. In syphilitic aortic disease 1.0 mega unit of benzylpenicillin should be given daily for 14 days with steroid cover to minimise a Herxheimer reaction.

DISSECTING ANEURYSM OF THE AORTA

This occurs in an aorta already damaged by *atheroma* or by *cystic necrosis* the cause of which is not known but it frequently complicates Marfan's syndrome. There is also an association with scoliosis. The blood forces its way between the layers of the aortic wall and splits it for a variable distance, often occluding various branches of the aorta. The blood in the false passage may re-enter the lumen, leaving the patient with a 'double-barrelled aorta', but more often it ruptures externally into pericardium, mediastinum, or retroperitoneal space and the patient does not long survive.

Clinical Features. The patient is seized by a sudden severe pain usually in the chest and often extending to the back. The attack is associated with collapse and may prove rapidly fatal. Examination usually shows a severely ill patient in great pain and a clue to the diagnosis may be provided by finding absent or unequal radial or femoral pulses. If the dissection involves the thoracic aorta it may produce acute aortic incompetence or a left-sided bloody effusion. Occlusion of the spinal arteries may cause focal neurological signs.

The ECG shows no specific change. The diagnosis can be confirmed by aortography. If the patient survives the acute episode radiological examination shows widening of the aorta.

Treatment. The immediate treatment of a dissection is bed rest and relief of pain, and diamorphine will usually be required. A surgical opinion should be sought early as surgical treatment improves the outlook especially in patients with a proximal dissection (arising from the root of the aorta). Patients with a distal dissection (arising below the origin of the left subclavian artery) usually fare better with medical treatment. It is important to lower the blood pressure in those with hypertension and this should be done rapidly (see page 171).

β adrenergic blocking drugs have been shown to improve the prognosis in those who survive the acute episode, presumably by reducing the stresses on the aorta.

Although the immediate prognosis is poor (about 30–50% of patients die within a short time of admission to hospital), a few survive for remarkably long periods—over ten years has sometimes been recorded.

ANEURYSM OF THE ABDOMINAL AORTA

An aneurysm of the abdominal aorta is nearly always due to atheroma. It may cause abdominal pain which is often quite severe and is due to pressure on the vertebral column and neighbouring organs. The diagnosis can be confirmed by palpation and by ultrasound. If rupture occurs it causes severe lower abdominal pain with a mass in the lower abdomen. Large aneurysms should be treated if possible by resection and replacement by graft.

CARDIOMYOPATHIES

Cardiomyopathy occurs in several diseases and affects primarily myocardium, although the endocardium or pericardium are also sometimes involved. It may complicate such generalised diseases as amyloidosis, scleroderma, systemic lupus erythematosus or leukaemia, or may appear as an isolated phenomenon.

There are two main types:

(1) *Congestive Cardiomyopathy*. This is essentially a dilatation of the heart with failure of the myocardium. The main clinical features are congestive cardiac failure frequently with arrhythmias. The heart is enlarged, often with a triple rhythm and sometimes functional mitral and tricuspid incompetence.

(2) *Obstructive Cardiomyopathy*. The essential feature is hypertrophy without dilatation. This leads to resistance to filling of the ventricles in diastole and to obstruction to outflow in systole producing a picture similar to aortic stenosis. The clinical course may be prolonged over many years but sooner or later congestive failure develops. Angina of effort may occur and sudden death is not uncommon.

Propranolol is effective in relieving the outflow obstruction and increasing diastolic filling; if this fails, removal of a segment of the hypertrophied muscle may be necessary.

Alcoholic Cardiomyopathy. Prolonged and heavy drinking can damage the heart muscle. Early symptoms are dyspnoea on effort and palpitation. There are no specific physical signs but tachycardia, ectopic beats, or atrial fibrillation may occur and the electrocardiogram may show T wave changes. At this stage the condition is probably reversible. If drinking continues, a state similar to beri-beri may develop with oedema and cardiac enlargement and with signs of a high cardiac output.

Endomyocardial fibrosis is largely confined to East Africa. There is fibrosis with thrombosis often affecting both sides of the heart and obstructing both inflow and outflow. The clinical picture is one of severe congestive failure with valve involvement and sometimes systemic emboli.

VIRAL MYOCARDITIS

Some involvement of the myocardium is quite common in a variety of viral infections including those due to Coxsackie A and B, adenovirus, echovirus and influenzal viruses, it is not usually clinically important and only produces transient ECG changes. Occasionally, however, myocardial involvement is more serious, causing cardiac arrhythmias or failure occurring either with the acute infection or delayed for a week or two.

Clinical Features. It is usually a disease of young men and there may be a history of vigorous exercise being taken during the viral infection. The picture is that of cardiac failure perhaps with a pericardial effusion, various arrhythmias including conduction defects and often a triple rhythm. Chest pain may be prominent due to an associated pericarditis.

Sometimes the disease takes a subacute course with recurrent attacks of congestive failure and arrhythmias and sometimes the disease appears to burn itself out but leaves varying degrees of residual damage. Whether these varieties are due to a virus is not known.

Treatment is symptomatic and includes relief of the cardiac failure and control of the arrhythmias. Provided the patient survives the acute stage, recovery is usually but not always complete. Precise diagnosis depends on serial measurement of viral antibodies in the plasma.

ATRIAL MYXOMA

The benign tumour usually develops in the left atrium and produces symptoms and signs similar to those of mitral stenosis. Peripheral emboli may occur. The treatment is surgical removal.

Echocardiography is particularly helpful in diagnosis.

THE HEART AND THYROID DISEASE

Thyrotoxicosis

Thyrotoxicosis frequently affects the heart, particularly in the older age groups. The action of increased thyroid hormone is to raise the cardiac rate and output. In young subjects tachycardia with a full bounding pulse, high pulse pressure, warm extremities and an overactive heart are the chief signs in the cardiovascular system. In older patients these signs may be complicated by various arrhythmias, particularly atrial fibrillation, and by heart failure. The heart failure and atrial fibrillation of thyrotoxicosis are difficult to control adequately with digitalis and the addition of a β blocker is useful. The thyrotoxicosis itself should be treated as quickly as possible; after this is relieved the heart usually returns to normal and if atrial fibrillation persists it can nearly always be easily reversed.

Myxoedema

Myxoedema may also have effects on the heart. Bradycardia, sometimes extreme, is fairly uncommon. Patients with myxoedema have a high incidence of coronary artery disease. In addition, myxoedema is occasionally complicated by a pericardial effusion, the cause of which is not clear.

The *electrocardiogram* is characteristic, showing low voltage QRS complexes in all leads, with flat T waves.

HEART DISEASE AND PREGNANCY

Pregnancy produces a number of changes in the circulation which throw an increased strain on the heart and which may be wrongly interpreted as evidence of heart disease. These changes begin during the second month of pregnancy, increase until about the thirty-second week and then diminish. The chief changes are:

(1) an increase in cardiac output;
(2) some retention of sodium and water.

Clinically there is tachycardia, a full pulse and warm, flushed and pulsating extremities. There may be some ankle oedema, although this may also be a sign of toxaemia. The apex beat is rather forcible and may in the later months of pregnancy be displaced a little to the left. The jugular venous pressure is slightly raised. The increased cardiac flow produces pulmonary and aortic systolic murmurs. A physiological third heart sound is not uncommon due to rapid ventricular filling.

Fitness for Pregnancy. The decision as to whether a patient with heart disease is fit for pregnancy is not always easy and when there is any doubt expert advice should be sought.

Generally speaking the following rules will be found useful:

(1) Patients with no symptoms or evidence of cardiac enlargement will usually go through a pregnancy without trouble.
(2) Patients who have had heart failure or who have severe effort intolerance should be advised against pregnancy; if they have already conceived, the pregnancy should be terminated in the first three months.
(3) The middle group present the main difficulty. This includes those with moderate dyspnoea on effort and some cardiac enlargement. Each of these cases will have to be judged on its own merits.

Cardiac Surgery and Pregnancy. If the patient has some lesion which can be corrected surgically this should be done before pregnancy or, if the patient is already pregnant, within the first three months.

General Management during Pregnancy. All patients with heart disease should be carefully observed by both physician and obstetrician.

Patients who have symptoms before pregnancy or those who develop some dyspnoea during pregnancy must have a full night's rest and in addition should rest during the afternoon. The earliest signs of cardiac failure are the development of pulmonary congestion causing cough and dyspnoea with râles at the bases of the lungs and X-ray evidence of congestion. Filling of the neck veins and the presence of slight ankle oedema are often misleading as these may occur normally in pregnancy.

If failure develops it should be treated in the usual way (p. 143).

Management of Labour. In most patients natural delivery assisted perhaps by forceps in the second stage is quite satisfactory. Caesarian section is rarely required except perhaps in coarctation of the aorta where there is a risk of rupture. During the period of labour and for four days afterwards amoxycillin 500 mg four times daily should be given as there is a risk of infective endocarditis.

Post-Partum Period. Rest is important in the post-partum period and the long-term problem of looking after a child and a home must be considered before embarking on a further pregnancy.

Mitral Stenosis in Pregnancy. The majority of patients with heart disease and pregnancy have rheumatic heart disease, usually mitral stenosis.

The main danger in these patients is the rapid development of pulmonary congestion with attacks of pulmonary oedema, which may be fatal. This usually starts early in pregnancy and is an indication for an emergency mitral valvotomy. In addition, atrial fibrillation may start in pregnancy and produce a rapid onset of cardiac failure.

With the fall in the incidence of rheumatic valve disease, congenital heart disease is relatively more common. Pulmonary hypertension, whether as part of Eisenmenger's syndrome or as an isolated phenomenon carries a bad prognosis for both mother and foetus and may well be an indication for termination of the pregnancy. In general expert guidance will be required for these patients.

Heart Disease and the Pill. Oral contraception should be avoided in patients with systemic or pulmonary hypertension, with coronary artery disease or with a history of venous thrombosis or pulmonary embolism.

CONGENITAL HEART DISEASE

Congenital heart disease may be classified as follows:

Acyanotic	**Cyanotic**	
Without shunt	*With right to left shunt*	
Coarctation of the aorta	Fallot's tetralogy	
Dextrocardia	Eisenmenger's syndrome	
Bicuspid aortic valves	Pulmonary atresia	Very rare
Pulmonary stenosis	Transposition of the great vessels	Very rare
Congenital aortic stenosis		
With shunt (left to right)		
Persistent ductus arteriosus		
Atrial septal defect		
Ventricular septal defect		

This list is by no means exhaustive, but covers the commoner congenital lesions. *Some types of congenital heart disease are diagnosed in infancy and their investigation and management is a specialised subject and will not be considered here.*

ACYANOTIC GROUP

COARCTATION OF THE AORTA

In coarctation of the aorta there is a narrowing of the aorta usually just below the origin of the left subclavian artery.

The narrowed aorta is partially bypassed by a collateral circulation between branches of the subclavian and axillary arteries and the intercostal and superior epigastric arteries.

Clinical Features. The condition may remain asymptomatic in early life and adolescence. It may present as hypertension; as heart failure, which usually develops between the ages of thirty and forty years; or as a subarachnoid haemorrhage due to rupture of a congenital berry aneurysm of the circle of Willis, which is a common (15 %) associated condition.

Examination shows a raised blood pressure in the arms; the mean blood pressure in the legs is usually normal, but with a low pulse pressure. The *femoral pulses* are either absent or feeble and delayed. There is often conspicuous *arterial pulsation in the neck*. The heart may show evidence of left ventricular enlargement and there is a widespread *systolic murmur* heard over the praecordium and at the back. This murmur is due to blood passing through the coarctation and also through the collaterals. A small number of cases are complicated by bicuspid aortic valves and these may have the characteristic murmur of aortic regurgitation. Careful examination will show pulsation in *collateral vessels*, particularly around the scapula. A radiograph of the chest will often show *notching of the ribs* due to erosion by the large and tortuous intercostal arteries.

Prognosis and Treatment. The prognosis is variable, but few patients with untreated coarctation live beyond middle age. Surgical relief of the stenosis should be recommended for the majority of these patients, the optimum age for operation being between seven and fifteen years. The operative mortality is about 5 %.

DEXTROCARDIA

Dextrocardia is often associated with transposition of the abdominal viscera. It is of no importance clinically except that if its presence is unrecognised it may lead to misdiagnosis.

BICUSPID AORTIC VALVES

These may remain symptomless throughout life, but are especially liable to severe atheromatous change and to infective endocarditis. They may be associated with coarctation of the aorta and may become incompetent.

CONGENITAL AORTIC STENOSIS

Congenital aortic stenosis is considered under aortic stenosis (p. 185).

PULMONARY STENOSIS

Simple congenital pulmonary stenosis is usually valvar and rarely infundibular.

Clinical Features. A round face is a common finding. In mild pulmonary stenosis there may be no symptoms and the diagnosis is suggested by finding a *systolic ejection murmur and thrill* over the pulmonary artery, usually in the second or third left intercostal space. It may be associated with an *ejection click*.

Severe cases usually develop cardiac failure by early adult life. The venous pulse in the neck shows a *large 'a' wave*; there is evidence of right ventricular hypertrophy with a *systolic ejection murmur and thrill* in the pulmonary area. The *second sound in the pulmonary area is usually single*, because the pulmonary component is delayed and often inaudible.

If the foramen ovale is patent and the pressure rises in the right atrium during the course of severe pulmonary stenosis, there will be a shunt from the right to the left atrium with the subsequent development of central cyanosis.

An ECG shows evidence of right ventricular hypertrophy, and an X-ray shows diminished vascularity of the lung fields with post-stenotic dilatation of the pulmonary artery.

Prognosis and Treatment. Severe cases of pulmonary stenosis rarely reach middle age and all cases run the risk of infective endocarditis. All but the mildest cases should be offered relief of the stenosis by valvotomy.

PERSISTENT DUCTUS ARTERIOSUS

The ductus joining the left pulmonary artery and aorta usually closes at birth or soon afterwards. If it persists, there is a shunt from the aorta to the pulmonary artery, with a consequent increase in pulmonary artery flow and in the output of the left ventricle.

Clinical Features. The condition is often symptomless when it is discovered. Infective endocarditis develops in about one-third of the patients who reach middle age. Cardiac failure is another complication which is found in the third and fourth decades, although in a proportion of patients with a large ductus it may occur even in infancy.

Examination may show a *collapsing pulse* with a low diastolic blood pressure. The apex beat is forcible and suggests some left ventricular hypertrophy. The '*machinery*' *murmur* which is characteristic of persistent ductus is best heard in the second left intercostal space. It is more or less continuous, starting in early systole, becoming louder in late systole and dying away towards the end of diastole. It may be associated with a thrill. If the pulmonary artery pressures increase, the murmurs may be confined to systole when the pressure gradient is greatest.

In addition over a third of subjects with a persistent ductus have a *mitral diastolic murmur* which is presumed to be due to increased blood flow through the mitral valve.

The second sound may be normally split on inspiration. With a large ductus the left ventricle may be overloaded and the aortic component of the second sound delayed so that normal splitting does not occur.

A proportion of patients with a persistent ductus arteriosus develops pulmonary hypertension, with reversal of the blood flow through the duct and the development of cyanosis.

An ECG may show some left ventricular hypertrophy and radiography some enlargement of the pulmonary vessels with a well-marked aortic knuckle.

Prognosis and Treatment. Persistent ductus arteriosus is amenable to surgical closure and this should be advised for all patients except those with pulmonary hypertension.

ATRIAL SEPTAL DEFECT

Atrial septal defect (ASD) is commonly due to a failure of development of the septum secundum. More rarely the septum primum fails to fuse and this defect is usually accompanied by a deficiency in the mitral valve causing mitral regurgitation. Half or more of the blood which enters the left atrium passes through the defect into the right atrium and thus back through the pulmonary circulation. Usually the increased flow can be accommodated by the pulmonary circulation without a rise in pulmonary artery pressure. Rarely changes occur in the pulmonary vessels with a rise in pressure and a reversal of the atrial shunt.

Clinical Features. ASD does not as a rule produce much in the way of symptoms until middle age when it usually presents as cardiac failure. *Examination* will show some right ventricular enlargement. The apex beat is not obvious and is sometimes described as 'tapping' in quality. The increased pulmonary blood flow may be detected as marked pulsation in the enlarged pulmonary artery, palpable in the second and third left intercostal space. The majority of patients have a *systolic murmur* in the pulmonary area due to increased blood flow from the right ventricle into the dilated pulmonary artery. The *second sound* in the pulmonary area is *widely split*. This split is not altered by respiration and is due to delay of the pulmonary element and is an almost constant feature of the disorder. Sometimes a diastolic murmur is present at the lower end of the sternum and is due to a very high flow rate through the tricuspid valve in diastole, and occasionally a pulmonary regurgitant murmur can be heard if pulmonary hypertension is present. In ostium primum defects there may be an apical pansystolic murmur due to mitral regurgitation.

On a *radiograph of the chest* there is marked dilatation of the pulmonary arteries, which can be seen to pulsate on screening (hilar dance). The right ventricle is enlarged and the aortic knuckle is small.

The ECG shows some evidence of right ventricular enlargement with characteristically an RSR pattern (right bundle branch block) in lead VI.

If pulmonary hypertension develops there may be reversal of the shunt through the defect leading to venous blood entering the left side of the heart and producing cyanosis.

Prognosis and Treatment. Most patients with ASD eventually develop cardiac failure, which should be treated along the usual lines. Surgical repair of the defect should be undertaken if possible.

VENTRICULAR SEPTAL DEFECT

The volume of the shunt between the left and right ventricles depends on the size of the defect and the pulmonary artery pressure and may vary considerably. It may be an isolated defect or may be complicated by other defects (see Fallot's tetralogy).

Clinical Features. *Small Defect* (*Maladie de Roger*). A small defect gives rise to no symptoms unless infective endocarditis supervenes. It is suggested by finding a *pansystolic murmur and thrill* in the third or fourth left intercostal space.

The prognosis is good and the patient should live his normal span.

Large Defect. If the left to right shunt is large so that the pulmonary blood flow may be three or four times the systemic flow there is overloading of the pulmonary circulation and the output of the left ventricle is increased. Heart failure may present in middle age, or more commonly pulmonary hypertension may develop with reversal of the shunt and consequent central cyanosis. The *heart is enlarged*, with a forcible left ventricular type of apex beat. *Marked pulsation over the pulmonary artery* in the second and third interspaces will be palpable. A *pansystolic murmur and thrill* in the third and fourth interspaces will be found, together with a *functional mitral diastolic murmur* due to the high flow rate through the mitral valve.

An ECG may show evidence of some left ventricular hypertrophy and if pulmonary hypertension is present some right ventricular hypertrophy as well.

A *radiograph of the chest* may show dilated pulmonary arteries, which will be seen to pulsate on screening.

Prognosis and Treatment. With small defects the prognosis is good and surgery is not indicated. The main risk is the development of infective endocarditis. Large defects, however, causing a marked increase in pulmonary blood flow reduce life expectancy and closure may be necessary, particularly if there is cardiac enlargement or a rising pulmonary artery pressure.

CYANOTIC GROUP

FALLOT'S TETRALOGY

Fallot's tetralogy is the commonest cause of cyanotic congenital heart disease. The tetralogy consists of pulmonary stenosis (valvar or subvalvar), ventricular septal defect, overriding of the aorta so that it lies over both ventricles, and right ventricular hypertrophy. As a result of the obstruction of outflow from the right ventricle due to the pulmonary stenosis venous blood passes into the aorta. The size of the shunt will depend on the severity of the pulmonary stenosis and the pressure in the aorta.

Clinical Features. *Central cyanosis*, with polycythaemia and clubbing of the fingers, is usually present from birth or soon after. In severe cases the patient is undersized. *Dyspnoea* is a prominent symptom. The patient often adopts a characteristic *squatting position* which decreases the right to left shunt by increasing the peripheral resistance and thus the pressure in the aorta.

The heart usually shows minimal right ventricular enlargement and the apex is tapping in quality. There is a *systolic murmur*, often accompanied by a thrill, in the second or third left intercostal space. The pulmonary second sound is single.

An ECG shows marked right ventricular hypertrophy.

On *radiography of the heart* the cardiac apex is often elevated with a deep pulmonary bay, giving rise to the classical 'cœur en sabot'. The *lung vascular markings are much reduced.*

Prognosis and Treatment. Patients with Fallot's tetralogy rarely reach adult life. Operative treatment is now available, either the Blalock operation which aims at increasing the pulmonary blood flow by an anastomosis between a systemic artery and the pulmonary artery, or preferably by the Brock operation which directly relieves the pulmonary stenosis. More recently total correction of the deformity has been undertaken with relief of the stenosis and repair of the septal defect. This will probably become the treatment of choice ultimately.

There are a number of other causes of cyanotic congenital heart disease but they are rare and will not be discussed.

Eisenmenger's Syndrome

This group of disorders consists essentially of a right to left shunt coupled with pulmonary hypertension. The shunt is usually via a VSD, ASD or patent ductus, though more complicated congenital lesions may be involved. Whether the pulmonary hypertension is present at birth or is the result of the large pulmonary blood flow is not known.

Clinical Features. The age of onset of symptoms depends on the underlying lesion. With an ASD it is usually in middle age but with other lesions they may develop considerably earlier in life or even in infancy.

The patient is cyanosed with clubbing and complains of dyspnoea. The signs are those of *pulmonary hypertension* (p. 226) with a *systolic murmur* from the shunt. Cardiac failure may develop.

Treatment. There is no specific treatment and closure of the shunt is contraindicated. Heart failure is treated in the usual way when it arises. Death usually occurs by middle age.

INFECTIVE ENDOCARDITIS

Patients with congenital heart disorders are at risk of developing infective endocarditis although this risk varies with different lesions. Operations, etc. should be covered with the appropriate antibiotic (see p. 221).

ISCHAEMIC HEART DISEASE

The following conditions may cause cardiac ischaemic pain:

(1) coronary artery disease;
(2) aortic valve disease;
(3) syphilitic aortitis;
(4) severe anaemia;
(5) paroxysmal tachycardia (occasionally).

ATHEROMATOUS CORONARY ARTERY DISEASE

One of the most striking changes in the twentieth century in the pattern of disease which affects the Western world has been the emergence of coronary artery disease as one of the most common causes of death, particularly amongst middle-aged men. The reason for this increase is not clear, but several factors may be involved, including a high intake of animal fat, and excessive smoking.

Coronary artery disease starts with narrowing of the arteries by plaques of atheroma which contain cholesterol. Obstruction of the blood flow eventually becomes so severe that when exercise increases the oxygen consumption of heart muscle, not enough blood can pass through to supply it. The muscle, therefore, becomes ischaemic and produces the characteristic pain of angina of effort.

The next stage of the disease is the development of a thrombus on the plaque of atheroma, which cuts off the blood supply to an area of heart muscle and produces a cardiac infarct. This may be fatal, but often healing occurs with fibrosis and scar formation. If collateral circulation is good, however, the muscle will survive. It can be seen therefore that thrombosis is not necessarily followed by infarction, although the terms coronary thrombosis and myocardial infarction are often used synonymously.

It must be realised that some atheroma of the coronary arteries is present in all men and most women over the age of thirty and that the coronary circulation has great powers of opening collateral channels and thus circumventing narrowed arteries. Whether or not symptoms develop depends on the rate of progress of the atheromatous process and the ability of the coronary circulation to open up adequate collateral circulation.

It is now realised that spasm of the coronary arteries may produce symptoms of ischaemia. Spasm may occur in normal vessels or may complicate atheromatous deposits. The mechanism is not known.

The Background to Coronary Disease. It seems probable that clinical coronary disease is the result of a number of factors and processes. Many of these factors are now known, although the whole picture is not complete. A knowledge of these factors may be important in that some of them can be avoided, and therefore it may be possible to diminish the risk of developing coronary disease.

The most important factors so far discovered are:

(1) *Elevation of the Plasma Lipids.* Elevation of the plasma cholesterol is a major risk factor. The levels of cholesterol in the blood correlate well with the amount of saturated fat in the diet.

The distribution of cholesterol among the lipoprotein fractions of plasma may also be important and there is accumulating evidence that the ratio of high density lipoprotein (HDL) cholesterol to total lipoprotein or to low density lipoprotein cholesterol is relevant. A high HDL cholesterol/total cholesterol ratio has a protective action against atheroma.

Triglycerides have also been implicated but they are not as important as cholesterol.

There is little evidence at present that alteration of diet influences the course of developed coronary artery disease. It seems logical, however, to treat those with elevated plasma cholesterol levels. This requires the treatment of obesity, if present, and the replacement of saturated fats with unsaturated fats in the diet. The place of clofibrate is doubtful and its use is associated with an increased incidence of gall stones.

(2) *Hypertension.* A raised blood pressure carries with it an increased incidence of coronary disease. Although evidence is still conflicting, it seems probable that lowering the blood pressure, particularly by the use of β blockers, decreases the risk of infarction.

(3) *Cigarette Smoking.* There is a correlation between smoking and coronary disease, especially in the younger age groups. The risk decreases if smoking is stopped.

(4) *Other Factors. Obesity*, unless excessive, is only weakly linked to coronary disease if dietary factors are excluded. In diabetes but not the nephrotic syndrome there is a high incidence of atheromatous disease. *A personality type* (type A) has been depicted as having a high risk, the important characteristics being aggression, punctuality and urgency. *Lack of exercise* has been implicated from time to time, but it is unlikely that it is of much importance.

On the information available it seems that a considerable change in national habits is required if the incidence of atheroma and coronary disease is to be reduced. This will include a diet in which fewer calories are obtained from animal fat and sugar, control of the blood pressure in those with hypertension and the exclusion of cigarette smoking. These should be associated with moderate regular exercise.

ANGINA OF EFFORT (Angina Pectoris)

Clinical Features. The patient with angina of effort usually has few complaints apart from his pain. This is described as constricting, or as a heavy feeling, a pressing feeling, an ache or tightness. It is usually substernal and may radiate down the inside of the left arm or both arms or up into the neck or jaw. It may be felt only in the back. *It is brought on by effort and relieved within a few minutes by rest.* It is more easily provoked in cold weather, after a heavy meal, or with emotional upsets.

Anginal pain may be associated with some dyspnoea. This is believed to be due to temporary deterioration in left ventricular function with a rise in end-diastolic filling pressure.

The onset of the attacks of pain may be gradual or it may appear quite suddenly one day. A sudden onset of severe angina of effort should always raise the suspicion that the complaint has gone beyond a narrowing of the coronary arteries and that an actual coronary thrombosis with infarction has occurred. The course of the disease is variable. The symptoms may become progressively more severe, they may remain stationary or rarely they may improve. At any time a coronary thrombosis may supervene and this may be fatal.

Examination of the patient rarely reveals any abnormality. Occasionally a third or fourth heart sound is heard or there may be signs of mitral incompetence secondary to ischaemic damage to the papillary muscle. The exception to this is when angina is secondary to aortic valve disease when the characteristic signs will be found. Usually the diagnosis depends on an accurate history which may be supported by the relevant tests.

The *electrocardiogram* may be very useful in confirming the diagnosis (Fig. 4.18). The following may be found:

(1) Some 50% of patients with angina have a normal ECG at rest. After exercise or pacing at a high rate with an electrical pacemaker, the ECG may show S-T depression. However, even a normal effort test does not exclude the pain being due to ischaemia. It does however

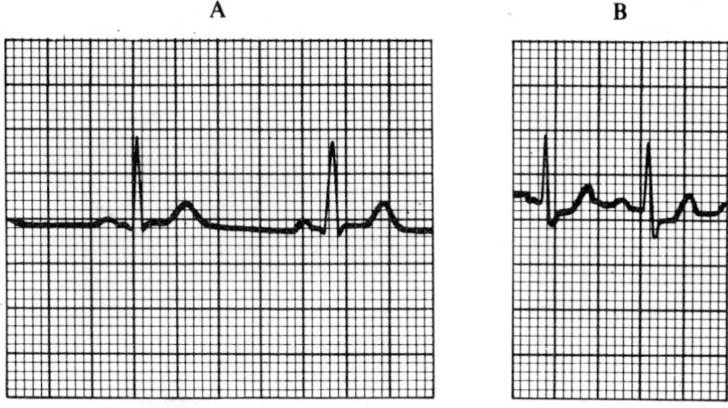

Fig. 4.18 ECG Lead V6. (**A**) Rest. (**B**) After exercise showing S-T depression.

suggest that the obstruction to the coronary circulation is more likely to be due to intermittent spasm rather than a fixed stenosis. It should also be remembered that S-T depression can occur on the ECG without the patient experiencing any pain.

(2) The resting ECG may show evidence of ischaemia with S-T depression or T wave inversion.

(3) There may be evidence of actual infarction.

Isotope Scanning

Two types of scanning can be used to demonstrate ischaemic heart disease:

(1) *Thallium Scanning.* The uptake of thallium by the myocardium depends on coronary perfusion. In patients with ischaemic heart disease there is a diminished uptake of the nucleotide in those areas of muscle supplied by obstructed or partly obstructed arteries, thus it is possible to obtain a functional picture of myocardial perfusion and deduce which arteries are narrowed.

(2) *Technetium 99 Scanning* (*Multiple Gated Scan*). Technetium is injected and pictures can be obtained of the cavities of the heart at the end of systole and at the end of diastole, thus allowing the following to be assessed:
   (a) The left ventricular ejection fraction.
   (b) The presence of a ventricular aneurysm.
   (c) The kinetic behaviour of the ventricular muscle.

If the heart is stressed by immersing the hands in ice-cold water, by exercise or by isometric contraction, the ischaemic areas of the myocardium do not contract in the normal manner and become relatively akinetic, and thus provide useful evidence of the presence and distribution of coronary obstruction.

Coronary Angiography

Radio-opaque material is injected into the coronary vessels and recorded by cineradiography. This allows the site and extent of the atheromatous obstructive lesion to be determined. Its main use is as a prelude to surgery. It is not particularly useful in the differential diagnosis of chest pain as the extent of coronary atheroma and the presence or absence of symptoms do not correlate closely.

Prognosis and Treatment. Depression and anxiety often follow a patient's discovery that he has angina, which is understandable since the probability of sudden death at a relatively early age is common knowledge. Considerable reassurance is therefore required as many of these patients live full and useful lives for ten, fifteen or more years.

The patient's mode of life must be organised to fit both his disease and his temperament. Strenuous exercise must be prohibited, but moderate exercise is not harmful provided it does not produce pain and it may perhaps be beneficial. The patient should if possible continue in his occupation, but overwork or work which keeps him under continued pressure must be avoided. If he is overweight then weight must be reduced. Smoking undoubtedly reduces coronary blood flow and all patients with angina should be advised to abstain from it. Some patients improve remarkably on giving it up.

Nitrites are the most useful drugs for relieving the attacks of pain. *Glyceryl trinitrate* in doses of 0.5 mg should be sucked or chewed and will relieve angina within two to three minutes. The drug should be used whenever the pain occurs but is more effective if used to prevent attacks of pain when some effort is required. Their most important effect is to lower blood pressure and thus cardiac work, rather than to increase coronary flow.

Long-acting coronary vasodilators can be used particularly in patients who have frequent attacks of angina; *isosorbide dinitrate* 10–40 mg orally is given three or four times daily.

β blockers are useful in angina for reducing the sympathetic drive to the heart. Atenolol 50–100 mg daily or metoprolol 50–100 mg two or three times daily are satisfactory.

Nifedipine 10 mg three times daily, and increased if necessary, reduces the oxygen requirements of the myocardium and is a vasodilator. It is useful in some patients with angina particularly if coronary spasm is suspected.

There have been many attempts to improve coronary circulation by *surgical measures*. The introduction of coronary angiography has made possible better delineation of the extent of the coronary obstruction. *Saphenous vein grafting* should be seriously considered in patients whose symptoms are not controlled by medical treatment, particularly those under 60. There is now some evidence that the prognosis is improved by surgical treatment (see p. 216).

Variants of Angina

There are several types of angina which do not conform to the classical pattern. The introduction of coronary angiography has also made it clear that occasionally there can be ischaemic pain without coronary obstruction. To some degree the variants given below overlap.

Unstable Angina (Acute Coronary Insufficiency)

A number of patients present with severe anginal pain, occurring at rest, lasting 20–30 minutes and not relieved by trinitrin. In others, after a period of stable angina, attacks become frequent, more easily provoked and more prolonged. In such patients the ECG may show transient depression of the S-T segment and T wave changes. The enzymes are not raised. In spite of the alarming symptoms, the prognosis is quite good. A small proportion of these patients develop a frank infarct, but in the rest the condition stabilises.

Treatment. These patients usually respond well to bed rest combined with a vasodilator such as isosorbide dinitrate and/or nifedipine and a β blocker. When the acute symptoms are controlled the patients should be treated as for angina; some will require coronary angiography and possibly venous graft.

Coronary Artery Spasm

The introduction of coronary angiography has shown that spasm of the artery may be a causative factor in some patients with angina. It is sometimes possible to precipitate a spasm during angiography by the injection of ergometrine. Spasm should be suspected clinically where the anginal pain has an unusual pattern, particularly if it occurs at rest. In these patients β blockers may exacerbate symptoms and they are best treated by trinitrin, long-acting nitrites and nifedipine.

Prinzmetal's angina variant is commoner in women and may start at a relatively early age. The pain although similar in nature and distribution to classical angina is not related to effort, and is associated with elevation of the S-T segment on the ECG rather than S-T depression. In many patients, particularly those in the younger age group, coronary angiography shows no evidence of obstruction. It has been suggested that the pain is due to ischaemia following a transient spasm of the coronary artery.

MYOCARDIAL INFARCTION

In subjects with coronary atheroma, there is always the danger that a thrombus may form on the atheromatous plaque, thus suddenly cutting off the blood supply to an area of heart muscle; in other words, a coronary thrombosis may occur leading to myocardial infarction.

When a large coronary artery is obstructed by thrombosis the patient may suddenly fall down dead; indeed this is the only cause of really sudden death. More often the patient survives but suffers some decline in left ventricular function. This may produce no symptoms or signs but with more extensive infarction there will be a fall in cardiac output and the development of pulmonary congestion. About 10% of patients develop shock and/or pulmonary oedema. Over the next few weeks the dead heart muscle is absorbed and replaced by a fibrous scar.

This scar may be firm and strong, but occasionally, particularly if the infarct has been a large one, the scar may become stretched and produce an aneurysm of the heart wall. The functional ability of the heart may be near normal after recovery from an infarct; but sometimes after a large infarct, the loss of infarcted muscle so encroaches on the reserve power of the heart that congestive failure occurs, or the patient may be left with crippling angina of effort.

Clinical Features. A myocardial infarct may occur at any time of the day or night, at rest or on exercise. The onset is usually sudden with severe substernal pain, of the same type and distribution as angina pectoris. It can be distinguished from angina by the fact that it often comes on when the patient is at rest, and, unlike angina, which is relieved by a few minutes' rest, it persists for several hours. Some patients will have noted that for a few days before the acute attack they have had mild and short-lived attacks of substernal pain, the so-called 'warning pains', while in other patients the only complaint may be the rather sudden onset of severe angina.

Rarely, other symptoms may overshadow the chest pain, for example sudden onset of left ventricular failure, abrupt loss of consciousness due to transient cardiac arrest or arrhythmia, or severe vomiting. These may all be presenting symptoms and only careful questioning will elicit a history of substernal pain. Generally speaking, however, the history is typical and the diagnosis obvious.

Examination in typical cases shows the patient to be anxious, pale, sweating, and with a rapid pulse and low blood pressure. In milder cases these signs may be missing and it is worth remembering that the blood pressure may not fall markedly for some hours after the acute attack. Cardiac arrhythmias of any type may occur with a coronary thrombosis, one of the most common being ventricular extrasystoles; these may herald the onset of a dangerous ventricular tachycardia or even ventricular fibrillation. Auscultation of the heart shows a triple rhythm in about half the cases. Sometimes it may be possible to hear transient apical systolic murmurs due to functional mitral regurgitation. If the heart is examined daily after the acute attack it is often possible to hear a pericardial friction rub on about the third or fourth day. Pericarditis should also be remembered as a cause of persistent chest pain after a cardiac infarct.

During the first week there is often a rise in temperature, a polymorphonuclear leucocytosis, and a rise in the sedimentation rate, all indications of the inflammatory reaction around the damaged myocardium.

The serum levels of aspartate transaminase (AST, formerly known as glutamic oxaloacetate transaminase or GOT) and creatine kinase (CK) are raised in most patients after an infarct. The enzymes are released by breaking-down heart muscle.

Serum levels of enzymes are raised in damage of other organs such as the liver, pancreas and skeletal muscle. The creatine kinase concentration is so sensitive to tissue damage that even an intramuscular injection can produce some elevation. A method is available to detect the appropriate isoenzyme of creatine kinase.

Table 4.4 Enzyme levels in myocardial infarction

	Upper Limit of Normal	*Period of Elevation*
Aspartate transaminase	35 Karmen units/ml	24 h–5 days
Creatine kinase	100 units/litre for men 60 units/litre for women	8 h–3 days

The ECG should be used to confirm the diagnosis and define the position and extent of the infarct. The following changes may be found:

(1) *The Classical Picture of Cardiac Infarct*

(a) *Anterior infarction* produces a large Q wave and raised S-T segment in lead I and in the anterior chest leads with S-T depression in lead III. This changes during the next few weeks to a Q wave with marked T wave inversion in lead I and the anterior chest leads and the return of the S-T shift to the isoelectric level.

(b) *Inferior infarction* with a large Q wave and raised S-T segment in leads II and III and a VF with S-T depression in lead I. This also changes in the next few weeks to Q wave with marked T wave inversion, in leads II and III and a VF and return of the S-T shift to the isoelectric level.

(c) *True posterior infarction* does not show pathological Q waves but may be identified by tall R waves combined with tall and symmetrical T waves in leads VI and V2.

(2) *Lesser Changes*

Symmetrical inversion of T waves without large Q waves or S-T segment shift.

A number of other minor changes in the ECG have been described which alone do not necessarily indicate myocardial infarction, but taken in conjunction with such a history as outlined above, are good enough evidence of an infarct.

It must be remembered that a full 12-lead ECG must be taken and must be repeated at frequent intervals as the changes after a small infarct may be confined to one lead and may be quite transitory.

Immediate Complications of Cardiac Infarction

(1) *Cardiac Failure.* It is quite common to find a mild and transient rise in venous pressure or some pulmonary congestion in the days following an infarct. It usually resolves rapidly but after a very large infarct the patient may be left in chronic failure. Rupture of a papillary muscle can lead to mitral regurgitation with failure.

(2) *Cardiac Arrhythmias.* Some 80% of patients develop some type of arrhythmia after cardiac infarction. These may be transient and last

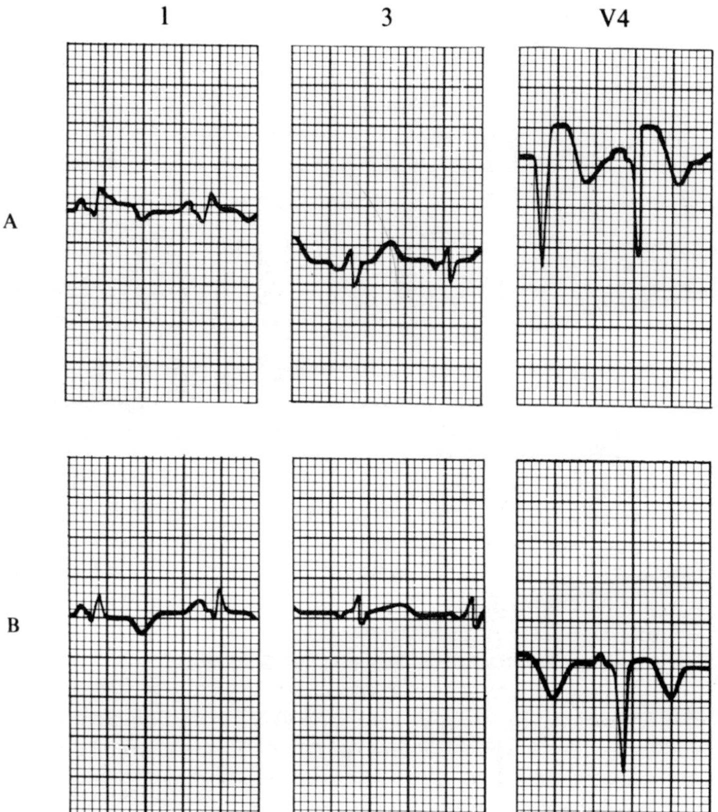

Fig. 4.19 Anterior Infarct. (**A**) Immediate changes. (**B**) After several months.

no more than a few seconds, or may be prolonged and may seriously decrease cardiac output. The arrhythmia may be of any type. They tend to disappear as the infarct heals, although atrial fibrillation and varying degrees of heart block may persist indefinitely.

(3) *Thromboembolic Phenomena.* Patients lying immobile after a coronary thrombosis are very liable to deep vein thrombosis in the calf veins with the attendant risk of pulmonary embolism. A thrombus may form on the endocardium over the infarcted area. A piece of clot may break off and obstruct arteries in the systemic circulation, particularly those of the brain.

(4) *Hypotension.* Hypotension may complicate cardiac infarction; it may be due to a fall in cardiac output subsequent to extensive myocardial damage or sometimes to a prolonged arrhythmia which interferes with cardiac function. The clinical picture is one of acute circulatory failure (see p. 136) with peripheral vasoconstriction, cold extremities and

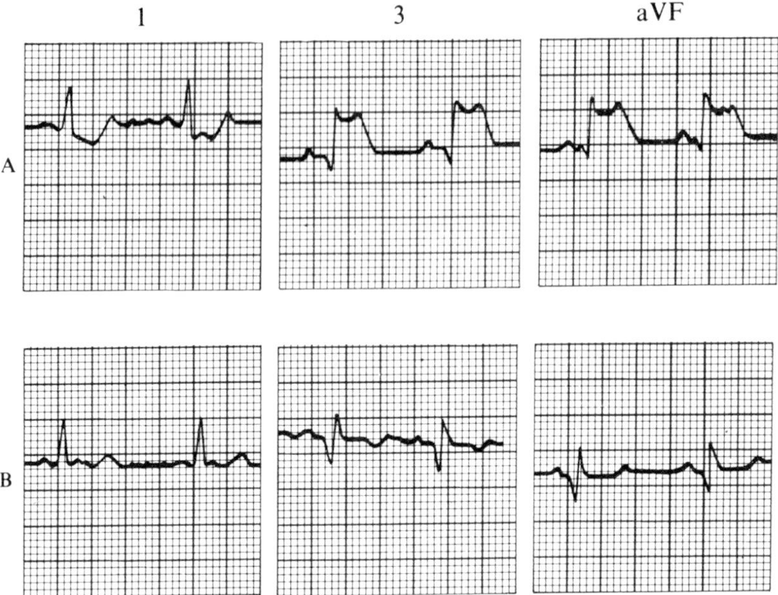

Fig. 4.20 Inferior Infarct. (**A**) Immediate changes. (**B**) After several months.

mental clouding. If this state is prolonged oliguria will develop. Sometimes, however, the cardiac output may in fact be higher than normal, but the peripheral resistance is lowered by vasodilation. Such patients usually have extremities of normal colour and temperature.

It is not uncommon for patients to develop vasovagal attacks with bradycardia, sweating, hypotension and nausea, and in some but not all such patients these symptoms appear to be precipitated by the administration of opiates.

(5) *Rupture of the Heart.* Sudden exertion in the week immediately after an infarct may cause a fatal rupture of the heart. This risk can be diminished by careful mobilisation.

Treatment. In the early stages bed rest is important but should not be prolonged. Mobilisation can usually start at three days in patients with uncomplicated infarction, and thereafter a graded return to activity should be made. A commode should be allowed from the day of infarction but no special effort should be made to get the bowel open during the first few days; however, it is worth giving a gentle laxative to prevent undue constipation. For most patients an ordinary light diet is satisfactory. Smoking should be forbidden.

Severe pain is a prominent feature of cardiac infarction and should be treated by diamorphine 2.5 mg IV, and the dose and frequency of administration should be titrated to keep the patient comfortable. This should be combined with prochlorperazine 12.5 mg IV to reduce nausea and vomiting. If pericarditis develops, the pain can be relieved by aspirin 600 mg every 6-hourly. Full anticoagulation is now rarely used after cardiac infarction. Heparin 5000 units subcutaneously is given twice daily until mobilisation is started to prevent venous thrombosis and thrombosis on the endocardium, and it is common practice to insert a 'butterfly' catheter in case prompt IV injection is required in an emergency; 500 units of heparin is given four times daily via the catheter to prevent its becoming blocked.

In patients with persistent pain or those with a poor cardiac output it is sometimes helpful to give a vasodilator to lower afterload and improve cardiac function. Isosorbide dinitrate 10–20 mg four times daily orally or by intravenous infusion with a starting dose of 4.0 mg/hour and increasing as required.

If the patient is anxious diazepam 2.0–5.0 mg t.d.s. orally is useful.

Home Management or Hospitalisation

It is now realised that cardiac arrhythmias are a frequent cause of circulatory failure and sudden death in the two or three days following cardiac infarction. If patients are continuously monitored by ECG during this period it should be possible to diagnose these arrhythmias immediately and to give appropriate treatment. This is the main reason for the development of the coronary care unit which is found in most major hospitals throughout the world. Unfortunately, dangerous arrhythmias are very liable to occur immediately after infarction and before medical help is available. This in turn has led to the creation of ambulance flying squads and even to the teaching of elementary resuscitation to the ordinary citizen.

Whether intensive monitoring during the period immediately following cardiac infarction actually decreases mortality is still the subject of debate in spite of numerous trials which have compared management at home with that in hospital.

Elderly patients who are taken ill at home may be treated there when the attack does not appear severe and there is no evidence of shock or arrhythmias, provided that the facilities are good. It is still possible that such patients will develop a fatal arrhythmia in the hours immediately following the infarct, but there is little evidence that admission to hospital will make a significant difference. Patients with more serious infarction or with arrhythmias should be sent to hospital as quickly as possible so that they may be monitored and have the benefit of intensive care.

Treatment of Arrhythmias

Prevention. Various regimes have been tried to prevent arrhythmias developing in the post-infarction period. In the present state of knowledge the only step worth taking is to keep the plasma potassium level above 4.5 mmol/l as lower concentrations appear to predispose to arrhythmias. General measures such as the treatment of hypoxia (if present) and the relief of pain and anxiety are important.

Developed Arrhythmias

Bradycardias

Sinus bradycardia, sometimes complicated by arrest or by escape ventricular arrhythmias, usually responds to atropine 0.3 mg IV every five minutes until the pulse rate is above 50 beats per minute (the maximum dose of atropine is 2.4 mg/h). Digoxin and verapamil will increase bradycardia and should be avoided. Pacing is rarely required.

The prognosis and management of *atrioventricular block* depends largely on the site of the damage. With an inferior infarct the block is in the region of the A-V node (intranodal) and recovery is usual. With an antero-septal infarct the damage is to the bundle branch system (infranodal) and the myocardium and the prognosis is poor.

Mobitz type I A-V block (see p. 159) is intranodal with a good prognosis and pacing is only required if the ventricular rate is too low. Mobitz type II A-V block often progresses to complete A-V block and pacing is required (see below).

Complete A-V block complicating an inferior infarct has a narrow QRS complex on the ECG; recovery is to be expected and pacing is required only with low ventricular rates or with Stokes–Adams attacks. Complete A-V block with an anterior infarct implies serious damage and the prognosis is poor. Temporary demand pacing is indicated; a rate of 65–75 beats per minute will prevent escape ventricular arrhythmias but in a severely damaged heart output is rate dependent and it may be necessary to increase the rate and titrate it against the haemodynamic response.

Bundle Branch Block. The importance of bundle branch block is that it may progress to a more serious conduction defect. Right bundle branch block when complicated by either left anterior or left posterior hemiblock (see p. 162) may progress to complete heart block and prophylactic pacing is required. In other types of heart block opinions differ and generally pacing is only required if the rhythm becomes unstable.

Tachycardias

Ventricular Ectopics occur very frequently. It is commonly held that if they are:

(a) frequent,
(b) multifocal,
(c) close to the T wave (R on T),

it heralds the onset of ventricular fibrillation, although it probably occurs in no more than 10% of patients showing this type of change. Often serious ventricular arrhythmias can develop without any warning.

If ectopics show the above characteristics, 100 mg of lignocaine should be given IV followed by an infusion of 4.0 mg/min for 30 minutes, followed thereafter by 1.0–2.0 mg/min. In cardiac failure, the metabolism of lignocaine is slowed and the dose should not exceed 1.0 mg/min. Monitoring of plasma levels may be helpful if facilities are available.

Ventricular Tachycardia. If the attack is well tolerated and the ventricular rate below 160 beats per minute, it should be treated with lignocaine as detailed above. If this fails, disopyramide 100 mg IV given over 15 minutes may be tried. In patients who tolerate the arrhythmia poorly, DC cardioversion should be used and followed by a continuous infusion of lignocaine.

Atrial fibrillation or flutter is treated with digoxin. The addition of verapamil 0.1 mg/kg IV given at a rate of 1.0 mg/min will augment the slowing action of digoxin and may be useful. Cardioversion is occasionally required.

Hypotension and Cardiac Failure

Hypotension may be due to vagal overactivity, perhaps exacerbated by diamorphine or to a low cardiac output (pump failure) secondary to myocardial damage or to an arrhythmia.

Vagal overactivity should respond to atropine and arrhythmias can be given the appropriate treatment (see above).

In circulatory failure the foot of the bed should be raised as long as this does not precipitate pulmonary oedema. Many patients have a low arterial oxygen saturation due to disorganisation of ventilation/perfusion in the lungs and should be given oxygen 2 l/min by MC mask (approximately 40–60%).

Attempts to raise cardiac output are not usually very successful. Dopamine can be given by IV infusion in a dose of 5–15 μg/kg/min; it has an inotropic effect on cardiac muscle and may also increase renal perfusion and is thus sometimes useful. Prolonged hypotension carries a bad prognosis.

If cardiac failure with pulmonary oedema develops, it is treated in the usual way with diuretics (see p. 146).

Subsequent Management

When the period of rest has finished the patient is gradually allowed up, but should not return to work for at least two months after the acute attack. If possible the patient should return to his normal employment. If, however, his job is exceptionally heavy or if he is severely crippled by cardiac failure or angina of effort, then some change will be necessary.

Some patients will require considerable encouragement and support in the months following an infarct. They may become depressed, anxious, and irritable, and it is the doctor's job to show them that it is possible to lead a normal and useful life, even if they have had a heart attack.

Prevention of Recurrence

Following cardiac infarction the overall mortality is about 25 % and death usually occurs in the first 48 hours. About 15 % of patients leaving hospital die in the first year and thereafter about 5 % per year. A number of measures have been tried to diminish the incidence of further infarction and improve survival rates. These can be divided into the use of drugs, surgical correction of the coronary arteries and general measures.

Drugs. Some trials using β blockers have been shown to improve survival after cardiac infarction, but results are not unanimous. If the patient is hypertensive, β blockers should certainly be included in the treatment regime, as long as heart failure is not a risk. Whether they should be used in normotensive post-infarction patients requires further evidence. Sulphinpyrazone in doses of 200 mg four times daily has been shown to reduce mortality up to the seventh month after infarction. The mechanism of this action is not clear and as with β blockers further confirmation is required.

Surgery. Coronary artery bypass grafting (CABG) has now become commonplace, but the selection of patients for operation is more controversial. It is impossible to be dogmatic and the opinions expressed here should be modified by the facilities available and by further experience.

The method widely used at present for patients under sixty is an ECG effort test, performed either one week or six weeks after their infarct. A high proportion of those showing ischaemic changes have persistent coronary narrowing which can then be confirmed by coronary angiography. The evidence so far available suggests that patients with ischaemic symptoms following infarction and who have obstruction of one or three of the main coronary vessels benefit from surgery. It is not yet certain which treatment is best for patients who have no symptoms but have some obstruction of the coronary arteries. It seems probable that surgery is indicated if the obstruction is severe.

General measures consist of stopping smoking, reducing weight if necessary, graduated exercise and correcting lipid abnormalities if present. It seems that these measures alone will reduce the incidence of sudden death after infarction.

Long-Term Complication of Cardiac Infarction

(1) **Post-infarction Aneurysm of the Ventricle**. This is an area of fibrous tissue in the ventricular wall which follows a transmural infarct,

usually due to occlusion of the anterior descending branch of the left coronary artery.

Symptoms and Signs. The common symptoms are persistent left ventricular failure associated with dyspnoea and sometimes angina.

On examination it may be possible to feel the systolic thrust of the aneurysm and there may be a triple rhythm. The ECG will show monophasic Q waves over the aneurysm and the S-T segment may remain elevated. X-ray of the heart usually shows cardiac enlargement and sometimes a bulge. The diagnosis is confirmed by left ventricular angiography with coronary arteriography and possibly by isotope scanning.

Treatment. In patients with marked symptoms relief can be obtained for the majority by surgery consisting of resection of the aneurysm and by-pass vein grafting of the coronary artery if possible.

(2) **Dressler's Syndrome.** In the two months following cardiac infarction 3–4% of patients develop a fever which is usually combined with pleural or pericardial pain. A friction rub may be heard and a pericardial effusion is found in about half of those affected. Radiology of the chest often shows increased size of the cardiac shadow and patchy consolidation at the lung bases. The disorder is self-limiting and recovery is the rule although relapses may occur. In severe cases the symptoms can be controlled by steroids or aspirin. Anticoagulants should be avoided as they may cause bleeding into the pericardium. A similar syndrome may follow cardiotomy.

CORONARY EMBOLISM

In a small number of patients who present with the symptoms of cardiac infarction, obstruction to the coronary circulation is due to an embolus. This usually arises as a complication of:

a) Infective endocarditis
b) Cardiovascular disease or from valve prostheses
c) Recurrent arrhythmias

Clinical features are essentially those of cardiac infarction with similar ECG changes. Coronary angiography if performed at the time of the attack will show arterial obstruction but the embolus rapidly lyses so that angiography some weeks after the incident is normal.

Treatment. The management of the acute attack is as for coronary thrombosis (see above). The patient should, however, be anticoagulated and in most cases this should be continued indefinitely.

ENDOCARDITIS

ACUTE INFECTIVE ENDOCARDITIS

This usually occurs in the course of septicaemia due to organisms of high virulence, frequently the staphylococcus pyogenes. The endocardium is affected and the heart valves may be spared.

SUBACUTE INFECTIVE ENDOCARDITIS

Infective endocarditis is due to infection of the endocardium by organisms of moderate virulence. The most common infecting organism is the *Streptococcus viridans* which is often an inhabitant of the mouth and throat of normal people. However, in recent years there has been an increase in infective endocarditis due to other organisms, particularly *Streptococcus faecalis*, the micro-aerophilic streptococci, the staphylococci and *Coxiella burneti*.

Infective endocarditis starts on the heart valves, usually the aortic valve. It most commonly occurs on valves damaged by previous rheumatic fever. It may complicate various congenital lesions including ventricular septal defect, pulmonary and aortic stenosis, persistent ductus arteriosus and bicuspid aortic valves and may develop on various types of prosthetic valves. It is very rare in syphilitic aortitis and atrial septal defect. There is a group of patients, usually over fifty, who appear to develop infective endocarditis on an apparently normal heart. The infecting organism is frequently *Str. faecalis*.

The starting point of infective endocarditis is often a transient bacteraemia. This may follow dental extraction or filling, when the organism is usually *Str. viridans*; or after operations on the urinary tract or bowel, when infection with *Str. faecalis* is more common. This emphasises the need for penicillin 'cover' if these operations are performed in a patient with damaged heart valves. The bacteria settle on the damaged valve, set up an inflammatory reaction which is followed by deposits of fibrin and the formation of a vegetation which often spreads from the valve to adjacent endocardium.

Clinical Features. The most constant clinical feature is a persistent *low grade fever*, and this diagnosis should be considered in any patient with rheumatic heart disease who develops a pyrexia for which there is no other obvious cause. Increasing *malaise*, *tiredness*, and *breathlessness* are common symptoms. In some patients sweating and vague point pains may suggest a recurrence of rheumatic fever. After the first week or two *anaemia* develops and the patient begins to lose weight. The fingers become *clubbed* and in patients left untreated generalised pigmentation occurs; this combined with the anaemia causes a characteristic coloration, sometimes described as the '*café au lait*' appearance.

The bacteraemia gives rise to antigen-antibody complexes which cause widespread vascular damage, which show as:

(1) *Osler's nodes.* Small, tender, red round areas most commonly seen on the pads of the fingers and lasting 24–28 hours.
(2) *Splinter haemorrhages.* Found under the nails.
(3) *Purpura.* Most commonly found on the chest and neck.
(4) *Renal damage.* An increased number of red cells in the urine is a common feature. In addition, there may be widespread glomerular lesions which in time may progress to renal failure.
(5) *Involvement of cerebral vessels* which may give rise to neurological signs or even a confusional state.

In addition, emboli may break off from the vegetations on the diseased valves, and 30 % of patients will have major infarcts in the brain, liver, spleen, intestines, or limbs. Retinal involvement produces typical 'boat-shaped' haemorrhages.

The *spleen* is usually moderately enlarged, from the chronic septicaemia which is a feature of the condition. Infarction may lead to an acute attack of pain in the splenic area.

The *heart* shows signs of the underlying valve lesion and, rarely, changes in the character of the murmurs can be detected. Heart failure may develop and it will be of acute onset if it is due to rupture of a valve.

When infective endocarditis occurs in congenital heart disease with a left to right shunt such as a patent ductus arteriosus, the emboli are swept into the pulmonary circulation and lead to infarcts of the lung. This produces rather a different clinical picture, with recurrent episodes of fever, pleurisy, and patchy consolidation of the lungs, so that an erroneous diagnosis of recurrent pneumonia may be made.

Special Investigations. Examination of the blood reveals a moderate anaemia with a slight leucocytosis. The sedimentation rate is nearly always raised. The urine in the great majority of cases shows an increased number of red cells, although these may be only detected on microscopy.

The *diagnosis* is confirmed by isolation of the organism on *blood culture*. At least four samples of blood must be taken for culture before antibiotic treatment is started and incubation should continue for three weeks. If organisms are isolated, their sensitivity to various antibiotics must be determined. It is best if blood for culture is taken at the height of the fever. If the patient is very ill and the diagnosis is suspected on clinical grounds, the blood cultures should be taken at short intervals so that the start of treatment is not delayed. There is rarely need to await the report on the blood cultures before giving antibiotics.

About 30 % of patients will have a persistently negative blood culture. In these patients a fungal or rickettsial infection should be considered, and appropriate serological test carried out. It may be necessary to give a full course of treatment without the diagnosis being confirmed by a positive culture.

Complications. (1) *Rupture of a Valve.* The aortic valve may be weakened and finally rupture during the course of infective endocarditis. When this occurs it may lead to sudden death or to the rapid development of cardiac failure. Examination shows the characteristic, loud, regurgitant murmur (*cooing dove*).

Less commonly, mitral incompetence may develop as a result of a ruptured chorda, and both these complications are an indication for immediate surgery with valve replacement.

(2) *Mycotic Aneurysm.* Mycotic aneurysms may develop due to small emboli in the vessels supplying the walls of the large arteries. They may require surgical treatment.

Treatment. The patient must be in bed and be given full nursing care. The specific treatment will depend on the infecting organism.

(a) *Streptococcus viridans.* 2.0 mega units of benzylpenicillin IM four times daily, is usually adequate if the organism is sensitive. If there is no response, or if the organism proves to be partially resistant to penicillin the dose can be increased to 20 mega units of penicillin or more daily. Owing to the bulk of the injection, it is necessary to give it by continuous IV drip. Blood levels can also be increased by giving probenecid 0.5 g four times daily.

(b) *Streptococcus faecalis.* 4.0 mega units of benzylpenicillin q.i.d., plus gentamicin 80 mg t.d.s. The dose of antibiotics should be modified according to response, sensitivity tests and, in the case of gentamicin, also the plasma concentration.

(c) *Staphylococcus aureus.* The antibiotic programme will depend on sensitivities. Usually two antibiotics will be required and benzylpenicillin or flucloxacillin plus gentamicin or fucidin are useful combinations.

(d) *Patients with persistently negative blood* cultures should be treated with penicillin and gentamicin in the first instance.

(e) *Endocarditis on prosthetic valves* may be caused by unusual organisms including *Staphylococcus albus* and fungi. Treatment will depend on the causative organism but may have to include valve replacement.

Treatment should aim at abolishing the fever, stopping all embolic phenomena and restoring the ESR and urine to normal. Blood cultures should of course be negative after treatment. The earlier treatment is started in the course of the disease, the better the chance of effecting a cure. Antibiotic therapy must be given for at least 6 weeks.

With these measures it is possible to eradicate infection in the majority of patients with subacute infective endocarditis. In spite of this mortality is still about 25 %. This is due to delayed diagnosis leading to extensive damage to the heart valves and chronic heart failure. In addition the production of immune complexes may cause widespread vascular disease particularly affecting the kidney. All patients must be carefully followed up as relapse or re-infection may occur.

Prevention of Infective Endocarditis

In patients with valve disease or congenital heart disease, dental operations, including extractions, should be covered by an antibiotic. Amoxycillin 3.0 g given orally one hour before the procedure is satisfactory. For patients who are sensitive to penicillin, erythromycin 1.5 g orally followed by 500 mg four times daily for 2 days can be given.

With genitourinary and similar cases when *Str. faecalis* may be involved, ampicillin 1.0 g + gentamicin 100 mg should be given intramuscularly just before operation and 12 hours afterwards.

PERICARDITIS

The following types of pericarditis may be encountered:

(1) benign (probably viral);
(2) rheumatic;
(3) pyogenic;
(4) tuberculous;
(5) malignant;
(6) subsequent to a cardiac infarct or cardiotomy;
(7) associated with uraemia;
(8) systemic lupus erythematosus.

Pericarditis may be dry or may be associated with an effusion.

DRY PERICARDITIS

Clinical Features. Dry pericarditis may occur from any of the above causes. Pain is a frequent, but not a constant, symptom. It may be praecordial or referred to the shoulder or neck region. It may be constant or made worse by movement or by respiration. The patient may also complain of symptoms which are related to the disease underlying the pericarditis.

Examination will usually show a pericardial friction rub; this may be either loud or soft; it usually sounds rough and rather superficial. It may be heard anywhere over the praecordium and may be either systolic and/or diastolic in timing.

ECG Changes. In the early stages the ECG shows elevation of the S-T segment, the elevated segment being concave upwards. This is followed by the return of the S-T segment to the isoelectric line and flattening or inversion of the T waves. These changes, unlike those of cardiac infarction, can be recorded from both the anterior and posterior aspects of the heart at the same time.

PERICARDIAL EFFUSION

The symptoms and signs of a pericardial effusion depend on the underlying cause and on the size of the effusion. Small effusions may be indistinguishable from a dry pericarditis. When the size of the effusion increases rapidly the pressure within the pericardial sac rises, interfering with the venous return to the heart, a state known as *cardiac tamponade*. This in turn reduces the cardiac output and thus seriously interferes with cardiac function.

Clinical Features. The patient often appears restless and ill and complains of praecordial discomfort and dyspnoea. If the effusion is large, examination will reveal *pulsus paradoxus* (p. 123). The venous pressure will be raised, and the apex beat may be felt within the outer limit of cardiac dullness to percussion, which is increased. A pericardial friction rub can often be heard on auscultation, in spite of the presence of an effusion.

A radiograph of the heart shows a pear-shaped cardiac shadow with sharper margins than usual; this is because they have moved less during exposure of the film. *Echocardiography* is very useful for showing even small effusions.

Treatment. Effusions large enough to endanger life are rare. A high venous pressure and low arterial pressure are indications for tapping the effusion. It must be remembered that the high venous pressure found with pericardial effusions is necessary to maintain diastolic filling of the heart and attempts should not be made to lower venous pressure by venesection or by diuretics. Otherwise the treatment is that of the underlying conditions.

Varieties of Pericarditis

Viral Pericarditis. Benign pericarditis can probably be caused by several viruses including coxsackie, mumps and influenza. It is most common in young adults and there is often a history of a recent upper respiratory tract infection. The onset is sudden with fever, malaise, and pericardial pain. Small effusions sometimes develop. Recovery is the rule within a few weeks, but a number of cases relapse.

Treatment is symptomatic.

Rheumatic Pericarditis. Pericarditis develops during the course of acute rheumatic fever in about 10 % of patients and provides definite evidence of cardiac involvement. It may or may not be associated with an effusion. Treatment is as for rheumatic fever.

Pyogenic Pericarditis. Pericarditis may occur as a complication of pneumonia or may complicate a septicaemia. It should be vigorously treated with antibiotics. Surgical drainage is rarely required.

Tuberculous Pericarditis. Tuberculous pericarditis is not common. It usually presents as a subacute pericarditis with effusion and some general malaise with evening fever. The effusion is a clear yellow fluid, occasionally bloodstained, and may be found on culture to contain tubercle bacilli.

Treatment consists of prolonged rest, with rifampicin, isoniazid, and ethambutol (see p. 299).

If the effusion is large, aspiration may be required and streptomycin 0.5 g should then be injected into the pericardial sac.

A number of patients subsequently develop constrictive pericarditis (see below).

Cardiac Infarction. A pericardial friction rub can often be heard transiently over the infarcted area within a few days of a coronary thrombosis.

Post-Cardiotomy and Post-Infarction (Dressler's Syndrome). Pericarditis may develop in the weeks after the occurrence. It responds to steroids.

Uraemia. A pericardial rub may be heard in the terminal stages of uraemia.

Malignant Pericarditis. Involvement of the pericardium by new growth may give rise to an effusion which may require tapping. This is a common terminal complication of bronchial neoplasms.

CHRONIC CONSTRICTIVE PERICARDITIS

Chronic constrictive pericarditis is due to previous tuberculous pericarditis or may follow viral or bacterial infection. The heart is encased in a shell of fibrous tissue which may be calcified, and as a result the heart is unable to expand in diastole and venous filling is greatly impeded.

Clinical Features. The patient is usually in adult life and complains of some dyspnoea on effort associated perhaps with oedema of the ankles and swelling of the abdomen. Orthopnoea is not a feature and the degree of dyspnoea is often slight in comparison with the evidence of gross venous congestion.

Examination sometimes may show a pulsus paradoxus and there often is atrial fibrillation. The venous pressure is high, but falls sharply during diastole (the 'y' descent) when the tricuspid valves open. The heart is not usually much enlarged and auscultation may reveal a third heart sound or may be normal. Enlargement of the liver, ascites, and oedema of the ankles are often present. Long-standing disease may have caused chronic hepatic congestion sufficient to end in cirrhosis of the liver.

A radiograph of the heart usually shows a normally sized or slightly enlarged heart and calcification may be seen in the pericardium in about half the cases, provided lateral as well as postero-anterior radiographs are taken.

An *electrocardiogram* usually shows decreased voltage in the QRS complexes with widespread flattening or inversion of T waves.

Treatment. Treatment consists of surgical removal of the constricting pericardium. The operation is a major undertaking, but the results are usually satisfactory.

ADHERENT PERICARDIUM

Occasionally following rheumatic pericarditis the heart may become attached to surrounding structures. This may be diagnosed clinically by systolic retraction of the lower left ribs posteriorly (Broadbent's sign), fixation of the apex beat and systolic retraction of intercostal spaces. There is no evidence that an adherent pericardium has any effect on cardiac function and if heart failure supervenes in these cases it is due to the associated valve disease.

PULMONARY HEART DISEASE

PULMONARY EMBOLISM

A pulmonary embolus arises most commonly from deep-vein thrombosis in the leg or pelvis (p. 232). Rarely it may arise from an intracardiac thrombosis following atrial fibrillation or cardiac infarction. Phlebothrombosis in the legs occurs particularly in obese middle-aged or elderly patients who have been confined to bed, often with heart disease, but also with other medical conditions, pregnancy, or after major surgical operations. Occasionally it occurs in apparently healthy people, particularly women taking an oral contraceptive.

Clinical Features. *A large pulmonary embolism* causes dilatation of the right ventricle with a drop in right ventricular output, and a rise in systemic venous pressure. This results in a fall in cardiac output which is accompanied by peripheral vasoconstriction. A massive embolism may cause sudden death but more commonly the patient complains of the abrupt onset of substernal tightness, or pain, dyspnoea and a sudden call to stool. He is sweating, pale and slightly cyanosed. The pulse is small and rapid, the blood pressure low, the cervical venous pressure is raised and frequently there is a gallop rhythm. X-ray of the chest may show a segment with diminished vascular marking and the diagnosis can be confirmed by pulmonary arteriography or lung scan.

The ECG is variable. It may show a deep S wave in lead I with a Q or inverted T wave in lead III. The chest leads may show T wave inversion in lead VI-V3, or more rarely there may be a right bundle branch block pattern. The changes are usually transitory.

Smaller pulmonary emboli cause pulmonary infarction, the symptoms of which are often so slight that it is the most commonly overlooked serious respiratory lesion. When the infarct extends to the surface of the lung there may be acute pleuritic pain, and about 40 % of patients have a haemoptysis; but frequently the only clinical features are sudden shortness of breath or unexplained rise of temperature and/or pulse rate.

With a small embolus, X-ray may show a shadow due to the infarct which is classically but by no means always segmental. Other changes include a pleural infusion.

Lung Scan. Perfusion scans within a day or two of a pulmonary infarct show defects in perfusion, and if this is combined with a ventilation scan the combination of normal ventilation and impaired perfusion is diagnostic of an infarct.

It should also be remembered that repeated small pulmonary emboli may seriously obstruct the pulmonary vascular bed and lead to pulmonary hypertension and right ventricular failure.

Treatment. A patient who has had a pulmonary embolus should be nursed fairly flat in bed because the cardiac output and blood pressure may be low. In severe cases oxygen should be given. If the patient is in pain or distress a small dose of morphine 5.0–10 mg can be given. Care must be taken to avoid respiratory depression and there is a danger of further decreasing cardiac output by the venodilating properties of morphine. If morphine is used or if there is evidence of respiratory depression nikethamide 500 mg can be given IV and repeated as required. *Anticoagulants* should be started with IV heparin 10 000 units 6-hourly. When heparin is given in this way for only 48 hours, control of dosage is not required. If however treatment is continued for longer periods the *kaolin-cephalin time* should be estimated before each dose to ensure that a progressive build-up of heparin is not occurring. Heparin may also be given by continuous infusion following an initial bolus of 5000 units, and this requires daily estimation of kaolin-cephalin time to determine and modify the dose. The anticoagulant effect of heparin is almost immediate.

At the same time treatment should be started with an oral anticoagulant. This group of drugs acts by suppressing the formation in the liver of prothrombin and Factor VII, which are necessary for the coagulation of blood.

Warfarin is commonly used. There are several methods of dosing but the easiest is to give 9 mg as a single dose each day. Smaller doses will be required in the elderly, the very ill, the malnourished and those with liver disease. Twelve hours after the third dose the prothrombin time is measured and thereafter the dose is adjusted to keep the prothrombin time between 1.7–3.0 times the normal value. *Before starting anticoagu-*

lants it is wise to obtain base line figures for kaolin-cephalin and prothrombin times.

The most important side-effect of oral anticoagulants is bleeding from overdosage, a common site being the urinary tract. If this occurs the drug must be stopped. The coagulability of the blood can be restored by giving Vitamin K_1 (phytomenadione) IV; it is important to use the smallest effective dose or there may be an abrupt fall in prothrombin time with further clotting. The dose usually lies between 2.5–20 mg.

Anticoagulants should rarely be used in the very elderly and in those in whom there is a risk of haemorrhage, e.g. from a duodenal ulcer.

There is a large number of drugs which interact with oral anticoagulants. A short list is given below but it is wise to consider this possibility if any drug is given to this group of patients.

(1) Aspirin—risk of gastric bleeding.
(2) Liquid paraffin—enhances effect by blocking Vitamin K absorption.
(3) Phenylbutazone, clofibrate, sulphonamide and phenytoin—enhance effect by decreasing plasma protein-binding.
(4) Barbiturates, rifampicin—enhance breakdown of anticoagulant in the liver.

The clot can be lysed by using *streptokinase*. However its control is more difficult, although a short course at the beginning of treatment has its advocates especially after a large embolus. Streptokinase is given for about five days and then anticoagulation is started with heparin and warfarin (see above).

Anticoagulants are usually continued for at least six weeks, and many authorities consider they should be continued up to six months or sometimes for life, particularly if there is any evidence of recurrent embolism.

Rarely in patients with massive pulmonary embolism and where facilities are available *embolectomy* may be performed within a few hours of the acute episode.

PULMONARY HYPERTENSION

Physiology

In health the pulmonary circulation is a low pressure system (range = 15/5–30/15 mmHg). It seems probable that at rest in the upright position the main blood flow is through the lower parts of the lungs. With increased flow as occurs on exercise, vasodilatation occurs and more blood passes through the upper zones. The pulmonary artery pressure rises only with flow rates above 15 litres per minute.

In man there is evidence that active vasoconstriction of the pulmonary arteries can occur, although its mode of production is unknown.

This may be in response to:

(1) increased pulmonary blood flow;
(2) a rise in left atrial pressure;
(3) hypoxia and perhaps hypercarbia.

Clinical Types of Pulmonary Hypertension

(1) **Idiopathic (Primary) Pulmonary Hypertension**
Idiopathic pulmonary hypertension is due to structural narrowing of the pulmonary arteries, the arteries showing medial thickening and arteritis. It is a disease predominantly of young women and the cause is unknown.

(2) **Secondary Pulmonary Hypertension**

(a) Pulmonary hypertension may be due to progressive obliteration of the pulmonary arteries by repeated thrombosis or embolism. This often follows a phlebothrombosis in the puerperium. Early symptoms are dyspnoea on effort, cough and sometimes haemoptysis. Chest X-ray reveal areas of oligaemia which is confirmed by perfusion scan. Early diagnosis is important as at this stage the process may be reversible by anticoagulants.

(b) It may be secondary to increased blood flow through the lungs such as occurs in *atrial* or *ventricular septal defects* or with a *persistent ductus arteriosus*. In these conditions the pulmonary artery can usually accommodate the increased flow without a rise in pulmonary artery pressure. Sometimes, however, active constriction of the pulmonary arteries eventually develops and pulmonary artery pressure may even exceed the systemic pressure, with reversal of the shunt and the development of central cyanosis.

(c) In *mitral valve disease* there is usually a small passive rise in pulmonary artery pressure transmitted back from the left atrium. In a small proportion of cases there is in addition active pulmonary vasoconstriction with a considerable rise in pulmonary artery pressure.

(d) Pulmonary hypertension and heart failure may complicate *chronic lung diseases*, commonly chronic bronchitis or emphysema, or rarely pulmonary fibrosis due to silicosis, sarcoidosis or other causes. It is due to obliteration of the pulmonary artery bed by the lung disease; in addition there may be active vasoconstriction due to hypoxia and perhaps hypercapnia. The clinical features and management of *cor pulmonale* are considered on p. 261.

Clinical Features. Dyspnoea is common and other symptoms are cough and syncope. Early signs are evidence of right ventricular hypertrophy, a short systolic murmur and a systolic click over the pulmonary artery and a loud pulmonary element to the second heart sound. Later a giant 'a' wave in the jugular venous pulse, triple rhythm and cardiac failure with functional tricuspid incompetence may develop. The ECG shows right ventricular hypertrophy and strain.

Treatment. With repeated pulmonary emboli, long-term anticoagulant therapy may reverse the process. In mitral stenosis, relief of the stenosis will frequently release the vasoconstriction.

In those with increased pulmonary flow repair of the shunt with reduction of flow has proved disappointing.

DISEASES OF THE ARTERIES

Diseases of the peripheral vasculature may be subdivided into:

(1) Chronic obliterative arterial disease due to
 (a) Atherosclerosis;
 (b) Buerger's disease.
(2) Acute obstruction to the arterial circulation by embolism or thrombosis.
(3) Venous thrombosis, which may affect either the superficial or deep veins.
(4) Raynaud's syndrome.
(5) Acrocyanosis.

PERIPHERAL VASCULAR DISEASE

ATHEROSCLEROSIS

This occurs most frequently over the age of 50. Predisposing factors are lack of exercise, raised plasma cholesterol and smoking. There is a marked association with coronary artery disease. The atherosclerotic lesions are found mainly in the large and medium sized vessels, particularly the aorta and the iliac and femoral arteries. The upper limb is rarely affected.

Clinical Features. The symptoms are to some degree dependent on the site of the obstruction and two syndromes can be defined:

(a) *Femoropopliteal Obstruction.* This is the commonest type, the occlusion is in the femoral artery, just below the origin of the profunda femoral branch. The earliest symptom is *intermittent claudication*, a cramp-like pain felt in the calf and causing the patient to limp. It may be bilateral or unilateral but is usually worse on one side, it is brought on by walking and quickly relieved by rest. As the disease advances the pain may occur at rest when it is usually felt in the feet, and is most troublesome at night when it may become almost unbearable. Examination of the limb will reveal absent or reduced pulses in the limb, the skin may be shiny and hairless and the nails atrophic.

When the circulation to the limb is severely impaired areas of gangrene may appear. They often follow trauma especially round the nail bed and over the heel. In the most advanced cases gangrene may extend to the whole foot and to the leg.

(b) *Aorto-iliac Occlusion.* The main obstruction is in the lower aorta at its bifurcation and in the iliac arteries. Claudication in the calf is an early symptom but the pain spreads to the thighs and buttocks. This may be associated with impotence (Leriche's syndrome). On examination the femoral pulses are reduced or absent and there may be wasting of the buttock and thigh muscles. The blood pressure in the legs will be lowered and may drop almost to zero on exercise.

Auscultation over the abdominal aorta and iliac vessels may reveal a murmur due to stenosis.

Investigation. If surgical treatment is contemplated arteriography is essential to define the position and extent of the occlusive disease. An ECG is also useful as concurrent coronary artery disease is common.

Prognosis and Treatment. For the majority of patients with intermittent claudication the condition is relatively benign and symptoms may last for years without progression and without the development of gangrene. In some patients symptoms may actually improve due to the opening up of collaterals. For the elderly patient with a mild to moderate disability, treatment should be conservative. Patients should be told to avoid trauma to the feet and the assistance of a chiropodist should be enlisted to help with care of the toe-nails and to deal with callouses, etc. Under heat or cold should be avoided as far as the feet are concerned, but the body should be kept warm to produce as much reflex vasodilation as possible. Various vasodilator drugs are used to try and improve the peripheral circulation; tolazoline 25 mg t.d.s. is popular but there is no evidence that it has a therapeutic effect. Alcohol may be of value in moderate doses.

Tobacco reduces peripheral blood flow and should be avoided by all patients with vascular disease.

Indications for Surgery

Femoropopliteal Obstruction. Surgery in this group is disappointing; patients under 60, with apparent unilateral disease and severe or progressive symptoms should have an arteriogram and if the disease is proved to be unilateral and limited, and if they are in good general health, operation, usually a by-pass graft is justified.

Aorto-iliac Obstruction. Patients in this group do better with surgery, and it should be offered to those with severe symptoms.

In a few patients, lumbar sympathectomy may be successful, but it is difficult to predict which patients will be helped by this operation. Finally, severe rest pain or gangrene may make amputation necessary.

DIABETIC PERIPHERAL VASCULAR DISEASE

There is a strong association between diabetes mellitus and vascular disease. The reason for this is not entirely understood but changes in plasma lipids, platelet stickiness and vascular permeability have been suggested. An important additional factor in the diabetic is neuropathy and necrosis is particularly liable to occur over pressure points such as the heel.

Clinical features are those of atherosclerotic vascular disease often developing at a relatively young age. Infection with ensuing gangrene is liable to occur and may be difficult to treat. Diabetic atherosclerotic disease is usually progressive and amputation often necessary.

Treatment consists of rest, the best possible control of the diabetes and keeping the ulcerated areas clean with systemic antibiotics and local applications.

BUERGER'S DISEASE

Buerger's disease is very rare. It occurs almost exclusively in men, usually starts between the age of 25 and 45, and is associated with heavy smoking. The lesions begin in the small arteries in the feet and lead to progressive obliteration from the periphery of the arteries of the lower limbs. Involvement of arteries in the arms and elsewhere is very rare.

Clinical Features. The disease usually starts in the foot with recurrent arterial thromboses. In addition, superficial venous thrombophlebitis develops in the legs and sometimes in the arms. The disease is slowly progressive.

Treatment. Treatment consists of care of the extremities, giving vasodilator drugs, and avoiding tobacco. Anticoagulants should be used for acute thrombophlebitis. Sympathectomy may produce prolonged relief of symptoms, particularly in the earlier stages of the disease. Amputation may be necessary in advanced cases.

ACUTE ARTERIAL OCCLUSION

Acute arterial occlusion may be caused by an embolus arising from the left side of the heart, usually in a patient with mitral stenosis or subacute infective endocarditis. Mural thrombi overlying infarcted areas may similarly become detached. Alternatively, thrombosis on an atheromatous plaque may occur *in situ* as a complication of atheromatous obliterative arterial disease.

Clinical Features. The onset is sudden with severe pain, pallor, coldness, loss of sensation, and weakness in the affected limb. The arterial pulses disappear below the level of the obstruction.

(a) The patient and the affected limb should be kept at room temperature.
(b) Heparin 10 000 units should be given intravenously and anticoagulation continued in the usual way (see p. 225).
(c) There is some evidence that 500 ml of dextran 40 solution given over 6 hours daily is helpful.
(d) Analgesics will probably be required.

A careful watch should be kept for the appearance of gangrene; amputation may sometimes be necessary. When obstruction is due to an embolism, embolectomy as soon as possible is the treatment of choice and an early surgical opinion should be sought.

RAYNAUD'S SYNDROME

This is produced by spasm of the digital arteries. It may be the result of a variety of causes:

(1) *Idiopathic Raynaud's disease*, believed to represent hypersensitivity of the digital vessels to cold and responsible for about 50% of cases.
(2) *Autoimmune disorders*, especially systemic lupus erythematosis and scleroderma.
(3) *Occupational* in butchers, fishmongers, and people handling vibrating tools.
(4) *Other arterial diseases*, atheroma, Buerger's disease.
(5) *Blood disorders*, polycythaemia vera, haemolytic anaemias.
(6) *Thoracic outlet syndromes*, cervical ribs, prefixed plexus.
(7) *Diseases of the nervous system*, syringomyelia.
(8) *Phaeochromocytoma.*
(9) *Drugs* including β blockers and methysergide.

Clinical Features. The idiopathic form is common in young women. On exposure to cold the change begins distally and spreads proximally. First the fingertips, then the fingers and even the hands become cold and white, and sensation and fine movement are impaired. The radial pulse however remains palpable. Recovery is in the reverse order, and causes painful paraesthesiae in the affected areas, which become patchily discoloured red, white and blue. It may be followed by reflex vasodilatation, so that the hand is red and warm, and the pulse bounding. Rarely the nose and more frequently the toes may be affected. Early in the disease there is no evidence of permanent changes but after some years gangrene of the tips of the fingers may develop.

Treatment. The patient should avoid exposing the hands to cold and the whole body should be kept as warm as possible to promote reflex vasodilation. Vasodilator drugs are sometimes useful and tolazoline, 25mg t.d.s., or nifedipine 10mg t.d.s. can be tried. Sympathectomy is indicated if medical treatment fails but relapse usually occurs after a few years.

ACROCYANOSIS

This is a condition of unknown cause found in young people, characterised by painless cyanosis of the hands and feet, sometimes with swelling. The condition is harmless and treatment is unsatisfactory.

VENOUS THROMBOSIS

DEEP VEIN THROMBOSIS (Phlebothrombosis)

There are many factors which may lead to a deep vein thrombosis and the positive risk factors are given below:

Immobility—particularly after abdominal or hip operations;
Postoperative sepsis;
Obesity—diabetes mellitus;
Increasing age;
Myocardial infarction or other thrombotic disease;
Heart failure;
Pregnancy or oral contraceptives;
Occult malignant disease (particularly carcinoma of the pancreas or bronchus);
Varicose veins;
Intravenous cannulae;
Polycythaemia/Buerger's disease/Behçet's disease;
Occasionally they occur for no apparent reason.

Studies using phlebography and measuring the uptake by the thrombus of ^{125}I-labelled fibrinogen suggest that up to 35% of patients have venous thrombosis after major surgery, although nearly all of them show no clinical evidence of disease. The danger of a deep vein thrombosis is that a portion of the clot may break off and be swept through the right side of the heart to the lungs to produce a pulmonary infarct (p. 224). This occurs in about 10% of patients with deep vein thrombosis. It is unlikely if the thrombosis is confined to the calf, but becomes more frequent with extension to the popliteal or femoral veins.

Clinical Features. The symptoms of a deep vein thrombosis are often slight. There may be a slight rise of temperature with a leucocytosis and the patient may complain of pain in the calf. Examination will show perhaps slight swelling of the ankle, tenderness of the calf and dorsiflexion of the ankle will be painful (Homans' sign). Sometimes a pulmonary embolism will be the first indication of a deep vein thrombosis. With obstruction of the main venous return from the leg, the whole leg will become swollen and occasionally gangrene of the toes develops, thus leading to an erroneous diagnosis of arterial block.

Physical signs may be unreliable, but the following methods of investigation are available:

(1) *Venography*. This is the most accurate method of diagnosis. It is however, moderately invasive and takes time. It is useful when the diagnosis is in doubt.
(2) *Injection of* ^{125}*I-labelled Fibrinogen* which becomes incorporated in the thrombus and can thus be detected. It is easy to perform and useful for screening.
(3) *Doppler Ultrasound Effect*. This measures the rate of flow of blood in the femoral vein on compressing the calf. It will only detect thrombosis in the popliteal, femoral or iliac veins.

Treatment. The patient and the affected limbs should be rested and slightly elevated. Active movements are best avoided in the early stages in case a clot is dislodged, but gentle passive movements are allowed to prevent stagnation of blood. As soon as the acute stage has settled a crepe bandage should be firmly applied to the leg and the patient should be encouraged to walk.

Anticoagulants should be given (p. 225) and continued for four weeks after the patient has become ambulant. Surgery is required only for extensive thrombosis or repeated pulmonary emboli which have failed to respond to anticoagulants. Thrombectomy can be carried out after the extent of the obstruction has been defined by venography. With repeated pulmonary emboli the inferior vena cava or femoral vein should be ligated or plicated as a life-saving manoeuvre.

In a number of patients some swelling of the lower leg persists and is particularly noticeable towards the end of the day. Elastic stockings which are put on before getting up help to reduce oedema.

Prevention. It would obviously be most satisfactory to prevent the development of phlebothrombosis, particularly in patients at risk following surgery. Intermittent stimulation or compression of calf muscles during operation may be helpful. Although early leg exercises in the postoperative period are widely used, there is no good evidence that they are effective. There is now considerable evidence that heparin given subcutaneously in doses of 5000 units half an hour before operation and then 12-hourly for the next seven days reduces the incidence of deep vein thrombosis and pulmonary emboli and it should be given to those showing positive risk factors.

Superficial Vein Thrombosis

Thrombosis may occur in the superficial veins, particularly of the lower limbs. The vein becomes painful and on examination the thrombosis can be palpated as a tender cord. The skin over the thrombosis may be red. Superficial vein thrombosis may occur as a result of injury or as a complication of varicose veins. It should be remembered that it occasionally indicates a deep-seated neoplasm. There is little risk of pulmonary embolism.

Treatment consists of firmly bandaging the limb and allowing the patient to walk as much as is comfortable. Phenylbutazone in doses of 100 mg three times daily for a few days will often reduce inflammation and discomfort.

Iliac Vein Compression

Obstruction of the venous return from the lower limbs by the right common iliac artery is an occasional cause of swollen legs. Usually in such patients the left common iliac vein is compressed (68 %) but the lower end of the inferior vena cava (16 %) and the right common iliac vein (16 %) may also be affected. The condition is twice as common in women as in men, and is believed to be a major factor in the occurrence of acute venous thrombosis after childbirth or surgical operations (p. 232), which may be followed by life-long oedema of one or both limbs. In other patients no such acute episode is recorded, the patient presenting with aching and swelling of one or both legs.

Swelling occurs three times as commonly on the left as the right, and the whole of the affected limb is swollen. Pain in the limb on exertion is the rule, and has been termed '*venous claudication*'. It differs from arterial claudication (p. 228) in that it takes longer to appear and is less quickly relieved by rest. It usually affects the calf, but may spread to the thigh. Sometimes there are recurrent episodes of thrombosis, and chronic varicose ulcers may occur.

The diagnosis is proved by combined phlebography and arteriography, and treatment is surgical.

Thrombosis of the Axillary Vein

This occasionally occurs in young, fit adults, particularly following trauma to the vein such as produced by carrying a rucksack. There is a swelling of the arm and the axillary vein is tender. An embolism is rare and the arm should be rested until the condition subsides.

FURTHER READING

Cantwell, J. D., *Modern Cardiology*, Butterworth, London, 1977.

Joint working party of the Royal College of Physicians of London and the British Cardiac Society, Prevention of Coronary Heart Disease, *J. Roy. Coll. Physicians*, **10**, 214 (1976).

Krikler, D. M. and Goodwin, J. F., (eds.), *Cardiac Arrhythmias*, W. B. Saunders, Philadelphia and London, 1978.

Oram, S., *Clinical Heart Disease*, 2nd edition, Heinemann, London, 1981.

Schamroth, L., *Introduction to Electrocardiography*, 6th edition, Blackwell, Oxford, 1982.

CHAPTER 5

THE RESPIRATORY SYSTEM

ANATOMY AND DEFENCE MECHANISMS

The upper respiratory tract consists of the nose, nasopharynx and larynx and the lower respiratory tract comprises the trachea, bronchi and lungs. The air passages are lined with ciliated epithelium down as far as the respiratory bronchioles, and the rich blood supply of the lining membrane enables it to warm and moisten the inspired air. A thin film of mucus is secreted by the submucosal glands in the larger bronchi and by the goblet cells extending throughout the respiratory tract. It is kept continuously moving away from the lungs by the sweeping action of the cilia—the so called ciliary escalator—and this is a most effective filter in removing particulate matter from the air before it reaches the lungs. The other local defence mechanisms include the cough reflex, whereby foreign matter is expelled explosively (p. 244); the synthesis of immunoglobulin (secretory IgA) by plasma cells in the submucosa and its passage through the epithelium, together with the presence of alveolar macrophages, provide mechanisms for destruction and phagocytosis of infecting agents and particulate matter. Disease states occur when any of these defence mechanisms are deficient. For example, patients with the *immotile cilia syndrome* (*Kartagener's syndrome*) (p. 265) invariably suffer from rhinitis, sinusitis and chronic bronchitis, and recurrent respiratory infections occur in patients with *IgA deficiency*.

ANATOMY OF THE BRONCHIAL TREE

The bronchi to the separate lobes of each lung arise from the main bronchi on their respective sides. The primary subdivision of the lobar bronchi, together with the segments of lung which they supply, form the *bronchopulmonary* segments. The segmental bronchi are regarded as the first generation of the subdivisions of the intrapulmonary bronchi which continue to divide and subdivide to produce some 15–20 generations. By definition, once cartilage is lost from the wall, the airway becomes a *bronchiole*. The *terminal bronchiole* is the last airway proximal to the *respiratory bronchioles* which in turn open directly into the *alveoli*. The alveoli are lined by type I and type II pneumocytes, the latter probably being responsible for production of surfactant which is of importance in lowering surface tension of the alveoli and terminal airways.

The pulmonary and the bronchial arteries follow the pattern of the branching airways, the former supplying the alveoli and the latter the bronchi and bronchioles. Blood from lung tissue and the airways drains into the pulmonary veins which enter directly into the left atrium. The bronchial veins drain blood from the proximal bronchi only, as well as the hilar structures, and enter the azygous veins. Thus, an anastomosis between systemic and pulmonary circulation occurs in the lungs.

Lymphatics exist in the connective tissue of the lung, in the pleura and in the interlobular septa which occur at the lung edges. Oedema or prominence of the lymphatics of the septa (such as occurs for example in mitral stenosis, left ventricular failure, pneumoconiosis and lymphangitis carcinomatosa) produce *Kerley B* (septal) lines on the chest X-ray; they are short (less than 2 cm), horizontal lines extending from the pleural surface and are most marked at the lung bases. Lymphatic drainage of the lungs mostly follows the bronchovascular pattern, but some lymphatic vessels course irregularly through the lungs, and when prominent from distension or infiltration produce *Kerley A* lines; these are more central, not connected to the pleura and are some 2–4 cm in length.

Surface Markings of the Lobes

The upper and lower lobes of the left lung are separated by the oblique fissure. The right lung is composed of three lobes and the right oblique fissure separates the lower lobe from the upper and middle lobes. On each side the oblique fissure extends from the anterior end of the 6th rib and runs upwards and backwards round the chest wall, usually along the line of the 5th or 6th rib to the vertebral column. Its surface marking roughly corresponds to the position of the medial border of the scapula when the hand is placed on top of the head. The horizontal fissure separates the right upper lobe from the middle lobe. Its surface marking starts at the fourth right costal cartilage and runs horizontally around the chest to join the oblique fissure in the midaxillary line. The segment of the left lung which occupies the position corresponding to the middle lobe is called the lingula, and it is part of the left upper lobe.

The Bronchopulmonary Segments (Fig. 5.1)

A proper knowledge of the anatomy of the bronchopulmonary segments is essential to the understanding of the localisation and spread of many diseases of the lung. Many lung infections spread via the bronchi and the distribution of the infection is determined by the segments which these bronchi supply. The segments of each lobe are named after their corresponding bronchi.

The Upper Lobes. The right upper lobe bronchus divides almost immediately into anterior, apical, and posterior branches. The anterior

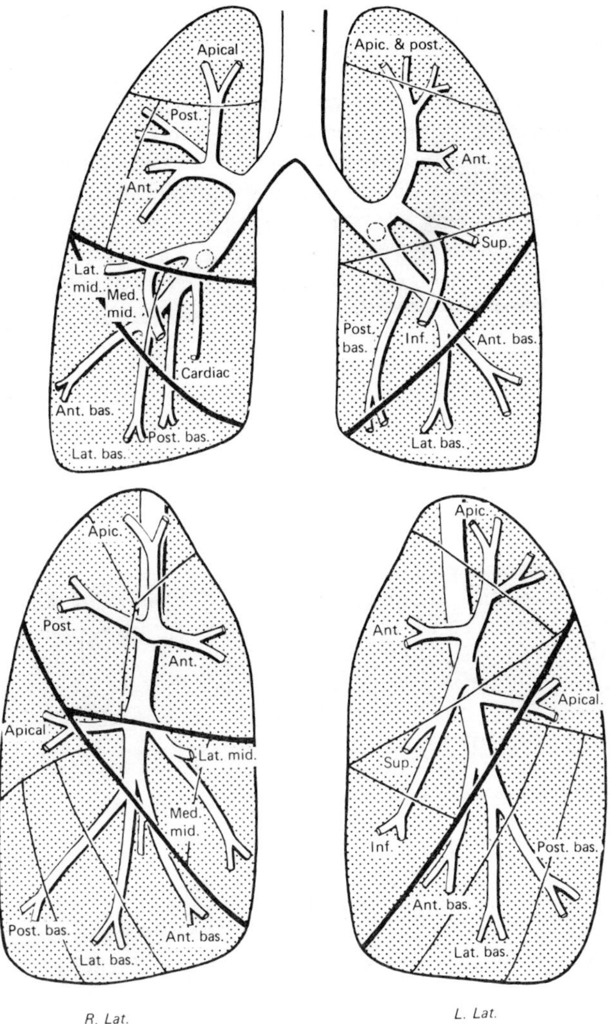

Fig. 5.1 The bronchopulmonary segments.

and posterior bronchi have axillary branches which supply the lateral part of the upper lobe.

The left upper lobe bronchus quickly gives origin to the lingula bronchus which runs downwards and forwards, subdividing into superior and inferior branches. It then gives off branches to the anterior, apical, and posterior segments of the lobe, but differs from the right side in having a common apico-posterior bronchus.

The Middle Lobe bronchus is only present on the right side and runs downwards and forwards dividing into lateral and medial divisions.

The Lower Lobes. The right lower lobe bronchus gives off an apical branch which arises opposite the middle lobe bronchus and runs backwards to the apical segment of the lower lobe. The basal bronchi consist of anterior, lateral, and posterior branches and, in addition, a medial basal (or cardiac) bronchus supplies a small segment in the medial aspect of the lower lobe.

On the left side the arrangement is similar, but the medial basal is usually insignificant or absent.

LOOKING AT THE CHEST X-RAY

A chest radiograph is an integral part of the examination of a patient suspected of lung disease, and indeed in many conditions radiological abnormalities are present long before the development of physical signs.

The film should be examined in a systematic, rather than haphazard, manner. Firstly it should be ensured that the film has been taken straight by observing that the medial ends of the clavicles are equidistant from the centre of the spine. Undue rotation can produce abnormal looking appearances of the mediastinum and the hilar shadows, as well as gross differences in the opaqueness of the two lungs. The trachea should be central; displacement may be due to rotation, shift of the mediastinum (see palpation, p. 250) or due to a superior mediastinal swelling (p. 317). The diaphragms should next be examined; flattening of the diaphragms occurs with over-inflated lungs and undue elevation of a diaphragm may be due to diminished lung volume on that side, to diaphragmatic paralysis or be due to pathology below the diaphragm. The right diaphragm is normally higher than the left and the costophrenic angle should be clear and at an acute angle, filling-in being due to fluid or pleural thickening. The lung fields are then examined by comparing one side with another; the apices of the lungs above the clavicles are first compared and then coming down the chest X-ray and using the anterior ends of the ribs as markers one interspace is compared with the other on the opposite side. In this way small focal lesions can be detected. In addition, the pulmonary vascular markings should be examined and an assessment made as to whether there is any diffuse shadowing in addition to the normal markings. The position of the horizontal fissure should be noted. The hilar regions should be examined; enlargement may be due to a prominent pulmonary artery, pathological enlargement of the pulmonary artery, enlarged lymph glands or hilar mass. Starting with the first ribs, and comparing one side with another, both the posterior and anterior parts of the ribs should be examined for abnormalities. A lateral chest X-ray will be necessary for full interpretation of a lesion and for correct anatomical localisation (see Bronchopulmonary Segments p. 236), and in addition a lateral film is essential for a suspected lesion in the left lower lobe as it may be obscured in the straight X-ray by the heart shadow.

Tomograms may give additional information by defining lesions and cavitation more exactly and by demonstrating narrowing of major bronchi. Both A-P and lateral tomograms may be undertaken.

CT scan, when available, is more likely to pick up small intrapulmonary or pleural lesions (such as secondary deposits) not shown by conventional radiology. It is also of particular value in demonstrating abnormalities in the mediastinum.

RESPIRATORY FUNCTION TESTS

Tests of respiratory function aid the clinical assessment of a patient, for they provide a quantitative method of estimating the respiratory ability. They may be helpful, for example, when thoracic surgery is being considered and serial recordings are of value, both in assessing the effectiveness of a form of treatment and in following the progress of a disease. In addition, they may indicate the nature of underlying disease, either causing an *obstructive ventilatory defect*, as in asthma, chronic bronchitis and emphysema, or a *restrictive ventilatory defect*, as in fibrosing alveolitis and kyphoscoliosis.

Some tests are easy to perform and others require skill and complicated apparatus. Each has its limitations and it may be necessary to test several aspects of function before reaching a satisfactory conclusion. It is proposed to discuss the principles involved, rather than the technical aspects.

TESTS OF VENTILATION

Figure 5.2, which is self-explanatory, illustrates the various subdivisions of the lung volume. The *tidal volume* is the volume of air breathed in or out at rest. The *minute volume* is the product of the tidal volume and the number of breaths per minute. They provide useful information in suspected cases of hypoventilation, as with respiratory depression from drugs. They are measured by the patient breathing through a small portable instrument called a 'Wright's respirometer', which can also be connected to an endotracheal or tracheostomy tube.

The *functional residual capacity* (FRC) is the resting expiratory volume of the lung and the *total lung capacity* (TLC) is the maximum volume of gas in the lungs after a full inhalation. A full unhurried

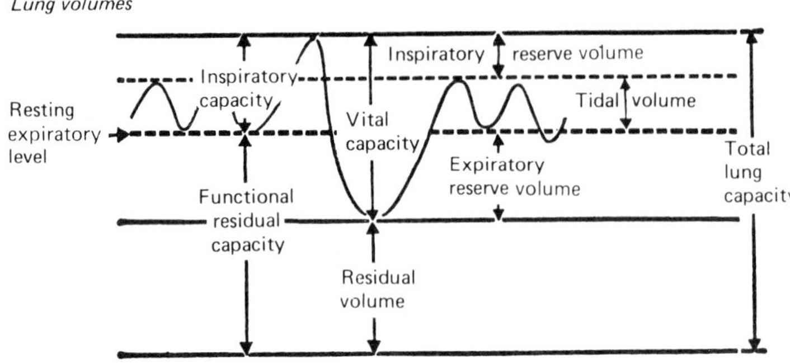

Fig. 5.2 Tests of pulmonary ventilation.

exhalation from the TLC gives the *vital capacity* (VC). A reduction in all of these volumes indicates a *restrictive ventilatory defect*, and is a feature of many disorders of the lung, pleura and thoracic cage where there is stiffness, deformity or weakness.

The residual volume (RV) is the volume of gas remaining in the lungs after a full unhurried exhalation and its proportion of the TLC is fairly constant. Up to the age of 30 years, it forms 20–25 % of the TLC but it then increases with age. The RV/TLC ratio is abnormally increased in those diseases where there is airflow obstruction, and consequently over-inflation of the lungs, as in asthma and emphysema. However, neither RV nor TLC can be measured by normal spirometry but require body plethysmography or helium dilution techniques for their estimation. Airflow obstruction is best measured when the vital capacity is determined with reference to speed. For this, the robust and portable 'Vitalograph' can be used. The *forced vital capacity* (FVC) is the volume of a maximal exhalation carried out as rapidly as possible following a maximal inhalation to TLC. The volume expired during the first second of the FVC is termed the *forced expiratory volume in one second* ($FEV_{1.0}$). The percentage of the FVC expired during this first second is termed the *Forced Expiratory Ratio* (FER) and is normally 75 % or more. A reduction in both the $FEV_{1.0}$ and FER occurs in those disorders with an *obstructive ventilatory defect* (see Fig. 5.3). Improvement of the $FEV_{1.0}$ occurring five minutes after an inhalation of a bronchodilator, such as salbutamol, helps to distinguish a reversible airflow obstruction (asthma) from an irreversible airflow obstruction (as in emphysema or chronic bronchitis). Alternatively, in a patient with normal spirometry but suspected of having asthma, an exercise test can be performed to demonstrate the development of airways obstruction.

The *peak expiratory flow rate* is the maximal expiratory flow rate

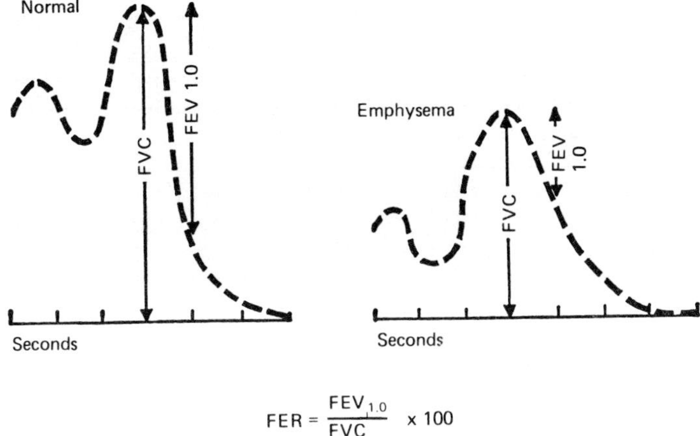

$$FER = \frac{FEV_{1.0}}{FVC} \times 100$$

Fig. 5.3 Timed volume studies.

achieved during a maximal forced exhalation. It is measured with a 'Wright's peak flow meter' which is small, portable and easy to operate. Although measuring rather different aspects of airflow, both the *peak flow* and $FEV_{1.0}$ are reduced in the diseases causing airflow obstruction.

All the measurements described are determined by the patients's race, sex, age and size, being larger in males than females, increasing until adulthood, then declining with age. The predicted values for any individual have a large normal range. For example, for a man of 39 years, who is 1.79 m (5 ft 11 in) tall, the normal ranges are:

Forced Expiratory Volume in one second	($FEV_{1.0}$)	2.9–4.7 litres
Forced Vital Capacity	(FVC)	4.0–6.0 litres
Forced Expiratory Ratio	(FER)	63–92%
Peak Expiratory Flow Rate	(PEFR)	482–722 litres/minute

BLOOD GAS ANALYSIS

Measurements of the oxygen and the carbon dioxide tensions in arterial blood can be used to assess the efficiency of alveolar ventilation and also the matching between ventilation and perfusion of the lung. Normally the arterial partial pressure for CO_2 ($Paco_2$) is 40 mmHg (5.3 kPa) with a range of 36–44 mmHg (4.8–5.9 kPa) and for O_2 (Pao_2) is 90 mmHg (12 kPa) with a range of 70–110 mmHg (9.3–14.6 kPa).

Alveolar hypoventilation leads to arterial oxygen desaturation and retention of carbon dioxide in the blood with a consequent rise in its arterial partial pressure ($Paco_2$) and the development of a respiratory acidosis. This state of affairs may be **precipitated** by any complication producing severe impairment of ventilation, such as poliomyelitis or respiratory depression from drugs, or it may be **persistent** in patients with chronic chest disease.

'Mismatching' between ventilation and perfusion occurs when there is filling of the air space (as in pulmonary oedema or pneumonia), with infiltration of the lung or with emphysema. In these conditions there are areas of the lung in which perfusion continues but ventilation is prevented. This effectively results in venous blood passing straight through the lung without being oxygenated, as in intracardiac right to left shunts. There is a resulting reduction in the partial pressure of arterial oxygen (Pao_2) but as carbon dioxide is about twenty times more diffusable than oxygen, unless the mismatch is very severe there is no increase in the partial pressure of carbon dioxide ($Paco_2$). Indeed, hyperventilation is often present at rest, which may produce an increased excretion of carbon dioxide by the lungs with a reduction in the $Paco_2$, and the development of a respiratory alkalosis. At rest, the reduction of the partial pressure of arterial oxygen (Pao_2) depends on the severity of the condition, and the compensatory hyperventilation, but after exertion it falls sharply with a further reduction $Paco_2$.

In chronic hypoxic states, the respiratory centre depends on the hypoxia for its stimulation. Relief of severe hypoxia by oxygen therapy is an important part of the treatment of cor pulmonale for example, but this may release the respiratory centre from its 'hypoxic drive' and depress ventilation. The patient may thus be relieved from hypoxia, but the additional reduction in alveolar ventilation leads to further retention of carbon dioxide. Mental disturbance usually occurs when the arterial pH is less than 7.2 or the $Paco_2$ higher than 100 mmHg (13.3 kPa), and coma usually supervenes with arterial levels of pH below 7.1 or the $Paco_2$ above 120 mmHg (16.0 kPa). The serial estimation of the $Paco_2$ from arterial puncture or the mixed venous blood by the Campbell rebreathing technique are thus valuable in ensuring the proper control of oxygen administration in such patients.

GAS TRANSFER

In certain conditions the predominant physiological defect is one of impairment of transfer of gases between the pulmonary capillaries and the alveoli. This occurs in such diseases as fibrosing alveolitis, asbestosis, infiltration of the lungs with sarcoid granulomata, carcinomatosis lymphangitis, and pulmonary oedema. The abnormality can be determined by measuring the *transfer factor* of the lung for carbon monoxide (TLCO). There are various methods for its measurements, but the most usual is to measure the uptake of carbon monoxide from the lung after a single full inhalation to TLC of a gas mixture containing a low concentration of carbon monoxide. In the above conditions, hyperventilation may be present even at rest, and the impaired gas transfer may be reflected in a lowered $Pa\text{O}_2$ and a normal or low $Pa\text{CO}_2$, these changes becoming more marked after exertion (see 'mismatching' between ventilation/perfusion in Blood Gas Analysis above). In the conditions described, in addition to the blood gas changes and reduced TLCO, if the pathological changes are sufficiently advanced, then there will be a restrictive ventilatory defect with reduction in FVC and FEV_1, but the FER and the PEFR are usually normal. In contrast, although the TLCO is lowered in emphysema, because the area of the alveoli available for gas transfer is reduced due to destructive dilatation of the alveoli, the FER and the PEFR are also reduced indicating the associated airflow obstruction.

THE WORK OF BREATHING AND COMPLIANCE

The measurement of the work involved in breathing requires the summation of various complicated physiological processes. These include such aspects as the oxygen requirements of the respiratory muscles and the mechanical effects of overcoming airway resistance, tissue resistance and lung elasticity. Most of these are difficult to test but lung elasticity, or *lung compliance*, can be measured fairly simply by recording the negative intrathoracic pressure through an oesophageal catheter, at the same time as ventilatory volumes. The lung compliance is the inspiratory volume which is produced by a change in negative pressure 1 cmH_2O and in the normal is 0.09 to 0.33 litres/cmH_2O.

The normal values have been related to the functional residual capacity (FRC) as they are influenced by the size of the lungs. The compliance is *reduced* in conditions which produce abnormally stiff lungs. Examples of such conditions are pulmonary venous congestion from *mitral stenosis* or *chronic left ventricular failure*, and *diffuse fibrotic or infiltrative lesions of the lungs*.

FLOW VOLUME CURVES

Decreases in flow rate at different lung volumes are easily seen when flow is displayed against volume in a maximal expiratory flow-volume loop; this is constructed by use of a spirometer or an integrated pneumotachograph. From a point soon after peak flow the configuration is relatively independent of effort. Flow rates at low lung volumes may reflect particularly the function of smaller airways and it has been suggested that they may be used to detect early chronic bronchitis. With the addition of a maximal inspiratory phase the shape of the flow-volume loop is useful in evaluating obstruction in large airways. Any fixed obstruction cuts off peak inspiratory and expiratory flows; a variable obstruction in an extrathoracic airway predominantly affects inspiratory flow while in an intrathoracic airway it predominantly affects expiratory flow.

LUNG SCANNING

Scanning of the lung is of value in the diagnosis of pulmonary embolism. Perfusion scan is performed after the intravenous injection of macroaggregates of albumin labelled with radioactive technetium and ventilation scan after the inhalation of radioactive krypton. With pulmonary embolism and a normal chest X-ray there are segmental defects of perfusion with a normal ventilation scan. With lung disease defects of perfusion and ventilation are matched in the areas involved.

SYMPTOMS AND SIGNS OF LUNG DISEASE

Types of Cough and Sputum

A forced expiration against a closed glottis produces a high pressure in the trachea and bronchi and the sudden opening of the glottis is followed by the explosive discharge of air, producing the characteristic barking noise of a cough. This removes secretions and foreign particles from the air passages. The cough reflex is stimulated by irritation of nerve endings in the larynx, trachea, bronchi, and even the pleura.

In the early stages of respiratory tract infections, inflammatory swelling of the mucous membrane causes the cough to be dry and unproductive. With the later development of inflammatory exudate, the cough produces clear or whitish, sticky sputum. In *whooping cough* the exudate is particularly tenacious. The patient gives a series of quickly repeated coughs during one expiratory movement in an effort to dislodge the sputum, and this is followed by an inspiratory 'whoop' through a partially closed glottis. The cough typically occurs in paroxysms and is not always associated with a 'whoop'.

A yellow or greenish colour to the sputum signifies that it is purulent. This occurs with secondary pyogenic infection during respiratory tract infections. Purulent sputum is also expectorated in patients with *bronchiectasis*. With change of posture when waking in the morning, the patient coughs up the infected sputum which has collected in the dilated bronchi during the night. The quantity of sputum depends on the degree of infection and extent of the disease. It may amount to several ounces per day and is sometimes very offensive in smell due to the action of putrefactive bacteria. Purulent sputum tends to be more fluid than other types as enzymes from the pus cells liquefy the mucus.

The cough in *bronchial carcinoma* is at first persistent and unproductive due to invasion of the mucous membrane. When partial bronchial obstruction develops distal infection produces mucopurulent sputum which may be blood-stained.

In *pulmonary tuberculosis* there may be no sputum in the earlier stages of the disease. If sputum is produced it is clear or white and very sticky, so that it remains in separate lumps in the sputum pot (nummular sputum).

During the early stages of *pneumococcal pneumonia* the patient may cough up very viscid sputum tinged with blood which gives it a rusty colour.

Cardiac asthma (p. 140) is due to acute pulmonary venous engorgement. In extreme cases oedema fluid exudes into the alveoli and the attack is associated with the expectoration of a large quantity of clear, frothy sputum, which is sometimes pinkish in colour due to the presence of red cells. In *bronchial asthma*, however, the sputum consists of firm, whitish pellets, which can sometimes be unravelled in water into spiral ribbons (Curschmann's spirals). These represent casts of the bronchial tubes in which they have formed.

Haemoptysis

The coughing up of blood must be distinguished from haematemesis, the vomiting of blood.

(1) Blood from the lungs is usually bright red, frothy, and mixed with sputum. That from the stomach is usually dark in colour, having been altered to acid-haematin by the hydrochloric acid; it is often mixed with food.
(2) Many patients can state definitely whether the blood has been coughed up or vomited.
(3) Often there will be symptoms or signs which point to disease of the lungs or the alimentary tract.

The common causes of haemoptysis are:

Respiratory	*Cardiovascular*
Carcinoma of the bronchus	Pulmonary infarct
Pulmonary tuberculosis	Mitral stenosis
Acute or chronic bronchitis	Acute left ventricular failure
Bronchiectasis	
Lung abscess	

Although there may be an isolated haemoptysis in carcinoma of the bronchus, characteristically the ulcerated area leads to repeated daily blood-streaking of sputum. An early lesion of pulmonary tuberculosis sometimes presents with an haemoptysis of an ounce or more of bright-red blood, not associated with sputum. Colonisation of an old tuberculous cavity with *Aspergillus fumigatus* to form a mycetoma may produce persistent or profuse haemoptysis. Blood-streaking of sputum from inflamed bronchial mucosa is very common in respiratory tract infections and ulceration of bronchial arteries in bronchiectasis sometimes produces severe haemoptysis. Haemoptysis may be the first evidence of pulmonary embolism in a woman who is pregnant or taking the contraceptive pill.

Every patient presenting with haemoptysis should be fully examined and have a chest radiograph, particularly to exclude bronchial carcinoma and pulmonary tuberculosis. A normal chest radiograph does not exclude a bronchial carcinoma, and ideally bronchoscopy should be performed to exclude this possibility. However, unless there are good clinical grounds for suspecting a bronchial carcinoma, bronchoscopy is often not justified at this stage and it is sufficient for the patient to be followed up carefully with fairly frequent chest radiographs. Cytological examination of the sputum for malignant cells can also be carried out. The majority of such patients do not develop any serious disease and in nearly half of all patients presenting with a small haemoptysis, no definite cause is found.

Pain in the Chest

Acute pleuritic pain from pleurisy is sharp and stabbing in character and aggravated by coughing or deep breathing. The pain is usually localised to the site of the pleurisy, but it may be referred to the abdominal wall and be confused with an acute abdominal condition. With diaphragmatic pleurisy the pain is referred to the tip of the shoulder, as the skin in this situation has the same sensory nerve supply (C3, 4, and 5).

Lesions of the chest wall, such as fractures or secondary deposits in the ribs, may cause severe local pain and tenderness. The aetiology of *Tietze*'s *syndrome* is uncertain, but it is a painful condition, usually involving one of the upper costochondral junctions. Chest pain may also be referred from the thoracic spine. The seventh cervical nerve supplies the pectoralis major and pain referred from this root may be felt in that muscle as well as in the arm. Intrathoracic structures, other than the lungs, can produce pain in the chest, common examples being pain from ischaemic heart disease and from oesophageal spasm and hiatus hernia.

Types of Respiration

Respiration in men is mainly diaphragmatic in type and in women it is mostly costal. Inspiration is a more powerful muscular movement than expiration, the latter depending on elastic recoil of the lungs and relaxation of the diaphragm and intercostal muscles. Obstruction to the large air passages produces a prolonged inspiratory phase with stridor, as inspiration is the more powerful movement. The bronchi and bronchioles normally dilate on inspiration and narrow on expiration, so that obstruction of the airways, as in asthma, leads to prolonged, wheezy, and difficult expiration.

Respirations in *pneumonia and pleurisy* are rapid and shallow, the inspirations being abruptly stopped, often with an audible grunt, as soon as the pleuritic pain is felt. Normally, expiration immediately follows inspiration and there is then a pause before the next breath. In pneumonia this rhythm is sometimes reversed, the pause taking place between inspiration and expiration.

The acidosis which occurs with uraemia and diabetic ketosis causes very deep breathing, known as *air hunger*, or *Kussmaul's breathing*, due to marked stimulation of the respiratory centre. *Cheyne–Stokes breathing* is a characteristic respiratory arrhythmia occurring when the respiratory centre has a diminished sensitivity to carbon dioxide in the blood. The amplitude of respiration progressively deepens until a maximum is reached and then diminishes until there is a period of apnoea. During the period of apnoea, the carbon dioxide in the blood rises to a level high enough to stimulate the respiratory centre. There is then an exaggerated response producing the period of hyperventilation, which washes the carbon dioxide out of the blood until the stimulus to respiration is removed and apnoea occurs. The whole cycle lasts two or three minutes and is then repeated. This type of breathing occurs with left ventricular failure and with various cerebral causes of depression of the respiratory centre.

Clubbing of the Fingers

The earliest change is a filling in of the angle between the skin at the base of the nail and the base of the nail itself, the skin becoming swollen and shiny. The base of the nail may be fluctuant. Later increased curvature of the nails occurs and finally the pulps of the fingers become enlarged. Clubbing has many unrelated causes:

Cardiovascular

(1) Infective endocarditis.
(2) Cyanotic congenital heart disease.
(3) Arteriovenous communications in the arm.

Respiratory

(1) Carcinoma of the bronchus.
(2) Chronic suppuration in the chest, such as bronchiectasis, lung abscess, and empyema.
(3) Chronic fibrosing alveolitis.

At times clubbing is familial and there is no underlying disease. More

Table 5.1 Examination of the chest

Condition	*Inspection*	*Palpation*	*Percussion*	*Auscultation*
*CONSOLIDATION	Respiration rate increased. Movement decreased on affected side.	Mediastinum central. TVF increased over consolidation.	Dullness over consolidation.	Bronchial breathing Bronchophony WP Late crackles. } Over consolidation.
ABSORPTION COLLAPSE	Movement diminished on affected side.	Mediastinum shifted to affected side. Absent TVF over collapsed segment.	Dullness over collapsed area.	Breath sounds diminished or absent. Voice sounds diminished or absent.
FIBROSIS	Flattening of the chest and diminished movement on affected side.	Mediastinum shifted to affected side. Increased TVF over fibrosis.	Dullness over fibrosis.	Bronchial breathing Bronchophony WP } Over fibrosis. Early coarse crackles due to concomitant bronchiectasis.

Condition	*Inspection*	*Palpation*	*Percussion*	*Auscultation*
FLUID	Movement diminished on affected side.	If large, mediastinum shifted to opposite side. TVF absent over fluid.	Stony dullness over fluid, the line tending to rise in the axilla with moderate effusions.	Absent breath sounds and voice sounds over fluid. Sometimes bronchial breathing, WP, and aegophony above upper level of fluid.
PNEUMOTHORAX	Movement diminished an affected side.	If large, mediastinum shifted to opposite side.	Normal or hyper-resonant. Diminished cardiac dullness of the left and liver dullness on right.	Breath sounds and voice sounds diminished or absent. Sometimes if large, bronchial breathing, WP, and positive coin sound.

* These signs are only heard over a considerable area of consolidation. With small patches of pneumonia, or when the pneumonic process has not reached the surface of the lung, signs may be scanty and are often confined to a small area of inspiratory crackles.

rarely it is associated with cirrhosis of the liver, steatorrhoea, or polyposis of the colon.

EXAMINATION OF THE CHEST (Table 5.1)

Inspection

(1) The General Contours

(a) *Kyphosis* and *kyphoscoliosis* may be developmental in origin. If gross, they may in later years give rise to severe impairment of lung function and heart failure. Abnormalities of spinal curvature may also occur secondary to intrathoracic disease.
(b) *Funnel-shaped depression of the sternum* (pectus excavatum) may occur in varying degrees. Deep depression may displace the heart to the left and lead to the erroneous diagnosis of cardiac enlargement.
(c) *Over-inflation of the lungs*, such as occurs with asthma and emphysema, leads to increase in the antero-posterior diameter of the chest and the shoulders are held high.
(d) *Unilateral flattening* of the chest occurs with long-standing pulmonary or pleural fibrosis.

(2) The Respiratory Movements

(a) The respiratory rate is increased in many conditions, including acute and chronic lung disease, cardiac failure, and anxiety. It is decreased with depression of the respiratory centre, as in narcotic poisoning and with various cerebral lesions.
(b) The accessory muscles of respiration may be used if there is severe respiratory distress, as in an asthmatic attack.
(c) Decreased movement on one side of the chest indicates disease of the lung or pleura of that side.
(d) The respiration may have a special character (see p. 246).

Palpation

The position of the mediastinum is assessed by determining the position of the apex beat and the trachea. Shift of the mediastinum towards the side of the lesion indicates shrinkage of the lung due to collapse or fibrosis. Displacement away from the lesion occurs with fluid or air in the pleural cavity. Displacement of the trachea alone is more likely with contraction of an upper lobe and shift of the apex beat alone in a lesion of a lower lobe.

Tactile vocal fremitus (*TVF*) is decreased with air or fluid in the pleural cavity and with pulmonary collapse. Increased tactile vocal fremitus occurs with conditions which also produce bronchial breathing.

Percussion

Normally the lungs are resonant to percussion and there are areas of dullness over the heart and liver. In emphysema and pneumothorax, hyper-resonance is sometimes found and cardiac and liver dullness are either diminished or absent. Impaired resonance is found over consolidated, collapsed or fibroid lung, or with pleural thickening. A flat, dull note is found over pleural fluid.

Auscultation

(1) The Breath Sounds

The breath sounds heard over the chest wall are in part the result of turbulence of airflow in the more peripheral airways together with a component of filtered and attenuated sound transmitted from the central airways.

The normal breath sounds are rustling, with a long inspiratory phase followed by a short expiratory phase. Over the lung roots the normal breath sounds take on a bronchial character. The breath sounds are diminished or absent with fluid or air in the pleural cavity and with impaired inflation of the lung, as in emphysema and collapse. In *bronchial breathing*, the breath sounds have a harsher quality and the expiratory phase is longer than the inspiratory, with a short gap between the two. Bronchial breathing is heard in the normal by listening with a stethoscope over the larynx or trachea. When bronchial breathing is heard over the lungs, it indicates a pathological process which is enhancing the transmission of the tracheal sound to the chest wall. It occurs with pneumonic consolidation, with fibroid lung (fibrosis plus bronchiectasis), and over a large cavity. It also occurs sometimes above the upper level of a pleural effusion and over a large pneumothorax, which acts as a resonating chamber. Bronchial breathing is always accompanied by whispering pectoriloquy and by increased TVF and bronchophony.

(2) The Voice Sounds

Normally, when the stethoscope is placed over a peripheral part of the lungs the spoken voice comes through in a modified form so that the consonants are blurred and indistinct; the whispered voice cannot be heard at all. Transmission of the spoken and whispered voice in an unmodified bronchial form (such as can be heard in the normal subject by listening over the trachea, though it is not necessarily as loud as this) is called respectively *bronchophony* and *whispering pectoriloquy* (WP). They occur under the same circumstances as bronchial breathing.

Aegophony is the peculiar nasal quality to the voice sounds heard above the upper level of an effusion.

(3) Wheezes (Rhonchi)

A wheeze is a musical squeak produced by air passing through an airway on the point of closure; vibrations of the wall act like the reed of a musical instrument. Polyphonic wheezing occurs in obstructive airways disease when expiration produces dynamic compression and sequential narrowing of the larger airways. Also in bronchitis and asthma wheezing occurs from narrowing of the airways from spasm, mucosal swelling or exudate and it is more marked on expiration. A bronchial neoplasm may produce a persistent monophonic wheeze.

(4) Crackles (Râles)

Crackles are popping noises due to explosive equalisations in air pressure which occur with the sudden opening of airways; they are most marked on inspiration. When associated with bronchitis or bronchiectasis they are low pitched and start early in the inspiration, with regular spacing between the crackles due to boluses of air passing through at regular intervals. With pulmonary oedema, pneumonia and fibrosing alveolitis the crackles are high pitched and start later in inspiration, as sequential opening of abnormal alveoli begins at this phase of respiration. Late crackles are heard at times at the lung bases in normal people who have been breathing quietly, when they are the result of partially deflated alveoli opening, but they should disappear after a few breaths.

DISEASES OF THE RESPIRATORY TRACTS

HAY FEVER AND PERENNIAL RHINITIS

These are allergic disorders characterised by bouts of sneezing, profuse watery nasal discharge, and smarting and watering of the eyes. Hay fever is due to sensitivity to grass and tree pollens and occurs during the months of April to August; a type I (anaphylactoid) hypersensitivity reaction occurs (see Asthma, p. 267). Perennial (vasomotor) rhinitis is due to sensitivity to a variety of allergens, such as house dust mite and may occur throughout the year. They may be associated with nasal polyps.

Treatment. *Hay fever*: A course of desensitisation injections may be given if skin testing confirms pollen sensitivity (see asthma p. 267). At least three yearly courses are required for a prolonged effect. *Antihistamines* are of considerable value during an attack. Usually one preparation can be found to suit the patient. Among the most valuable are chlorpheniramine, 4.0 mg twice daily or promethazine, 25 mg once or twice daily; the latter often causes troublesome drowsiness. *Sodium cromoglycate* or *beclomethasone* inhaled into the nose are both valuable in the treatment of hay fever. In severe cases where there is much disability monthly injections of a depot corticosteroid, such as methyl prednisolone, may be justified.

Perennial rhinitis: Precipitants such as house dust, pets, or feathers should be avoided. Skin testing is seldom helpful as the patient is often sensitive to many allergens. Antihistamines may be tried, but are not usually as successful as in hay fever. Good symptomatic relief may be obtained with *betamethasone* (0.1 %) nasal drops or with *beclomethasone* spray. Surgical treatment, e.g. submucous resection, should be avoided unless there is a very definite indication.

VIRUS INFECTIONS OF THE RESPIRATORY TRACT

The following are some of the viruses which affect the respiratory tract:

Rhinovirus
Adenovirus
Influenza virus
Parainfluenza virus
Respiratory syncytial virus
Coxsackie } Enteroviruses
ECHO }

All the above viruses have a nucleic acid content of RNA, with the exception of the adenovirus which contains DNA. An increasing number of serotypes are being identified with some of the above viruses; for example, there are more than 90 serotypes of the rhinovirus and 33 of the adenovirus. The enteroviruses, ECHO and Coxsackie A and B, also produce respiratory infections as well as other illnesses such as pericarditis and meningitis (pp. 222, 365). The influenza virus consists of types A, B and C; influenza A virus is the cause of pandemics and major epidemics, B virus causes smaller epidemics and is a less virulent type of infection and influenza C is principally endemic producing a fairly trivial respiratory infection. Major changes in the antigenic nature of influenza A virus occur about every ten to fifteen years, but minor changes may occur during the intervening years—the so-called 'antigenic drift'. For this reason effective vaccines against influenza should contain type B virus and the latest strain of type A. The development of effective vaccines against the other respiratory viruses has not been possible because of the large number of viruses involved and because there would be no cross-protection between the different serotypes in the same group.

Generally speaking each type of acute respiratory illness can be produced by a number of different viruses. A cold, for example, can be caused by the rhinovirus and the adenovirus, and the latter virus may also be responsible for a sore throat, in influenza-like illness or pneumonia.

CORYZA (The Common Cold)

Coryza is an infection of the mucous membrane of the nose and nasopharynx. The majority of cases are due to infection with the rhinoviruses, but any of the other respiratory viruses may be responsible—in particular the adenoviruses. It is spread by droplet infection, particularly in crowded places such as buses, trains, and cinemas. There is a high level of endemic infection during the autumn and winter and chills and dampness seem to be predisposing factors. After sneezing and profuse watery nasal discharge for a few days, secondary bacterial infection often occurs and the secretions become thick and yellow. Infection may spread causing:

(1) *Acute sinusitis*, with fever, headache or pain in the face, and localised tenderness may be present over the frontal or maxillary sinuses. Chronic sinusitis may result.
(2) *Acute otitis media* with fever, deafness, and earache.
(3) *Tracheitis bronchitis, or pneumonia.*

Treatment. A day or two in bed usually cuts short the course and prevents complications. It also helps to limit spread of the infection to others.

Soluble aspirin 0.6 g 6-hourly, often alleviates the minor discomforts. Inhalation of tinct. benzoin and menthol, one teaspoonful in a jug of hot water, may relieve the nasal congestion.

ACUTE LARYNGITIS AND LARYNGOTRACHEO-BRONCHITIS

Acute laryngitis occurs with the common cold and in young children with parainfluenzal virus infection. Tracheitis and bronchitis often occur at the same time. The throat is sore, the voice is at first hoarse and then reduced to a whisper and there is a dry, painful cough. In small children, swelling of the mucous membrane of the larynx may cause serious obstruction, the condition known as 'croup'; breathing becomes noisy and laboured and alarming paroxysms of coughing occur.

Treatment. If feverish the patient should be in bed in a warm room where the atmosphere is not too dry. The dryness of central heating, electric and gas fires should be prevented by using a steam kettle. The patient must not talk, since the larynx needs rest. Smoking is forbidden. Steam inhalations containing tinct. benzoin co., one teaspoon to one pint of boiling water, given for ten minutes three times a day, often give great relief; hot gargles and frequent hot drinks make the throat more comfortable. Linctus codeine, 5–10 ml, may help to suppress an irritating cough.

CHRONIC LARYNGITIS

Chronic laryngitis is more common in men than in women and is particularly liable to occur with untrained over-use of the voice. Hence the term 'clergyman's throat', though costermonger's throat would be more apt, as excessive use of tobacco and alcohol are often predisposing factors. Chronic sinus infection may also play a part.

Clinical Features. The voice is hoarse and weak. Examination of the larynx shows congestion with thickening of the vocal cords, either generalised or confined to the posterior third.

Presistent hoarseness for more than three weeks demands expert examination of the larynx. It may be due to papilloma, carcinoma, laryngeal palsy, or more rarely tuberculosis or syphilis.

Treatment. Complete rest of the voice is important. The patient should not speak above a whisper for several weeks. Nasal infection should be treated if present and tobacco and alcohol forbidden.

DISEASES OF THE BRONCHI

ACUTE TRACHEITIS AND BRONCHITIS

Acute tracheitis and bronchitis may complicate colds, influenza, measles, and other virus infections, and are particularly liable to occur in cold, damp and foggy weather. After the first few days, secondary bacterial invasion commonly occurs. Broncheolitis in infants is due to the respiratory syncytial virus.

Clinical Features. Acute tracheitis causes a dry, painful cough with soreness behind the sternum. Spread of infection to the bronchi produces tightness of the chest, with wheezing and difficulty in breathing. At first there is a little sticky, mucoid sputum, but secondary bacterial infection soon makes it yellow and more profuse. The severity and duration of the fever and of the general malaise are very variable; usually the illness is a mild one, lasting a few days. It may be serious and lead to pneumonia in young children, in the elderly or debilitated, or in patients with chronic bronchitis.

The signs of acute bronchitis are moderate fever, raised respiratory rate, particularly in children or in those with underlying lung disease, widespread wheezes and often crackles.

Treatment. The patient should be kept in bed. The room should be warm and the atmosphere not too dry. A steam kettle or steam inhalations reduce the soreness and aid expectoration. A dry, troublesome cough is helped by linctus codeine 5–10 ml t.d.s. or elixir diphenhydramine 10–20 ml; the latter also aids sleep.

After a few days the fever settles and the cough disappears. Convalescence is advisable after an attack of acute bronchitis, as early return to work with exposure to cold and a smoky atmosphere may delay complete recovery. Antibiotics are not required in mild, uncomplicated acute bronchitis. They are required where the risks of bronchopneumonia are greater:

(1) In a patient with severe bronchitis.
(2) In children and in the elderly and infirm.
(3) In the presence of complicating disease, such as heart disease.
(4) In patients with chronic bronchitis or bronchiectasis.

In these circumstances ampicillin or tetracycline (250 mg four times daily), or co-trimoxazole (Bactrim or Septrin) two tablets twice a day are usually effective.

CHRONIC BRONCHITIS

Great Britain has higher mortality rate from chronic bronchitis than any other country in the world. It is a major cause of chronic disability and death, particularly in men over middle age. It is related to air pollution, cigarette smoking and the liability to viral respiratory tract infections, and is most common in outdoor manual workers in urban districts. It is a complication of the pneumoconioses (p. 302), and obesity is an aggravating factor.

Chronic bronchitis is defined as productive cough occurring on most days for three months or more of the year, for at least two consecutive years. In the early stages there is hypertrophy of the mucous glands of bronchi, even when there is no inflammatory cell infiltration of the mucosa. In addition goblet cells replace the normal peripheral bronchial epithelium. Later, inflammatory changes in the mucosa occur with micro-abscesses and ulceration of the alveolar walls. When the sputum is mucoid bacteriological study is unrewarding. With persistently purulent sputum, and in acute exacerbations of bronchitis, *Haemophilus influenzae* and the pneumococci are the most common pathogens isolated.

Clinical Features. The earliest symptom is probably the 'smoker's cough', with the early morning production of non-infected mucoid sputum. This causes no disability and the patient is unlikely to seek medical advice. Later the patient complains of a winter cough with sputum, often with wheezing. At first these symptoms may only occur in episodes after a cold, which is slow to clear. Later they persist throughout the whole winter and eventually during the summer as well. There is usually a moderate amount of sputum, which may be mucoid or purulent; the latter nearly always occurs during an acute exacerbation of bronchitis, but sometimes the sputum is persistently purulent. A large volume of sputum should arouse suspicion of concomitant bronchiectasis.

After some years increasing dyspnoea, due to progressive airways obstruction and the development of emphysema, becomes an even more urgent symptom. The patient becomes too breathless to work and finally becomes completely disabled. There is considerable variation in the degree of disablement as many patients go throughout life with chronic cough and sputum and little dyspnoea, whereas others may become complete respiratory cripples within a few years.

Examination shows wheezes due to airways narrowing; if the lungs are over-inflated with poor breath sounds the wheezing may be heard best by listening over the trachea. Early inspiratory crackles may also be heard particularly at the lung bases. As emphysema develops it produces additional signs (p. 259). *A chest radiograph* in chronic bronchitis may show no abnormality until emphysema is present.

Treatment. This is generally disappointing, but in certain cases considerable symptomatic improvement can be achieved. The progress of the disease may be slowed by stopping smoking and by preventing, as far as possible, acute exacerbations of bronchitis and by treating them vigorously when they occur. This is more rewarding in the early case where destructive changes are not advanced and symptoms are minimal.

General Management. The smoky atmosphere of the city and dusty work should be avoided. This ideal is difficult to achieve as most patients, for financial and social reasons, cannot move to a healthier district or change their occupation. They can give up smoking and should be strenuously urged to do so. They should be advised to sleep in a warm bedroom, with the windows closed in the winter and they should stay at home in foggy weather and when they have a cold. A cold must be taken seriously, and the patient should be given a prophylactic antibiotic (see below) without delay.

Bronchodilators. Some degree of bronchospasm is often present and may be relieved by oral salbutamol or aminophylline or inhalers containing salbutamol or orciprenaline.

Prednisolone may be tried in some severely disabled patients in whom persistent bronchospasm is thought to be an important feature. Eosinophils in the sputum and a family history of allergy may be useful guides. This steroid therapy should be continued only if there is striking improvement within a week; it is then given on the same lines as for chronic asthma or alternatively a corticosteroid inhaler, such as beclomethasone, may be used.

Expectorant mixtures aim at loosening and aiding the expectoration of sputum. Pharmacological evidence suggests that in the dosage usually prescribed they have no effect on the volume or characteristics of the sputum expectorated. However, many bronchitic patients and doctors find such mixtures helpful and they continue to be prescribed. The reader is referred to the National Formulary for suitable prescriptions.

Sedative cough mixtures are used to suppress a troublesome cough at night, or to enable a patient to attend a social meeting in comfort. Examples are linctus codeine (NF) 4–8 ml and linctus pholcodine (NF) 4–8 ml.

Prophylactic antibiotics do not prevent colds, but are used to prevent the secondary bacterial infection and to cut short, or prevent, acute exacerbations of bronchitis. In a small group of patients with persistent purulent sputum considerable improvement can be achieved by prolonged treatment with antibiotics, from November to March. However, the majority of patients are best treated by giving them a supply of antibiotics so that they can start a course, on their own initiative, at the first signs of a cold. As *Haemophilus influenzae* and the pneumococci are the common pathogens, tetracycline 1 g daily, ampicillin 1.0 g daily, or co-trimoxazole (Bactrim or Septrin) in a dose of two tablets twice daily, are preferred to penicillin.

Breathing Exercises.

Heart failure in chronic bronchitis is quite common; it may be due to concurrent hypertension or coronary artery disease, or to true cor pulmonale (p. 261), or to a combination of factors.

EMPHYSEMA

Emphysema may be defined as a condition of the lungs in which there is pathological enlargement of the distal air spaces. Emphysematous bullae, which are cystic spaces of varying size, may develop and at post-mortem the lungs appear bulky as they fail to deflate. The numerous pathological classifications of emphysema are both complex and confusing. There are two main types:

Panacinar Emphysema. There is a dilatation or destruction of the acinus. This is the lung tissue distal to the terminal bronchiole and includes the respiratory bronchioles, alveolar ducts, atria and alveoli.

Centrilobular Emphysema. The dilatation or destruction is more proximal and involves the respiratory bronchioles. The emphysema is present in the centre of the lobules with the more distal part remaining unchanged. Bronchiolitis is probably the main causative factor.

Aetiology. Emphysema most commonly occurs with long-standing disease of the bronchi, namely chronic bronchitis or chronic asthma, or a combination of the two. At times it may be related to an occupational cause such as exposure to dust, and in coal miners' pneumonoconiosis (p. 303) there is characteristically a centrilobular emphysema ('focal' emphysema). Occasionally it develops as a primary disease without any previous history of bronchitis and familial cases of mainly basal emphysema are now recognised where there is a hereditary deficiency of alpha-l-antitrypsin in the blood.

The actual mechanism of production of emphysema is debated; 'air-trapping' due to widespread narrowing of the bronchioles, and weakening of the respiratory bronchioles and the alveolar walls from inflammation are both likely factors. The proteolytic enzymes released from leucocytes in the presence of inflammation are more likely to be destructive to the tissues when there is deficient activity of the principal enzyme inhibitor, namely *alpha-1-antitrypsin*. This may be produced by inhalation of cadmium fumes and also by tobacco smoke.

Effects on Lung Function. Emphysematous lung loses its elasticity and thus expiration requires a muscular effort on the part of the patient. Apart from the increased work involved, the forced expiration produces early closure of the airways and thus enhances the diffuse airflow obstruction already present. The chronic over-inflation of the lungs leads to an increase in the fixed volume of gas in the lungs, the residual volume, with the result that the mixing of inspired air in the lungs is less efficient. Reduction in the total surface area of the alveoli impairs the transfer of gases between the alveoli and the pulmonary capillaries (p. 242). However, blood gas abnormalities and cor pulmonale are less likely in 'pure' emphysema. Compensatory hyperventilation may enable the patient to sustain a relatively normal $Pa\text{O}_2$ (*pink puffers*); and because of the irregular nature of the pathological changes there is a mismatching between ventilation and perfusion (p. 241) for there are areas of comparatively normal lung where the hyperventilation prevents a rise in the $Pa\text{CO}_2$. Blood gas changes and cor pulmonale can occur in advanced states of emphysema, and where there is accompanying chronic bronchitis, being a particular feature of this disease (*blue bloaters*).

Clinical Features. The major symptom is dyspnoea. When emphysema is not too advanced there is likely to be only moderate shortness of breath on exertion. With progression of the disease the patient eventually becomes unable to walk more than a few steps. Quite frequently the breath is exhaled through pursed lips. The rate of progress of the disease is variable. Frequently it is slow, the patient reaching old age with only moderate disability. Sometimes it is rapid, the patient becoming a complete respiratory cripple by middle life. Occasionally the onset of severe disability is apparently sudden. This is usually precipitated by fog or a respiratory tract infection, the patient not admitting to significant symptoms beforehand.

With well-established emphysema, the chest appears over-inflated, with thoracic kyphosis, increase in the antero-posterior diameter of the chest, and horizontal ribs—a *'barrel' chest*. Chest expansion is diminished, the chest being lifted up by the accessory muscles of respiration rather than expanded. The percussion note is hyper-resonant and the areas of cardiac and liver dullness are diminished. The breath sounds are faint, often with prolonged expiration. Wheezes and crackles may be present if there is accompanying bronchial disease such as asthma, bronchitis or bronchiectasis.

Respiratory function tests show impaired ventilation with irreversible airflow obstruction (p. 240), increased residual volume (p. 239), impaired gas transfer (p. 242) and an abnormal shape to the flow-volume loop (p. 243). In advanced cases, particularly when associated with chronic bronchitis, blood gas abnormalities occur (p. 241) and the presence of cor pulmonale produces additional signs (p. 261).

The *chest radiograph* may be normal unless emphysema is well developed. In such cases the lung fields appear unduly translucent with atrophy of the peripheral vessels. The main pulmonary arteries are large and the heart thin and vertical. Bullae may be visible as localised areas of increased translucency. The ribs are horizontal and the diaphragm depressed and flattened. The lateral film shows an enlarged retrosternal 'window' of air.

Treatment. There is no specific treatment for emphysema, and breathlessness, once developed, will persist. The patient should stop smoking in an attempt to prevent progression of the disease. Improvement in airways obstruction may be achieved by treatment of bronchial infection (p. 258) and bronchospasm (p. 257) when they are present.

Breathing exercises may help to teach the patient to breathe in a more relaxed manner and to use the lower chest and diaphragms more effectively.

Surgical treatment of large bullae in patients with generalised emphysema is problematical, as the end result is usually impossible to predict.

Spontaneous pneumothorax should be suspected if there is sudden deterioration in a patient with emphysema, and dealt with accordingly (p. 316).

Compensatory Emphysema

When a section of lung contracts by fibrosis or collapse, or is removed surgically, the rest of that lung expands by over-inflation to fill the space. This is known as compensatory emphysema and is not usually associated with any defect of function.

Unilateral Emphysema

Unilateral translucency of a lung may be due to a large bulla or cyst, or be due to compensatory emphysema as a result of a totally collapsed lobe in the lung on that side. It also occurs when there is over-inflation of a lung due to partial obstruction of a major bronchus; this can produce a 'ball-valve' mechanism so that air enters on inspiration but is trapped in the lung on expiration. This is likely to be due to a bronchial neoplasm in an adult and to pressure from tuberculous glands in a child.

Unilateral emphysema (*Macleod's syndrome*) may follow an obliterative bronchiolitis occurring in early childhood; this arrests development of the lung which normally proceeds until the age of 8 years. The affected lung over-inflates rather than budding with the result that it has impairment of both ventilation and perfusion; the chest X-ray shows a hypertranslucent lung with attenuated vessels and a small pulmonary artery, and an expiration film shows failure of the lung to deflate with shift of the mediastinum to the opposite side. The patient often presents in middle age at the time of coincidental bronchitis; other presenting symptoms include unexplained chest pain on that side and haemoptysis, the latter probably related to an increased bronchial circulation. The signs are those of diminished breath sounds over the affected lung and late inspiratory crackles at the base resulting from the opening of poorly ventilated, partially deflated alveoli.

RESPIRATORY FAILURE

The function of the lungs may be so impaired by various diseases that there is a failure to maintain normal arterial gas tensions; this is respiratory failure. It occurs when the Pao_2 is below 60 mmHg (8.0 kpa) and the $Paco_2$ is above 50 mmHg (7.7 kpa) and is associated with central cyanosis and with respiratory acidosis. It may be due to *depression of the respiratory centre* by poisons, drugs, anoxia or cerebral disease; to *failure of the respiratory muscles* as in poliomyelitis, acute infectious polyneuritis and myasthenia gravis; to *loss of functioning lung* as in extensive pneumonia, pulmonary collapse, pneumothorax or following surgical lung resection; to *obstruction of airways* as in status asthmaticus or severe bronchitis.

Patients with chronic lung disease are especially prone to respiratory failure with any of the above complications, which may occur separately or in combination.

Respiratory failure can occur independently of cor pulmonale, although it may precipitate it.

Treatment is directed at the underlying cause. *Respiratory stimulants* (p. 263) are indicated when there is depression of the respiratory centre. *Oxygen therapy* (p. 263) and some form of *assisted respiration* in the form of positive-pressure ventilation with cuffed endotracheal tube may be essential to maintain life. *Tracheostomy* may be required. Such treatment needs careful management and it is only feasible in specialised units. One of the disadvantages of assisted respiration is that it may not be possible to wean patients with chronic lung disease from the respirator or the tracheostomy.

COR PULMONALE

This is heart disease secondary to disease of the lungs. It occurs most commonly with chronic obstructive lung disease; also with bronchiectasis and cystic fibrosis and with diffuse fibrotic lung disease from its many causes such as sarcoidosis, the pneumoconioses and fibrosing alveolitis. It may follow the long-standing deficient ventilation of severe kyphoscoliosis; or hypoventilation syndromes associated with sleep apnoea such may occur in association with obesity (*Pickwickian syndrome*), and possibly occurring in some chronic bronchitics who become 'blue bloaters'.

It is mostly precipitated by respiratory infection but drugs such as hypnotics, tranquillisers and β blockers may be important precipitants. *Hypoxia* and carbon dioxide retention (*hypercarbia*) occur and the abnormal gases produce impairment of renal function with retention of sodium and water, increase in blood volume and at first a rise in cardiac output. The systemic arterioles are dilated with warm extremities and bounding pulse, and dilatation of the cerebral vessels may produce headache and even papilloedema. The effect of the hypoxia on the pulmonary arterioles, however, is to produce active vasoconstriction. This, combined with obliteration of these vessels by disease and with the increase in cardiac output, produces pulmonary hypertension. It is only in the later stages of the disease, if pulmonary hypertension becomes severe or if the heart muscle is seriously affected by anoxia, that the cardiac output falls.

Clinical Features. The patient is cyanosed, with signs of chronic bronchitis and often emphysema. The extremities are warm but cyanosed, and the pulse full. The venous pressure in the neck is raised, the liver enlarged and there is dependent oedema. The heart sounds are often difficult to hear due to the overlying over-inflated lung, but it may be possible to detect triple rhythm. With gross enlargement of the right ventricle a right ventricular heave may be palpable and the systolic murmur of functional tricuspid incompetence be heard, with systolic pulsation of the neck veins. Proteinuria and a raised blood urea may be present. If the cardiac output falls, the extremities become cold and the pulse small and venous congestion and oedema increase.

An electrocardiogram shows the large sharply pointed P waves of right atrial hypertrophy and there may be signs of right ventricular hypertrophy. The heart is usually vertical.

Radiography shows dilatation of the main pulmonary arteries with cardiac enlargement. The lung fields may show evidence of emphysema but at times the lung fields appear congested.

Treatment is primarily directed at improving alveolar ventilation.

Bronchial infection should be treated with an effective antibiotic such as ampicillin, amoxycillin or co-trimoxazole, and if the patient's condition warrants it antibiotics should be given parenterally.

Physiotherapy is of prime importance to encourage the patient to cough properly and to clear the peripheral and central airways. It should be carried out frequently and if necessary during the night when hypoventilation is also likely to occur.

Respiratory stimulants may be given if respiratory depression occurs. These arouse the patient, increase the ventilation and induce coughing. Nikethamide is effective, and is given intravenously usually by intermittent injections (2 ml). Too large a dose may produce twitching or convulsions. Alternatively doxapram can be given by continuous IV infusion in a dose of 1–4 mg/min, depending on the patient's response.

Bronchospasm can be treated with aminophylline, either orally, by rectal suppository or intravenously—250 mg over the course of 10 minutes or by IV drip of 500 mg over 6 hours. Salbutamol inhalations can be given regularly either by using a pressurised aerosol inhaler or by using salbutamol solution and a nebuliser. A course of oral corticosteroids or IV hydrocortisone may be indicated.

Oxygen Therapy. In patients with cor pulmonale and chronic carbon dioxide retention the respiratory centre may depend on oxygen lack for its stimulation and treatment with high concentrations of oxygen may produce respiratory depression with increasing CO_2 retention, the patient becoming drowsy or comatose. For this reason it is best to use oxygen in a concentration of 24% in the first place using a mask employing the Venturi principle (e.g., Ventimask), or by using nasal cannulae with a flow rate of 2 litres/minute. This method should produce a $Pa\text{O}_2$ level of above 50 mmHg (6.7 kPa), which is usually considered safe. Even this method of oxygen administration can cause increasing CO_2 retention during the first few days, and a watch must be kept for CO_2 narcosis; estimations of blood gases and pH are invaluable.

Assisted Ventilation. Intermittent positive pressure ventilation (IPPV) with cuffed endotracheal tube or occasionally with tracheostomy may be life saving. The decision to initiate this treatment is likely to be made because of lowering of the level of consciousness, deterioration in the blood gases, the inability to cough and the general exhaustion of the patient; it will be influenced by knowledge of the patient's exercise tolerance prior to the current illness. The treatment is not justified for uncomplicated chronic lung disease, as it may be impossible to wean the patient from the ventilator.

Diuretics should be given for dependent oedema and may improve alveolar ventilation by eliminating pulmonary oedema. The blood urea and electrolytes should be monitored.

Digoxin is indicated if atrial fibrillation is present. It is otherwise disappointing in cor pulmonale and may induce dysrhythmias.

Vasodilators have been used to lower pulmonary hypertension but their place in cor pulmonale is not certain.

Polycythaemia. In patients who develop severe secondary polycythaemia with a PCV of 60 or more great clinical improvement can occur after adequate venesection to lower the PCV to normal levels. This is best done with simultaneous infusion of dextran or Hartmann's solution into the other arm so that there is little disturbance of the circulating volume at the time of the venesection.

Sedation. All hypnotics are potentially dangerous because of the liability of producing respiratory depression. Morphia is contraindicated. Treatment should be directed at relieving anoxia which is the cause of restlessness and mental confusion. However, when these symptoms are severe chloral hydrate is comparatively safe.

BRONCHIECTASIS

The essential pathological change in bronchiectasis is dilatation of the bronchi. It usually results from pulmonary collapse or as a complication of various types of pneumonia. In many patients the disease follows an attack of pneumonia complicating one of the childhood fevers, particularly whooping cough or measles. Plugging of some of the bronchi by sticky mucus leads to absorption collapse; dilatation of the bronchi in the related portion of the lung occurs, as a result of increased tractive forces on the bronchial walls. At this stage the process is reversible if the obstructing plugs of mucus are removed by vigorous physiotherapy, that is by firm percussion on chest wall combined with postural drainage and 'assisted' coughing. If the bronchial plugging is allowed to persist for any length of time, however, inflammatory changes develop in the walls of the dilated bronchi and lead to permanent bronchiectasis.

Bronchiectasis also develops distal to a chronic *bronchial obstruction*, such as bronchial carcinoma or bronchostenosis, say from a foreign body. Pressure of tuberculous nodes on a bronchus, from childhood primary tuberculosis (p. 295), may lead to bronchiectasis in later life. This most commonly affects the middle lobe, producing the *middle lobe (Brock) syndrome.*

Pulmonary infection which involves the bronchial walls and which heals by fibrosis also produces bronchiectasis. It is particularly seen in *pulmonary tuberculosis* which is a common cause of bronchiectasis of the upper lobes.

Proximal bronchiectasis may result from plugging of the bronchi which occurs with *allergic aspergillosis.*

Congenital bronchiectasis is associated with maldevelopment of acini so that there is retention of secretions with subsequent infection in poorly ventilated blind airways.

Sometimes an infective bronchiolitis results in a progressive form of the disease in the absence of pulmonary collapse. A similar widespread bronchiectasis commonly develops from a suppurating bronchiolitis in patients with fibrocystic disease of the pancreas.

Kartagener's Syndrome (Immotile Cilia Syndrome)

In Kartagener's syndrome there is transposition of the viscera (situs inversus), poorly developed paranasal sinuses and most of the patients have rhinitis, sinusitis and chronic bronchitis; about half have bilateral basal bronchiectasis. It is inherited as an autosomal recessive and is due to immotility of the cilia; electron microscopy of ciliary structure has demonstrated an absence of dynein arms to the microtubules. In the normal, ciliary movement in the primitive foregut of the foetus favours rotation to the left. Absence of ciliary activity means that there is an even chance of rotation to the right and causes a generalised respiratory tract disorder due to failure of normal transport secretions (p. 235). Male patients with this disorder are infertile, as the tails of spermatozoa have the same structure as cilia and are also immotile.

Clinical Features. The clinical features of bronchiectasis are variable and depend on the extent of the disease and the degree of infection in the affected bronchi.

(1) *Classical Bronchiectasis.* There is a history of recurrent episodes of pneumonia in childhood—the first often occurring after an attack of whooping cough or measles. The patient has a cough productive of a considerable volume of purulent sputum which may sometimes contain blood. In the winter there are exacerbations of the condition with increased cough and sputum and with fever, and recurrent attacks of pneumonia may occur. Examination shows a thin patient who looks ill. Dyspnoea and cyanosis are present if sufficient volume of lung is involved. The fingers are often clubbed. Examination of the chest usually shows signs of fibrosis and of retained bronchial secretions over the affected lobe or lobes. The physical signs may be few, perhaps only an area of persistent crackles, if healthy lung separates the diseased segments from the chest wall. If the patient is encouraged to cough, large quantities of sputum may be expectorated, and the breath and sputum may smell foul if secondary anaerobic infection is present (see p. 286). Such is the picture of gross bronchiectasis which nowadays is rare, and the majority of patients with this disease present in less dramatic form.

(2) *Other Types of Bronchiectasis.* Some patients with bronchiectasis have no symptoms at all, particularly those with bronchiectasis of the upper lobes where drainage is continuous. Such bronchiectasis is frequently the result of old tuberculous infection. In other recurrent haemoptysis, sometimes profuse, is the only symptom. Sometimes infection occurs only in the winter following upper respiratory infection and for the rest of the year the patient is well. In such patients there may be no physical signs, or simply persistent crackles over the bronchiectatic lobes.

Complications of Bronchiectasis. Patients with persistent infected sputum are liable to develop changes of chronic bronchitis. Patients are also prone to recurrent attacks of pneumonia either in the affected lobe or in another part of the lung due to 'spill-over' of infected sputum. Spread of bronchiectasis and lung fibrosis may follow. Lung abscess and empyema may also occur. Haematogenous spread, from infected thrombus in a pulmonary venous radicle, may lead to cerebral abscess. If infection has been extensive and prolonged, amyloid disease may develop, but is now rarely seen.

Diagnosis. The chest radiography may show no abnormality; more commonly there is some increased striation in the bronchiectatic lobe due to bronchial wall thickening and crowding of the blood vessels and cysts with fluid levels may be seen. Abnormal shadowing will be present if there is much associated fibrosis, with compensatory emphysema in the surrounding lung. The diagnosis of bronchiectasis can be confirmed and its extent determined by *bronchography*. Radio-opaque iodised oil is introduced into the bronchi to make them opaque to X-rays. The right bronchial tree is outlined first and both straight and lateral views are obtained. The left lung is then filled and an oblique view taken. The diseased bronchi appear dilated, their walls are often irregular and their outline blurred.

Treatment. Management depends on the careful assessment of the patient's history and the extent of the bronchiectasis.

Surgical Treatment. This is rarely indicated. Young patients with a history of severe chronic infection which is not controlled by medical means can be considered for surgical treatment. The disease should be confined to one lobe and complete bronchograms are required to exclude bronchiectasis in other parts of the lung. Surgery is contraindicated if the disease is too widespread, if there is coincident asthma or chronic bronchitis or if there is impaired ventilatory capacity.

Medical Treatment. In many cases the disease is not severe enough to warrant surgical treatment. In others the bronchiectasis is too extensive for resection, or the remaining lung is too damaged by chronic bronchitis and emphysema. Sometimes the patient's age or general health make operation impossible. In such cases medical treatment is usually remarkably effective, though clearly it cannot be curative.

The severity of the symptoms is not always directly related to the anatomical extent of the bronchiectasis. They can nearly always be satisfactorily controlled and the complications largely prevented by regular and competent *postural drainage*. The patient is taught the position in which secretions will drain from the bronchiectatic area towards the main bronchi and the trachea. This enables sputum to be coughed up. The lower lobes are affected in the majority of patients. Postural drainage for this lobe is achieved by leaning face downwards over the side of the bed with the hands on the floor. Alternatively the foot of the bed is raised on 18-inch blocks, the patient lying on his face or side, according to the segments affected. Postural drainage of the right middle lobe is achieved by placing the patient on his back with a pillow under the right side of the chest and the foot of the bed is slightly raised. With upper lobe bronchiectasis, drainage will take place if the patient is sitting up, leaning towards the unaffected side. The appropriate position must be adopted for at least 10 minutes twice a day, and forcible coughing should be continued until no more sputum will come up. Drainage of the secretions can often be improved by 'clapping' on chest over the affected lobe. The physiotherapist or the nurse may carry out this procedure, but later the patient's relatives will have to be instructed. Postural drainage should be carried out first thing in the morning as sputum collects in the dilated bronchi during the night. It should also be performed before retiring to bed and it may be necessary to repeat it before the midday and evening meals. A hot drink given before each treatment may increase expectoration.

A course of ampicillin or tetracycline, 250 mg 6-hourly or co-trimoxazole two tablets twice a day for one or two weeks may be given if the purulent sputum becomes more profuse, particularly if the patient also has fever and malaise. Sometimes continuous suppressive antibiotic treatment over the winter months may be considered. In patients with foul sputum there is often infection with anaerobic organisms and penicillin and metronidazole are the antibiotics of choice. No treatment is necessary in patients whose bronchiectasis is symptomless and without evidence of infection.

ASTHMA

Patients with bronchial asthma suffer attacks of wheezing and difficulty in breathing due to bronchospasm, mucosal swelling and sticky secretions; at times these symptoms may be persistent with intermittent acute exacerbations. The cause of the disease is complex and in most patients multiple factors operate.

Extrinsic (Allergic) Asthma

The extrinsic form of asthma is most likely to start in childhood or early adult life. There may be a previous history of eczema or hay fever as well as a family history of allergic disorders. An atopic individual is prone to develop increased amounts of reaginic antibody (IgE) which becomes attached to cells in the bronchial mucosa, in particular to the mast cells. Inhaled allergen combines with IgE and damage to mast cells releases inflammatory agents and spasmogens such as histamine, bradykinin and slow reacting substance of anaphylaxis (SRS-A), now identified as the leucotrienes. This is a *Type I (anaphylactoid) hypersensitivity reaction.*

There are a large number of substances to which the asthmatic may be allergic. They are most often inhaled; common examples are pollens and spores from plants and moulds (such as grasses, *Aspergillus fumigatus* (p. 301) and dry rot), dusts of various kinds (such as the house dust mite,

Dermatophagoides pteronyssinus which lives on the scales of human skin) and animal danders. Ingested allergens are less often to blame; champagne is the classical example.

Eosinophilia suggests that allergy is important but may also be present with intrinsic asthma. The history is the best guide to the part that allergy plays. If attacks occur in the spring and early summer it is reasonable to suspect that pollens are responsible; attacks in the winter months may be related to infection or to bronchopulmonary aspergillosis (p. 301); or attacks may be induced by proximity to a domestic animal such as a cat or a horse.

Skin sensitivity tests can be performed. Drops of specially prepared solutions of a range of suspected allergens are placed on the skin of the forearm and superficial pricks made through the drops. The result is positive if a raised wheal appears within 15 minutes. A positive skin test does not necessarily imply that the asthma is related to that particular antigen, and is only of significance if it coincides with the history. Skin tests are not affected by sodium cromoglycate or corticosteroids, but they are by antihistamines.

In addition to allergy, the following may play a part in the aetiology:

(a) *Infections* of the respiratory tract commonly precipitate asthma, and in some patients they may be the main cause.

(b) *Reflex Factors.* Various stimuli may induce attacks by a reflex vagal mechanism; examples are sudden exposure to cold, laughing and physical exertion (see below).

(c) *Psychological factors* play some part in a large number of asthmatics, and quite often anxiety or depression appear to be mainly responsible, if not in starting the asthma, at least in maintaining it.

(a) (b) (c) above may produce their effect by reducing the stability of mast cells.

(d) *Pharmacological Causes.* β blockers, given for angina or hypertension, may precipitate asthma. Aspirin-induced asthma, which occurs in a small number of patients, is probably the result of a pharmacological effect on the prostaglandin pathway; it is usually associated with nasal polyps and occurs most often in patients with intrinsic asthma (see below).

Intrinsic (Late-onset) Asthma

The intrinsic form usually occurs for the first time in later life. Although mast-cell instability may be present, allergic factors are not evident in the history or demonstrable by skin testing or by increased IgE production. It is more often associated with bronchitis and psychological factors. It may occur for the first time after a respiratory infection, and persistent cough and wheezing may be misinterpreted as chronic bronchitis. It tends to be more intractable and response to bronchodilators may be disappointing.

Special Types of Asthma

There are various special types, which may give rise to diagnostic difficulties.

(1) *Exercise-induced Asthma.* Although exercise may induce asthma in most asthmatics, in some patients asthma is produced almost exclusively by exertion. Hyperventilation and cooling of the airways seems to be the trigger mechanism; it probably stimulates the vagus which in turn increases mast-cell activity, for the asthma can be prevented by prophylactic use of sodium cromoglycate, as well as by salbutamol inhalation.

(2) *Paroxysmal Cough and Early Morning Asthma.* It may not be appreciated that a paroxysmal cough may be an early feature of asthma; or asthma occurring in the early hours of the morning (at the time of the early morning 'dip' in peak flow) may be dismissed as there are no abnormal signs when the patient sees the doctor later in the day.

(3) *Late-onset asthma superimposed on chronic bronchitis and/or emphysema* is likely to be misinterpreted as a progressive worsening of the chronic condition. Furthermore, reversibility of the airways obstruction to inhalation of a bronchodilator may not be present as quite often there is poor response to bronchodilators in this type of asthma; reversal of the airways obstruction may, however, be achieved by a therapeutic/diagnostic course of corticosteroids. Clinical clues to the existence of this state of affairs are marked fluctuations in the degree of wheezing and disability; response to inhalation of a bronchodilator when it occurs; a family history of asthma; eosinophilia or eosinophils in the sputum.

(4) *Occupational Asthma.* The inhalation of organic dusts, fumes or vapours may induce an *immediate (Type I)* attack of asthma in atopic subjects. The immediate asthmatic reaction can also occur in non-atopic individuals if the concentration of the inhalant is high and the exposure is prolonged.

The relationship of asthma to an occupational cause may be overlooked when there is 'late' asthma occurring some 4–6 hours after exposure. It is associated with a *Type III immune response* and extrinsic (allergic) alveolitis is usually present; precipitins to the specific allergen are present in the blood. Examples are inhalation of spores of *Micropolyspora faeni* in mouldy hay (*Farmers' lung*) and dust containing avian protein (*Bird fanciers' Lung*) (p. 308).

Some inhalants may produce both immediate and late asthma; for instance isocyanates used in the production of polyurethanes and enzymes produced by *Bacillus subtilis* used in 'biological' soap powders.

Clinical Features. There may be no abnormal signs at the time a patient is seen and the diagnosis depends on the history of attacks. During a typical attack the patient complains of tightness in the chest, difficulty in breathing and wheeziness. There is often cough, dry at first but towards the end of an attack sticky, tight little pellets or strings of clear mucus may be produced. The sputum is yellow when infection is present or when it contains large numbers of eosinophilia. On examination at the time of an attack the chest is over-inflated and there are widespread wheezes, most marked on expiration. Tests of respiratory function show impaired ventilatory capacity due to airways obstruction (p. 240).

Treatment

(1) *For an Attack*

Most patients can abort or cut short an attack themselves by using a pressurised aerosol containing a β_2 receptor stimulator, such as *salbutamol*. The patient must be carefully instructed in its use; after breathing out fully, release of the metered dose should be timed with the start of a deep inspiration, when the breath is then held for a short time to allow absorption to take place. Although the effects on the heart are less than with a β_1 receptor stimulator (isoprenaline), it is usual to restrict the dosage of salbutamol to two puffs (0.2 mg) 4-hourly. With more severe or prolonged attacks, salbutamol can also be given by inhalation of 1–2 ml of 0.5% solution using a nebuliser, and bad asthmatics can be provided with this for use in the home. If the patient finds he needs medical help to relieve a severe attack *intravenous aminophylline* 0.25–0.5 g in 10–20 ml sterile water is a valuable drug. Regular *oral salbutamol* 2–4 mg up to q.d.s. *or slow release aminophylline* preparation 200 mg b.d. may help to suppress a background of wheeze and to prevent attacks. Tremor may occur as an unwanted side-effect of salbutamol therapy due to over-stimulation of β_2 receptors in striated muscle.

(2) *Status Asthmaticus*

This implies that a severe attack has lasted more than a day or so and is resistant to conventional bronchodilator therapy; it is potentially fatal and the patient should be admitted to hospital. Although there may be exhaustion through lack of sleep and the effort of breathing, under no circumstances must morphine or any other opium derivature be given as it is liable to cause death. A persistent tachycardia is often a good indication of the severity of the condition and pulsus paradoxus may be present. Dehydration should be corrected and corticosteroid therapy is indicated. Its effect is not immediate and the most rapid response is obtained by IV hydrocortisone 200–300 mg given as bolus injections 4–6-hourly until improvement occurs. Oral prednisolone is also started, giving 60 mg on the first day, 40 mg the next day and 30 mg subsequently, tailing off over the next 8–10 days depending on clinical improvement. Intravenous aminophylline can be given by intermittent injections of 250 mg over the course of 10 minutes or by intravenous drip of 500 mg over 6 hours. Inhalations of salbutamol 0.5% solution may be very effective given by a nebuliser. Status asthmaticus is likely to be associated with infection, either as a precipitant or as a secondary feature, and an appropriate antibiotic such as ampicillin is indicated. Failure to respond to treatment and a rising $P\text{aco}_2$ are indications for considering intermittent positive pressure ventilation (IPPV), either using a tight face mask or cuffed endotracheal tube.

Patients known to have severe asthma should have open access to hospital and medical help; speed is of the essence as severe and potentially fatal asthma may develop very rapidly.

(3) *General Management*

Attacks of asthma need treatment as they arise, but the main aim of management should be to prevent asthma occurring. The patient, if required, must be prepared to take prophylactic treatment regularly. Once fully established in a good phase for a reasonable period of time, the treatment can be gradually tailed down to nothing. Recurrence of symptoms as treatment is reduced means that the patient should continue with the minimal dosage required to keep free of asthma for a further period, before another attempt at reduction is made.

(a) *Extrinsic Asthma.* Allergic subjects should avoid contact with known allergens as far as possible. When there is sensitivity to house dust the bedroom should be spartan and furnishings which harbour dust should be avoided; the bedclothes should be changed at frequent intervals to eliminate exposure to skin scales and the *dermatophagoides*. Feather quilts should not be used and sorbo rubber substitutes should replace feather pillows and hair mattresses. When there is clear-cut allergy to pollen, *specific desensitisation* may be attempted. This is done by giving a series of 7–9 subcutaneous injections of a suitable preparation of allergen, such as Alavac-P, at weekly or fortnightly intervals, starting with a very small dose and gradually increasing it until the patient is able to tolerate quite a large dose, or in other words has become desensitised. The patient must be kept under observation for at least half an hour after each injection. Syringes containing 1 : 1000 adrenaline must be available, and an injection of 0.5 ml of adrenaline and 10 mg of chlorpheniramine given at once if the patient develops any reaction, such as wheezing or faintness. If a reaction occurs at the next injection the dose is reduced slightly, and then steadily increased again over the following weeks. Desensitisation against pollens must be completed before the end of April, as severe and even fatal reactions may occur if injections are given when pollens are present in the atmosphere. Repeated courses over three consecutive years are usually necessary to produce a prolonged effect.

Sodium cromoglycate inhibits release of spasmogens from mast cells, and its regular use may be of great value in the prevention of allergic asthma. It is administered by inhalation, using a Spinhaler, up to one capsule (20 mg) four times a day or by use of a pressurised aerosol (Intal inhaler) two puffs four times a day; if effective the frequency of administration can be progressively reduced to the minimum required to keep the patient free of asthma.

If response to cromoglycate is poor, asthma may be well controlled by using a corticosteroid aerosol, such as *beclomethasone*, two puffs (100 μg) four times a day. This type of corticosteroid is poorly absorbed, thus systematic side effects are avoided. To achieve maximal inhalation of beclomethasone it is helpful to precede it on each occasion by 1–2 puffs of salbutamol. Once the asthma is suppressed the frequency of administration can be gradually reduced to the minimum necessary. Regular oral salbutamol or aminophylline may be indicated (p. 270). If asthma remains chronic in spite of the above measures then oral corticosteroids are indicated, either in 'booster' courses or on a long-term basis (see below).

(b) *Intrinsic Asthma.* Dust and fumes should be avoided, although allergic features are not usually important. States of anxiety or depression should be treated if severe, and persistent infection if present should be suppressed with antibiotics. Sodium cromoglycate is usually ineffective but may be tried. Response to bronchodilators is often only partially successful, and the asthma tends to be intractable. Often the only effective treatment is some form of corticosteroid therapy. In a good number of patients the asthma can be suppressed by regular inhalations of beclomethasone (see above). Those who continue to have disabling symptoms can be controlled only by oral steroids; in them the dangers of such treatment are outweighed by the benefits. Initial dosage of 30–40 mg prednisolone daily is gradually reduced to the minimum effective level; once the dosage has reached 10 mg daily, further gradual pruning of the dosage can be achieved by using 1 mg tablets. Regular beclomethasone inhalations should be continued as they have a systemic steroid-saving effect. The final dose of prednisolone required may be very small, and it may be possible for the patient to tail off the oral treatment completely. Further 'booster' courses of prednisolone may be required at times of exacerbation of asthma, for example with a respiratory infection. Starting, say, with 30 mg on the first day, the daily dose can then be progressively reduced by 5 mg each subsequent day.

CARCINOMA OF THE BRONCHUS

This disease has become much more common in recent years. It is now the commonest type of cancer in men, in whom it occurs four or five times more frequently than in women. The reports from the Royal College of Physicians and others have emphasised the importance of cigarette smoking as a cause of bronchial carcinoma. There is also some evidence that the incidence is higher in those who live in the polluted atmosphere of industrial areas. An increased incidence is reported in miners exposed to dust from chromium, nickel, and radioactive ores, and there is a greatly increased incidence in association with pulmonary asbestosis. It may also arise in scar tissue from pulmonary tuberculosis or diffuse lung fibrosis, when it is most commonly adenocarcinoma. About half the tumours arise within an inch or two of the bifurcation of the trachea. The remainder are peripheral. Histologically they are squamous adeno- or anaplastic carcinomas (the latter group including the small cell or oat cell carcinoma).

Clinical Features. A dry cough is the commonest early symptom. Recurrent haemoptysis may result from ulceration and sometimes this is the presenting symptom. Mucopurulent sputum occurs as increase in size of the growth produces progressive bronchial obstruction, then distal infection and shortness of breath develop with collapse of the lung segment supplied by the affected bronchus. A persistent wheeze due to the narrowed bronchus and dull deep-seated pain are not uncommon symptoms. Some patients are symptom-free when the disease is discovered by mass radiography or remain so until one of the **complications** occurs. These are:

(1) *Pneumonic Infection.* The segment of lung beyond the bronchial obstruction is particularly liable to infection. Patients may present with a segmental pneumonia, which either fails to resolve satisfactorily or recurs repeatedly in the same area of lung. Such events should always raise suspicion of an underlying carcinoma.

(2) *Lung Collapse.* Complete obstruction of a bronchus by carcinoma produces collapse of the lung segment supplied by that bronchus. The collapsed lung may become infected causing fever and toxaemia, but there may be little or no sputum because of total bronchial obstruction. Collapse may be associated with a pleural effusion on the same side, with the result that there is no mediastinal shift. A chronic empyema may develop.

(3) *Lung abscess* may develop in an area of pneumonic infection (see above). When the growth is in the periphery of the lung its centre may become necrotic and be coughed up. This produces a ragged abscess cavity with walls which are composed of carcinomatous tissue, and which characteristically are thick and irregular when seen on a radiograph.

(4) *Superior vena caval obstruction* may occur from pressure of a growth in this situation. The patient complains of fullness in the head and face and may be in acute discomfort. There is oedema of the face and upper limbs, with gross distension of the neck veins and anastomotic veins over the upper part of the chest. Other causes of this syndrome are aneurysm of the ascending aorta, malignant mediastinal glands, malignant thymoma and haemorrhage into a retrosternal thyroid.

(5) *Local Spread and Pleural Effusion.* Carcinoma cells may invade the mediastinal lymph nodes and the pleura, giving rise to a pleural

effusion which is often, but by no means invariably, blood-stained.

(6) *Cardiac Involvement.* Atrial fibrillation may occur due to direct infiltration of the atria, and it is sometimes the presenting symptom. Spread of growth to the pericardium may produce a pericardial effusion or malignant pericardial constriction.

(7) *Distant Metastasis.* Bronchial carcinoma may metastasise to the liver, the bones, the suprarenals, the brain, the skin, and the lymphatic glands, the deposits causing symptoms and signs referable to the organs affected. When secondary neoplasm is suspected and the primary focus is not apparent, the lungs are a prime area of suspicion and the chest should be examined clinically and radiologically.

(8) *The Nervous System.* Tumours occurring at the apex of the lung may involve the first rib and the lower part of the brachial plexus producing Horner's syndrome together with pain down the arm with weakness and wasting (Pancoast's tumour). Both laryngeal and diaphragmatic palsy may occur due to invasion of the recurrent laryngeal and phrenic nerves. Lung cancer may present with cerebral metastases, and a chest radiograph should always be taken when a cerebral tumour is suspected.

(9) *Non-Metastatic Syndromes*

(a) *Endocrine.* Occasionally tumours may produce polypeptides which have a hormone-like activity (p. 597).

Ectopic ACTH syndrome occurs with oat cell carcinoma, as well as with tumours of the thymus and pancreas. Because of the rapidity of the growth, the classic features of Cushing's syndrome may not have time to develop; muscle weakness with potassium depletion, oedema and hypertension with sodium retention and marked pigmentation may occur. Blood cortisol levels are often extremely high and fail to show diurnal variation.

Inappropriate secretion of antidiuretic like hormone (ADH) also occurs with oat cell carcinoma, producing water retention, hyponatraemia and mental confusion.

Hypercalcaemia may be due to a parathormone-like substance usually produced by a squamous carcinoma. More commonly hypercalcaemia is due to extensive deposits in bone.

Polypeptides producing thyrotoxicosis and gynaecomastia have been reported.

(b) *Cardiovascular. Thrombophlebitis migrans*, with spontaneous thromboses occurring in the veins of the legs and arms, is a complication of adenocarcinoma; less common is *thrombotic non-bacterial endocarditis* which may present with systemic emboli.

(c) *Nervous System.* Various disorders of nervous tissue and muscle may develop in association with lung cancer, usually with oat cell carcinoma. They may appear some considerable time before the tumour is evident. They include encephalopathies, in particular cerebellar degeneration; neuropathies; myopathic-myasthenic syndromes; polymyositis and dermatomyositis.

(d) *Skeletal. Hypertrophic pulmonary osteoarthropathy* usually occurs in association with gross clubbing of the fingers, and is most commonly seen with squamous carcinoma of the lung; there is pain and swelling of the ankles and the lower shin and around the wrists; it may be confused with rheumatoid arthritis but the radiograph shows typical subperiosteal new bone formation. It remits if the tumour is resected.

(e) *Renal.* Nephrotic syndrome, with albuminuria and oedema, may occur as the result of immune complexes produced by lung carcinoma.

Physical Signs. There may be no abnormal signs in the chest in spite of well-marked symptoms or obvious metastases. The changes when present may be those of collapse, pneumonia, lung abscess, or pleural effusion. A combination of effusion with collapse is not uncommon. A stridor with deep breathing or a monophonic wheeze may be present. Clubbing of the fingers is frequent. A careful examination should be made for secondary deposits in the liver and the lymphatic glands, particularly cervical and supraclavicular.

Diagnosis. A patient presenting with any of the above features should have radiological examination of the chest. This will confirm the presence of collapse, consolidation, effusion, or abscess cavity, or may show a mass spreading out from the hilum, or a peripheral mass. It should be emphasised that a carcinoma may be present in spite of what appears to be a normal chest X-ray.

If the diagnosis remains in doubt the patient should be bronchoscoped, and a biopsy of the suspected lesion removed for microscopy. The fibre-optic bronchoscope enables biopsy and brushings to be carried out on peripheral lesions. If this is unrewarding percutaneous needle biopsy under fluoroscopic control may be undertaken. Biopsy of scalene nodes or of clinically enlarged glands may confirm the diagnosis. Bronchoscopy will be essential if surgery is contemplated in order to assess the extent of the growth and its operability and mediastinoscopy or mediastinotomy may be necessary. Expert examination of the sputum for cancer cells is positive in 80% of cases.

Treatment. The main hope of cure lies in *surgical removal* of the affected lobe or lung. Unfortunately, many patients cannot be treated in this way, either because the carcinoma has already metastasised or is too extensive, or because the patient is not fit enough to withstand the operation. With successful removal the 5-year survival rate is about 20% and is best with lobectomy for squamous carcinoma.

Radiotherapy can be used to produce a remission in patients unsuitable for surgery, and for oat cell carcinoma it is probably just as effective as surgery. It is extremely unlikely to destroy the growth, although occasional cures do occur. More commonly it is used to relieve symptoms. It is of value in patients with superior mediastinal obstruction, and in those with haemoptysis, persistent cough or severe pain from bone metastases. It is best avoided in patients generally ill with advanced disease, or with large tumours, as it is likely to make them worse.

Chemotherapy for lung cancer has on the whole been disappointing. Various regimes of intermittent treatment using multiple cytotoxic drugs are being assessed with regard to producing worthwhile remission, particularly for small cell (oat cell) carcinoma. Many regard this tumour as being a systemic disease and more suitable for chemotherapy rather than radiotherapy.

The average survival time of patients without treatment is about nine months from the onset of symptoms.

MESOTHELIOMA

The rising incidence of this tumour is believed to be related to the increased risk of exposure to asbestos dust. It may present as a pleural opacity or as a blood stained effusion which rapidly recurs after aspiration. Pleural masses may be visible when fluid has been removed. Malignant cells may be detected in the fluid or on pleural biopsy. The tumour is often associated with severe pain as it invades the chest wall and it may grow through needle tracks or sites of pleural biopsy.

Treatment is universally ineffective for the tumour shows little response to radiotherapy or to cytotoxic drugs. Cases with recurring effusion are best treated by pleurodesis.

ALVEOLAR CELL CARCINOMA

Alveolar cell carcinoma is an uncommon tumour of the lung. Pathologically it appears as an adenocarcinoma which is arising from the epithelium of the alveoli or bronchioles. It may develop in lungs previously damaged by fibrosis. An area of tumour may remain static for some time and then spread widely throughout the lungs via the bronchi and lymphatics. Profuse bronchorrhoea from excessive mucus production is dramatic but rare. When the disease is advanced the patient suffers severe breathlessness and finally respiratory failure. The X-ray changes may be those of nodular shadows confined to a segment or lobe or of confluent areas of consolidation; they may be unilateral or bilateral.

ADENOMA OF THE BRONCHUS

The term adenoma of the bronchus is a misnomer as the great majority are carcinoid tumours. They are mostly benign but a proportion become malignant and metastasise locally. The systemic symptoms which arise from gut carcinoid with liver metastases do not occur with a bronchial lesion. A small number of adenomas are due to an adenoid cystic carcinoma (cylindroma), which is a low-grade malignant tumour, or due to an adenoma of the mucous glands. Bronchial adenoma is much less common than carcinoma and occurs rather more often in women. A rounded opacity may be seen on chest X-ray or tomograms, and the majority of the tumour may be extrabronchial as a dumb-bell extension. More commonly the chest X-ray shows collapse/consolidation of a segment or a lobe. It may present as recurrent haemoptysis or as bronchial obstruction with segmental infection. Diagnosis is confirmed by bronchoscopy and biopsy; the histology may be misinterpreted as oat cell carcinoma. The adenoma should be removed surgically, either bronchoscopically or by bronchotomy or lobectomy.

HAMARTOMA

This benign tumour of the lung is composed of a mixture of tissues normally present in the lung, particularly cartilage. It usually produces no symptoms and is discovered on the chest radiography as a rounded opacity with clear-cut edges, a 'coin' lesion. There may be areas of calcification, best seen on tomography, when it may be impossible to distinguish it from a tuberculoma. Calcified glands and calcified lesions in other sites of the lung will be in favour of tuberculoma. Otherwise the likely differential diagnoses are an isolated secondary deposit or a peripheral carcinoma of the lung. Surgical resection may be the only certain way of establishing the nature of the lesion.

THE PNEUMONIAS

Classification can be based both on the nature of the *infecting organism* and on the *anatomical distribution* of the pneumonia.
Infecting organisms which may produce pneumonia include the following:

Bacteria	*H. influenzae* *Strep. pneumoniae* *Staph. pyogenes* *Klebsiella pneumoniae* *Legionella pneumophila* *Mycobacterium tuberculosis*

Viruses	Influenza Para-influenza Adenovirus Respiratory syncytial virus Cytomegalovirus
Other Organisms	*Mycoplasma pneumoniae* Chlamydiae *Coxiellia burneti*
Protozoa	*Pneumocystis carinii*
Fungi	*Aspergillus fumigatus*

In general, leucocytosis above 15 000 per mm strongly suggests a bacterial infection. Identification of the organism should be attempted by direct examination of the sputum with Gram staining, and if necessary by Ziehl–Neelsen stain. Culture of the sputum and antibiotic sensitivities should be performed. Blood cultures are of value in severe pneumonias.

Blood for serological tests can be taken if Legionnaire's pneumonia, psittacosis, Q fever, viral or mycoplasma pneumonia are suspected. A four-fold rise in antibody titre over a two-week period is significant, but suffers the disadvantage that it is by then a retrospective diagnosis.

Not infrequently there is a failure to identify the infecting organism in spite of every attempt to do so, in which case antibiotic therapy is directed at the infection most likely to be present in a given clinical setting.

Anatomical Distribution

The chest X-ray will demonstrate the distribution of the pneumonia. There are, however, no absolute diagnostic radiological appearances which will reveal the nature of the infecting organism upon which treatment should be based.

(1) Bronchopneumonia

This is consolidation occurring in patches around infected terminal bronchi. It may be confined to a small segment of lung or it may be widespread throughout both lungs, tending to be more marked at the bases. It is often the result of secondary bacterial infection following an acute viral bronchitis; organisms such as streptococci, *Haemophilus influenzae* and pneumococci which may be present normally in the upper respiratory tract can spread down the air passages to infect terminal bronchi. It has a greater tendency to occur in the very young, the elderly, in those with established heart and lung disease, and the debilitated. It is often the terminal event in a seriously ill patient.

Influenza may at times cause a fulminating bronchopneumonia with super-added bacterial infection usually with *Staph. pyogenes*.

Tuberculosis by bronchogenic spread throughout the lung, may produce a widespread bronchopneumonia.

(2) Segmental Pneumonia

(a) *Inhalation Pneumonias*. The aspiration of infected material into the lungs may give rise to pneumonia. The distribution of the consolidation depends on the quantity of material inhaled and its nature. If large amounts of highly infected or irritating material are inhaled, as when an anaesthetised patient inhales vomit, a widely distributed and severe bronchopneumonia involving both lungs may result. If a smaller amount of highly infected material is inhaled into a segment of lung it will result in pneumonic consolidation of the segment and unless aspirated material is coughed up or sucked out and the infection controlled, the consolidation may proceed to abscess formation.

(b) *Aspiration Pneumonitis*

Clinical Features. This is the commonest type of pneumonia seen in general practice. It is due to bronchial obstruction by mucus, with subsequent infected lobular or segmental collapse. The mucus is aspirated from the upper respiratory tract at the time of a cold or sinus infection, or it may have a bronchial origin at the time of a bronchitis. Aspiration pneumonitis may also occur due to the inhalation of anaerobic organisms from the oropharynx. The clinical picture varies considerably depending on the nature of the accompanying bacterial infection. At one extreme the pneumonitis may be discovered by chance on radiography at the time of a cold, there being no localised or constitutional symptoms. With virulent organisms, however, the clinical picture resembles that of the specific bacterial pneumonias. Most commonly, a few days after a cold or bronchitis, the patient's general condition becomes a little worse and there is malaise, cough, continuing fever and sometimes pleuritic pain. Usually the only physical sign is a patch of crackles over the affected area. Radiography of the chest shows an opacity due to an area of segmental collapse and consolidation.

Treatment with ampicillin 500 mg four times daily combined with simple postural therapy is usually satisfactory.

(3) Lobar Pneumonia

Lobar consolidation bounded by the fissures and with the normal size of the lobe maintained is characteristic of infection with virulent strains of *pneumococci*. It diffusely involves one or at times more lobes of the lung. It also occurs with *Klebsiella pneumoniae* (Friedländer's pneumonia), in which case the lobe may be so distended with inflammatory exudate that there is bulging of the fissure—the so-called 'heavy' lobe; lung sloughing and cavitation may occur. Cavitation also occurs with infections with *Staph. pyogenes* and *M. tuberculosis* which may also produce lobar or lobular pneumonia.

It should be remembered that segmental or lobar pneumonia with collapse/consolidation may be due to an obstructive lesion such as carcinoma of the bronchus.

Viral and *mycoplasma* infections produce hazy lobular or lobar shadowing, which may be extensive.

BACTERIAL PNEUMONIAS

Pneumococcal Pneumonia

Clinical Features. Pneumococcal lobar pneumonia may occur at any age; it is quite a common terminal event in the lives of the elderly or infirm, but it may equally attack people in the prime of life. It is more common in the winter months, and usually occurs sporadically. It is due to infection with virulent strains of pneumococci.

The onset is usually sudden with shivering or even a rigor and sometimes vomiting. The temperature rises abruptly and fever remains continuous. The face is typically hot and flushed and cyanosis may be marked. The respiration rate rises out of proportion to the temperature. An acute dry pleurisy develops over the affected lobe leading to severe pain on respiration, so that the breathing becomes rapid, shallow, and sometimes grunting. The development of herpes on the lips completes the classical picture. A painful cough is common at this stage of the disease and the sputum may have a 'rusty' tinge.

Examination of the chest at the onset usually shows little except diminished movement on the affected side together with reduced breath sounds, and perhaps some crackles or a pleural rub. After the first 24–48 hours, the signs of consolidation appear; dullness, bronchial breathing, whispering pectoriloquy, and bronchophony over the consolidated lobe. There is a polymorphonuclear leucocytosis.

In the days before antibiotics were available recovery occurred by crisis at about the seventh day, the temperature falling quite rapidly and the patient's general condition taking a sudden turn for the better. Antibiotic treatment modifies the course of the disease and the patient's condition usually begins to improve within 48 hours of starting treatment. As the signs of consolidation disappear they are replaced by coarse crackles due to the liquefying inflammatory exudate.

In the elderly, lobar pneumonia may not produce the dramatic picture outlined above. There may be little fever and the diagnosis depends on finding signs of consolidation.

Chest radiography confirms the presence of lobar consolidation.

Complications

(1) *Delayed Resolution.* The time taken for the lung to return to normal, with disappearance of physical signs and radiological clearing, varies a good deal in different patients. If resolution is delayed for more than two or three weeks the possibility of some underlying condition such as carcinoma or bronchiectasis must be investigated. Alternatively the pneumonia may be due to organisms resistant to the antibiotic in use, such as the tubercle bacillus. This will require careful and perhaps repeated examination of the sputum. Bronchoscopy and bronchography may be required. Pneumonia responds slowly to treatment in patients with diabetes, cirrhosis, chronic alcoholism, or nephritis.

There remains a small group of patients in whom the pneumonia instead of resolving proceeds to fibrosis and chronic suppuration. Postural drainage and inhalations should be used, but the affected lobe may require surgical resection.

(2) *Effusions.* Since the advent of chemotherapy, empyemata have become uncommon but serous pleural effusions appearing about one to two weeks after the onset of the pneumonia continue to occur. Treatment is by daily aspiration with infusion of 500 000 units of benzylpenicillin into the pleural cavity until the fluid subsides. The pleural fluid should be cultured for organisms and systemic antibiotics should be continued. The site of the aspiration is determined by the position of the physical signs and by radiography. The majority of serous effusions subside within a week or so of treatment.

(3) *Empyema.* In a small proportion of patients the effusion becomes purulent and the patient's condition deteriorates. Fever recurs and becomes remittent in type. The patients looks ill and suffers from anorexia, malaise, and drenching sweats. Examination of the chest reveals signs of fluid (p. 249). A white count shows considerable polymorph leucocytosis. The diagnosis is confirmed by aspirating pus from the pleural cavity. Empyema is considered further on p. 314.

(4) *Heart Failure.* Cardiac failure complicated perhaps by cardiac arrhythmia, particularly atrial fibrillation, may occur in elderly patients. For treatment see p. 143.

(5) *Other complications* include pericarditis, endocarditis, and meningitis. Certain patients have severe headache and some neck stiffness in the early stages of pneumonia, although the cerebrospinal fluid is normal. The syndrome is called meningismus.

Staphylococcal Pneumonia

Clinical Features. Staphylococcal pneumonia may occur at any age. It can occur as a primary infection but more commonly as a complication of influenza. It can be part of a staphylococcal septicaemia and there may be a history of a recent boil or some other staphyloccal infection. Pulmonary infarcts may be secondarily infected with staphylococci.

The onset is often acute with malaise, vomiting, anorexia, and rigors. Pleurisy may occur. The sputum is purulent and may be blood-stained. Fever is characteristically remittent.

The *physical signs* are variable and often inconspicuous. They are often bilateral with patches of impaired resonance, reduced breath sounds and crackles. Bronchial breathing may be present. *Radiography* of the chest confirms the presence of consolidation which often cavitates to form an abscess. Alternatively thin walled abscesses may occur which are distension cysts typical of staphylococcal pneumonia, particularly when part of a septicaemia. Empyema and spontaneous pneumothorax may also occur.

It is often striking that a lung riddled with pneumonia and abscesses can resolve completely with antibiotic treatment, but residual areas of fibrosis and cyst formation are not uncommon. The lung abscesses and pleural infection rarely require surgical treatment.

At times staphylococcal pneumonia complicating influenza becomes a fulminating infection (p. 284).

The *diagnosis* is confirmed by sputum culture or by direct examination of the sputum with Gram staining. The sensitivity of the organism to various antibiotics should be determined, as it may be widely resistant.

Friedländer's Pneumonia

Clinical Features. Pneumonia due to Friedländer's bacillus (*Klebsiella pneumoniae*) is not common. It usually presents acutely as lobar consolidation although at times it may have an insidious onset when it may mimic tuberculosis or carcinoma. Friedländer's pneumonia has a tendency to progress to lung sloughing with abscess formation and fibrosis. The mortality rate is considerable. The diagnosis is confirmed by culturing the organism in the sputum, or more immediately by identification of the Gram-negative bacilli on direct examination.

Treatment of Specific Bacterial Pneumonias

General. Severe pleuritic pain is best treated with an injection of intramuscular pethidine 100 mg or subcutaneous morphine 15 mg. The beneficial effects of these drugs in promoting rest far outweigh the dangers of respiratory depression. A persistent unproductive cough may be relieved by linctus pholcodine 10 ml.

If the patient becomes cyanosed, oxygen should be given. An oxygen mask may frighten or distress the patient and careful explanation and reassurance are important. Care should be taken on administering oxygen to patients with chronic lung disease because of the danger of CO_2 retention.

Patients severely ill with pneumonia are not infrequently dehydrated and need adequate fluid intake, either orally or intravenously.

Most patients can be allowed up five to seven days after the temperature has become normal, but this will be influenced by the patient's age and the severity of the illness. Breathing exercises should begin when the temperature falls and should be continued through convalescence, the length of which depends on the occupation and the home environment.

Specific Treatment. In practice it is not always easy to be sure of the nature of the organisms and culture of the sputum takes time or may be impracticable.

Pneumococcal Lobar Pneumonia responds satisfactorily to treatment with ampicillin 500 mg 6-hourly.

The patient usually responds, within 48 hours, but treatment should be continued for one to two weeks. If clinical response is satisfactory the dosage can be reduced to ampicillin 250 mg 6-hourly.

Other antibiotics are occasionally required when the patient is sensitive to ampicillin or when the organisms are resistant, such as may occur in pneumonia complicating chronic bronchitis or bronchiectasis. In these patients it is often advisable to use a 'broad spectrum' antibiotic, such as co-trimoxazole 2 tablets twice-daily or tetracycline 250 mg four times a day.

Staphylococcal Pneumonia. Quite frequently, infection is due to penicillin-resistant organisms and if the patient is severely ill, there is no time to await the result of sputum culture or the clinical response to benzyl-penicillin. Under these circumstances IV flucloxacillin 500 mg 6-hourly with sodium fusidate 500 mg three times daily should be given. Subsequent antibiotic treatment will depend on the response of the patient and the result of sensitivity tests, and it is advisable to continue treatment for several weeks because of the liability to relapse. If clinical response is satisfactory, flucloxacillin can be given orally.

Recovery is usual in these severe cases but when staphylococcal infection is associated with *fulminating influenzal pneumonia*, the outlook is grave (see below).

Friedländer's Pneumonia is resistant to penicillin but responds to gentamicin 60–120 mg 8-hourly. Many strains of *Kl. pneumoniae* are also sensitive to co-trimoxazole and cefotaxime. The sensitivity of the organism to antibiotics should be determined whenever possible. If abscess formation or fibrosis ensues, surgical treatment may be required.

Legionnaires' Disease

This unusual type of pneumonia occurs sporadically. It is due to a Gram negative aerobic organism (*Legionella pneumophila*) which can be growth on blood agar with additives. The reservoir for the organism is probably in humid and wet situations. In the early stages malaise, myalgia, headache and fever, with rigors, predominate. Respiratory symptoms of dry cough and pleuritic pain may then be overshadowed by gastrointestinal and central nervous system symptoms—namely vomiting and diarrhoea and mental confusion. Laboratory findings include moderate leucocytosis (usually less than 15×10^9/litre); proteinuria and haematuria; hyponatraemia (serum Na less than 130 mmol/litre); and abnormal liver function tests. Examination of the chest reveals crackles only. The chest X-ray shows segmental or lobar pneumonia which may be widespread and which is slow to clear. Pleural effusions may be present. Diagnosis can be confirmed by detection of antibodies by an indirect fluorescent antibody test or by culture of the organism. The illness varies from a mild pneumonia to a severe illness with respiratory failure and a generalised disorder involving the central nervous, renal and gastrointestinal systems, and fatalities occur.

Treatment is with erythromycin in full doses. Rifampicin, in a dose of 600 mg b.d., is also effective against the organism, but should never be given on its own because drug resistance develops rapidly.

Tuberculous Pneumonia

Tuberculosis may rarely present with lobar pneumonia or widespread bronchopneumonia, associated with severe constitutional symptoms. It will fail to respond to penicillin. The sputum of every patient with pneumonia which does not respond to ordinary antibiotic treatment must be examined, and the diagnosis of tuberculous pneumonia will be established by finding the organism.

Treatment is along the usual lines for tuberculosis.

Pneumonia Complicating Influenza

Influenza is sometimes complicated by pneumonia; this is rare when influenza is sporadic, but may become common during epidemics and accounts for the majority of deaths which occur.

Any type of pneumonia may complicate influenza. The most common is a localised aspiration pneumonia (see p. 279) and staphylococcal pneumonia also occurs. Of particular importance is the severe infection called *fulminating influenzal pneumonia.* There is an overwhelming toxaemia due to a combination of infection with the influenzal virus and *Staphylococcus aureus.*

Clinical Features. The onset of severe pneumonia complicating influenza is rapid, often alarmingly so. The patient has a simple attack of influenza which appears to be progressing in the usual way when over a few hours the condition deteriorates rapidly. The respiration rate becomes rapid, cyanosis appears, sometimes with a typical greyish blue colour (*heliotrope cyanosis*). There may be evidence of circulatory collapse with rising pulse rate and falling blood pressure. Pleuritic pain is uncommon. Examination of the chest shows evidence of patchy consolidation with scattered crackles and perhaps an occasional area of bronchial breathing. Leucopenia is common.

Treatment. In *fulminating influenzal pneumonia* treatment must be started before the results of sputum culture are available. Antibiotics are therefore used which are active against both the staphylococcus and other unknown organisms. Flucloxacillin 500 mg 6-hourly should be used because of the possibility of penicillin-resistant organisms. There is also a good case for giving a broad spectrum antibiotic in addition until the nature of the infecting organism has been established, for example gentamicin or one of the newer cephalosporins such as cefuroxime. Once staphylococcal infection has been identified, sodium fusidate 500 mg 8-hourly, or IV diethanolamine fusidate, may be given as a second antistaphylococcal agent in severely ill patients. Erythromycin should be used in any case in patients known to be allergic to penicillin.

Oxygen therapy may be indicated and circulatory collapse with a falling blood pressure can be treated with IV hydrocortisone 200 mg 4-hourly until improvement occurs.

VIRUS PNEUMONIAS

Most cases of so-called virus pneumonia have, in fact, an area of collapse-consolidation occurring at the time of a viral respiratory tract infection. This is the result of blockage of a bronchus with sputum with superimposed secondary bacterial infection (see Aspiration Pneumonitis p. 279). Infections with viruses, such as the adenovirus and influenza can affect the lungs producing pneumonia, but the roles of primary virus infection and bacterial infection are often in doubt. In these circumstances it is reasonable to give antibiotic treatment as for bacterial infection. Respiratory syncytial virus causes bronchiolitis in infants and cytomegalovirus produces pneumonia in immunosuppressed patients (p. 287).

PNEUMONIAS DUE TO OTHER ORGANISMS

Mycoplasma Pneumonia

The organism *Mycoplasma pneumoniae* has features of both a virus and a bacterium. Although it is small and has no cell wall, at the same time it does not require a living organism for culture and is sensitive to the tetracycline group of drugs. It is not sensitive to the penicillins as these depend on their action on the bacterial cell membrane for their antibiotic effect.

Clinical Features. The disease starts with the general symptoms of a virus infection, namely malaise, anorexia, headache, backache, and sometimes depression, followed within a day or two by cough and sometimes pleurisy. Venous thromboses may occur and severe cases may develop haemolytic anaemia, myocarditis, pericarditis and pleural effusions. Examination of the chest usually shows only a patch of râles or perhaps an area of impaired resonance and bronchial breathing. Radiography reveals an area of consolidation having a rather ground glass appearance and of varying distribution. There is no leucocytosis and the blood contains cold agglutinins. Serological tests will show a fourfold increase or more in the antibody titre over a two-week period.

Treatment. Tetracycline or erythromycin should be given in full dosage of 500 mg 6-hourly.

Anaerobic Infections

Anaerobic infections of the lung usually follow the inhalation of mixed organisms from the oropharynx. In most cases there is infection of the gums, but the absence of teeth does not exclude the diagnosis. Other predisposing factors include alcoholism and epilepsy, and loss of consciousness from coma, drug overdose or general anaesthesia. Defective cough due to neurological disease and dysphagia from any cause may also predispose to inhalation. The types of infection include aspiration pneumonitis (p. 279), a necrotising pneumonia (to be distinguished from tuberculosis and from staphylococcal or klebsiella pneumonia), lung abscess and empyema. The infection is likely to be sited in the most dependent parts of the lung at the time of inhalation (see Lung Abscess p. 287). In addition, anaerobic organisms may secondarily infect bronchiectasis and devitalised lung, as with pneumoconiosis and emphysematous bullae, and obstructive pneumonitis from carcinoma. The sputum and the breath are characteristically extremely foul (putrid or fetid) with anaerobic infections, due to the presence of short chain fatty acids produced by the organisms.

Treatment. The infection responds to treatment with benzylpenicillin and metronidazole. The most effective cephalosporin against anaerobes is latamoxef but it is expensive and the above treatment is usually satisfactory.

Ornithosis (Psittacosis)

The organism (*Chlamydia psittaci*) occurs widely among many species of birds and is intermediate between a virus and a rickettsia. The illness is caught mainly from parrots, budgerigars and canaries. It is an influenza-like illness and the patient may develop patchy consolidation in the lungs. Splenomegaly is common and rose spots resembling those seen in typhoid fever may be found. At times a severe fulminating pneumonia with considerable mortality may develop.

In the early stages the organism can be cultured from the blood or sputum and at a later stage a rising titre of serum antibodies can be demonstrated.

Treatment. The organism responds to tetracycline which should be given in full doses of 500 mg four times daily.

Q Fever

The organism (*Coxiella burneti*) is known to infect domestic animals such as sheep, cows and goats. Human infection probably occurs through drinking raw milk, from inhaling animal dust or from ticks. It is characterised by fever, toxaemia, cough and 'atypical' pneumonia. Q fever endocarditis may also occur.

Treatment. Tetracycline in full doses is effective but response is slow. Treatment may have to be prolonged, particularly with endocarditis when it may have to be continued for six months to a year.

OPPORTUNIST LUNG INFECTION

Lung infection is a not infrequent complication when immune responses are impaired. This may result from disease, such as reticulosis or leukaemia, or because of drug treatment, such as cytotoxic therapy, immunosuppressant drugs or corticosteroids. Bacterial pneumonia or tuberculosis may occur but at times infection may occur with organisms not commonly pathogenic to the lungs; these include protozoa (*Pneumocystis carinii*), viruses (*Cytomegalovirus*), yeasts (*Cryptococcus neoformans* and *Candida albicans*) and fungi (*Aspergillus fumigatus*). Pneumocystis infection responds to co-trimoxazole in large doses. Invasive aspergillosis (p. 301) can be treated with intravenous amphotericin B or in combination with flucytosine, and possibly ketoconazole in addition. Cryptococcal infections are discussed on p. 301, and candidal infections on p. 302.

LUNG ABSCESS

An abscess in the lung develops when an area of consolidated lung breaks down to form an infected cavity. Among the many causes are:

(1) *Inhalation of infected material* into the bronchial tree from the upper respiratory tract, particularly gross paradontal infection. It is liable to be inhaled when the cough reflex is suppressed during sleep, or when the patient is in a coma or under anaesthesia. Infected pus and blood clots may also be inhaled at the time of dental extractions or tonsillectomy. The material is inhaled into a bronchopulmonary segment and leads to segmental pneumonia which breaks down to form an abscess. The contents are coughed up leaving a chronic abscess cavity usually infected with a mixed group of organisms. If they include anaerobic organisms, the pus becomes foul-smelling and lung abscesses

are classified into *putrid* and *non-putrid* on this basis. Sometimes the breakdown of lung tissue is very rapid and the state is sometimes called *gangrene of the lung*. The site of inhalation lung abscess is influenced by gravity. As the unconscious patient usually lies on his side or back the most dependent segments in these positions are the segments supplied by the axillary branches of the upper lobe bronchi, the posterior segment of the upper lobe and the apex of the lower lobe. Inhalation of foreign bodies, food or vomit may also cause lung infection leading to abscess formation.

(2) Secondary to breakdown of peripheral carcinoma or to bronchial obstruction from carcinoma or other causes.

(3) Abscesses may develop in the course of various *specific pneumonias*, namely staphylococcal pneumonia, Friedländer's pneumonia and tuberculosis.

(4) Rare causes include extension of an amoebic abscess of the liver through the diaphragm, actinomycosis, infected hydatid cyst, and abscesses developing during the course of a pyaemia.

(5) In a small proportion of patients with lung abscesses, *no cause* can be found.

Clinical Features. These depend on the underlying cause of the abscess. With 'putrid' lung abscess, onset of symptoms is usually acute. There may be a history of coma or an anaesthetic in the presence of paradontal infection, or of dental extraction or some other operation on the upper respiratory tract one to three weeks previously. The patient complains of fever, shivering, night sweats, malaise, and anorexia. Pleurisy is quite common. There is usually a cough with mucoid sputum; after some days, the abscess discharges into a bronchus and the patient coughs up large quantities of foul purulent sputum. This may be preceded by a foul smell to the breath and is pathognomonic of lung abscess.

When the abscess has discharged, the patient's general condition may improve but unless adequate treatment is given he continues to cough up large quantities of purulent sputum sometimes mixed with blood. If the abscess is allowed to become chronic there is the risk of cerebral abscess, of blocking of the abscess cavity with rapid deterioration in the patient's condition. The abscess may rupture into the pleural cavity leading to an empyema.

Clubbing of the fingers develops. The *signs* over a lung abscess are variable. Usually there is impairment to percussion together with crackles and sometimes bronchial breathing; a pleural rub may also be heard. Both postero-anterior and lateral chest radiographs must be taken; the exact segment of lung involved will then be apparent. In the early stages the affected segment is opaque, but when discharge of the abscess has occurred a cavity can be seen containing a fluid level and sometimes a slough. The radiograph of a breaking-down peripheral carcinoma is characteristic, the walls of the abscess cavity being thick and irregular.

The white count shows a polymorphonuclear leucocytosis. The sputum should always be examined bacteriologically as the lung abscess may be secondary to a specific bacterial infection, such as the *Staphylococcus aureus*, Friedländer's bacillus, or *M. tuberculosis*.

Treatment. Treatment is initially by antibiotics and correct postural drainage. It is usual to start with intramuscular benzylpenicillin but this may have to be changed or added to depending on the result of the sputum examination or if there is a poor clinical response. Metronidazole is also effective against anaerobic infections. The position for postural drainage is determined by the site of the affected segment; treatment must be intense, 4–6 times daily, and the patient must sleep so as to give the abscess dependent drainage.

With this treatment the lung abscess usually resolves. When the response is not satisfactory or when drainage is not occurring freely, bronchoscopy is required to exclude any obstruction to drainage, such as a carcinoma of the lung. External drainage is rarely required.

In a small proportion of patients in whom the abscess fails to heal and who are left with a grossly damaged lobe, resection may be necessary.

PULMONARY COLLAPSE

Collapse of the lung may occur in two ways:

(1) *Absorption Collapse*. If a bronchus either to a whole lung or to a segment of lung becomes completely blocked, then the air in that segment is absorbed into the blood stream and the segment collapses to a smaller size. The space formerly occupied by the collapsed lung is filled by any combination of the following:
   (a) The diaphragm is elevated.
   (b) The mediastinum moves towards the side of the collapsed lung (see Palpation p. 250).
   (c) The remaining lung becomes hyperinflated, a condition known as compensatory emphysema.

(2) *Pneumothorax and Hydrothorax*. If air or fluid is introduced into the pleural space then the elastic tissue in the lung will contract and the lung will collapse to a smaller size, the degree of collapse depending on the volume of air or fluid in the pleural cavity. The mediastinum may be displaced to the opposite side if the pneumothorax or effusion is large.

Absorption Collapse

Bronchial obstruction may be due to several causes; the more important are:

(1) *Bronchial carcinoma*, or more rarely bronchial adenoma.
(2) *Foreign material* in the bronchial tree. Mucus or inflammatory exudate may collect following an operation, but also occurs in asthma, bronchitis, bronchiectasis, measles, and whooping cough. Sometimes foreign material may be inhaled, for instance blood clot from the mouth following dental extraction, or foreign bodies such as beads, peanuts, or pieces of bone.
(3) *Compression of the bronchus from outside* may occur from enlarged lymph nodes in tuberculosis, sarcoidosis or Hodgkin's disease, or occasionally may be due to aortic aneurysm.

Both bronchial carcinoma and external compression of the bronchus usually cause collapse of major segments of lung. Mucus may also cause collapse of a major segment, but if inhaled into the smaller bronchi may cause multiple small areas of collapse. Absorption collapse is usually followed by some degree of infection and sometimes this may be severe enough to lead to abscess formation (see p. 287). If the lung is not re-expanded within a month, permanent changes are likely to occur and the lung does not return to normal.

Clinical Features. The symptoms of collapse depend on the extent of lung involved. They may also be overshadowed by the symptoms of the underlying lung disease.

Obstruction of a large bronchus usually gives rise to dyspnoea, sometimes severe, and to a feeling of tightness across the chest. If infection occurs, there will be fever. Examination shows an increase in the pulse and respiration rate and perhaps also some cyanosis. There will be mediastinal shift towards the lesion with dullness to percussion and absent breath sounds over the collapsed area. Smaller segments of collapse may give rise to little in the way of symptoms or physical signs and can only be diagnosed by radiography. The interpretation of radiographs in this condition depends on a knowledge of the anatomy of the bronchopulmonary segments; both postero-anterior and lateral films of the chest are required to localise the collapsed segment.

Treatment. This is directed towards relieving the bronchial obstruction and controlling any pulmonary infection. This in turn depends on the underlying pathology, for often it is due to carcinoma of the bronchus.

In those cases occurring with bronchitis or asthma, where bronchial obstruction is due to a mucus plug, the patient should be positioned so that drainage from the obstructed bronchus is aided by gravity. The chest wall over the collapsed lung should be percussed and the patient encouraged to cough. Using these methods the plug is usually dislodged. At times, aspiration through a bronchoscope is required.

Postoperative Absorption Collapse is due to blocking of a bronchus by a mucus plug. A number of factors render this likely to occur:

(1) It is more common after abdominal and chest operations, for these

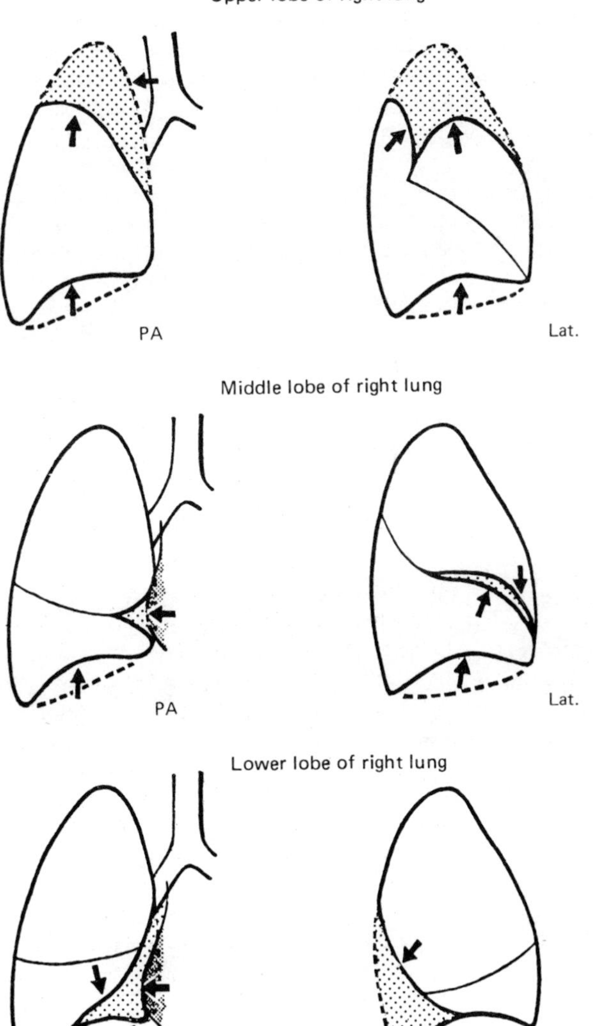

Fig. 5.4 Diagram of radiographic appearances of lobar absorption collapse.

make coughing painful and thus interfere with the clearing of mucus from the bronchi.

(2) Infections of the respiratory tract, such as a cold or bronchitis at the time of operation, increase bronchial secretions.

(3) The excessive use of atropine makes the sputum viscid and more difficult to clear from the bronchi.

Clinical Features. Postoperative collapse usually occurs within two or three days of operation. The symptoms and signs are those described under collapse (see p. 290).

The subsequent course will depend on the adequacy of treatment for if the condition is allowed to persist there is a danger of bronchiectasis and pulmonary fibrosis developing.

Treatment

Preventive

(a) No subject with an acute respiratory tract infection should be given a general anaesthetic except in an emergency.
(b) Patients with chronic respiratory disease should receive breathing exercises, rostural drainage and, in some cases, antibiotics before a general anaesthetic. Smoking should be forbidden.
(c) Infected teeth and sinuses should be treated before an anaesthetic.
(d) Immediately after the operation the patient should be encouraged to clear sputum from the bronchi by coughing and the position in bed should be changed regularly to prevent stagnation of secretions in one part of the lung.

Curative

(a) The patient should be postured so that drainage of the blocked bronchus is assisted by gravity.
(b) Coughing should be encouraged. This causes pain from the operative incision which can be controlled by supporting the wound when the patient coughs, and by giving IM morphine 10 mg. The chest over the collapsed lung should be percussed rapidly and further coughing encouraged.
(c) If these measures are not followed by improvement in the patient's condition over the next few hours, the mucus should be aspirated by bronchoscopy.
(d) Oxygen must be given to those patients who are cyanosed and distressed.
(e) Ampicillin 250–500 mg 6-hourly should be given to deal with any associated infection.

CYSTS OF THE LUNG

Cysts of the lung may be classified as follows:

(1) Congenital Cysts

Congenital cysts of the lung are due to maldevelopment of part of the primitive lung buds. They are lined with epithelium similar to that of the respiratory passage. They may be single or multiple.

Clinical Features. Congenital cysts are commonly symptomless. *In infancy* a single congenital cyst may develop a valve-like mechanism so that air is sucked in during inspiration, but cannot be expired. The cyst expands until it interferes with respiration, causing distress and cyanosis. The situation can be temporarily relieved by inserting a needle into the cyst and connecting it by a tube to an underwater seal. Further treatment is surgical.

Congenital cysts are also liable to become infected. Single cysts then present a picture similar to that of lung abscess and multiple cysts may be mistaken for bronchiectasis. Although antibiotics may control the infection and constitutional upset, postural drainage of the cyst is usually unsatisfactory due to inadequate bronchial connections; surgical excision of the infected cyst is therefore advisable when practicable.

(2) Acquired Cysts

These are much more common than congenital cysts of the lung. They have a variety of causes, but are basically due to stretching and breaking down of alveoli; they are not lined with respiratory epithelium. The chief causes are:

(a) *Acute lung infection*, particularly staphylococcal pneumonia (p. 281).
(b) *Pulmonary tuberculosis* may lead to cavities with a stop valve connection with a bronchus. They become distended and take on the characteristics of cysts.
(c) *Emphysema*. Localised or generalised cysts of the lung may occur.

Clinical Features. Large bullae interfere with respiratory function, for they decrease the total alveolar surface of the lung, diminish mixing of respiratory gases and may interfere with the normal stretch reflexes arising in the lung.

Generally the alveolar over-distension and cyst formation are so widespread in both lungs that no specific treatment is possible, but bullae can occasionally be resected or plicated.

PULMONARY TUBERCULOSIS

General Considerations

Infection with the tubercle bacillus in a subject who has never previously experienced contact with the organism is called *primary tuberculosis*; reinfection after the primary lesion is called *post-primary tuberculosis*. The disease follows different courses in the two instances, the difference being attributed to the acquisition of a delayed hypersensitivity reaction (Type IV) in response to the primary lesion.

In Great Britain and the USA, and most of the other countries of the Western Hemisphere, infection is almost entirely with the human bacillus. In less economically developed countries milk still serves as a vehicle for infection with the bovine organism, and primary abdominal tuberculosis and its sequelae may occur.

The human bacillus is spread almost exclusively by droplet infection and lesions other than in the lung are uncommon. There is a wide range of susceptibility to the disease. Negroes, and dwellers in isolated communities, have little natural resistance. It is not a hereditary disease, but increased susceptibility may be inborn; if one of a pair of identical twins develops tuberculosis the other has a greatly increased chance of being affected, even if living in a totally different environment. Resistance may also be conditioned by such factors as alcoholism, diabetes, malnutrition, overwork, and lack of sleep. The risks of infection are much increased by proximity, either from overcrowding of housing, or individual exposure, for example in dentists, and in doctors or nurses working with tuberculous patients.

Deaths from tuberculosis of all forms fell steadily in all civilised communities from the turn of the century. The rate of decline was so regular, with the exception of the war years, in the British Isles that it may be concluded that it was little influenced by any passing fancy in therapy and that the improvement was more likely to be due to public health measures. Since the introduction of effective chemotherapy death rates have declined precipitously.

PRIMARY TUBERCULOSIS

Characteristically the initial lesion is small and the local lymph nodes bear the brunt of the infection.

Pulmonary. A small pneumonic lesion (Ghon focus) may be situated in any part of the lungs. Lymphatic spread soon occurs and the local lymph nodes become enlarged. The radiographic appearance of a small shadow in the lung associated with hilar lymphadenopathy is known as the *primary complex*. It is accompanied by a change in the tuberculin reaction to positive (see p. 298). There is usually little upset in health and the natural tendency is to heal by fibrosis and calcification. In the past, primary tuberculosis commonly occurred in young people and up to 1950 over 95% of urban dwellers had unknowingly healed such lesions before reaching adult life. Not all primary lesions heal spontaneously and without complications. As tuberculosis is now less common, an increasing proportion of children reach adult life without infection and it is these for whom protection is sought by vaccination with BCG (see p. 300).

Complications. Sometimes the lung lesion increases in size to spread through the lobe, and rarely it may cavitate. This is more liable to occur in young adults, who are also prone to develop primary *tuberculous pleural effusions* (see p. 311).

In infants and young children particularly, the enlarged hilar lymph nodes may cause compression of a bronchus with segmental collapse, producing the radiographic appearance known as *epituberculosis*. This may lead to permanent bronchiectasis, such as the *middle lobe syndrome* (p. 264). An infected lymph node may also rupture through the wall of a bronchus, the caseous material being discharged into the bronchial tree and causing a widespread *tuberculous bronchopneumonia* (p. 279). Alternatively, the nodes may erode blood vessels so that blood-borne tuberculosis may occur in such sites as bone, joints, kidney, epididymus, Fallopian tubes, brain, or meninges. Tuberculous pericarditis may develop as a result of direct spread of infection from mediastinal glands.

Miliary Tuberculosis

Miliary tuberculosis is due to widespread haematogenous dissemination. In primary tuberculosis it usually results from a caseous lymph node eroding a bronchial vessel, but it also occurs at times with post-primary lesions and in the elderly.

Clinical Features. The onset is usually insidious with general malaise, pyrexia, loss of weight, and sweats. Children often become listless and lose interest in their toys. Evidence of miliary spread through the lungs is not obvious early in the disease but later cough develops, with little sputum or dyspnoea. In some cases meningeal involvement is the most prominent feature and the patient presents with a tuberculous meningitis (p. 364).

Chest signs are either absent or confined to scattered fine crackles. The spleen is often just palpable and careful examination of the retina may show choroidal tubercles. They are greyish-white lesions about one third the size of the optic disc. A chest radiograph shows the typical fine mottling of miliary tubercles throughout the lungs.

Treatment. This is along the usual line with chemotherapy (see p. 299). The prognosis is quite good provided meningeal involvement is not too advanced.

Primary Abdominal Tuberculosis

Bovine organisms gain access to the gut in infected milk. Small ulcers form in the small intestine and the infection spreads through lymphatics to the abdominal lymph nodes (*tabes mesenterica*). The nodes usually heal with calcification, but sometimes the infection spreads to the peritoneum (*Tuberculous peritonitis*). Miliary tuberculosis can result from involvement of abdominal blood vessels.

Tuberculous Cervical Lymphadenitis

The initial infection occurs in the tonsillar crypts and spreads to the cervical lymph nodes. These may become chronically enlarged and heal by fibrosis and calcification. They may undergo caseous necrosis, the pus tracking through the fascial planes to form a superficial cold abscess at some distance from the nodes (*'collar stud' abscess*).

Both the above are now uncommon in the UK, except in immigrants.

POST-PRIMARY TUBERCULOSIS

General Considerations. The infection is almost invariably pulmonary and usually occurs in the upper lobes or the apical segment of the lower lobe. The early lesion consists of an area of tuberculous bronchopneumonia which radiographically appears as soft shadowing. Spread is initially by direct extension to adjacent lung. Later *caseation* occurs and the necrotic centre of the lesion is discharged into a bronchus, producing a cavity in the lung, and cough with sputum. The infected sputum may be inhaled into other parts of either lung, producing new tuberculous lesions by *bronchogenic spread.* These may follow the same course. Peripheral lesions may cause *pleurisy*, which may progress to tuberculous *effusions* or empyema (p. 311). *Haemoptysis* occurs with erosion of blood vessels. *Tuberculous bronchitis* may produce a valvular obstruction to the bronchi draining a cavity, so that it distends to form a *tension cavity*. A *tuberculoma* is a blocked cavity with thick walls and full of inspissated material. It shows on the chest radiograph as a rounded opacity with clear-cut edges and may show areas of calcification.

The rate of progress of the disease is variable. It is rapid at times, but more commonly it is slow, the early lesion taking some years to develop into widespread tuberculosis. It depends on the extent and severity of the original infection and on the patient's resistance. The disease may become arrested at any stage, either permanently or temporarily, due to spontaneous healing by resolution, fibrosis, and calcification, or as the result of treatment. Alternatively widespread tuberculous bronchopneumonia, miliary tuberculosis, or metastatic tuberculosis may supervene. As opposed to *acute tuberculosis*, with infiltration and cavitation, a state of *chronic fibrocaseous* or *fibroid tuberculosis* may develop with gross fibrous contraction of the upper lobes and emphysema of the lower lobes. Respiratory reserve is then diminished and dyspnoea becomes a prominent symptom.

The expectoration of infected sputum may cause *tuberculous tracheitis, laryngitis,* or *tuberculous ulcers on the tongue*. Swallowed sputum may cause gastritis or tuberculous ulcers in the lymphoid patches of the *ileum*. The colon is usually spared, but tuberculous *fistula-in-ano* is common.

In patients with long-standing extensive disease, secondary amyloidosis may develop.

Clinical Features. Most patients with early tuberculosis of the lungs are free of symptoms but some present with haemoptysis.

The disease is usually well advanced by the time symptoms have developed. Classically they are chronic ill health, cough with mucoid sputum, low-grade fever, anorexia, tiredness, progressive weight loss, and night sweats. In advanced cases the patient appears ill, sweating and has lost weight, and the continual coughing up of infected sputum may spread infection and lead to further symptoms. Tracheitis causes retrosternal soreness, and laryngitis hoarseness and dysphagia. Tuberculous ulcers in the mouth, usually around the edge of the tongue, are extremely painful. Gastritis from swallowed sputum causes dyspepsia. As this may be a presenting symptom, pulmonary tuberculosis must always be considered in the differential diagnosis of dyspepsia. Tuberculous ileitis causes diarrhoea, and occasionally symptoms from bleeding, perforation, or obstruction. Fistula-in-ano causes a sero-sanguineous peri-anal discharge.

There are no abnormal signs from an early lesion. The first physical sign to appear is usually a small area of persistent crackles at one or other apex, but by this time lung involvement is considerable. With more extensive disease there will be impairment to percussion, more widespread crackles and sometimes areas of bronchial breathing if consolidation or cavities are near the chest wall. Fibrosis of an upper lobe leads to shift of the trachea towards the lesion, flattening and diminishing movement of the upper chest with impaired percussion note, bronchial breathing, and crackles.

Signs of fluid will be present if there is an associated pleural effusion or empyema.

Investigations

Radiography is essential for diagnosis, to assess the extent and nature of the disease, to detect cavities and to follow progress. Both postero-anterior and lateral views are required at the start, and tomograms may be helpful to demonstrate cavities and delineate the extent of the lesion.

It is difficult to judge the activity of a lesion from a single radiograph. Cavitation means activity and soft fluffy opacities are usually of recent onset. Hard and calcified shadows suggest healing and inactivity. Serial films provide the best way of judging both the activity and progress of the disease.

There is no radiological appearance which is diagnostic of tuberculosis, although cavitating disease involving the upper lobes is extremely suggestive of it. Often the diagnosis depends on exclusion of other diseases or the confirmation of tuberculosis by sputum examination.

Sputum examination is essential in a patient suspected of having pulmonary tuberculosis. The finding of tubercle bacilli confirms the diagnosis and indicates that the disease is active and the patient infectious. Relatives and close contacts must be radiographed, sometimes repeatedly.

A random sample of sputum, stained by the *Ziehl–Neelsen technique*, may be examined by direct microscopy, or a 24-hour collection may be made, concentrated, and similarly examined. The sputum should also be cultured, as this increases the chance of finding tubercle bacilli and sensitivity tests to chemotherapeutic agents may be made. Gastric washings, laryngeal swabs, and pleural fluid may be similarly examined. In general, the ease of finding the organism and the number found are indications of the extent of the disease.

Sedimentation Rate. A normal ESR does not exclude an active lesion. A raised ESR may be additional evidence of activity, and serial measurements are useful in following the progress of the disease.

Tuberculin Test. A delayed cell-mediated hypersensitivity reaction (Type IV), initiated by lymphocytes in the tissues, develops in response to infection with the tubercle bacillus, and this hypersensitivity state persists after the infection has become inactive. There are rare exceptions to this; for instance, in some cases of overwhelming miliary tuberculosis. The delayed hypersensitivity can be demonstrated by injecting intradermally an antigen prepared from dead tubercle bacilli (tuberculin). A local reaction occurs in the skin, producing an area of redness and swelling and rarely ulceration. A *positive result* is judged as a papule larger than 5 mm which appears within 2–4 days of injection. False positive results appear in the first 48 hours and last only a day or two. The test may be carried out by using a Tine test or a Heaf multipuncture test. In the Mantoux test, 0.1 ml of a solution of PPD (purified protein derivative) containing 5 TU is injected intradermally. If negative, increasing concentrations containing 10 TU or 100 TU can be injected. A positive result simply indicates previous exposure; it is not a measure of activity. A negative result would indicate that a radiographic pulmonary opacity is not tuberculous.

Treatment. Active disease requires treatment, whereas healed disease only requires observation. It is not always easy to decide if a lesion is active, but it must be regarded so in the following circumstances:

(a) Clinical evidence of disease, i.e. fever and weight loss.
(b) Tubercle bacilli in the sputum.
(c) Radiological evidence of spread of the disease. Comparison with past chest X-rays is invaluable in this respect.
(d) The presence of cavities.

The *principles of treatment* are well established and include general measures to raise resistance, specific treatment, and local measures to the lung.

(1) **General.** With effective chemotherapy prolonged hospital treatment or bed rest is no longer required, but the patient should be kept in bed if he is ill with fever or toxaemia. Good food is essential. This means adequate, but not excessive calories, plenty of protein, with sufficient vitamin and mineral content. Iron and vitamins may be given as a

supplement if necessary. The aim should be to regain, but not exceed, the normal body weight.

(2) **Chemotherapy.** Some general principles governing drug therapy may be stated:

(1) Chemotherapy is indicated if the disease is active.
(2) It should be continued for a prolonged period.
(3) No drug should be given alone. Combinations of the drugs should be used to avoid the emergence of drug-resistant strains of tubercle bacilli.

Treatment is started with three of the drugs to obtain a maximum therapeutic effect and to cover the possibility that the organism is resistant to one of the drugs. Sputum culture and tests of the organism's sensitivity to the drugs will subsequently determine this.

The standard treatment used in the UK at the present time is:

Ethambutol 15–20 mg/kg body weight daily
Rifampicin 450–600 mg (10 mg/kg body weight) daily
Isoniazid 300 mg daily.

All three drugs can be given together in a single dose before breakfast, as rifampicin is best absorbed on an empty stomach. Rifampicin and isoniazid are best taken combined in a single tablet. It is usual to add pyridoxine 10–20 mg daily to prevent neuropathy developing in patients on long-term isoniazid.

All three drugs are given for the first 2 months of treatment; ethambutol is then stopped and rifampicin and isoniazid are continued as long-term therapy. A course of 9 months is usually satisfactory for pulmonary tuberculosis but treatment may be continued for 12 months or more for disease elsewhere.

Rifampicin is relatively free from side-effects. It may cause a transient disturbance of liver function tests, which can be disregarded; but hepatitis with jaundice, which is more likely to occur with intermittent high dose therapy and those whose liver function is already impaired, is an indication for stopping the drug. Patients should be warned that rifampicin produces a reddish colour in the urine and reduces the efficacy of the contraceptive pill.

Isoniazid causes neuropathy in high doses and particularly those who inactivate the drug slowly.

Ethambutol in a high dosage can cause optic neuritis, so that patients taking it as long-term therapy should have their visual acuity tested before treatment and thereafter at regular intervals, and patients should be warned to report any impairment in vision.

Pyrazinamide is being used increasingly and can be added to the regime for 1–2 months. It is bactericidal for tubercle bacilli and used in the recommended small doses rarely causes liver damage but liver function should be measured regularly whilst on treatment. It is particularly useful in tuberculous meningitis and tuberculous lymphadenopathy, where it can replace ethambutol. It is given in divided doses orally:

Body Weight	*Dose*
50 kg	1.5 g daily
50–74 kg	2.0 g daily
75 kg	2.5 g daily

The older regime of *streptomycin*, *PAS* and *isoniazid* is now rarely used. It is an effective regime but more troublesome for the patient. It has, however, the advantage of being cheap and is, therefore, useful in the Third World countries.

Corticosteroids are of value in acute tuberculosis with severe toxaemia which is not responding quickly enough to chemotherapy alone.

Resection. Surgical resection and chemotherapy were both introduced at approximately the same time. It is now realised that with adequate longer-term chemotherapy, resection is not necessary; it is reserved for certain occasional selected cases.

(a) Patients with localised cavitation which persists in spite of adequate rest and chemotherapy.
(b) Some cases infected with tubercle bacilli resistant to chemotherapy.

Prophylaxis

This includes measures to raise standards of hygiene and to improve nutrition and living conditions, and the detection of both early and infectious cases of pulmonary tuberculosis by routine radiography in countries where tuberculosis is still common.

Efforts have been made to increase individual resistance by vaccinating susceptible (tuberculin negative) subjects with an attenuated strain of the tubercle bacillus (*Bacille Calmette–Guérin; BCG*). Freeze-dried BCG is the most reliable preparation. An intradermal injection of 0.1 ml of the vaccine is made and the appearance of a papule at the site of the injection within 10–14 days indicates a successful vaccination. Conversion of the tuberculin test to positive should occur between the 6th and 8th week after vaccination. Complications include abscesses and persistent ulceration at the site of injection, and enlargement of the axillary lymph glands; they may require treatment with rifampicin and ethambutol.

The World Health Organisation have used BCG vaccination on an enormous scale in India, Africa, and some parts of Asia with few ill effects and benefits that are variable. It is available at chest clinics, school medical clinics and infant welfare centres in the UK, but because of the declining incidence of tuberculosis mass BCG vaccination is of doubtful value; it is best reserved for those exposed to tuberculous infection and contacts.

OPPORTUNIST MYCOBACTERIAL INFECTION

Acid-fast bacilli distinct from *M. tuberculosis* may at times produce a lung infection which mimics an indolent form of tuberculosis. These different 'atypical' mycobacteria can be distinguished on cultures by their rate of growth and ability to produce pigment. *M. kansasii*, the commonest variety seen in this country, produces a yellow pigment when cultures grown in the dark are exposed to light. *M. xenopi* and *M. avian intracellulare* are also prone to infect emphysematous lungs.

Treatment. The organisms invariably show resistance to many of the drugs on *in vitro* sensitivity tests. Response to treatment is slow and it may have to be continued for up to two years. *M. kansasii* is usually sensitive to rifampicin and ethambutol and partially sensitive to isoniazid. It may also be sensitive to streptomycin, ethionamide and pyrazinamide. *M. xenopi* infection usually responds to treatment with rifampicin, isoniazid and streptomycin. *M. avian intracellulare* is usually resistant to most of the antitubercular drugs but clinical response to rifampicin, isoniazid, ethambutol and pyrazinamide may occur in spite of drug resistance being demonstrated by *in vitro* tests.

FUNGUS INFECTIONS

Histoplasmosis, coccidiodomycosis and *blastomycosis* are fungus diseases of the lungs occurring in the USA, but they are not endemic in this country.

Torulosis. Sporadic cases occur and it may arise as an opportunist lung infection (p. 287). It is due to infection with the yeast *Cryptococcus neoformans*. Pulmonary lesions may develop into cavitating granulomas, or into tumour-like masses. Infection may spread by the blood stream to the meninges mimicking tuberculous meningitis, even when the pulmonary lesions are small.

Treatment consists of surgical resection, where feasible, combined with intravenous amphotericin B. Cryptococcal meningitis has also been successfully treated with flucytosine.

Aspergillosis

Mycetoma. The fungus *Aspergillus fumigatus* is not pathogenic to the normal respiratory tract. It may infect pulmonary infarcts, and cysts or cavities which have resulted from such diseases as tuberculosis, sarcoidosis, staphylococcal pneumonia or ankylosing spondylitis. A solid ball of fungus (*mycetoma*) grows free in the cavity. On tomography a crescent of air may be seen above the opacity, which can be seen to move its position when the patient is tipped. Precipitins to aspergillus can be detected in the blood. Recurrent haemoptyses may occur and the sputum may be thick and purulent.

An invasive necrotising pneumonia may occur as part of an opportunist lung infection (p. 287), and haematogenous spread to the brain, meninges and other organs may occur.

Bronchopulmonary allergic aspergillosis. A different and distinct syndrome results from hypersensitivity to aspergillus in atopic subjects. It produces asthma, radiographic changes and eosinophils in the blood and sputum (see Pulmonary Eosinophilia, p. 304).

Treatment. Invasive aspergillus pneumonia can be treated with intravenous amphotericin B, but treatment has to be prolonged and there is a risk of nephrotoxicity. It can be combined with flucytosine and possibly ketoconazole in addition.

A mycetoma responds poorly to this treatment. Ideally it is best removed surgically, but this is rarely possible because associated severe lung disease precludes operation. Allergic bronchopulmonary aspergillosis is dealt with on p. 304.

Moniliasis. The yeast *Candida albicans* is a normal saprophyte found in the respiratory tract and in the intestines. The administration of antibiotics may encourage its growth so that it may be abundant in the sputum but not necessarily pathogenic. It may, however, invade the mucosa, causing *thrush* in the mouth and pharynx, and at times in the oesophagus and in the trachea and bronchi; it may also cause diarrhoea and anogenital pruritus. It is debatable whether monilial infection of the lung itself occurs. Rarely, in debilitated patients and in patients on treatment with antibiotics, steroids and cytotoxic drugs (with such diseases as leukaemia and reticuloses), blood stream infection and meningitis may occur (p. 304).

Treatment. Nystatin by mouth, 5 ml t.d.s. (100 000 units per ml), is the drug of choice. Inhalations of nystatin or brilliant green may be used for bronchial moniliasis. In the rare systemic infections intravenous amphotericin B or oral flucytosine or clotrimazole may also be used.

DUST DISEASES OF THE LUNGS (The Pneumoconioses)

Silicosis

Silicosis is due to the inhalation of fine particles of free silica. It occurs in coal miners, and in the granite and sandstone industries, in metal foundries, in various grinding processes in which sandstone is used and in the pottery industry.

The earliest change is the development throughout the lungs of fine, fibrotic nodules around the particles of silica. As the disease develops these nodules increase in size and coalesce until finally there are large areas of fibrosis. Tuberculosis may complicate the picture.

Clinical Features. In the early stages there are no symptoms or signs and the diagnosis depends on the radiographic picture of diffuse mottling combined with a history of exposure.

The first symptom is dyspnoea on effort and later cough with mucoid sputum develops. Eventually the patient becomes severely disabled and death occurs from bronchopneumonia, tuberculosis or cor pulmonale.

Prevention consists of adequate exhaust ventilation, damping down the dust and personal protection by means of masks. All people exposed to silica dust should have regular chest radiographs.

Treatment. There is no specific treatment and those showing evidence of the disease must be removed from exposure to dust.

Asbestosis

The inhalation of asbestos fibres, which are silicates, causes a progressive diffuse fibrosis of the lungs, particularly the lower lobes. The disease progresses in spite of removal from exposure. Blue asbestos (crocidolite) is more destructive than white asbestos (chrysolite). The chief symptoms are cough and dyspnoea and the clinical picture is that of fibrosing alveolitis (p. 308); *asbestos bodies*, formed of asbestos fibres and fibrin, can be found on microscopy of the sputum. Preventative measures are similar to those used in silicosis. Carcinoma of the bronchus is a common complication and malignant mesothelioma of the pleura also occurs. Calcified pleural plaques and acute pleural reactions also occur in workers exposed to asbestos dust.

Coal Miners' Pneumoconiosis

A special type of pneumoconiosis affects miners who inhale coal dust, rather than rock dust which produces silicosis. In this country it is most prevalent in the South Wales coal-fields. There are two types:

(1) *Simple Pneumoconiosis.* Radiographically there are diffuse linear shadows at first. Later scattered small nodules up to 5 mm in diameter develop, often with surrounding emphysema. The disease is only progressive if the worker remains exposed to dust.
(2) *Progressive Massive Fibrosis.* Radiographically there are large dense shadows mostly in the mid and upper zones, with surrounding emphysema. It probably represents a massive fibrotic response to low grade inflammation. At times the centre undergoes necrosis and is coughed up to leave a shaggy-walled cavity. Although tuberculous infection or infection with opportunist mycobacteria may be suspected, there is no evidence that they play a part in the aetiology. It is progressive even if the subject is no longer exposed to coal dust.
(3) *Caplan's Syndrome.* This consists of discrete fibrotic nodules, some 3 cm or more in diameter, occurring in a patient with coal miners' pneumoconiosis and rheumatoid arthritis. The rheumatoid factor is present in the blood. The rheumatoid arthritis may precede the development of the lung lesions or develop some years later.

Clinical Features. There are no symptoms in the early stages. In the later stages of simple pneumoconiosis and with massive fibrosis dyspnoea on exertion is a prominent symptom. Cough and sputum, sometimes blackened by coal dust, develop and recurrent bronchitis is common. In advanced cases the patient becomes grossly disabled and death from cor pulmonale is usual.

Prevention. Of importance are adequate ventilation and reduction of dust by damping it down with water, by wet drilling and wet cutting. Masks are not very satisfactory as they interfere with the performance of heavy work. Chest radiographs at regular intervals should be carried out on all workers at risk, and those showing evidence of pneumoconiosis should be removed from further exposure to coal dust.

Byssinosis

Byssinosis is due to exposure to dust arising from the processing of cotton. It is believed to be an unusual allergic reaction of the bronchi to cotton dust. In the early stages of the disease the patient complains of dyspnoea, a constricted feeling in the chest, and cough which characteristically occurs on Mondays when the patient returns to work. Later the dyspnoea and cough become permanent and finally emphysema develops. Prevention is by adequate ventilation.

PULMONARY EOSINOPHILIA

There is a group of conditions characterised by a varying degree of constitutional upset, cough, transient infiltration of the lung and eosinophilia in the blood.

The *chief causes* of this syndrome are:

(1) *Worm and Parasite Infiltration.* Pulmonary infiltration and eosinophilia may result from the migration through the lungs of the larvae of *Ascaris lumbricoides* (see p. 682).

(2) *Asthma.* Some patients develop pulmonary eosinophilia at the time of an attack, perhaps associated with an infection, and at other times the cause is unknown. *Allergic bronchopulmonary aspergillosis* occurs in patients with extrinsic asthma (p. 267) and is more likely to arise during the winter when high spore counts are prevalent. It produces asthma, changing shadows on the chest X-ray and a high eosinophil count in the blood and sputum. Precipitins are present in the blood and the skin prick test to aspergillus antigen is positive. The patient may cough up plugs of yellow sputum in which the mycelia may be detected. The radiographic appearances are those of fluctuating areas of consolidation or collapse, or the proximal bronchi, distended with tenacious sputum, may be seen as band-like shadows or their inflamed walls visible as tram-line shadows. Chronic changes may develop with proximal bronchiectasis visible as tubular or ring shadows and fibrosis of the upper lobes may develop, mimicking tuberculosis.

Treatment with oral prednisolone usually resolves the asthma and clears the X-ray changes rapidly and a small suppressive dose may be required to prevent relapse. A course of oral di-iodohydroxyquinoline 1500–1800 mg a day has been reported to produce worthwhile remission in a proportion of cases.

(3) *Tropical Eosinophilia.* This is a well-defined clinical entity, occurring in tropical countries, particularly India and Pakistan, and due to microfilarial infestation. The symptoms may be acute or chronic with fever, cough, malaise, and attacks of dyspnoea. Radiography may show miliary mottling and there is always a high eosinophilia.

The condition usually responds to diethylcarbamazine in oral doses of 4.0 mg/kg body weight, t.d.s. for four days.

(4) *Cryptogenic Pulmonary Eosinophilia.* General symptoms of malaise and fever are associated with radiographic changes of diffuse shadowing around the periphery of the lungs – a 'reversed bat's wing', but the appearances may change rapidly from day to day. There is marked eosinophilia and a high ESR, and eosinophils are present in the sputum. Intrinsic asthma may be present or may develop later and some patients develop polyarteritis nodosa.

Treatment. The condition rapidly resolves with prednisolone, and after a prolonged remission it may be possible to tail off the treatment completely without relapse.

(5) *Polyarteritis.* Hypersensitivity arteritis, a variant of polyarteritis nodosa, may produce asthma and transient infiltration in the lung with eosinophilia.

(6) *Drug Reactions.* Some drugs, in particular nitrofurantoin but rarely others such as antituberculous drugs and sulphonamides, may produce pulmonary infiltration and blood eosinophilia.

SARCOIDOSIS

Sarcoidosis is a granulomatous disease in which epithelioid cell tubercles, without caseation, are present in all the affected organs. The lesions may resolve spontaneously but the older lesions become converted to hyalinised fibrous tissue, and if they involve vital organs such as the eye, lungs, heart or nervous system severe impairment of function may result. A similar granulomatous lesion is sometimes seen on biopsy, for example, of skin or lymph node, in quite unrelated conditions such as carcinoma or reticuloses. This *sarcoid reaction* must be distinguished from the disease sarcoidosis.

The aetiology of sarcoidosis is not known but there is an immunological defect present due to impairment of T cell lymphocytes. There is depression of the cell-mediated delayed type of hypersensitivity response (Type IV), with a negative tuberculin test.

A few patients develop frank tuberculosis.

Clinical Features. The three commonest clinical presentations are:

(1) *Erythema nodosum* with *bilateral hilar node enlargement, fever* and often *polyarthritis*.
(2) *Routine chest radiography*. The patient is commonly symptom free and an apparently healthy young adult. The radiograph may show hilar node enlargement, or hilar nodes with pulmonary mottling, or mottling alone. If the patient is breathless it is likely that long-standing fibrotic sarcoid will be present.
(3) *Uveitis*. This may be symptomless and found on slit-lamp examination of the eye. It is commonly acute and transient. It may, however, be insidious and persistent with keratic precipitates forming in the anterior chamber, adhesion of the iris to the lens and obstruction of the angle of the anterior chamber leading to glaucoma. The choroid and retina may also be involved.

Other organs which may be involved include the *spleen, lymph nodes, liver* and *salivary glands*. *Skin lesions* are characteristically few, sharply defined, brownish in colour with a predilection for the face. They may persist for months or even years; they are benign, do not ulcerate and involute spontaneously, leaving either no trace or a pigmented or atrophic scar. *Lupus pernio*, a chilblain-like condition which affects the nose and at times the fingers may occur. *In the nervous system* a granulomatous basal meningitis may produce pituitary lesions or cranial nerve lesions. Diabetes insipidus or hypopituitarism may develop. Cerebral deposits may occur occasionally. *Cystic bone change* may occasionally occur, usually in the heads of the metacarpels and phalanges. *Hypercalcaemia* may be present resulting from an abnormal sensitivity to Vitamin D and be more marked in the summer months. Rarely the *heart* is involved, leading to arrhythmias, congestive failure, or sudden death.

Investigations

Chest radiograph is essential. Pulmonary involvement is one of the main features of the disease, and it can only be assessed by following the changing radiological picture.

Tuberculin Reaction. A negative tuberculin reaction supports the diagnosis. However, as one third of the patients with proved sarcoidosis give a positive reaction to 10 TU (1 : 1000 old tuberculin), a positive reaction does not exclude it. If a patient with sarcoidosis and a negative tuberculin reaction is treated with corticosteroids, the reaction then becomes positive; this is almost diagnostic of sarcoidosis.

Plasma Proteins. In approximately one third of cases there are raised α_2 and/or γ globulins present. This probably indicates activity of the disease.

Kveim Test. The intradermal injection of a saline suspension of sarcoid tissue obtained from spleen or lymph node of patients with active sarcoidosis is followed by the development of a nodule in the skin within the next six weeks. Biopsy of this nodule will show sarcoid histology. The test is positive in about 70% of cases of sarcoidosis; a negative result does not exclude sarcoidosis.

Angiotensin converting enzyme (ACE) is produced by granulomata and raised serum levels of ACE indicate active sarcoidosis and certain other granulomatous diseases.

Biopsy of skin lesions or affected glands will confirm the diagnosis. Liver biopsy is positive in about 50% of patients with sarcoidosis, even when there is no clinical evidence of involvement of the liver.

Respiratory function tests are only abnormal when there is marked pulmonary mottling, when the main defects are those of *compliance* (p. 243) and *gas transfer* (p. 242). In the later stages of pulmonary fibrosis impairment of *ventilation* may be marked.

Progress and Treatment

There is no evidence that antituberculous chemotherapy influences the course of the disease.

Steroids are indicated in uveitis because of the danger to sight, and local instillation of drops is usually sufficient. Steroids are also indicated with hypercalcaemia, because of the danger of renal failure.

Erythema nodosum and hilar node enlargement carries a good prognosis. With hilar node enlargement the great majority of patients improve spontaneously; the remainder develop pulmonary infiltration. With pulmonary infiltration 50% of patients improve spontaneously; if this has not occurred within two years then it is unlikely to remit subsequently. The infiltration may then remain unchanged with little or no disability to the patient, but in a proportion it progresses to severe fibrosis with associated bronchiectasis and bullous change. These patients become respiratory cripples and eventually succumb to cor pulmonale (p. 261).

No specific treatment is indicated in patients with hilar node enlargement. Steroids are usually indicated in patients with pulmonary mottling showing no sign of resolution after a year. It often produces symptomatic relief and hastens resolution, and is aimed at preventing the development of severe fibrosis. Prednisolone 20 mg daily is a satisfactory starting dose. A daily maintenance dose of 5 to 10 mg may be required for several years, as relapse may occur if treatment is too short. Steroids have no effect on the lungs in the fibrotic stage but may help to relieve symptoms.

Once the disease has remitted it is unlikely to recur.

PULMONARY FIBROSIS

Generalised Pulmonary Fibrosis

This is relatively uncommon. The causes are:

(1) The pneumoconioses (p. 302).
(2) As an end result of infiltration of the lungs by a variety of pathological processes, including sarcoidosis (p. 305), and some of the generalised lipoidoses.
(3) Fibrosing alveolitis.

Fibrosing alveolitis

This is a generalised disorder of alveolar walls in which inflammatory changes advance to progressive fibrosis.

Extrinsic allergic alveolitis results from inhalation of organic dusts which produce a Type III hypersensitivity reaction in alveolar walls with the formation of sarcoid-like granulomata; these progress to fibrosis. A large number of allergens have now been identified as causing the disease. These include spores in mouldy hay (*Micropolyspora faeni*) causing *Farmer's lung*, and avian proteins producing *Bird fancier's lung*. Precipitins to the allergen can be detected in the patient's blood.

Clinical features. In the acute stages 'late' asthma (p. 268) may occur some hours after intermittent exposure, as in Farmer's lung. It is less likely if the exposure is more continuous, as in those keeping birds as pets. Breathlessness is the predominant symptom. Cough may be present but it is usually unproductive. Fine inspiratory crackles are best heard at the bases. Clubbing may be present in chronic cases. The chest X-ray shows diffuse mottling and in long-standing cases fibrosis develops mainly in the upper zones. Respiratory function tests indicate that the main defect is that of gaseous exchange across the alveolar membrane (see Gas Transfer, p. 242).

Treatment. Known allergens must be removed from the patient's environment. A course of corticosteroids may be very effective in tiding a patient over an acute episode; they are helpful but less effective with chronic changes. *M. faeni* is sensitive to tetracycline.

Cryptogenic fibrosing alveolitis. In this condition there is no evidence of an allergic alveolitis and the cause is often not known. The inflammation in the alveolar walls is not associated with granulomatous changes. It may occur in association with the collagen diseases such as systemic sclerosis, SLE and rheumatoid arthritis. Rheumatoid factor and antinuclear factor may be present in the blood.

Clinical features. Many of the features are similar to those of allergic alveolitis. Breathlessness on exertion is the striking symptom. It is associated with late inspiratory crackles without sputum, most marked at the bases, and at times associated with an inspiratory wheeze. In advanced cases the patient becomes hypoxic on exertion and even at rest. Clubbing of the fingers is common. The chest X-ray shows diffuse fibrotic changes most marked at the lung bases, with diminished lung volumes and at times honeycombing of the lungs. Respiratory function tests show a restrictive defect of ventilation without airway obstruction and impaired gas transfer (p. 242). Advanced cases become respiratory cripples with respiratory failure and cor pulmonale.

Treatment. Corticosteroids may give symptomatic treatment and are usually required on a long-term basis. They are less effective the more advanced the condition is. Oxygen in the home and portable oxygen produces symptomatic relief.

Localised Pulmonary Fibrosis

Fibrosis of the lungs is commonly localised to one or more lobes, or even a segment of a lobe. It is usually the result of inflammation and common causes are tuberculosis, unresolved pneumonia, chronic lung abscess and long-standing collapse. Bronchiectasis invariably develops in such fibrotic segments or lobes. Persistent infection is not common with fibrosis of the upper lobes because drainage is adequate.

Clinical Features. In some patients there are no symptoms, except perhaps the history of the original illness which led to the fibrosis. This is often the case with healed, fibrotic tuberculosis of the upper lobes, and no treatment is required.

In others the clinical picture is that of the accompanying *infected bronchiectasis*, both with regard to symptoms and complications (see p. 265). Diagnosis and treatment are also discussed under this section.

The physical signs of fibrosis include flattening of the chest overlying the lesion with diminished movement, impaired percussion note, bronchial breathing, whispering pectoriloquy, and bronchophony. The mediastinum is shifted towards the side of the lesion and coarse crackles are present with associated bronchiectasis.

DISEASES OF THE PLEURA

PLEURISY

Inflammation of the pleura may be *dry* or associated with *effusion*, the former often proceeding to the latter.

DRY PLEURISY

It may be due to:

(1) *Pneumonia* either bacterial or viral.
(2) *Pulmonary infarct* (p. 224).

(3) *Tuberculosis.* This variety nearly always progresses to pleurisy with effusion.
(4) *Lung abscess.*
(5) *Epidemic pleurodynia* (Bornholm Disease). This is a Coxsackie virus infection which may occur in outbreaks. It affects the muscles of the chest wall and produces a primary pleurisy without lung involvement.
(6) *Injury* to the chest and lungs.

Clinical Features. The cardinal symptom of dry pleurisy is *pain*, described on p. 246.

On examination the respirations may be short and grunting, for severe pleuritic pain limits inspiration. The diagnosis is confirmed by finding a *pleural rub*, which is a superficial grating or crunching sound related to respiratory movements. It appears to arise just under the stethoscope, which indeed it does, and characteristically comes and goes. Occasionally a pleural rub may be heard in a patient who makes no complaint of pain.

Chest radiography may reveal underlying disease if present, but shows no specific sign of dry pleurisy. Screening may show diminished movement of the chest and diaphragm on that side.

Treatment. Bed rest and analgesics are required. Tabs. codeine co.2 4-hourly, pethidine 50–100 mg IM or hypodermic morphine 15 mg may all be used, depending on the severity of the pain. Some patients obtain relief by applying a hot-water bottle over the area. Specific treatment is that of the underlying lesion, and subsequent management will depend on this.

PLEURISY WITH EFFUSION

Fluid in the pleural cavity may represent a transudate or an exudate.

Transudates occur when the osmotic pressure of the plasma is reduced (the nephrotic syndrome or cirrhosis of the liver) or when the venous pressure is high (congestive cardiac failure or constrictive pericarditis). The fluid in a transudate is usually clear and of low specific gravity. It contains less than 2.0 g protein per 100 ml.

Causes of pleural transudates are:

(1) *Cardiac failure.*
(2) *Nephrotic syndrome.*
(3) *Cirrhosis of the liver.*

Exudates occur in the presence of inflammation or neoplasm. They are of high specific gravity and contain more than 2.0 g protein per 100 ml. Exudates may be clear (tuberculous, neoplastic disease). Cloudiness may be due to blood (neoplasm, pulmonary infarct) or pus cells (pneumonia or lung abscess).

Causes of pleural exudates are:

(1) *Tuberculosis.*
(2) Complicating *pneumonia.*
(3) *Neoplasm.*
(4) *Subphrenic abscess*, and complicating other inflammatory lesions outside the chest.
(5) *Pulmonary infarction.*
(6) During the course of some *collagen diseases*, notably systemic lupus erythematosus and rheumatoid arthritis.
(7) Complicating fibroma of the ovary (*Meigs' syndrome*).

Tuberculous Pleural Effusion

(1) **Effusion Associated with Primary Tuberculosis.** This is the common type of tuberculous effusion and usually occurs between the ages of fifteen and thirty and within a year of tuberculin conversion. It is believed that at this stage the tissues are sensitised to the tubercle bacillus, and if bacilli reach the pleura there is an acute inflammatory reaction with an outpouring of fluid into the pleural cavity.

Clinical Features. The onset is variable. Sometimes it is acute with fever, malaise, sweating, and severe pleuritic pain. Other patients have little pain but complain of vague ill-health and dyspnoea on effort. Occasionally an effusion may be found on routine examination or chest radiograph in a patient with no symptoms.

Examination shows the typical signs of effusion (see p. 249). If it is large there is mediastinal shift to the opposite side, with stony dullness on percussion and absent breath sounds over the effusion.

Chest radiograph shows the effusion as an opacity at the base of the hemithorax. It obliterates the costophrenic angle and rises up into the axilla. The mediastinum may be displaced to the opposite side. It is unusual to see any intrapulmonary lesion even when the effusion has cleared.

Diagnosis is confirmed by aspiration of a sample of fluid. It is straw-coloured and contains cells, most of which are lymphocytes, although in the early stages polymorphs may predominate. Tubercle bacilli can be isolated from the fluid by culture in about 50% of cases. Pleural biopsy, using an Abrams needle stands a good chance of confirming the tuberculous histology. It is positive in about 70% of cases.

The *course* is usually towards resolution. There is a potential danger of the infection spreading and occasionally miliary tuberculosis, renal tuberculosis, or tuberculous meningitis occur. Slow absorption of a large effusion may lead to pleural fibrosis, with subsequent restriction of lung expansion and contraction of the chest wall—a 'frozen' chest. Before chemotherapy was available about 25% of patients developed frank tuberculous lesions in the lungs within five years of an effusion.

Treatment. The aims are to eradicate the infection and to prevent serious residual pleural fibrosis by encouraging rapid clearing of the effusion.

Antitubercular drugs should be given for 12 months, starting with triple chemotherapy (p. 299). Unless the effusion appears to be disappearing rapidly aspiration should be carried out every 2 or 3 days until no further fluid can be removed. Half to one litre should be removed at each aspiration. Fluid should be removed without delay if there is much mediastinal shift or if the patient is short of breath. Effusions which do not resolve, or which keep reforming in spite of these measures, may be treated in addition with corticosteroids. The steroid therapy need not be prolonged and must be combined with chemotherapy; prednisolone 20 mg daily reducing to a maintenance dose of 10–15 mg daily for 6 weeks is satisfactory.

Bed rest is best continued until the effusion has cleared usually within a few weeks. The patient should then make a gradual return to full activity and should remain off work for 2 to 3 months. Follow-up supervision with chest radiographs is essential as with other forms of tuberculosis.

Effusion with Post-primary Tuberculosis

Effusions may develop with post-primary pulmonary tuberculosis and usually indicate severe tuberculosis. Because of the underlying lung disease they resolve more slowly than effusions associated with primary tuberculosis, and may develop into tuberculous empyemata.

Treatment. Half to one litre of pleural fluid should be aspirated every other day until the pleural cavity is dry.

The subsequent management depends on the nature of the underlying lung disease, and will require bed rest and systemic chemotherapy (see p. 299).

Neoplastic Pleural Effusion

Malignant effusion is most commonly due to carcinoma of the bronchus. It also occurs with mesothelioma and with spread of extrathoracic growth to the pleura, such as carcinoma of the breast, stomach, kidney, ovary, or testicle. Pleural effusions are not uncommon in Hodgkin's disease.

Clinical Features. The degree of general ill-health is variable and depends on the extent and nature of the primary neoplasm. The effusions are often of insidious onset, but as they usually become large dyspnoea is a common symptom. The fluid usually reaccumulates rapidly after aspiration; it is often blood-stained and may contain malignant cells. Malignancy may be confirmed by pleural biopsy using an Abrams needle, or by biopsy taken at thoracoscopy.

Treatment. The patient must be kept comfortable by repeated aspiration; usually large quantities can be removed without danger. It is often possible to prevent reaccumulation of fluid by producing a chemical pleurodesis. This may be achieved by injecting irritants such as cytotoxic drugs, talc or mepacrine into the pleural cavity and draining off the fluid by a chest drain. It is most effectively carried out by performing thoracoscopy (when biopsies can be taken) and talc pleurodesis, followed by adequate drainage of the effusion to ensure that the pleural surfaces become adherent to each other.

Effusions associated with breast carcinoma may respond to hormone treatment.

Blood-stained Pleural Effusions

Blood-stained effusions are not uncommon. The chief causes are:

(1) Neoplasm, commonly bronchial carcinoma but any neoplastic effusion may be responsible (see above).
(2) Pulmonary infarct.
(3) Rarely tuberculosis.
(4) A haemothorax which has been diluted by a pleural exudate may have the appearance of a blood-stained effusion.

HAEMOTHORAX

Haemothorax may follow trauma to the chest wall. It also occurs with a spontaneous pneumothorax, due to bleeding from the tear in the lung or from tearing of pleural adhesions; it is then a haemopneumothorax. An aneurysm may leak into the pleural cavity.

Blood in the pleural cavity clots rapidly and fibrin is deposited on the pleural surfaces. Pleural reaction also occurs, with outpouring of further fluid. If the blood is left in the pleura, organisation with pleural fibrosis occurs with subsequent serious interference with lung function.

Clinical Features. If the pleural bleeding is large and rapid the patient will be shocked and collapsed, with rapid pulse and respiration. There may or may not be evidence of trauma to the chest. There are *signs* of pleural fluid (p. 249) or in those cases complicating a pneumothorax the signs are those of both fluid and air in the chest.

Diagnosis is confirmed by aspiration of blood from the pleural space. It is important to distinguish between a frank haemothorax and a blood-stained effusion.

Treatment. The general treatment for internal haemorrhage should be given. Morphine may be required, the patient's blood group should be determined and a transfusion given when necessary.

The effusion should be aspirated and the pleural space kept as dry as possible by further daily aspiration. Antibiotics should be given during the period of aspirations as there is a danger of secondary infection, usually staphylococcal.

Severe bleeding or serious damage to the chest wall will require surgical treatment. Thoracotomy is also necessary when the blood cannot be evacuated by aspiration.

EMPYEMA

Empyema may be defined as a localised collection of pus in the pleural cavity. It most commonly results from a pneumonia, usually pneumococcal lobar pneumonia, or it may be due to anaerobic infection. It may also be due to spread of infection from a lung abscess, from a subphrenic abscess, from mediastinal sepsis and from a chest wound. An underlying carcinoma may be present. Empyema may also result from tuberculous infection of the pleural cavity (see p. 315). Infected serous fluid may collect in the pleural cavity during the course of a pneumonia (*syn-pneumonic empyema*). It is not localised and it usually resolves with adequate treatment. It may, however, progress to become purulent and localised, and by this time the underlying pneumonia has resolved (*meta-pneumonic empyema*). When an empyema becomes loculated in the fissures between the lobes it is known as an interlobar empyema.

Clinical Features. Empyema most commonly arises one to two weeks after the start of a pneumococcal pneumonia. Instead of the temperature falling and the patient recovering, the temperature begins to rise again and takes on a remittent character. The patient looks ill, has drenching sweats and complains of malaise and anorexia. Examination of the chest shows the signs of fluid; the mediastinum will be shifted if the collection of fluid is large. There is dullness over the fluid; classically the upper limit of the dull area rises in the axilla, but this is not constant as the fluid is often loculated. Usually there are absent or diminished breath sounds over the fluid although, particularly in children, it is sometimes possible to hear bronchial breathing which may lead to an erroneous diagnosis of unresolved pneumonia.

It is important to take both postero-anterior and lateral radiographs of the chest so that the fluid may be exactly localised. The diagnosis is finally confirmed by needling the chest and withdrawing turbid fluid. In the early stages, the fluid will be thin and serous, but if a true empyema develops it will become thick and purulent. The fluid should be cultured for organisms.

Treatment

(1) *The Stage of Infected Pleural Effusion.* The infected effusion must be aspirated daily to keep the pleural cavity as dry as possible; following aspiration, 500 000 units of benzylpenicillin should be injected into the pleural cavity. At the same time systemic antibiotic treatment should be continued; benzylpenicillin, 500 000 units 6-hourly is satisfactory unless the infecting organism is resistant to penicillin, when the appropriate antibiotic should be used. With this treatment most effusions will

subside. Sometimes, however, the infection is not controlled and the aspirated fluid becomes progressively purulent.

(2) *True Empyema.* Treatment at this stage is surgical. Resection of a portion of a rib and the insertion of a drainage tube into the most dependent part of the empyema cavity ensures the best possible drainage. The aim is complete obliteration of the empyema cavity with the minimum of pleural scarring and fixation of the lung. It is therefore essential, once a true empyema has developed, not to delay surgical drainage or the wall of the abscess cavity may become so thick and rigid that it cannot be obliterated.

The drain is left in the empyema cavity until this space has disappeared. If the drain falls out before the cavity has been obliterated it must be replaced gently because of the danger of causing spread of infection to the brain (resulting in cerebral abscess). Breathing exercises are given to re-expand the lung and minimise fixation. Provided treatment is correctly carried out results are good. *Failure of empyema cavity to close* is usually due to:

(a) too long delay before a drainage.
(b) inadequate drainage with pocketing of pus; it will be necessary to radiograph the cavity, outlined with radio-opaque material, to determine the correct site for drainage of the most dependent part of the cavity.
(c) failure to recognise that it is a tuberculous empyema.
(d) presence of an underlying neoplasm.

An empyema cavity which fails to close owing to undue thickness of its wall will require permanent drainage with a tube; or surgical decortication of the lung with removal of the abscess cavity can be performed.

Tuberculous Empyema

Tuberculous empyema nearly always occurs in an effusion complicating post-primary pulmonary tuberculosis, and it is rare in a tuberculous effusion associated with a primary infection. It was a recognised complication of artificial pneumothorax, but this type of treatment for tuberculosis is not used now.

Clinical Features. The degree of constitutional upset varies. Some patients appear surprisingly well considering the chest is filled with tuberculous pus. Others have evidence of toxaemia with weight loss, sweating, and fever. If secondary infection occurs, particularly with *Staphylococcus aureus*, the patient becomes severely ill. This is especially likely to occur if there is bronchopleural fistula, such as may result from the rupture of a pulmonary cavity into the pleura. The signs are those of fluid in the chest. If a pneumothorax is also present the signs are those of fluid and air in the chest: an area of dullness below due to the fluid, with resonance above. It may be possible by tilting the patient to demonstrate shifting dullness.

Treatment. The patient requires the usual general treatment for tuberculosis, including a full course of antituberculous chemotherapy (see p. 299). The chest should be aspirated every other day until it is as dry as possible and streptomycin 1.0 g should be instilled into the pleural cavity after aspiration. Unless full expansion occurs, decortication, thoracoplasty or resection of part or all the lung may be required.

SPONTANEOUS PNEUMOTHORAX

Air collecting in the pleural cavity as a result of some pathological process is known as spontaneous pneumothorax. The artificial introduction of air, which was used as a form of therapy for pulmonary tuberculosis, is known as an artificial pneumothorax.

The commonest cause of spontaneous pneumothorax is the rupture of a small vesicle under the visceral plura which allows air to pass from the lung to the pleural space. This type of pneumothorax is common in young people and more common in men than women. It is not associated with any underlying lung disease. The patient is often slim with long fingers and high arched palate. In about 10 to 20 per cent of patients it recurs, sometimes repeatedly.

A spontaneous pneumothorax may also complicate lung disease such as emphysema and asthma. In addition, air may enter the pleural space from wounds of the chest wall or from a perforation of the oesophagus.

When the spontaneous pneumothorax is due to the rupture of a vesicle, the tear usually seals off rapidly and the air is absorbed from the pleural cavity over the next week or so. Occasionally a valve-like opening develops between the lung and the pleural space so that air can enter, but cannot leave the pleura; this leads to the accumulation of air in the pleural cavity and the development of a *tension pneumothorax*.

Clinical Features. The onset is usually sudden with pain in that side of the chest, and dyspnoea. The degree of constitutional upset is variable, but some patients may be quite shocked and collapsed. Occasionally the pneumothorax is found on routine examination and no history of chest pain can be elicited.

Examination of the chest may show diminished movement of the affected side. The degree to which the mediastinum is displaced away from the side of the pneumothorax is variable and depends on the size of the pneumothorax. Tactile vocal fremitus is decreased or absent. The note to percussion is either normal or hyper-resonant. On auscultation there are diminished breath sounds and absent voice sounds over the pneumothorax. An exocardial clicking sound may be heard over a small left-sided pneumothorax. A *coin sound* is sometimes present when there is a large or tension pneumothorax; this is a musical chiming heard through a stethoscope placed over the pneumothorax cavity when a coin laid on an adjacent part of the chest wall is tapped with another coin. The development of a *tension pneumothorax* is suggested by increasing dyspnoea, cyanosis, and distress. There will be signs of a pneumothorax with considerable mediastinal displacement. If the tension is not relieved, death may rapidly ensue.

Occasionally a spontaneous pneumothorax may be associated with a haemothorax due to the tearing of pleural adhesions or bleeding from the tear in the lung.

Chest radiograph shows air in the pleural cavity with a varying amount of collapse of the lung. There is rarely any evidence of lung disease.

Treatment. When a spontaneous pneumothorax is diagnosed within the first few hours after its onset, the patient is best moved to hospital if this is possible because of the slight but definite risk of a tension pneumothorax or haemopneumothorax developing. Rest at home for a short period is satisfactory if a pneumothorax has been present for a few days and is expanding satisfactorily. In the early stages some patients are shocked and in severe pain and require morphine 10–15 mg, perhaps repeated once or twice in the ensuing few hours.

No active treatment is required for a small or moderate sized pneumothorax. In all patients with a large or tension pneumothorax it is best to insert a catheter via a trochar through an intercostal space in the axilla into the pleural cavity, the other end being connected to an underwater seal. The patient is instructed to cough gently and thus slowly to expel the air from the pneumothorax; expansion of the lung will then take place. In an emergency, where a patient's life is threatened by a tension pneumothorax and hospital equipment is not at hand, a needle should be pushed through a cork and into the pneumothorax; the needle can then be fixed into position with strapping and attached by a rubber tube to an underwater seal.

Occasionally the pneumothorax persists in spite of these measures in which case continuous suction can be applied to the underwater seal to encourage the visceral pleura to become adherent to the chest wall. If this fails, thoracotomy may be required. With recurrent pneumothorax pleurodesis is indicated, either by painting the pleural surfaces with a solution of silver nitrate and thus allowing the visceral and parietal pleurae to become adherent, or by thoracotomy and pleurectomy of the parietal pleura.

MEDIASTINAL CYSTS AND TUMOURS

(1) Swellings in the Mid-mediastinum

(a) *Carcinoma of the Bronchus.* This is the commonest cause of a mediastinal mass. It may be due to direct extension of the growth or may result from infiltration and enlargement of lymph-nodes.

(b) *Enlarged Lymph Nodes*. These may be due to carcinomatous infiltration (commonly from the bronchus), Hodgkin's disease, lymphosarcoma, sarcoidosis, or tuberculosis.

(c) *Foregut Cysts*. Bronchogenic and enterogenous cysts may arise in the superior or lower mediastinum.

(2) Swellings in the Anterior Mediastinum

(a) *Retrosternal Goitre*. This is usually, but not always, associated with a goitre in the neck. It lies anteriorly behind the manubrium and may compress the trachea or other structures in the superior mediastinum.

(b) *Thymic tumours* lie in the upper anterior mediastinum. They are sometimes associated with myasthenia gravis. Some are malignant and may metastasise.

(c) *Dermoid cysts and teratomas* usually lie anterior to the upper part of the heart. Dermoids may become infected and form fistulae with surrounding structures. Both may undergo malignant change.

(d) *Pericardial Cysts* (*Spring-water Cysts*). These are found in the lower anterior mediastinum usually filling up the right cardiophrenic angle.

(3) Swellings in Posterior Mediastinum

Neurofibroma and Ganglioneuroma. These tumours usually lie on the paravertebral gutter. They seldom cause symptoms and are found on routine radiography, appearing as rounded opacities with clear-cut edges. Occasionally they extend into the spinal canal causing compression of the spinal cord. A neurofibroma of the first thoracic nerve often causes Horner's syndrome (p. 333).

Aortic aneurysm or aneurysmal dilatation of a pulmonary artery may appear as a mediastinal tumour.

Clinical Features. Mediastinal tumours and cysts may produce no symptoms and be found only on routine radiography. They may compress surrounding structures, causing a variety of symptoms and signs.

Investigation must always include postero-anterior and lateral radiographs of the chest. Tomography, bronchoscopy, and thyroid or CT scan may be required. Even with these investigations it is not always possible to make a definite diagnosis. Mediastinoscopy and thoracotomy may be required both for diagnosis and for treatment.

FURTHER READING

Bates, D. V. and Christie, R. V., *Respiratory Function in Disease*, 2nd edition, W. B. Saunders Co., Philadelphia and London, 1971.

Crofton, J. and Douglas, A., *Respiratory Diseases*, 3rd edition, Blackwell Scientific Publications, Oxford and Edinburgh, 1981.

D'Abreu, A. L., *Practice of Cardiothoracic Surgery*, 4th revised edition, Edward Arnold, London, 1976.

Forgacs, Paul, *Lung Sounds*, Baillière, London, 1979.

Parkes, W. Raymond, *Occupational Lung Disorders*, 2nd edition, Butterworth & Co., London, 1982.

Rubens, R. D. and Knight R. K., *A Short Textbook of Clinical Oncology*, Hodder and Stoughton, Sevenoaks, 1980.

CHAPTER 6

THE NERVOUS SYSTEM

INTELLECTUAL FUNCTION AND DEMENTIA

Tests of Intellectual Function

A formal psychometric analysis of intelligence provides quantitative information and can be used to follow progress. Simple bedside testing provides useful clinical information:

Orientation: The patient is asked the day of the week, the date, the month, the year, where he is at that moment and his home address.

Memory: Tests of memory are conveniently divided into three groups—

(1) Immediate recall. This is tested by asking the patient to repeat a sequence of random numbers, first forwards (normal more than six) and then backwards (normal four or more).

(2) The five-minutes memory test. This is usually carried out with a name, an address and a flower. The number of errors and the total number of words should be recorded.

(3) Long-term memory. Questions may include items from the patient's past or items of national importance and should be adjusted to the patient's educational level and social background.

Learning: The patient should be asked to learn the Babcock sentence by repeating it after the examiner as often as necessary to get it word perfect; this should be achieved in less than five attempts.

Calculation: Serial 7's. The patient is asked to subtract seven from a hundred and continue to subtract seven from the result, the time taken and number of errors should be recorded.

DEMENTIA (See also p. 53)

Dementia is a deterioration in the intellectual function of the brain as a result of organic disease. It is a sign and sometimes a symptom, but it is not a diagnosis.

About 50 % of elderly patients with dementia have Alzheimer's disease, about 15 % have cerebrovascular disease alone and about 20 % have a combination of these two degenerative diseases. The remaining 15 % are divided among a wide range of conditions, including syphilis, Jakob–Creutzfeldt disease, low-pressure hydrocephalus, Huntington's chorea, tumours, progressive multifocal leucoencephalopathy, toxic and deficiency diseases, including alcohol, Vitamins B_1, B_6 and B_{12} and myxoedema.

Although the chances of finding a treatable cause are small, it is important to attempt a precise aetiological or pathological diagnosis and to exclude the treatable conditions, particularly in younger patients.

Alzheimer's Disease (see also p. 54)

This progressive cerebral degeneration of unknown cause may occur at any age; it is more common in women and in the elderly. It presents with a very slow insidious onset of mental deterioration, often starting with memory impairment. The early signs may suggest lateralisation to the dominant or non-dominant hemisphere but focal deficits do not occur and epilepsy is unusual. Alzheimer's disease has a characteristic pathological appearance with neurofibrillary tangles and argyrophilic plaques.

Vascular Disease

Cerebrovascular disease rarely causes dementia under the age of 60 without clear evidence of generalised vascular disease, particularly systemic hypertension. Dementia may result from a stroke and the subsequent deterioration may be stepwise as further infarcts occur. Vascular disease may also cause a more insidious dementia without clinically evident infarcts. Men are much more frequently affected than women and insight is often preserved.

It is usually easy to identify patients with the typical features of these two principal causes of dementia, but in the elderly they often occur together and they are not mutually exclusive.

Investigation of Dementia

This should include a search for space-occupying lesions, toxic, metabolic and deficiency states and tests for syphilis. Special tests should include electroencephalography, skull X-ray, cerebrospinal fluid examination and CT scan. Where a CT scan is not available a gamma brain scan and an air encephalogram may be necessary. Exceptionally a brain biopsy is required to establish a diagnosis.

THE DOMINANT HEMISPHERE AND LANGUAGE

This is the left hemisphere in all right-handed patients and in about 50% of left-handed patients. The dominant hemisphere is concerned with all forms of language.

(1) **All language inputs** are processed in Wernicke's area, which is at the posterior end of the superior temporal gyrus. It receives input from the primary visual cortex for reading, semaphore and other visual forms of language and from the primary auditory cortex for speech, morse code and auditory forms of language. It may also receive information from the somatosensory cortex for the interpretation of Braille.

A lesion of the primary visual cortex causes blindness, but a lesion of the pathway between the visual cortex and Wernicke's area causes dyslexia; in patients with this condition, comprehension of the spoken word is preserved. Information going initially to the right hemisphere has to cross the corpus callosum to reach Wernicke's area, so that a lesion affecting the left visual cortex and the posterior part of the corpus callosum causes a right homonymous hemianopia and dyslexia because of interruption of information from the right visual cortex to Wernicke's area.

Wernicke's Aphasia (fluent, receptive or sensory aphasia)

Lesions of Wernicke's area cause loss of ability to understand any form of language input. The patient can still speak clearly and fluently, but since there is no auditory feedback, cannot understand what he is saying and is unaware of any errors he may make. This usually produces fluent nonsense.

(2) **All language output** arises in Broca's area and is then relayed to the motor cortex for speech and writing.

Broca's Aphasia (non-fluent, expressive or motor aphasia)

If the lesion is confined to Broca's area and Wernicke's area is intact, comprehension is preserved but the patient is unable to express himself. If he attempts a word and gets it wrong, he is immediately aware of the error and attempts to correct it. This produces a halting, non-fluent dysphasia, which in mild cases may consist of some hesitation only, while in the more severe cases there may be no speech at all.

Both Wernicke's area and Broca's area, together with their connecting pathways, are supplied by the middle cerebral artery and an infarct in this territory is the commonest cause of dysphasia; tumours are the next commonest cause. Anterior lesions are more likely to cause non-fluent dysphasia and posterior lesions cause fluent dysphasia.

Gerstmann's Syndrome

This is caused by a lesion of the dominant angular gyrus and consists of finger agnosia, right/left disorientation, dysgraphia, dyscalculia and dyslexia.

THE NON-DOMINANT HEMISPHERE AND SPATIAL ORIENTATION

The non-dominant hemisphere is concerned with spatial awareness, both personal and extrapersonal, at a higher level than the primary sensory cortex concerned with vision, hearing and somatosensory information. This is the reason why patients with a right hemisphere lesion may show a striking neglect of the left side of the body and ignore objects in the left visual field out of proportion to the sensory and visual loss. Lesions of the left hemisphere may cause some sensory extinction, but neglect or denial of the right side of the body is unusual. This loss of spatial orientation causes difficulty in dressing (dressing dyspraxia) and difficulty in finding the way in a familiar environment (topographical amnesia).

THE CRANIAL NERVES

THE OLFACTORY NERVE (I Cranial Nerve)

This is the only cranial nerve in the anterior fossa. Numerous small fibres arising in the mucosa in the roof of the nasal cavity pass through the cribriform plate to reach the olfactory bulb, which is continuous posteriorly with the olfactory tract lying in the olfactory groove. Just above the anterior clinoid processes there is a partial decussation. Lesions behind this decussation cannot cause a unilateral or complete loss of the sense of smell. The sensory cortex for smell is in the uncus on the medial aspect of the temporal lobe.

This pathway serves all smell and this includes all flavour—only the cruder sensations of salt, sweet, bitter and acid are relayed through the chorda tympani and glossopharyngeal nerves.

Apparent loss of the sense of smell may be due to nasal obstruction. It is important, therefore, to determine that the airway is clear before testing smell on both sides separately with a mild non-irritant odour. There may be temporary loss of smell as a result of acute or chronic rhinitis, but the commonest cause is head injury, particularly occipital head injuries. If the penetrating fibres through the cribriform plate are sheared, the loss of smell is permanent. If continuity exists they may recover. Unilateral or bilateral anosmia may be an early sign in tumours in the floor of the anterior fossa, in particular, olfactory groove meningiomas.

THE OPTIC NERVE (II Cranial Nerve)

Changes in visual acuity imply some abnormality of macula vision. There may, of course, be a distortion of information reaching the macula due to refractive errors or lens opacities. It is important, therefore, to test visual acuity with the refractive errors corrected. Impairment of visual acuity may also be due to a lesion affecting the macula fibres in the optic nerve. Lesions behind the chiasm always affect the vision in both eyes.

Lesions of the visual pathways causing visual field defects can be accurately localised due to the anatomical arrangement of the visual fibres as they traverse the length of the brain to the visual cortex.

(a) *Retinal Lesions.* The raised intraocular pressure associated with glaucoma first affects the superficial retinal fibres which come from the periphery, with resultant loss of peripheral vision (tunnel vision). Infarction of small bundles of retinal fibres cause arcuate scotomata.

(b) *Loss of one visual field* without any involvement of the other must be due to disease of the optic nerve. Small lesions cause unilateral scotomata or defects and are best delineated with a small red object. The commonest cause is retrobulbar neuritis (disseminated sclerosis).

(c) *Lesions Affecting the Chiasm.* Central compression damages the decussating fibres and causes a bitemporal field defect; in the early stages this may be bilateral temporal scotomata, which are often asymmetrical. Later the more typical bitemporal hemianopia develops. The commonest cause is a chromaphobe adenoma of the pituitary. There are usually some features of hypopituitarism or hypothalamic dysfunction, either clinically or on laboratory investigation. Eosinophilic tumours may also cause chiasmal compression but the clinical features of acromegaly are usually obvious. Basiphil adenomas produce florid Cushing's disease before they become sufficiently large to compress the chiasm. Craniopharyngiomas produce a similar visual field defect; calcification can often be seen in the tumour on plain X-ray.

(d) *Lesions of the visual pathways* behind the chiasm cause homonymous hemianopia. The nearer the visual cortex, the more congruous the defect. The fibres of the optic radiation are widely separated shortly after leaving the lateral geniculate ganglion, so that lesions of the temporal lobe may cause an upper quadrantic defect and lesions above the Sylvian fissure a lower quadrantic defect. Macula sparing may occur in vascular lesions of the cortex because the cortical area concerned with macula vision receives its supply from more than one main cerebral artery.

Ophthalmoscopy

The retina with its blood supply and the optic disc can be visualised directly.

Papillitis and Papilloedema

The optic disc may be oedematous and appear swollen. If this is due to an inflammatory process of the nerve head (the same pathology as retrobulbar neuritis) it is called papillitis and vision is affected early and severely. There are no other retinal changes and no haemorrhages. If the swelling is caused by raised intracranial pressure or systemic hypertension, it is called papilloedema and the vision is not affected apart from enlargement of the blind spot. In severe cases of papilloedema the pressure may occlude the arterial supply and cause attacks of amblyopia, which occasionally results in permanent blindness. The presence of hypertensive retinal changes and a markedly elevated systemic blood pressure or the presence of retinal haemorrhages with preservation of vision clearly distinguishes papilloedema from papillitis, but in many patients the appearance of the fundus is indistinguishable. Raised intracranial pressure may be accompanied by headache and vomiting and, if acute, by altered consciousness.

Optic Atrophy

Optic atrophy refers to an appearance of the optic disc, which loses its normal pink/yellow colour and assumes a grey/white appearance. There is usually reduced visual acuity or a field defect. The terms primary optic atrophy, secondary optic atrophy and consecutive optic atrophy are purely descriptive and have no pathological connotation. Primary optic atrophy implies a clearly demarcated pale disc with normal retina and blood vessels. It is caused by any lesion of the optic nerve, the commonest of which is retrobulbar neuritis, but it may follow compression by tumours or be the result of toxic (quinine, tobacco, methyl alcohol) or deficiency states (Vitamin B_{12}). Secondary optic atrophy implies a pale disc with a hazy outline, which follows swelling of the nerve head (papilloedema or papillitis). Consecutive optic atrophy implies a pale disc where the cause of the atrophy can be seen in the fundus (retinitis pigmentosa, syphilis).

III, IV AND VI CRANIAL NERVES AND EYE MOVEMENTS

Disorders of the oculomotor system can be divided into upper motor neurone lesions (disorders of gaze), lower motor neurone lesions (disorders of the III, IV and VI cranial nerves) and internuclear lesions (a mixture of upper and lower motor neurone disorders with vestibular or cerebellar components).

Gaze Palsies

Gaze palsies result from upper motor neurone lesions of the oculomotor system and, in common with all upper motor neurone lesions, it is the movement which is represented, not the action of individual muscles—in this case conjugate eye movement. There are centres concerned with gaze in both cortex and in the brain stem.

Cortex

There are two cortical gaze centres in each hemisphere.

(1) *The frontal eye field* in the premotor cortex—this area is responsible for scanning and roving eye movements and is the site of conscious voluntary control of eye movement. As with the control of other movements, one hemisphere is responsible for the opposite side of the body and the contralateral extrapersonal space; the left frontal eye field therefore directs eye movement to the right, and vice versa. The effect of destruction and excitation can therefore be predicted:

Destruction (e.g. infarction)—transient paralysis of gaze to the opposite side. Occasionally deviation of the eyes to the side of the lesion may be seen.

Excitation (e.g. epilepsy)—deviation of the eyes and usually the head to the opposite side (frontal adversive seizure).

Following and reflex eye movement are not affected by lesions of the frontal eye field and optokinetic nystagmus is normal.

(2) *The occipital eye field* in the visual association cortex. This area is responsible for following, pursuit and reflex eye movements. It is intimately associated with the visual pathways and lesions in this area are usually associated with a field defect. In destructive lesions (infarction or tumour) there is a full range of voluntary movements but inability to follow or locate objects. Examination is usually complicated by the associated field defect. Optokinetic nystagmus is impaired.

Brain Stem

There are two areas in the brain stem concerned with conjugate eye movement:

(1) *Upper midbrain and vertical eye movements.* There is no precise centre for vertical eye movement but the pathways concerned must lie at and above the level of the III nerve nucleus in the region of the posterior commissure. Lesions in the pretectal region (pinealomas) pressing on the superior corpora quadragemini cause defects of upward gaze (Parinaud's syndrome).

(2) *Pons and horizontal eye movement.* Clinical evidence strongly suggests the presence of pontine gaze centres for lateral eye movement and these areas appear to lie postero-lateral to the VI nerve nuclei on either side of pons and are responsible for gaze to the same side.

Examination for gaze palsies should include both voluntary and following movements as well as tests for optokinetic nystagmus.

The III, IV and VI Cranial Nerves

The III Cranial Nerve

The III cranial nerve nucleus lies ventrally in the periductal grey matter in the midbrain at the level of the superior corpora quadragemini and the red nucleus. It is a large nucleus with clear grouping of nerve cells responsible for the different muscles innervated. Nearby is the Edinger–Westphal nucleus whose parasympathetic fibres run with the III nerve. The nerve runs forwards through the red nucleus and the medical part of the basis pedunculi emerging close to the midline in the interpeduncular fossa. The two nerves pass on either side of the basilar artery between the posterior cerebral artery above and the superior cerebellar artery below. The nerve lies just below the posterior communicating artery throughout its length, passes laterally over the internal carotid artery to enter the cavernous sinus where it lies on the lateral wall. It passes through the superior orbital fissure and divides into two main branches—the superior branch to the superior rectus and levator palpebrae superioris and the inferior branch to the medial rectus, inferior rectus and the inferior oblique. The parasympathetic nerves travel with the inferior branch. A complete III nerve palsy comprises a fixed dilated pupil due to the unopposed action of the sympathetic, ptosis due to involvement of levator palpebrae superioris and the eye is fully abducted due to the unopposed action of VI nerve.

The IV Cranial Nerve

The IV cranial nerve lies ventrally in the periductal grey matter nearly at the junction of the midbrain and pons and at the level of the inferior corpora quadragemini. The nerve runs round the aqueduct and decussates in the superior medullary velum. The nerve then passes round the cerebral peduncle below the tentorium, the posterior cerebral artery lying just above the tentorium. Like the III nerve, it passes between the posterior cerebral artery and the superior cerebellar artery, crosses the apex of the petrous temporal bone just above and medial to Meckel's cave, and enters the cavernous sinus lying on the lateral wall below the III nerve; it then pàsses through the superior orbital fissure to supply the superior oblique muscle. A IV nerve palsy causes vertical diplopia, maximal on downward gaze with the affected eye adducted.

The VI Cranial Nerve

The VI cranial nerve nucleus lies in the lower pons close to the midline and near the floor of the 4th ventricle. The fibres of the VII nerve are wrapped around the VI nerve nucleus and this forms a small hump in the floor of the fourth ventricle, the facial colliculus. The nerve runs forward to merge at the pontomedullary junction near the midline. It runs up the clivus in front of the pons parallel to the basilar artery and then at the tentorial hiatus it turns forwards to enter the cavernous sinus where it lies below the internal carotid artery. From the cavernous sinus it passes through the superior orbital fissure to supply the lateral rectus muscle.

A VI nerve palsy causes horizontal diplopia, maximal on gaze to the affected side.

Lesions Affecting the III, IV and VI Cranial Nerves

Conditions Which May Affect All Three Nerves

All three nerves may be damaged by brain-stem tumours and vascular disease. The extramedullary part of the nerve trunks between the brain stem and the cavernous sinus are vulnerable to granulomatous meningitis (tuberculosis and sarcoid), meningovascular syphilis and nasopharnygeal carcinoma. The intracavernous course of these nerves may be damaged in cavernous sinus thrombosis, carotid aneurysm and pituitary tumours. The superior orbital fissure may be encroached by sphenoidal ridge meningiomas and the nerves may be damaged in the intraorbital part of their course by orbital tumours. In addition the nerves may be damaged by involvement of their vasa-nervorum in diabetes, hypertension and collagen vascular disease (polyarteritis nodosa and giant cell arteritis).

Lesions of the III Nerve

Intramedullary Lesions

Nerve nucleus—lesions of the nuclei are usually bilateral because they lie close together, the commonest cause is pressure from above by tumours of the pineal gland or gliomas (Parinaud's syndrome).

The nerve trunk and red nucleus (Benedikt's syndrome)—the combination of a III nerve palsy and a contralateral flapping tremor with ataxia of the arm and hand is usually due to vascular disease, disseminated sclerosis or a tumour.

Nerve trunk and cerebral peduncle (Weber's syndrome)—a combination of a III nerve palsy and a contralateral hemiplegia is usually of vascular origin.

Extramedullary Lesions

Bilateral III nerve palsies and tetraparesis may result from any large space-occupying lesion in the interpeduncular fossa. The III nerve may be damaged by aneurysm at either end of the posterior communicating artery although the internal carotid/posterior communicating aneurysms are very much more common.

Lesions of the IV Cranial Nerve

Isolated lesions of the IV cranial nerve are rare and usually due to trauma, diabetes, granulomatous meningitis, syphilis or collagen vascular disease.

Lesions of the VI Cranial Nerve

Lesions affecting the nucleus almost always involve the VII cranial nerve and since these nerves then follow quite separate pathways, a combination of a VI and VII lower motor neurone lesion is likely to be at this level.

VI cranial nerve and contralateral hemiplegia (Raymond–Cestan syndrome) is directly analogous to Weber's syndrome.

The nerve trunk is very vulnerable when it crosses the free edge of the tentorium and it may be damaged here if the brain stem is distorted by a space-occupying lesion in the opposite hemisphere (a false localising sign) or if there is displacement of the brain stem through the tentorial hiatus (coning).

Internuclear Ophthalmoplegias

A combination of upper and lower motor neurone lesions usually associated with evidence of cerebellar or vestibular involvement (nystagmus) is common because of the wide spatial separation of the III, IV and VI nerve nuclei from the upper midbrain to the lower pons, the separation of mechanisms controlling vertical and horizontal conjugate movement and the intimate relationship of vestibular and cerebellar function to eye movement. There are many possible combinations; patients may develop a series of different combinations of signs during the course of an illness particularly in progressive lesions such as pontine glioma. However, there are two principle combinations of signs:

(a) *Anterior internuclear ophthalmoplegia (superior or upper, Harris's sign)*. There is normal convergence but a failure to adduct on lateral gaze with nystagmus in the abducting eye. The lesion lies between the IV nerve nucleus and VI nerve nucleus and involves the medial longitudinal bundle. It is almost always due to disseminated sclerosis.

(b) *Posterior internuclear ophthalmoplegia (inferior or lower)*. This is the opposite of an anterior internuclear ophthalmoplegia and there is failure to abduct on lateral gaze with nystagmus in the adducting eye. The lesion lies at or just below the VI nerve nucleus.

The Analysis of Diplopia

The analysis of diplopia depends on a knowledge of the precise actions of the extraocular muscles. The medial walls of the two orbits are nearly parallel and the lateral walls are roughly at right angles to each other. Since the muscles are inserted into a fibrous ring at the apex of the orbit, the muscle cone is at an angle of about 23° to the optical axis. It is evident therefore, that the lateral and medial recti only move the eye in the horizontal plane, but the superior and inferior recti only become pure elevators or depressors when the optical axis is the same as the muscle-cone axis, that is when the eye is 23° abducted, so that the line of pull of the muscle lies over the optical axis of the globe. Similarly the superior and inferior oblique muscles are only pure elevators or depressors when the eye is adducted since the origin or effective origin of the oblique muscles is antero-medial to the eye. When the eye is abducted the oblique muscles produce rotation only around the optical axis but no vertical movement, and similarly the superior and inferior recti rotate the eye without elevation or depression when the eye is adducted.

The reason why the patients see double when one muscle is not functioning is that the normal eye moves to keep the image on the macula, but the image falls progressively further round the retina away from the macula in the palsied eye. The brain projects this false image further away from its true position and the degree of separation of the images is directly proportional to the distance from the macula. It follows, therefore, that the direction of maximal separation of the images is in the direction of action of the affected muscle and it also follows that the distal image is always the false one. In this context, distal means furthest away from a point straight in front of the eyes.

When a patient complains of double vision he should be asked the direction in which the separation of the images is maximal and whether the separation is in the horizontal or vertical plane. Since the distal image is always the false one, covering one eye will show which eye is giving rise to the false image. In horizontal diplopia, this will reveal whether the double vision is due to one medial rectus or the other lateral rectus. The situation is complicated in vertical diplopia because two muscles are used to elevate and two to depress the eye. First determine whether the diplopia is maximal on upward or downward gaze then determine which eye is responsible for the false image. This reduces the possibility to two muscles, then determine whether the diplopia is maximal with the affected eye abducted (a rectus palsy) or adducted (an oblique palsy).

Summary

(1) The direction of maximal separation of the images is the direction of action of the affected muscle.
(2) The peripheral image is always the false one.
(3) In vertical diplopia, separation of the images is maximal when the affected eye is adducted in oblique palsies and when abducted with rectus palsies.

The cause of diplopia is often obvious, such as a complete VI or III nerve lesion. But it may be difficult in partial lesions and in detecting multiple lesions without proper examination. The full range of movement should be tested with both eyes open and each eye separately with the cover test to determine which eye is fixing. When diplopia has been present for some time the false image may be suppressed and the patient loses the double vision. When there is already a marked disparity in the visual acuity of the two eyes, the patient may still prefer to fix with the eye with the better visual acuity, even if its movement is impaired.

Nystagmus

Accurate and stable eye fixation normally occurs despite constant movement of both the observer and the object. Fixation on a moving object while the observer remains still is achieved by the parieto-occipital eye field and ocular fixation. Compensation for movement of the observer is through a sensitive feedback mechanism from the vestibular system and to a lesser extent from the proprioceptive system via the cerebellum. A lesion affecting any one of these mechanisms, visual fixation, vestibular and cerebellar pathways can give rise to nystagmus.

(1) *Ocular Nystagmus.* This is due to a defect of fixation and is, therefore, seen with small central scotomata, general depression of visual acuity (usually congenital), miner's nystagmus and other defects of the macula. It usually takes the form of a fine oscillatory movement without clear fast and slow components, it is present in all directions of gaze, including gaze ahead, and may be only visible on ophthalmoscopic examination as a fine tremor (jelly nystagmus).

(2) *Vestibular Nystagmus.* Disturbance of the vestibular mechanism is the commonest and most important cause of nystagmus and may be due to a lesion of the vestibular end organ or its central connections. Nystagmus due to vestibular end organ disease is always associated with vertigo and habituates after a few weeks. Nystagmus not associated with any other features which persists for more than a few weeks must be due to a central lesion.

(3) *Cerebellar Nystagmus.* The cerebellum is concerned with the maintenance of ocular fixation and this is in part related to information from the proprioceptive system in the neck. Unilateral lesions of the cerebellum may produce nystagmus, particularly if it affects the deep nuclei. Midline and degenerative lesions usually do not cause nystagmus, probably because the balance between the two sides is not disturbed.

(4) *Brain Stem or Central Nystagmus.* Lesions of the vestibular and cerebellar pathways in the brain stem may cause nystagmus. This is often lateralised but may be bilateral and vertical nystagmus only occurs in brain stem lesions.

Examination. Nystagmus is the jerky eye movements due to a failure to maintain fixation; the eye drifts away from the object so that a rapid voluntary movement is required to regain fixation. The patient should be asked to follow an object, both vertically and to either side. The object must be held at or beyond the near point, so that the patient does not have to converge and the extremes of movement should be within binocular vision. Nystagmoid movements of no significance may be seen if these precautions are not followed. The direction of nystagmus is recorded as the direction of the quick component, even though the quick component is the voluntary overriding attempt at fixation and a slow drift to the resting position is the abnormal movement. If nystagmus is not present on gaze ahead but has to be elicited, it is always in the direction of gaze. The degree of nystagmus should be recorded: first-degree nystagmus to the left is nystagmus only on gaze to the left, second-degree nystagmus to the left is nystagmus to the left on gaze ahead, and third degree nystagmus to the left is nystagmus to the left on gaze to the right. In unconscious patients vestibular lesions or stimulation by caloric testing causes tonic conjugate deviation, because there is no conscious effort to override this.

THE PUPILS

The pupillary muscles are arranged both concentrically, the *sphincter pupilli*, which receives its parasympathetic nerve supply from the ciliary ganglion via the short ciliary nerves, and radially, the *dilator pupilli*, which is innervated by sympathetic fibres via the nasociliary nerve.

The Light Reflex

The pupil of one eye constricts when that eye is exposed to light (the direct reaction) and at the same time the pupil of the other eye also constricts (the consensual reaction). Dilatation occurs in the dark. The afferent pathway is via the optic nerve to the lateral geniculate ganglion and then relayed through the brain stem to the third-nerve nuclei on both sides. The efferent pathway runs from the Edinger–Westphal nucleus via the third nerve to the ciliary ganglion.

The Accommodation/Convergence Reflex

Fixation on an object within the near point requires convergence of the optical axes and this is associated with pupillary constriction. The afferent pathway is with the visual fibres to the occipital cortex, the efferent pathway is from the Edinger–Westphal nucleus.

Pupillary Abnormalities

(1) *Vascular and hyaline degeneration*, which is common in old age, may give rise to pupils which are small, unequal, irregular and relatively immobile.

(2) *The myotonic pupil* is dilated and shows a very slow reaction to light and convergence. It may be necessary to keep the patient in the dark for some time before testing the light reflex and to ask the patient to fix on

a near object for several minutes to show the contraction with convergence. This condition occurs much more commonly in women and is often of sudden onset. It is thought to be due to a post-ganglionic lesion in the efferent parasympathetic pathway. The defect is permanent but does not carry any other pathological connotation. The myotonic pupil may be found in conjunction with absence of tendon reflexes (*The Holmes–Adie Syndrome*).

(3) *Horner's Syndrome* consists of pupillary constriction, slight ptosis, and failure to sweat on the same side of the face. This syndrome results from a lesion anywhere in the sympathetic pathway from the hypothalamus down through the lateral part of the pons and medulla, and Clarke's column in the lateral column of the cervical cord. The fibres then emerge at the level of the first thoracic segment to relay in the cervical sympathetic ganglion and then pass up in a plexus on the carotid artery to be distributed throughout the territory of the external and internal carotid arteries. It is, therefore, a poor localising sign, but a good lateralising sign because the pathway does remain ipsilateral throughout its course.

(4) *Argyll Robertson pupils* are small, unequal, eccentric and irregular. They do not react to light but do constrict on convergence. The lesion is thought to affect the afferent pathway in the midbrain. It is almost always due to syphilis.

(5) *The afferent pupillary defect* is a useful sign in patients with an optic nerve lesion, such as retrobulbar neuritis. The ipsilateral direct reaction and the contralateral consensual reaction are impaired because of the lesion in the afferent pathway, but the consensual reaction following exposure of the other eye to light is brisk, since the efferent pathway functions normally. If a light is shone alternately into both eyes the affected eye will show only the consensual reaction and, therefore, follow the constriction and dilatation of the normal eye, so that when the light is moved from the normal to the affected eye the pupil is seen to dilate.

THE TRIGEMINAL NERVE (V Cranial Nerve)

The trigeminal nerve has three major peripheral branches:

(1) *Ophthalmic*, which supplies the eye via the nasociliary nerve, the forehead and the scalp as far back as the vertex. A small strip extends down the bridge of the nose. The fibres pass back through the roof of the orbit, through the superior orbital foramen, along the lateral wall of the cavernous sinus to reach the gasserian ganglion situated in Meckel's cave at the apex of the petrous temporal bone.

(2) *Maxillary*, which supplies the lower eyelid, the side of the nose, the cheek and the upper lip. It extends laterally only to a line approximately between the outer canthus of the eye and the side of the

mouth. The fibres pass through the maxilla and enter the antero-medial aspect of the middle cranial fossa via the foramen rotundum to reach the gasserian ganglion.

(3) *Mandibular*, which supplies the lower lip and chin, a thin strip lateral to the maxillary division but sparing an area of three fingers from the angle of the jaw; it supplies the upper part of the tragus and adjoining parts of the pinna and a variable area of adjacent scalp on the side of the head. The fibres pass back through the pterygoid fossa and reach the gasserian ganglion via the foramen ovale, which lies just below the ganglion.

The motor division travels with the mandibular branch and supplies muscles of mastication, particularly the lateral pterygoid.

Distal lesions usually affect one branch only because of the wide separation of the three main branches distal to the ganglion. Lesions of the nerve proximal to the ganglion, as it crosses the anterior end of the cerebello-pontine angle to enter the mid pons, affect all three divisions to some extent. The earliest sign of a lesion of the pathway between the main sensory nucleus and the gasserian ganglion is loss of the corneal reflex. Lesions below mid pons affect only the descending tract or its decussating fibres, which relay the sensations of pain and temperature. The arrangement of fibres in the descending tract results in 'onion skin' loss of sensation of the face from compressive lesions, with the snout area nearest the main sensory nucleus and the most peripheral of the 'onion skins' extending down into the upper cervical region. Lesions of the descending tract may cause diminution but not loss of the corneal reflex.

Intramedullary lesions affecting the trigeminal nerve include syringobulbia, demyelinating disease, tumours and infarcts. Extramedullary intracranial causes include lesions in the cerebellar pontine angle, such as acoustic neuromas, meningiomas and trigeminal neuromas, granulomatous meningitis (TB, sarcoid and syphilis) and nasopharyngeal carcinoma eroding the base of the skull.

Trigeminal Neuralgia (Tic Douloureux)

The cause of this condition is unknown, it may occur at any age but becomes more common with increasing age. In young patients it may be the first sign of multiple sclerosis. The characteristic features are:

(1) The pain is always *confined to the distribution of the trigeminal nerve*, usually affecting either the third or second divisions or both; involvement of the first division alone is rare. Involvement of both sides is exceptional.
(2) The pain is *paroxysmal* and usually described as a brief, stabbing, lancinating or shooting pain. It is usually extremely severe, lasting for a few seconds only but may be repeated frequently.

(3) The pain is always *precipitated* and patients may describe a trigger point which is particularly sensitive. Trigger stimuli include touch, washing or shaving, facial movement, eating and drinking hot or cold liquids, and during particularly severe bouts, patients may not be able to speak, eat or drink.

(4) Patients usually have frequent stabs of pain over a short period of time and may then have minutes or hours of freedom before the next bout. These paroxysms occur over several weeks before complete remission. The pain always returns but the interval may vary from months to years. The periods of remission tend to become shorter and bouts of pain more severe and longer. A few patients never show remission. The pain always remains paroxysmal and never becomes constant.

(5) There are *never any abnormal signs*. If abnormal signs are found it cannot be tic douloureux and there is an underlying abnormality such as disseminated sclerosis, a congenital vascular abnormality, a neoplasm in the cerebellar pontine angle or a nasopharyngeal carcinoma.

Treatment. The only effective medication is carbamazepine and this will control the pain in almost all patients, at least initially. Treatment should be started with 300 mg a day in divided doses and increased as required up to a total dose of 1200 mg a day. The development of a rash is an idiosyncratic side effect and the medication should be stopped. Dose-dependent side effects include unsteadiness, vertigo and nausea and these can be relieved by reducing the dose. In some patients this treatment is ineffective or becomes so with repeated exacerbations. For these reasons, or because the patient is unable to tolerate the medication, it may be necessary to destroy the trigeminal nerve. To be effective the lesion must be at or proximal to the gasserian ganglion as lesions distal to the ganglion cause only temporary relief of symptoms and are usually unsatisfactory. The ganglion may be reached through the cheek and foramen ovale and injected with phenol or alcohol, or destroyed with a radio-frequency probe or cryoprobe. The sensory root may be divided between the ganglion and the pons following craniotomy, in which case an attempt may be made to preserve the corneal reflex by a partial root section. If this is done properly, the analgesia and the relief of pain are permanent. After partial lesions a few patients complain of unpleasant sensations in the face (anaesthesia dolorosa). Most patients quickly become accustomed to a numb face, but they must always exercise great care to prevent corneal ulceration and should wear glasses with a side-piece to protect the eye. They should also be warned against nasal ulceration.

Trigeminal Neuropathy

Patients with this condition develop numbness, which may be confined to one of the divisions of the trigeminal nerve. The motor division is usually spared. The sensory deficit evolves over days or weeks and usually persists. In some patients the onset is associated with pain but this does not resemble trigeminal neuralgia. It is a benign condition but it is important to exclude other causes of trigeminal sensory loss.

THE FACIAL NERVE (VII Cranial Nerve)

The facial nerve nucleus lies in the floor of the fourth ventricle in the lower pons; the fibres pass round the sixth nerve nucleus forming a small hump in the floor of the fourth ventricle, the facial colliculus, and then run laterally to emerge from the pons near its lower border. They cross the cerebello-pontine angle with the nervus intermedius (secretomotor to the lacrymal gland and taste fibres from the anterior two-thirds of the tongue) and the eighth nerve. All three nerves pass through the internal auditory meatus into the internal auditory canal to the geniculate ganglion. The eighth nerve leaves at this point and shortly afterwards, the chorda tympani and the nerve to stapedius also leave the facial nerve, which finally emerges from the skull through the stylomastoid foramen. It divides in the parotid gland to supply all the muscles of facial expression.

Unilateral upper motor neurone lesions of the facial nerve cause quite marked weakness of the lower half of the face with the relative sparing of the upper half. This is because the supranuclear pathways for the muscles of the forehead and around the eyes are bilateral. Upper motor neurone lesions also cause greater impairment of voluntary movement than of involuntary and emotional movement. Strokes and hemisphere tumours are common causes.

Lower motor neurone lesions cause weakness of all facial muscles. The site of the lesion can often be accurately located because of involvement of associated structures.

(a) Lesions of the nuclei are nearly always associated with an ipsilateral sixth nerve palsy.
(b) Lesions in the cerebellar pontine angle are usually associated with eighth nerve and chorda tympani involvement. In addition the corneal reflex may be absent due to fifth nerve involvement and there may be cerebellar signs.
(c) Lesions in the internal auditory canal as far as the geniculate ganglion may also be associated with lesions of the eighth nerve and chorda tympani and there may also be hyperacusis due to paralysis of the stapedius muscle.

In the brain stem, tumours and vascular lesions are the commonest causes of seventh nerve damage. The facial nerve is the most frequently affected cranial nerve in the Guillain–Barré syndrome. It may also be damaged in operations on the parotid salivary gland and involvement with sarcoidosis may cause bilateral lesions. The commonest cause of a lower motor neurone lesion of the seventh nerve is, however, Bell's palsy.

Bell's Palsy

Bell's palsy is an acute lower motor neurone palsy of the facial nerve of unknown aetiology. The occurrence in some patients of hypercusis or loss of taste on the anterior two-thirds of the tongue implies that the nerve may be involved at different levels within the petrous temporal bone. The onset may be sudden or develop over several hours, rarely more than a day or so. The onset may be associated with some pain in or behind the ear. About 50% of patients make a complete recovery, although this may take weeks or months. Some patients start to improve within a few days but it is possible to make a complete recovery even if the improvement does not start for six to eight weeks. Some estimate of the prognosis can be made from electromyography after one month.

Treatment with steroids should be started within 24 hours of the onset of symptoms. Prednisolone 60–80 mg a day for two or three days, followed by a rapidly diminishing dose over two or three weeks is a suitable regime.

The Ramsay Hunt Syndrome. This is due to infection of the seventh nerve by herpes zoster. The syndrome consists of herpetic vesicles on the soft palate and in the external auditory meatus and may include deafness, facial palsy and trigeminal nerve involvement.

THE ACOUSTIC VESTIBULAR NERVE (VIII Cranial Nerve)

The acoustic and vestibular parts of the eighth nerve serve quite separate functions. The acoustic nerve arises in the cochlea and the vestibular nerve in the semicircular canals and otolith. Both pass down the internal auditory canal with the seventh nerve and chorda tympani, they cross the cerebello-pontine angle and enter the brain stem at the ponto-medullary junction. The nuclei are situated in the region of the inferior cerebellar peduncle.

From the cochlear nuclei some fibres decussate in the trapezoid body and ascend in the lateral lemniscus and some fibres ascend in the ipsilateral lateral lemniscus, so that there is bilateral representation of hearing at supranuclear level.

Hearing acuity should be tested and, if deafness is found, it is then necessary to determine whether this is due to middle-ear disease affecting the ear ossicles (conductive deafness) or whether it is due to a lesion of the nerve (perceptive deafness). Normally air conduction is better than bone conduction and this difference is preserved in perceptive deafness, but in conductive deafness bone conduction appears louder than air conduction because it by-passes the ear ossicles. Perceptive deafness due to intramedullary lesions is unusual and may be associated with other brain-stem or long-tract signs; lesions of the cerebello-pontine angle (acoustic neuroma, trigeminal neuroma, meningioma and cholesteatoma) may be associated with fifth and seventh nerve palsies and cerebellar signs; lesions in the petrous temporal bone (Paget's disease) may be associated with a facial palsy and impaired taste.

Vestibular nuclei are connected to the cerebellar hemisphere on the same side, to the third, fourth and sixth nerves via the medial longitudinal bundle, via the vestibular spinal tract to centres in the cord and via the ipsilateral lateral lemniscus to the cortex.

Vestibular function is assessed by the caloric test, in which the ear is syringed with water above and below body temperature. This stimulates movement of endolymph in the semicircular canals and causes nystagmus. A standard technique is used and should always be followed. The duration of the nystagmus is timed.

Acute vestibular lesions cause vertigo and disequilibrium. Vertigo which is solely related to changes in position indicates disease of the otolith, although it may occasionally occur in some posterior fossa lesions.

Vestibular neuronitis is an acute vestibular disturbance with nausea, vomiting and unsteady gait, which develops over a few hours and may be completely prostrating for a day or two before passing off over a few more days. Most patients have a liability to vertigo on rapid head movement for several weeks or even months.

Menière's Disease. Patients with this condition suffer recurrent attacks of vertigo with vomiting and prostration, associated with tinnitus, which is usually more persistent, and progressive deafness. During the acute attack, patients usually have nystagmus but this disappears during remission. The treatment is symptomatic with intramuscular or oral phenothiazines. The aetiology is unknown.

GLOSSOPHARYNGEAL NERVE (IX Cranial Nerve)

This is a mixed motor and sensory nerve, which arises in the medulla and leaves the skull through the jugular foramen with the vagus and the spinal accessory nerves and supplies the stylopharyngeus muscle. Sensory fibres carry all forms of sensation, including taste, from the posterior third of the tongue, the tonsillar fossa and the pharynx. Parasympathetic fibres from the inferior salivary nucleus also travel with the glossopharyngeal nerve but leave it within the skull to supply the parotid gland via the otic ganglion.

Isolated lesions of the glossopharyngeal nerve are rare, lesions at the jugular foramen also involve the vagus and accessory nerves.

Glossopharyngeal Neuralgia

This is a similar condition to trigeminal neuralgia but the pain is felt in the distribution of the glossopharyngeal nerve and is precipitated by eating and swallowing. Pain may also be felt deep in the ear. The treatment is also with carbamazepine. If this fails to control the pain, the nerve should be surgically divided.

THE VAGUS (X Cranial Nerve)

The nuclei of this motor and sensory nerve are situated in the medulla. The nerve leaves the skull through the jugular foramen and it lies in the carotid sheath in the neck. It is the motor supply to the pharyngeal and laryngeal muscles and it carries the parasympathetic supply to the thoracic and abdominal viscera. Sensory fibres carry sensation from the larynx. Lesions of one vagus nerve results in paralysis of the soft palate, the pharynx and the larynx.

SPINAL ACCESSORY NERVE (XI Cranial Nerve)

The nuclei of this motor nerve lie in the lower medulla and upper part of the spinal cord. The nerve emerges from the medulla and spinal cord in a continuous line of rootlets. The spinal rootlets unite to form a trunk which ascends through the foramen magnum to join the cranial rootlets. The nerve leaves the skull through the jugular foramen with the vagus. The cranial fibres are distributed to the pharynx and larynx. The spinal fibres descend to supply the sternomastoids and the upper fibres of trapezius.

THE HYPOGLOSSAL NERVE (XII Cranial Nerve)

The nucleus lies in the dorsal part of the lower medulla and the nerve leaves the skull through the hypoglossal foramen (the anterior condylar canal) and supplies the muscles of the tongue.

Lesions of the twelfth nerve cause wasting, fasciculation and weakness of the ipsilateral side of the tongue and the tongue deviates to the affected side on protrusion.

DYSARTHRIA

Dysarthria may occur in any lesion of the motor pathway to the bulbar muscles. Because the pathways are bilateral above the bulbar nuclei, a unilateral upper motor neurone lesion only causes temporary dysarthria. Dysarthria occurs in pseudobulbar palsy (upper motor neurone lesions) and in bulbar palsies (lower motor neurone lesions). Dysarthria may also occur in extra pyramidal and cerebellar lesions, myasthenia gravis and in some diseases of muscle.

It is necessary only to determine that the patient has dysarthria, since the physical signs will indicate the cause.

BULBAR AND PSEUDOBULBAR PALSIES

The lower cranial nerves (IX–XII) arise from a chain of motor nuclei in the medulla and emerge as an almost continuous line of rootlets. The ninth, tenth and eleventh nerves all leave the skull through the jugular foramen. This anatomical arrangement means that these nerves are often affected together.

A bulbar palsy is a lower motor neurone lesion affecting the cranial nerves whose nuclei lie in the bulb (the medulla), the commonest causes include syringobulbia, motor neurone disease and vascular lesions. The nerves may be affected outside the medulla in diphtheria and the Guillain–Barré syndrome. Tumours in the region of the jugular foramen may affect the ninth, tenth and eleventh nerves and these include nasopharyngeal carcinoma, meningioma and glomus jugulari tumours.

Patients with bulbar palsy complain of dysarthria and dysphagia, fluids may regurgitate through the nose when they attempt to swallow. Signs include loss of taste and sensation on the posterior third of the tongue and in the tonsillar fossa (IX), paralysis of the vocal chords (X), weakness of the sternomastoid and upper fibres of trapezius (XI) and, if the twelfth cranial nerve is involved, there may be wasting and fibrillation of the tongue.

Patients with *pseudobulbar palsy* have the same complaints and difficulties as patients with a bulbar palsy, but it is due to an upper motor neurone lesion of the bulbar muscles. The upper motor neurone pathways must be affected on both sides because the pathways are bilateral. Causes include motor neurone disease, vascular lesions, usually associated with hypertension, and multiple sclerosis. Signs include a brisk jaw jerk and a slow-moving spastic tongue. The plantar responses are usually extensor.

THE MOTOR SYSTEM

The motor system comprises the upper motor neurone pathways, the lower motor neurone, the myoneural junction and muscle.

CORTEX

The upper motor neurone pathway arises in the pre-central gyrus. Lesions strictly confined to the motor cortex give rise to a characteristic pattern of motor deficit. There is weakness of all movements of the affected part, there may be some wasting but there is no tone or reflex change (cortical pattern of motor deficit). Because of the wide extent of the motor cortex with the face/hand area laterally and the foot area medially, a single lesion only produces these signs in a relatively small part of the body, perhaps the hand or the foot. Large lesions necessarily involve subcortical structures and this produces a different pattern.

THE PYRAMIDAL TRACT

The upper motor neurone pathway descends from the precentral gyrus and is gathered into a compact bundle at the internal capsule, so that lesions at this level tend to produce a complete hemiplegia. Any lesion above the mid-brain will affect the cranial nerves on the same side as the hemiplegia. Some fibres cross the midline in the mid-brain, pons and upper medulla to supply the contralateral cranial nerve nuclei. A lesion, therefore, of a cranial nerve on one side, together with a contralateral hemiplegia, accurately locates the site of the lesion to the level of that cranial nerve nucleus. In the lower part of the medulla, just above the level of the foramen magnum, the pyramidal tract decussates from its anterior position in the brain stem to the lateral column of the cord on the opposite side.

Lesions of the pyramidal tract cause spasticity, which is an increase in muscle tone that is not uniform throughout the range of movement and does not affect both directions of movement equally. There may be flaccidity after an acute pyramidal tract lesion due to 'spinal shock' and spasticity may only develop later.

There is a characteristic distribution of muscle weakness. All the muscles may be weak on the affected side, but in the upper limb the extensors are much more affected than the flexors and in the lower limb the flexors are much more affected than the extensors. It is important therefore, to test shoulder abduction, elbow extension, wrist and finger extension and finger abduction in the upper limb and hip flexion, knee flexion, and ankle dorsiflexion in the lower limb.

The reflexes are all pathologically brisk. Reflexes which are normally only just obtainable may be very brisk, such as the digital reflex, and there may be clonus, particularly at the ankle. The cutaneous reflexes (the abdominal and cremasteric reflexes) are reduced or abolished on the affected side and the plantar response is extensor.

THE LOWER MOTOR NEURONE

The lower motor neurone, arising in the anterior horn cells of the spinal cord, is the final common pathway to muscle. Lesions anywhere in this pathway cause wasting, weakness and the reflexes are absent due to disruption of the efferent limb of the reflex arc. The nearer the lesion is to the spinal cord, the more likely is fasciculation to be found in the affected muscles. It is, therefore, very common in anterior horn cell lesions, frequently seen in root lesions and rare in peripheral nerve lesions (see under disorders of the peripheral nervous system).

MOTOR NEURONE DISEASE

This is a progressive degeneration of the motor pathways in the central nervous system. It may affect any part of the pathway from the motor cortex to the anterior horn cells. It usually occurs between the ages of 50 and 70 and affects men more often than women. It is extremely rare before the mid thirties. The clinical signs are strictly confined to the motor system and there are never any sensory signs or sphincter disturbance. The disease usually presents with one of three groups of symptoms—progressive bulbar palsy, amyotrophic lateral sclerosis or progressive muscular atrophy.

Progressive Bulbar Palsy

This is a progressive degeneration of the motor nuclei in the medulla, causing a lower motor neurone bulbar palsy (see p. 340). A wasted fibrillating tongue is the most important sign. This is the form with the worst prognosis and patients seldom survive more than a year after the diagnosis is made.

Amyotrophic Lateral Sclerosis

This is the most common presentation of motor neurone disease and, as the name implies, it is due to a combination of wasting and weakness, often most obvious in the hands, and pyramidal tract involvement, often most prominent in the legs. The finding of upper motor neurone signs with widespread fasciculation is a characteristic feature. The prognosis from diagnosis is usually less than five years and this is largely determined by the development of bulbar signs.

Progressive Muscular Atrophy

In this form of motor neurone disease there is a slowly progressive lower motor neurone involvement of the arms and legs with wasting and weakness. This is the form with the best prognosis and patients may survive from five to fifteen years; again, the length of survival depends largely on whether or not the bulbar muscles become involved.

The diagnosis is often clear on clinical grounds alone but it may be confirmed by electromyography.

No **treatment** is known which influences the course of the condition.

Kugelberg–Welander Syndrome (benign spinal muscular atrophy)

This is a genetically determined spinal muscular atrophy and most cases appear to be inherited by an autosomal recessive mechanism. It is now realised that most patients with 'limb girdle dystrophy' (see p. 346) have this condition. It presents at any age with wasting and weakness of the arms and legs and is very slowly progressive. Some patients show widespread fasciculation. The diagnosis can be confirmed by EMG and muscle biopsy, but secondary myopathic change commonly occurs and this confuses the EMG and biopsy findings.

THE NEUROMUSCULAR JUNCTION

The arrival of a nerve impulse at the neuromuscular junction causes the release of acetylcholine. The acetylcholine crosses the cleft between nerve and muscle and becomes attached to the acetylcholine receptor in the motor end plate, causing depolarisation and subsequent contraction of the muscle. The acetylcholine is rapidly destroyed by cholinesterase or taken up by nerve endings, and the motor end plate repolarises.

Procaine and botulinus toxins inhibit the release of acetylcholine, whereas guanidine increases the release of acetylcholine. Physostigmine, neostigmine and pyridostigmine destroy cholinesterase and allow the acetylcholine to accumulate, perpetuating its action. Curare, tubocurarine and galamine act as competitive inhibitors by reacting with the acetylcholine receptors on the end plate producing a conduction block.

MYASTHENIA GRAVIS

Myasthenia gravis is an immunological disease with damage of the acetylcholine receptors by antibody, which not only blocks the receptor sites but also causes degeneration of the receptors. The characteristic feature of this disease is abnormal fatiguability of striated muscle with rapid recovery after rest.

It may occur at any age but most commonly affects women in the second and third decades. Children born of myasthenic mothers may show evidence of myasthenia for some days after birth because the mother's antibodies cross the placenta. There is a much higher incidence of thyrotoxicosis in patients with myasthenia than can be accounted for by chance.

The condition does not affect all striated muscle equally and, although electromyography may show evidence of widespread disease, it may be quite localised clinically. It commonly affects the external ocular, bulbar, neck and limb girdle muscles. The onset is often gradual and fluctuating. Patients may complain of diplopia, dysphagia, dysarthria and difficulty in chewing and these symptoms may all show marked variability. Patients, for example, may have difficulty in completing a meal or only develop ptosis and diplopia in the evening.

Examination shows no wasting or fasciculation and the most striking feature is undue fatiguability which can be shown by asking the patient to raise the arm above the head 30 times and demonstrating the development of weakness as a result. Normal power returns after a few moments rest.

The diagnosis can be confirmed by intravenous edrophonium. This is a short-acting anticholinesterase drug which may give a dramatic response for up to two or three minutes. A test dose of 1 mg should be given and, if no undue reaction occurs, a further 9 mg should be injected IV. The response to edrophonium is often disappointing in ocular and bulbar myasthenia and a negative test does not exclude these varieties of myasthenia. Confirmation of the diagnosis may be obtained from electromyography, which shows the characteristic decrease in evoked response with Faradic stimulation. Single fibre recording shows an increase in jitter, demonstrating instability of neuromuscular junctions within one motor unit. Thyroid function tests should be carried out because of the association with thyrotoxicosis, and it is important to X-ray the chest with lateral views because of the association with thymoma. Skeletal muscle antibodies may be elevated and are almost always elevated if there is an underlying thymoma. Acetylcholine receptor antibody is usually elevated, but the level does not show an obvious relationship to the severity of the disease.

Treatment. Anticholinesterase drugs have been the basis of treatment since their use was first described in 1934 and remains the treatment of choice for limb myasthenia. Treatment should be started with pyridostigmine 60 mg t.d.s. and increased as necessary. Some patients require up to 600 mg a day. The half-life of pyridostigmine is about 4 hours. It may be helpful occasionally to use the shorter acting neostigmine bromide with a half-life of 1½ hours when a short lived boost is required, such as just before a meal in patients with bulbar myasthenia, but it is usually easier to stabilise the patient on pyridostigmine alone.

Although increasing the dose results in increasing strength initially, a plateau is soon reached and further increase results in progressive weakness due to conduction block. A patient who deteriorates while on treatment may be having either a myasthenic or a cholinergic crisis.

These can be distinguished by IV edrophonium, which can also be used to determine whether a patient is on an optimal dose of drugs. Ocular and bulbar myasthenia often respond poorly to anticholinesterase drugs and in these patients steroids are the treatment of choice. In contrast to the usual use of steroids, it is important to start with a small dose and make gradual increments until a therapeutic effect is achieved. Large doses given initially may precipitate a myasthenic crisis. It is usually possible to control symptoms satisfactorily with a modest dose of steroid, which may be given on alternate days to minimise the long-term side-effects.

If these measures fail to control the patient's symptoms, thymectomy should be considered and it is better to carry out this procedure sooner than later, particularly if immunosuppressive drugs are used in the treatment of limb myasthenia. Patients with a thymoma or thymic hyperplasia have a worse prognosis than those with a normal thymus. Thymectomy appears to make patients more responsive subsequently to anticholinesterase drugs and immunosuppression and this may be related to a reduction in the amount of circulating antibody. The amount of circulating antibody can be temporarily reduced by plasmapheresis and this may be helpful as a short-term measure while awaiting a response from immunosuppression. It may, for example, be enough to keep a patient off a ventilator during a critical time. If large doses of steroids are required to keep control or it is likely that this treatment would need to be continued for a long time, the steroid should be combined with an immunosuppressive drug such as azathioprine.

MYASTHENIC SYNDROME (The Eaton–Lambert Syndrome)

This condition usually complicates oat-cell carcinoma of the bronchus but it has been described with other carcinomata. The weakness may precede clinical evidence of the carcinoma by months or years. The patient complains of weakness after exertion but examination shows weakness of proximal limb girdle muscles which improves after exercise. The reflexes are almost always depressed or absent, unlike true myasthenia. The edrophonium test is usually positive but anticholinesterase drugs given therapeutically have little or no effect. The diagnosis can be confirmed by electromyography. The condition responds to guanidine hydrochloride given orally.

DISEASES OF MUSCLE

Diseases of muscle may be conveniently divided into the congenital genetically determined abnormalities, which carry the generic name of muscular dystrophy, and acquired lesions.

MUSCULAR DYSTROPHIES

These are classified according to their clinical picture and mode of inheritance.

(1) Sex-linked Pseudohypertrophic Muscular Dystrophy (Duchenne and Becker Dystrophy)

This is due to a sex-linked recessive gene or genes, although there is a high rate of new mutations. The abnormality becomes apparent at about the age of three with difficulty in walking and climbing stairs due to proximal leg weakness. Some pseudohypertrophy is very common and principally affects the calf muscles. Although termed pseudohypertrophy, there is, in fact, enlargement of individual muscle fibres. The condition is slowly progressive, patients become chairbound between the age of eight and ten and die at around the age of fifteen, usually from respiratory and cardiac causes. During the later years of his life the patient suffers progressive deformity, particularly of the chest. There is no treatment but female carriers can often be identified and, if they become pregnant, the sex of the child can be determined by amniocentesis.

The Becker type of muscular dystrophy is a more benign form of the Duchenne type and constitutes about 10 % of cases. The condition may develop at any age up to about the 25th year and patients may not become chairbound for another 25 years.

(2) The Autosomal Dominant Facioscapulohumeral Muscular Dystrophy

This condition affects both sexes equally and usually presents in adolescence with facial involvement, followed shortly by weakness of the shoulder girdle muscles. It may follow a very prolonged, low-grade course and the patients may never become chairbound.

(3) Limb Girdle Dystrophy

The majority of patients with this condition have the Kugelberg–Welander syndrome (see p. 343, Spinal Muscular Atrophy).

(4) Ocular Myopathy (Progressive Ophthalmoplegia)

Patients usually present with ptosis and subsequently develop bilateral external ophthalmoplegia over many years. The condition may be confined to the ocular muscles but some patients show weakness of facial and shoulder girdle muscles and others show evidence of degeneration in other parts of the nervous system.

(5) Myotonic Syndromes

Myotonia is the persistence of muscle contraction after voluntary effort has ceased and is well demonstrated by difficulty in relaxing the grip after vigorous contraction. A blow to a muscle belly causes a localised area of contraction, which relaxes slowly (myotonic dimpling).

(a) **Dystrophia myotonica** is a widespread dystrophic condition, not only affecting muscle. There is an autosomal dominant inheritance with onset usually in adolescence and early adult life. It appears to show the phenomenon of anticipation within a family, with each succeeding generation showing more widespread abnormalities.

The fully developed syndrome consists of frontal baldness, wasting of the masseter, temporal and sternomastoid muscles, facial weakness with ptosis, posterior capsular cataracts and a distal myopathy with wasting and weakness, starting in the hands and later involving the feet, gonadal atrophy—as shown by small testes in the male and menstrual irregularity in the female—and impaired production of thyroid hormone and insulin.

The first member of the family to be affected with this condition may have cataracts alone and the fully developed picture may not present for two or three generations.

(b) **Myotonia congenita (Thomsen's Disease).** Patients show widespread myotonia from birth. There is usually hypertrophy of muscles, giving the appearance of a Little Hercules. The condition is usually dominantly inherited.

ACQUIRED DISORDERS OF MUSCLE

These can be conveniently divided into primary inflammatory disorders of muscle (polymyositis) and those myopathies which complicate systemic disease, though this may be an artificial distinction.

Polymyositis

This is a group of conditions associated with weakness of proximal muscles which is usually painless and is probably due to an autoimmune mechanism. One muscle group constantly affected in polymyositis, which may be spared in other myopathies, are the neck extensors. It may occur at any age and usually follows a very prolonged relapsing and remittent course. *Raynaud's syndrome* is a common association in younger patients and there may be a characteristic rash (*dermatomyositis*). There is an association with occult neoplasm and this increases with age; there is usually a loss of reflexes in these patients. The diagnosis is made by the characteristic clinical picture, EMG and muscle biopsy. The ESR is usually raised. The majority of patients respond to corticosteroid medication and this may need to be continued for several years. Patients who require continued high-dose steroid medication may benefit from an alternate day regime or the addition of immunosuppressive drugs, such as azathioprine.

Myopathies Complicating Systemic Disease

Inflammatory conditions of muscle may complicate sarcoidosis, rheumatoid arthritis, polyarthritis nodosa, disseminated lupus erythematosus and scleroderma.

Polymyalgia rheumatica (See p. 433).

A proximal limb girdle myopathy may complicate steroid therapy, thyrotoxicosis and occasionally myxoedema. Diabetic amyotrophy is not a myopathy but describes the wasting that follows a neuropathy principally affecting the femoral nerve.

THE SENSORY SYSTEM

Pathways for the different modalities of sensation have separate courses in different parts of the nervous system, so that lesions at various levels produce characteristic patterns of sensory deficit.

Peripheral Nerve Lesions

The area of sensory loss in a peripheral nerve lesion is fairly constant, it may be associated with dysaesthesia, such as pins and needles, tingling or burning sensations. The triple response is abolished.

Root Lesions

The autonomous area of skin supplied by a single root may be extremely small, so that even a complete lesion may not produce any detectable sensory loss; this is because of overlap from adjacent dermatomes. Conversely, the rash of herpes zoster may be found over a relatively large area, since vesicles occur where there is any contribution from one nerve root.

Sensory Pathways in Spinal Cord

After entering the spinal cord through the dorsal root, there is a separation of fibres, with those responsible for pain and temperature crossing the midline to reach the contralateral spinothalamic tract in the anterior white matter of the cord, and those fibres concerned with touch and position sense travel in the ipsilateral posterior columns to the gracile and cuneate nuclei in the lower medulla. Fibres from these nuclei decussate to form the medial lemniscus and lie in close association with the spinothalamic tract; so that the pathways for all sensation lie on the same side of the brain stem. These pathways are joined by the fibres from the fifth nerve nucleus, the quintothalamic tract (see trigeminal nerve). The sensory pathways then pass up to the thalamus, where all sensory information from one half of the body is relayed to the cortex. The pain pathways above the thalamus are very extensive, so that localised lesions of the main sensory radiation cause marked loss of light touch and position sense with relative preservation of pain.

THE BASAL GANGLIA AND EXTRAPYRAMIDAL SYSTEM

There are two principal non-pyramidal systems concerned with control of movement, the cerebellum and the extrapyramidal system. Disorders of the basal ganglia and extrapyramidal system can cause a wide variety of movement disorders.

PARKINSON'S DISEASE

James Parkinson first described paralysis agitans in 1817. Its three principal characteristics are an increase in muscle tone (rigidity), slowness of movement (bradykinesia) and a characteristic tremor.

(a) *Rigidity*. This form of hypertonus must be distinguished from spasticity. In rigidity the increase in tone is present throughout the range of movement and in both directions.

(b) *Bradykinesia*. The slowness of voluntary movement is out of proportion to the degree of rigidity and patients have difficulty in initiating and carrying out coordinated movements.

(c) *Tremor* is present at rest and inhibited by movement. It may also be temporarily inhibited by conscious effort.

Parkinson's disease may develop at any age but is much commoner after the fifth decade. The patient may present either with rigidity and bradykinesia and little or no tremor or with an obvious tremor which may be confined to one limb with little or no rigidity and bradykinesia. All three features eventually develop. The condition is slowly progressive over many years. Early features include loss of facial expression, a monotonous speech and loss of associated movements, such as swinging the arms when walking.

The disease is caused by the degeneration of dopaminergic pathways in the basal ganglia, principally in the globus pallidus and substantia nigra. These structures are found to be relatively deficient in dopa in patients with Parkinson's disease.

Treatment. The aim of treatment is to increase the dopamine levels in the brain. Dopamine cannot be given orally because it does not cross the blood–brain barrier. Dopa is its immediate precursor but only the laevo form crosses the blood–brain barrier. More than 90% of an orally administered dose of dopa is destroyed outside the brain by dopa decarboxylase. It is usual, therefore, to administer L-dopa, together with a proportionate amount of a decarboxylase inhibitor, which itself does not cross the blood–brain barrier, but inhibits the extracerebral decarboxylation of L-dopa. This combination makes more L-dopa available in the brain and considerably reduces systemic side effects.

Two such preparations are available. Sinemet is a combination of L-dopa and carbidopa in a ratio of 10:1, tablets containing 100 and 250 mg of L-dopa combined with 10 and 25 mg respectively of carbidopa are available (Sinemet 110 and Sinemet 275); or in a ratio of 4:1 containing 100 mg of L-dopa and 25 mg of carbidopa (Sinemet Plus). These tablets are heavily scored so that it is easy to take whole or half tablets in any combination. Madopar is the combination of L-dopa and benserazide in a ratio of 4:1. When using lower doses of L-dopa it is usually necessary to use a preparation with a 4:1 ratio in order to achieve satisfactory peripheral decarboxylase inhibition. The 10:1 ratio gives a satisfactory inhibition in the majority of patients at higher dose levels. Treatment should be started with Sinemet Plus half a tablet t.d.s. and gradually increased according to response. Most patients achieve a satisfactory response on less than one tablet of Sinemet 275 t.d.s. Since the half life of L-dopa is only about four hours, a smoother response may be obtained by multiple divided doses.

The response to L-dopa is often dramatic and the patients may be able to return to a relatively normal life. It does not, however, alter the long-term prognosis and over the years it tends to become less effective, often producing unacceptable side-effects at a lower dosage. The principal dose-limiting side-effect is orofacial dyskinesia and other dystonic and choreiform movements affecting the limbs. This is dose-dependent and disappears with reduction in dosage. The reduction of the effect of L-dopa with time may be partly due to the loss of the enzyme which converts dopa to dopamine. This loss of response may occur after 5–7 years of treatment with L-dopa and has led to the suggestion that treatment in younger patients should be initiated with anticholinergic drugs and only changed to L-dopa when these become ineffective. In this way the problems associated with long-term L-dopa therapy may be postponed by several years.

Normally the dopaminergic pathways are in balance with the cholinergic pathways. If a satisfactory response cannot be obtained by increasing the dopa levels in the brain, the balance between these two systems may be restored by inhibition of the cholinergic system. The use of anticholinergic drugs is well established and was the mainstay of treatment before the advent of L-dopa. The most effective is benzhexol which is available in tablets containing 2 and 5 mg. It may be given in addition to L-dopa in a dose of between 6 and 15 mg a day. Orphenadrine may be better tolerated. Benztropine, methixene and procyclidine have similar properties. Side-effects include dry mouth and blurred vision, and commonly in older patients, confusion and hallucinations.

When these measures fail to control symptoms satisfactorily, the addition of the monoamine oxidase inhibitor selegiline may be useful; this delays the breakdown of L-dopa and is given as a single daily dose starting with 5 mg. Some additional response may be obtained by using the dopamine agonist, bromocriptine, which acts directly on dopaminergic receptors. The initial dose is 2.5 mg b.d. and this may be increased slowly to 40–60 mg a day according to response. Marked postural hypotension occasionally occurs after the initial dose so that a test dose of 1.75 mg given in the evening is recommended. When these two drugs are used it is usually necessary to reduce the dose of L-dopa. The antiviral agent amantadine is also beneficial in Parkinsonism. The dose is 100 mg b.d. Many patients find that the beneficial effect is short lived.

Physiotherapy can often result in considerable improvement in the performance of patients with Parkinson's disease and when combined with help and advice from occupational therapists, patients are often able to continue to lead an independent existence where this might otherwise not be possible.

Stereotactic Thalamotomy. This operation, once commonly performed, is now rarely necessary in view of the response of Parkinson's disease to L-dopa. However, it remains suitable for younger patients who have a unilateral tremor and little in the way of bradykinesia and rigidity and in whom there are no general medical contraindications to surgery, such as hypertension. Surgery does not affect the subsequent response to L-dopa.

Other Causes of the Parkinsonian Syndrome

In the 1920's there was a pandemic of encephalitis thought to be of viral origin although a virus was never isolated (encephalitis lethargica). This resulted in a very large number of patients with a Parkinsonian syndrome, post-encephalitic Parkinsonism. These patients had all the characteristic features of Parkinson's disease but in addition there was usually evidence of cortical damage from the encephalitis and this seems to make these patients peculiarly susceptible to L-dopa preparations, so that very small doses cause unacceptable mental confusion. They were also subject to oculogyric crises. Since no authenticated cases of this encephalitis have occurred since the 1920's, the condition is becoming extremely rare.

Vascular disease does not cause a true Parkinsonian syndrome, but extrapyramidal signs may occur in patients with vascular disease, often associated with pseudobulbar palsy.

CHOREA

Choreiform movements are involuntary movements which resemble part of a coordinated intended movement and patients may be able to disguise the fact that movement is involuntary.

(1) **Sydenham's Chorea** (see p. 175). This occurs in children in association with acute rheumatism. It is usually a benign condition and most patients recover within a few weeks.

(2) **Chorea Gravidarum.** A similar clinical picture may occur during pregnancy and some patients develop chorea on the contraceptive pill.

(3) **Chorea Following Stroke.** Choreiform movements may occur after cerebrovascular lesions, particularly in the elderly. There may be an obvious association with a stroke or the chorea may develop without such an obvious cause. The onset is sudden and unilateral. The chorea may persist but does not progress.

(4) **Huntington's Chorea.** This condition is inherited as an autosomal dominant and is characterised by chorea and progressing dementia. The new mutation rate is very low so that a positive family history is usually obtainable. Although evidence of the disease may appear at any age it is most common in middle age and usually after the reproductive period, so that patients often have children and grandchildren before the diagnosis is made. In children it may present with widespread rigidity mimicking an extrapyramidal disorder (rigid Huntington's).

The condition may present with either involuntary movements or with dementia, but the former is more common. If the family history is known to the patient, the depression associated with the development of involuntary movements is often mistaken for dementia. The combination of involuntary movement and dementia is strongly suggestive of this condition. The diagnosis is confirmed by obtaining a positive family history. There are no specific investigations but the CT scan or pneumoencephalography shows a characteristic dilatation of the lateral ventricles due to atrophy of the caudate nuclei. Tetrabenazine may be effective in reducing the abnormal movements.

Torsion Dystonia

This is a disorder of the basal ganglia of unknown aetiology. The onset is usually gradual, starting at any age, and the characteristic features are strong intermittent uncontrollable contractions of voluntary muscle. There is a wide spectrum of presentation from dystonia musculorum deformans presenting in childhood and resulting in considerable deformity over the years, to fragmentary forms, including spasmodic torticollis and writer's cramp. There is no effective treatment but anticholinergic drugs may be of some benefit.

THE CEREBELLUM

The cerebellar hemispheres are concerned with coordination of movement on the same side of the body. Coordination depends on the smooth contraction of one group of muscles (agonists), the equally smooth relaxation of the opposing muscles (antagonists) and the maintained contraction of other muscles to support the part of the body concerned. The central part of the cerebellum, the vermis, is concerned with equilibrium and maintains balance when the centre of gravity changes.

Signs of Cerebellar Disease

(1) *Nystagmus.* (see p. 331).
(2) *Dysarthria.* The coordination of the muscles of speech are affected (see dysarthria).
(3) *Intention Tremor.* Attempts at fine coordinated movement produce a tremor, which is worse at the completion of the movement and may be demonstrated by the finger/nose test and the heel/knee/shin test. Occasionally there may be a flapping tremor at rest. A cerebellar tremor on the same side as pyramidal tract involvement indicates a contralateral lesion between the red nucleus and the thalamus.
(4) *Disequilibrium.* This is caused by a lesion of the vermis or bilateral hemisphere disease. There may be a marked disturbance of gait without any evidence of ataxia or other physical signs.

Lesions of the Cerebellum and its Connections

The cerebellar pathways are frequently affected in disseminated sclerosis. Space-occupying lesions of the posterior fossa usually cause some cerebellar signs and there may also be involvement of the brain stem. The volume of the posterior fossa is relatively small, so that small lesions may obstruct CSF pathways and produce hydrocephalus.

The patients presenting with the slow insidious onset of a cerebellar syndrome may have a cerebellar degeneration. Usually no cause is found, but it may be a complication of myxoedema, alcoholism, some drugs (e.g. phenytoin) and as a non-metastatic manifestation of an occult neoplasm.

SPINAL CORD

The spinal cord is a segmental structure. The location of a lesion within the cord can be determined by finding the highest affected segment. This level may be motor, sensory or reflex. A motor level would give lower motor neurone signs at the affected segment due to involvement of the anterior horn cells and the emerging motor root, and upper motor neurone signs below this on the same side. A sensory level would give loss of all forms of sensation at the affected level due to involvement of the dorsal root and its entry zone, impairment of pain and temperature sense below this level on the opposite side due to involvement of the crossed spinothalamic tract and impairment of light touch and joint position sense on the same side due to involvement of the uncrossed posterior columns. A reflex level is the absence of a reflex at the level of a lesion due to interruption of the reflex arc and brisk reflexes below this on the same side with an extensor plantar response due to involvement of the pyramidal tract.

Hemisection of the cord would, therefore, produce lower motor neurone weakness, absent reflex and impairment of all forms of sensation at the level of the lesion on the same side. Below this level there would be ipsilateral pyramidal tract signs with brisk reflexes and impairment of touch and proprioception, while on the contralateral side there would be impairment of pain and temperature appreciation. This is the *Brown–Séquard syndrome* and is seldom seen in its complete form. Partial forms due to compression are quite common and usually associated with bilateral pyramidal involvement, often asymmetrical.

The causes of focal disease of the spinal cord may be conveniently divided into *extradural, intradural, extramedullary* and *intramedullary*. The commonest extradural cause is prolapse of an intervertebral disc in the cervical region. Cord compression occurs earlier in patients with congenital narrowing of the cervical canal and hypertrophy of the ligamentum flavum posteriorly may also narrow the canal. Other causes include vertebral collapse due to osteoporosis or metastases, myeloma, tuberculosis (Pott's disease) and subluxation.

Intrathecal extramedullary lesions include meningitis and arachnoiditis, meningioma and neurofibroma.

Intramedullary lesions include glioma, ependymoma, transverse myelitis, which may be caused by multiple sclerosis, radiation myelitis, vascular lesions (thrombosis of the anterior spinal artery) and herpes zoster.

Management. Any patient developing a focal lesion of the spinal cord must be assumed to have cord compression until proved otherwise. The patient should be investigated as a matter of urgency. Plain X-rays should be followed by myelography and this is preferably carried out in a neurosurgical unit so that decompression can follow the investigation immediately if a compressive lesion is found. In many patients a good recovery will occur if surgery is performed without delay.

SYRINGOBULBIA, SYRINGOMYELIA AND HYDROMYELIA

The majority of patients with syringomyelia have a developmental abnormality in the region of the foramen magnum with prolapse of the cerebellar tonsils through the foramen magnum (tonsillar ectopia), which obstructs the normal outflow of CSF from the fourth ventricle. This may be associated with adhesions which further impede the flow of CSF. The upper end of the central canal of the cord is kept patent by the normal pulse pressure waves in the ventricular system, and dilates. Eventually, the ependymal lining of the central canal ruptures and there is an extravasation of CSF into the surrounding central grey matter. These outpouchings dissect up and down to produce the typical syrinx seen on cross-section which may not obviously show a connection with the central canal. The first symptoms and signs are nearly always in the cervical cord and the condition may remain localised, but the whole cord may become affected. Rarely a syrinx will develop as a result of trauma to the cord and dissection occurs up or down from the level of the lesion.

The early involvement of the central grey matter interrupting the decussating pain and temperature fibres and the reflex arc determines the cardinal signs of syringomyelia, which are:

(1) Dissociated cutaneous sensory loss: loss of pain and temperature sensation with preservation of touch.
(2) Loss of reflexes.

As the lesion becomes more extensive, so there may be involvement of the anterior horn cells with wasting of the small hand muscles, involvement of the pyramidal tracts with development of upper motor neurone signs in the legs, involvement of Clarke's column with a Horner's syndrome and finally, in the late stages, involvement of the posterior columns. Syringomyelia is probably the commonest cause of Charcot joints in the upper limbs; this is a painless arthropathy due to loss of pain appreciation and results in gross disorganisation of joints. Despite this, pain is not an uncommon symptom in syringomyelia.

Upward dissection of a syrinx may extend into the medulla (syringobulbia) causing a bulbar palsy (see p. 340).

Treatment. If tonsillar ectopia can be confirmed by myelography, and there is no evidence of adhesions, the treatment of choice is decompression by enlargement of the foramen magum and a laminectomy of C1 and 2. The presence of adhesions is a contraindication to this procedure. Occasionally a syrinx may be drained by amputation of the filum terminale, allowing free drainage from below, or by a shunt.

SPINAL ROOT AND PERIPHERAL NERVE LESIONS

Lesions at different levels in the lower motor neurone produce characteristic patterns of neurological deficit.

The **motor distribution** of peripheral nerves is very constant, so that a lesion of one nerve causes weakness in a particular and specific combination of muscles. The level of the lesion can be predicted from the muscles affected and a knowledge of the levels of which the main branches arise; these may, of course, be affected without involvement of the main trunk. The motor distribution of roots is much less specific and most muscles receive some contribution from several roots; it is, however, important to know the principal contribution.

The **cutaneous distribution** of peripheral nerves is also fairly specific, although there is some variability and overlap. The cutaneous distribution of roots is extremely variable and there is considerable overlap. The autonomous area for a single root may be so small that a complete lesion may not cause any detectable sensory loss; whereas the rash of herpes zoster, which occurs wherever there is any contribution from the affected root, involves a relatively large area.

Principal 'Root Values' of Selected Muscles in the Arms and Legs

Root	*Muscle*	*Reflex*
C5	Deltoid	+
C5/6	Biceps	+
C6	Brachioradialis	+
	Extensor carpi radialis	
C7	Triceps	+
	Extensor digitorum	+
C8	The finger flexors	+
T1	The small hand muscles	
L1/2	Iliopsoas	
L2/3	Adductors	+
L3/4	Quadriceps	+
L4	Tibialis anterior	
L4/5	Tibialis posterior	
L5	Extensor hallucis longus	
L5/S1	Peronei	
S1	Gastrocnemius and soleus	+

ROOT LESIONS

Intravertebral Disc Prolapse and Osteophytes

A nerve root may be affected in the spinal canal by a lateral disc protrusion or as it enters the exit foramina by osteophytes and these are usually associated with chronic disc degeneration and a narrow disc space. These lesions occur at sites of greatest spinal mobility and are, therefore, frequently found in midcervical and lower lumbar regions. Thoracic disc prolapse is a rare cause of spinal cord compression and does not occur without plain X-ray changes. In the cervical spine the root emerges above the vertebral body of the same number and is affected by disc prolapse at the same level. For example, the C7 root is affected by the C6/7 disc. Since there are eight cervical roots and only seven cervical vertebrae, this relationship changes below C7 and in the thoracic and lumbar spine the root emerges below the corresponding vertebral body. In the lumbar spine a root is affected by the disc at one level above its exit. For example, the L5 root is affected by disc protrusion between L4 and L5, although it emerges between L5 and S1.

Disc herniation causing root compression may occur at any age and usually presents acutely with pain, which may be severe. The pain of a root lesion is felt in the myotome and not in the dermatome, so that the pain of a C7 root lesion is felt in triceps and in the forearm extensors and sometimes in pectoralis major. Numbness and dysaesthesia is felt in the dermatome. Depression or loss of a reflex at the appropriate level is an early sign in root lesions.

Radiography of the spine may show narrow disc spaces, osteophytes, subluxation or vertebral collapse, though the plain X-ray changes often do not accord with clinical evaluation or with the level of maximal compression as determined by *myelography*. In younger patients with acute disc prolapse, X-rays are usually normal. Myelography is only indicated if the diagnosis is in doubt or if surgery is contemplated. Surgery is indicated for pain or increasing neurological deficit. Painless stable deficit seldom improves after surgery.

Herpes Zoster (Shingles)

This may affect any root. Pain in the affected dermatome usually precedes the development of a rash by several days. The diagnosis is easy once the characteristic vesicular rash appears. The rash usually lasts a week or so and often leaves small permanent scars.

The cutaneous eruptions should be painted with idoxuridine but there is little merit in doing this after the first two or three days. Sufficient analgesia should be given to control the pain in the acute stage, since this may reduce the risk of continued pain afterwards.

Some patients suffer continued pain after the rash has resolved (*post-herpetic neuralgia*) and this is remarkably resistant to treatment. The best results at the moment are obtained from the use of a low-voltage electrical cutaneous stimulator.

Tumours affecting the cervical roots are rare. Neurofibromata (see p. 388) may occur and produce a characteristic enlargement of the foramina on plain X-rays.

Trauma. Cervical roots may be avulsed from the spinal cord by traction and the commonest cause of this is motor-cycle accidents. If the roots are completely avulsed there is a characteristic myelographic appearance and recovery does not occur. If continuity of the roots is preserved, some recovery is possible.

PLEXUS LESIONS

The Brachial Plexus

Lesions of the upper part of the brachial plexus (C5, C6 and the upper trunk) are usually traumatic.

(1) **Ruck sack palsy** is due to traction on the upper trunk from heavy and badly adjusted back packs. The nerves remain in continuity and recovery is usually complete.

(2) Any part of the plexus may be damaged by **trauma**. Lesions of the lower part of the plexus (C8, T1 and the lower trunk) are less often traumatic and usually due to malignant infiltration or to the thoracic outlet syndrome.

(3) **Malignant infiltration** may occur with apical lung carcinoma (*Pancoast's tumour*) or to local metastatic spread from mammary carcinoma. A slowly progressive weakness develops in the small hand muscles (T1) and spreads to involve the finger flexors (C8). There is often pain and sensory loss in the medial aspect of the forearm (T1). *Horner's syndrome* commonly occurs due to involvement of the cervical sympathetic ganglia.

(4) **Thoracic outlet syndrome.** The lower trunk of the brachial plexus may be angulated over a cervical rib, together with the subclavian artery. Patients may present with a neurological deficit or with vascular symptoms or a combination. Neurological signs and symptoms predominate with the small rudimentary ribs which continue into a fibrous band and vascular features predominate in the large well-formed bony cervical ribs.

Cervical ribs are quite common and only rarely cause symptoms. Neurological features commonly present in young women with the insidious onset of wasting and weakness of the small hand muscles, often accompanied by pain; a bruit may be heard over the subclavian artery. Other causes of a thoracic outlet syndrome include compression of the neurovascular bundle between scalenus anterior and the first rib.

(5) **Neuralgic amyotrophy (brachial neuralgia)** is an inflammatory neuropathy principally affecting branches of the brachial plexus. A characteristic feature is the dense involvement of some muscles and sparing of others within the same myotome. It commonly occurs in young adults and pain is usually a prominent feature at onset. A few days later weakness develops and later there may be quite marked wasting. The pain usually subsides in a week or so, but the weakness may persist for months, often with incomplete recovery, and some wasting may be permanent.

Lumbosacral Plexus

Malignant infiltration is by far the commonest cause, often due to spread from carcinoma of the cervix or uterus. It may also occur in the lymphomas. A radiculogram may be necessary to distinguish these conditions from intraspinal lesions. Lesions of the lumbosacral plexus are best demonstrated by a whole-body CT scan.

PERIPHERAL NERVE LESIONS

A *mononeuropathy* is a lesion of a single peripheral nerve. *Mononeuritis multiplex* is involvement of more than one peripheral nerve and this is often associated with some systemic disorder: causes include diabetes, polyarteritis nodosa, systemic lupus erythematosus and rheumatoid arthritis. *Polyneuropathy* (see p. 362) is symmetrical involvement of all peripheral nerves.

Peripheral nerves may be damaged by external compression or by internal entrapment. Other causes include trauma, fractures, operations, penetrating injuries and injections.

Compression usually occurs where a nerve lies between skin and bone, unprotected by soft tissue, for example, the ulnar nerve at the elbow and the common peroneal nerve at the head of the fibula. This anatomical arrangement means that some nerves are particularly prone to damage at certain sites, particularly if pressure is maintained for long periods without change in posture.

Entrapment usually occurs where a nerve passes through a fascial plane or down a fibro-osseous funnel. For example the *median nerve* in the *carpal tunnel* and the *lateral cutaneous nerve of the thigh* at the *inguinal ligament*.

Electromyography and nerve conduction studies may be helpful in localising the precise site of the lesion and quantify the severity of the lesion.

Peripheral Nerve Lesions in the Upper Limb

The Median Nerve

The Carpal Tunnel Syndrome. This is the commonest mononeuropathy and is due to compression of the median nerve as it passes through the carpal tunnel in the flexor retinaculum. The tunnel may be narrowed by rheumatoid arthritis, myxoedema, acromegaly, oedema, pregnancy and obesity. It is much more common in women and usually affects the dominant hand first. Patients complain of pain and paraesthesia which may wake them at night and they may shake the hand out of bed to obtain relief. Symptoms are brought on or aggravated by use, particularly activities which require gripping. In the early stages there may be no detectable deficit but, as the condition progresses, weakness of abductor pollicis brevis may develop with difficulty in fine manipulation. The earliest sensory deficit is usually widening of two point discrimination.

Abnormal signs are strictly confined to median nerve territory, but symptoms may occur in all digits and there may also be pain in the arm.

Treatment. Splinting, diuretics and local steroid injections may relieve the symptoms and may be the only treatment necessary to self-limiting conditions, such as pregnancy. In more severe cases, particularly if there is sensory loss or progressive weakness, surgical decompression is necessary. Pain and intermittent symptoms are relieved immediately, and the continuous symptoms may resolve with time but wasting of abductor pollicis brevis may never recover.

Anterior Interosseous Palsy. A lesion of the anterior interosseous nerve produces weakness of the flexor pollicis longus, flexor digitorum profundus 1 and 2 and pronator quadratus. There is no sensory loss. Spontaneous recovery usually occurs but the nerve should be explored if recovery is delayed beyond three months.

The Ulnar Nerve

Lesions of the ulnar nerve occur at four sites, behind the medial epicondyle, in the cubital tunnel, at the wrist and in the hand.

At the elbow, a classic site for a compressive lesion. Damage occurs if the groove is shallow and particularly if there has been damage to the elbow joint with a previous fracture. Sometimes the nerve may override the medial epicondyle in full flexion. These patients present with a slowly progressive deficit which may be predominantly motor or sensory. The nerve is usually thickened. Involvement of the ulnar innervated long flexors (flexors digitorum profundus 3 and 4) is rather variable; if it is affected, the lesion must be at the elbow.

In mild cases it may be sufficient to advise against full elbow flexion and leaning on the elbow. In more severe cases, or where the lesion is clearly progressing, it may be necessary to transpose the nerve anteriorly.

The cubital tunnel syndrome is an entrapment neuropathy of the ulnar nerve in the forearm flexor group. Clinically it is similar to the lesion at the elbow.

At the wrist the nerve may be compressed by a ganglion.

In the hand the deep motor branch may be compressed against the pisiform and the hamate if the hand is used as a mallet, the sensory branches are always spared and the motor supply to the hypothenar eminence may also be spared or less affected than the other ulnar innervated small hand muscles.

Radial Nerve

The commonest sites for radial nerve lesions are in the arm and in the extensor muscles affecting the posterior interosseous branch.

Lesions Above the Elbow. Crutch palsy is due to compression of the radial nerve above the spiral groove by long crutches when the weight is taken in the axilla.

Saturday-night palsy is due to compression of the radial nerve in the upper part of the arm and is caused by resting the arm against a sharp edge for a prolonged period; triceps is usually spared.

Both these lesions produce weakness of brachioradialis, wrist and finger drop and weakness of the long thumb extensors and abductor. There may be dysaesthesia in the distribution of the superficial radial nerve.

Posterior interosseous palsy is caused by entrapment of the posterior interosseous nerve in the forearm extensor group. It presents with weakness of finger and thumb extension but the radial wrist extensor and brachioradialis is spared and there is no sensory loss. These lesions usually do not recover spontaneously and should be explored.

Peripheral Nerve Lesions in the Lower Limb

The lateral cutaneous nerve of the thigh (*meralgia paraesthetica*) may be trapped under the lateral end of the inguinal ligament. Patients complain of an area of pain and paraesthesia with numbness on the lateral aspect of the thigh just above the knee. The area never extends across the midline anteriorly or below the knee. It is more likely to occur in obese, middle-aged patients and weight reduction may be the only treatment necessary. Local steroid injections are sometimes effective; decompression is occasionally required.

Femoral Neuropathy. A localised lesion of the femoral nerve may occur in diabetes (diabetic amyotrophy). Apparently spontaneous haematomas may also affect the femoral nerve and this occurs in patients with bleeding diathesis or in patients who are on anticoagulant treatment.

Sciatic Nerve Lesions

The sciatic nerve may be damaged by apparently spontaneous haematomas and misplaced injections.

Common Peroneal Palsy. The common peroneal nerve is relatively unprotected as it traverses the lateral aspect of the head of the fibula and may be compressed at this site. Patients present with a painless foot drop and may complain of numbness or paraesthesia on the lateral aspect of the foot. Examination shows weakness of dorsiflexion and eversion of the foot and weakness of extensor hallucus longus. Inversion and plantar flexion are normal and the ankle jerk is preserved. In the majority of patients, where the lesion is due to simple compression, recovery occurs within a few weeks. If the weakness progresses or fails to resolve in a month or two or if there is any obvious local lesion, surgical exploration may be required.

POLYNEUROPATHY

Polyneuritis or polyneuropathy is the term used to describe symmetrical involvement of all the peripheral nerves. The longest nerves are affected first so that signs and symptoms start in the feet and progress proximally, later involving the hands. The majority of patients have both motor and sensory signs and symptoms but some neuropathies are predominantly motor and others predominantly sensory.

Clinical Features. The earliest symptoms are usually persistent tingling and numbness of the hands and feet, accompanied by peripheral weakness. The signs accord with the symptoms with uniform distal weakness, absent reflexes and a characteristic 'glove-and-stocking' sensory impairment. In some patients the weakness is more proximal. Pathologically there are two main groups, the demyelinating neuropathies and the axonal neuropathies.

Demyelination of peripheral nerves results in slowing of conduction velocity and this is the striking feature of *demyelinating neuropathies.* Causes include diabetes, the Guillain–Barré syndrome, carcinomatous neuropathy, hypertrophic neuropathy, metachromatic leucodystrophy and diphtheria.

The Axonal Neuropathies. Nerve conduction velocity may be relatively preserved in the early stages of an axonal neuropathy due to normal conduction in unaffected fibres. Causes include alcoholism, porphyria, isoniazid, vincristine and thalidomide.

This differentiation is only valid in the early stages and eventually both myelin and axons are affected. This mixed pattern is commonly seen in diabetes and lead poisoning.

ACUTE INFECTIVE POLYNEURITIS (The Guillain–Barré–Syndrome)

This predominantly motor demyelinating neuropathy usually follows an upper respiratory tract infection by a week or so. The infection may be due to a wide range of organisms, including glandular fever, cytomegalovirus infection and mycoplasma infection. It may occur in either sex and at any age. It develops rapidly from onset, reaching its maximum within a few days. The paralysis may affect all four limbs and endanger respiration. Patients with progressive symptoms should be transferred immediately to a centre where artificial ventilation is available. Facial weakness occurs in most patients but any of the cranial nerves may be involved. There may be a retention of urine and, if the patient requires ventilation, it is usually convenient to catheterise the bladder.

It is unlikely that this is a single disease entity, but the diagnosis can be made on clinical grounds and supported by the demonstration of marked slowing of peripheral nerve conduction. CSF analysis shows characteristic changes with a markedly elevated CSF protein due to involvement of the spinal roots with a normal cell count. Sometimes the CSF pressure is high enough to produce papilloedema. Even in severe cases, it is not usually necessary to ventilate the patient for more than two or three weeks. With modern methods of artificial ventilation there is no reason why patients should not survive this critical period. Recovery can be quite prolonged, extending from six months to two years, but this is not incompatible with a complete restoration of function. Nerve conduction abnormalities usually persist. Temporary relapses may punctuate return to activity.

Treatment. Patients still progressing in the early stages must be transferred immediately to a unit where ventilation is available. Steroids have been the standard treatment of this condition for many years, but it is now known that they are of no benefit and there is some evidence that they may actually retard progress. However, they do seem to be of value in the chronic relapsing form of this disease.

INFECTIONS

Infections of the nervous system may be divided into acute and chronic infections of the meninges (meningitis) and of the brain parenchyma (encephalitis) and further divided into the bacterial or pyogenic infections, including fungal infections, and the viral infections.

ACUTE PYOGENIC MENINGITIS

Bacteria may reach the meninges and CSF via the blood stream consequent upon a bacteraemia, by direct spread from infected air sinuses and the middle ear or following rupture of a cerebral abscess into the CSF. Responsible organisms include meningococci, staphylococci, streptococci, pneumococci, *Haemophilus influenzae*, *E. coli* and cryptococci. A wide range of other organisms may cause meningitis, in patients on steroids or immunosuppressive therapy. The clinical features of acute meningitis are similar whatever the causative organism. The onset is usually acute with fever, headache and vomiting. Epilepsy is common in children but relatively rare in adults. Stupor or coma may occur in severe cases. The physical signs may be confined to neck stiffness and a positive Kernig's sign.

Management. The clinical diagnosis should be confirmed as soon as possible by examination of the CSF. There may be purulent fluid under pressure and analysis shows large numbers of polymorphs, a raised protein and a greatly reduced sugar. The responsible organism may be seen by direct stain and can usually be cultured. If the organism is identified from the smear the treatment is:

Meningococcal Meningitis. Although sulphadiazine is effective and penetrates well into the CSF, resistant strains are becoming common, therefore treatment should be started with benzylpenicillin 4.0 mega units given 4-hourly as an intravenous bolus which produces an adequate concentration in the CSF. If the organism is sensitive to sulphonamides, sulphadiazine 1.0 g 4-hourly by mouth can be added to the regime. Chloramphenicol is satisfactory for patients who are allergic to penicillin.

Pneumococcal Meningitis. Benzylpenicillin 4.0 mega units 4-hourly by intravenous bolus is the drug of choice, and treatment should be continued for two weeks. For patients who are allergic to penicillin, erythromycin 1.0 g IV 6-hourly has proved successful.

Haemophilus Influenzal Meningitis. Chloramphenicol in doses of 1.0 g given every 6 hours is the preferred treatment and may be combined with ampicillin 50 mg/kg IV 6-hourly.

If no organism is seen, the following should be given until the results of culture are available:

Benzylpenicillin 4.0 mega units IV 4-hourly +
Sulphadiazine 1.0 g 4-hourly +
Chloramphenicol 20 mg/kg IM 6-hourly.

Meningitis is one manifestation of a meningococcal septicaemia. Patients may show petechial, purpuric or maculopapular rashes; there is a marked polymorphonuclear leucocytosis and the organism may be cultured from the blood in the early stages. Conjunctivitis, pericarditis and arthritis may occur. Involvement of the adrenal glands may cause circulatory collapse (*Friderichsen–Waterhouse syndrome*).

CHRONIC MENINGITIS

Many organisms can cause a subacute or chronic meningitis and this may also be the consequence of inadequate treatment of organisms usually associated with acute meningitis. Tuberculosis, syphilis and torula are important causes.

Tuberculous Meningitis

In most patients this is the consequence of rupture of a small tuberculous brain abscess, which in turn is the result of blood-borne infection. A chronic granulomatous basal meningitis develops. Most patients have evidence of tuberculosis elsehwere, usually in the lung. Dissemination may occur spontaneously or the organism may be released by the use of systemic steroids. The onset is insidious, often with several weeks of vague ill health, sometimes with confusional episodes. Because of this, the diagnosis is often delayed. Eventually, the patient develops headache, often with vomiting, convulsions may occur and the patient becomes drowsy or even delirious. There is usually a low-grade fever. Papilloedema is a late development but choroidal tubercles may be seen quite early in the course of the illness. Cranial nerve palsies are quite common.

Lumbar puncture shows CSF under increased pressure; it is usually clear initially but on standing develops a fine 'cobweb clot'. Analysis shows a lymphocytosis with increased protein and a reduced sugar level. In the more acute forms there may be an initial polymorphonuclear leucocytosis, but this changes to a predominant lymphocytosis. A low CSF chloride, once thought to be characteristic of this condition, is a measure of the amount of vomiting. The tubercle bacilli may be found by direct staining and this, of course, confirms the diagnosis; but in the majority of cases the organism is not seen and culture may not be positive for several weeks, which often results in further delay in diagnosis and treatment.

It is usually necessary, therefore, to start treatment on the basis of a high index of clinical suspicion, rather than on a confirmed diagnosis.

Treatment. The difficulty of antibiotic treatment is the poor penetration of the most suitable agents into the CSF. Isoniazid in doses of 10 mg/kg/day, combined with pyridoxine 10 mg daily to avoid polyneuritis, is the most useful drug. This may be combined with streptomycin 1.0 g daily IM and rifampicin 12 mg/kg/day orally. In addition pyrazinamide 30 mg/kg (max 2.5 g) should be given orally daily for the first month of treatment. It penetrates well into the CSF but is hepatotoxic. Betamethasone 2.0 g q.i.d. is often given for the first few weeks of treatment to minimise reactive fibrosis in the meninges but its usefulness is unproven.

Torula Meningitis (Cryptococcus Neoformans)

Torula histolytica, a fungus, may cause a chronic meningitis, which may escape detection unless special stains are requested. Amphotericin B and 5-fluocytosine are effective treaments.

Sarcoidosis (p. 305), **syphilis** (p. 733) and **carcinoma** may all cause a chronic basal meningitis.

ACUTE VIRAL MENINGITIS (LYMPHOCYTIC MENINGITIS)

Viral infections are seldom confined to the meninges, hence the term meningoencephalitis. A very wide range of organisms may cause this clinical picture, including mumps, glandular fever, some Coxsackie and echo viruses, poliomyelitis and the virus of acute lymphocytic choriomeningitis. The clinical picture is similar with acute or subacute onset of meningitis. In the early stages CSF analysis shows both polymorphs and lymphocytes but, after a few days, it becomes purely lymphocytic and this is associated with a normal glucose level. There may be diagnostic difficulty in distinguishing this from tuberculous meningitis, when a tubercle has not been found in the CSF. The CSF sugar is not a reliable distinguishing feature. There may be other signs which help with the diagnosis, such as pharyngitis and lymphadenopathy in glandular fever and swelling of the salivary glands with mumps. There is no specific treatment, but the prognosis is good with the majority of patients making a complete recovery.

PYOGENIC ENCEPHALITIS (Brain Abscess)

Intracranial abscess may be extradural and secondary to osteitis of the skull or intracerebral, usually as a result of blood-borne infection. Subdural and subarachnoid abscesses are rare. Cerebral abscess due to spread of infection from middle ear disease was once common, but with effective early control of this condition, cerebral abscess is now a rare complication.

A cerebral abscess starts as a localised area of cerebritis, which later breaks down with pus formation. An encapsulated abscess then develops and may go on to act as a progressive space-occupying lesion.

Causes include spread from middle-ear disease, septicaemia, particularly in patients on steroids and immunosuppressive drugs, acute infective endocarditis and fractures of the skull. If the intracranial abscess is secondary to infection elsewhere, this is usually in the lungs. The onset may be acute or chronic, there is often evidence of infection elsewhere, there may be focal signs, there is usually headache and fever and there may be papilloedema. Most patients have a leucocytosis and the organism may be cultured from the blood. Patients may rapidly deteriorate and investigation and treatment is, therefore, a matter of some urgency. Lumbar puncture should be avoided because of the risk of herniation. The EEG is always abnormal and usually shows high amplitude slow activity over the abscess. Computerised tomography is the definitive investigation. The treatment is neurosurgical.

ACUTE VIRAL ENCEPHALITIS

A wide range of both DNA and RNA viruses may cause encephalitis. The onset may be acute or subacute with confusion, drowsiness, hallucinations and abnormal movements suggesting basal ganglia involvement. The EEG is always abnormal. The CSF may be either normal or show a lymphocytosis. The causative agent is identified by a rising antibody titre.

Encephalitis Lethargica

This was almost certainly viral in origin, although no organism was ever isolated. It was responsible for a pandemic between 1915 and 1925. It took the form of an acute encephalitic illness and was followed in a large number of patients by post-encephalitic Parkinsonism. No definite cases have occurred since then.

Herpes Simplex Encephalitis

Herpes simplex may cause an acute necrotising encephalitis which usually starts in one temporal lobe and a few days later affects the other temporal lobe. Epilepsy may be a presenting feature. The patient is usually seriously ill within a few days. The EEG is abnormal in the early stages and between the 2nd and the 12th day may show periodic complexes with relative attenuation of activity between; in severe cases this precedes marked flattening of the record on that side. Changes in the other temporal lobe follow the first affected side by a few days. CT scan shows low-density areas in the temporal lobe, indicative of oedema. The diagnosis can be confirmed by biopsy and the virus identified by immunofluorescence, electron microscopy and culture and also by the demonstration of a rising antibody titre, although this takes longer. Treatment should be started as soon as possible with the antiviral agent acyclovir and it may also be necessary to give betamethasone to reduce cerebral oedema. It was once thought that herpes simplex encephalitis was uniformly fatal, but it is now clear that milder causes do occur and the course of the illness may be modified by treatment. Patients are often left with a dense memory defect and dysphasia.

Poliomyelitis

The development of polio vaccines has dramatically altered the incidence of this disease, but outbreaks still occur from time to time. The portal of entry is thought to be the nasopharynx and there is an incubation period of about two weeks. In epidemics there is evidence that many patients are infected and have only a mild 'flu-like' illness; only a small proportion of patients develop paralysis, which usually progresses rapidly over a few days. The extent and the degree of the paralysis are extremely variable. The commonest cause of death is from respiratory paralysis, either as a consequence of bulbar nuclei involvement or from paralysis of the muscles of respiration. The mortality decreased considerably with the introduction of better methods of artificial respiration. Some recovery usually occurs but this is often incomplete.

Rabies (See p. 698)

Infection by the rabies virus may follow the bite of an infected animal because the virus is found in large quantities in the saliva and a bite is an effective innoculation. The disease is endemic in many parts of the world, including most of the continent of Europe. Although widespread among wild life, most cases of human infection are due to dog bites. The virus travels to the brain along nerve trunks, so that the incubation period depends on the distance from the bite to the brain, usually between one and two months. An early symptom is pharyngeal spasm brought on by drinking and this seems to lead to marked hydrophobia. The disease is invariably fatal. No cases of infection between human contacts have been reported.

CHRONIC VIRAL ENCEPHALOPATHIES

Subacute Sclerosing Panencephalitis

This disease is now known to be due to the measles virus and may develop months or even years after an attack of measles. It is slowly progressive over months or years and is nearly always fatal. Initially, there are signs of intellectual deterioration, accompanied by myoclonic jerks and occasionally by fits. The patient gradually becomes more demented. The EEG may show a repetitive burst suppression pattern. The diagnosis can be confirmed by finding an elevated measles antibody titre in the CSF.

Progressive Multifocal Leucoencephalopathy

This is an opportunistic viral encephalopathy which occurs in patients whose immunological competence is impaired. Associated conditions include the reticuloses and sarcoidosis. The infection causes foci of demyelination in the white matter of the brain. The clinical course is one of progression over months and the disease is usually fatal. Occasionally, patients survive for some years. The CT scan shows a characteristic appearance and the diagnosis can be confirmed by cerebral biopsy. Antiviral agents may be of value if given early.

Jakob-Creutzfeldt Disease (Subacute Spongiform Encephalopathy)

This is due to a slow virus whose transmissability has been demonstrated in humans. The incubation period is several years. Patients present with a rapidly developing dementia, associated with extrapyramidal features and myoclonus. The EEG is abnormal and may show a burst-suppression pattern. The condition is invariably fatal, usually within six months.

NEUROSYPHILIS (see p. 733)

The nervous system is involved in *secondary syphilis*. Invasion of the meninges by the spirochaete produces the symptoms of meningitis. Examination may show papilloedema and neck stiffness. These symptoms resolve, together with the other features of secondary syphilis, and there may be no further clinical manifestation. Less than 10 % of patients later develop tertiary neurosyphilis and this may follow the original infection by many years.

Tertiary neurosyphilis classically presents as one of three clinical syndromes; meningovascular syphilis, tabes dorsalis or general paralysis of the insane (GPI). In addition there may be gumma formation and optic atrophy. These typical and well-known presentations are relatively rare now and this may be because of the widespread use of penicillin. It is now more common to find positive serological tests for syphilis in patients with a wide variety of neurological signs and symptoms which are not immediately suggestive of this disease. It is important to carry out these tests in all patients with otherwise unexplained central nervous system disease, particularly as it is treatable.

Meningovascular Syphilis

This is due to an endarteritis affecting meningeal vessels and cerebral vessels. It may present as a basal granulomatous meningitis with cranial nerve palsies and obstruction to CSF pathways. Local syphilitic granulomas (gumma) may present as space-occupying lesions either in the subarachnoid space or in the brain itself.

Meningovascular syphilis affecting the spinal cord can cause a transverse myelitis. The CSF is abnormal with a raised protein and an increased immunoglobulin fraction, lymphocytosis and positive serological tests for syphilis.

Tabes Dorsalis

In this form of neurosyphilis there is progressive demyelination and atrophy of the posterior roots, the root entry zone and the posterior columns. The decussating pain and temperature fibres are also involved but the spinothalamic tracts do not show demyelination because they comprise second-order neurones.

The presenting symptoms include pain, paraesthesia, sensory ataxia and bladder disturbance. In more advanced cases there may be rectal incontinence, impotence, neurogenic ulcers and neuropathic joints (*Charcot joints*).

Lightning pains are common and characteristic. They occur without obvious provocation and are described as momentary sharp stabs of pain affecting one spot, as if stabbed by a knife. The affected spot is usually in the thigh, calf or ankle.

The pupils are usually small, irregular in outline and unreactive to light, but contract normally on convergence (*Argyll Robertson pupils*). Cutaneous hypoalgesia is often found in the legs and over the trunk anteriorly and down the medial aspects of both arms, as well as across the nose. The deep tendon reflexes are absent, there is loss of light touch, vibration and position sense, particularly in the legs, loss of deep pain appreciation and impairment of pain sensation, often accompanied by a prolonged delay in appreciating stimuli.

There may be trophic ulcers on the feet and neuropathic joints may develop due to loss of sensation; the shoulders, spine, hip, knees and ankles are commonly involved. There is gross disorganisation of the joint, which is nearly always painless. The CSF is usually abnormal.

General Paralysis of the Insane (GPI)

This is a chronic spirochaetal meningoencephalitis, and the spirochaete may be isolated from the brain. The presenting features are those of dementia and personality change, and epilepsy may be an early symptom. Examination shows the features of dementia, often associated with a dysarthria, tremors of the hands, lips, and tongue, a spastic paraparesis with extensor plantar responses, optic atrophy and Argyll Robertson pupils. The CSF is abnormal.

Syphilitic Optic Atrophy

This may occur as an isolated manifestation of neurosyphilis or it may accompany any of the other clinical syndromes. The funduscopic appearance may be that of a primary optic atrophy or there may be evidence of syphilitic choroidoretinitis.

Treatment. The treatment of all forms of neurosyphilis is by intramuscular procaine penicillin, 600 000 units daily for three weeks. A *Herxheimer* reaction is rare but can be prevented by covering the first few days of treatment with oral steroids.

SARCOIDOSIS (see p. 305)

Sarcoidosis may affect any part of the nervous system but the meninges and peripheral nerves are the most frequently involved. Sarcoid may cause a chronic granulomatous basal meningitis often associated with cranial nerve palsies. There may be hypothalamic, pituitary and chiasmal involvement.

Intracranial sarcoid granulomas are rare and tend to occur in the hypothalamus. The meningitis may result in obstruction of CSF pathways with raised intracranial pressure and papilloedema. There may be direct involvement of the optic nerve as well as retinal lesions and uveitis. The peripheral nervous system may also be affected with polyneuritis and there may be direct involvement of muscle (sarcoid myopathy).

Although neurological sarcoid is usually associated with evidence of sarcoidosis elsewhere, it may be confined to the nervous system. The CSF is usually abnormal, often with a markedly raised protein and a few lymphocytes.

The condition usually runs a fluctuating low-grade course and may be modified by steroids.

EPILEPSY

Epilepsy is the clinical manifestation of a paroxysmal electrochemical disturbance in the brain. The attacks are of sudden onset and brief duration. Heredity is an important factor and it may be that what is inherited is the epileptic threshold. Patients with the lowest threshold would be prone to spontaneous attacks and show the features of idiopathic (generalised, centrencephalic or major) epilepsy (see below). Those with a slightly higher threshold would only develop epilepsy if the brain was damaged by birth trauma, tumours, angiomas, head injury, infections, vascular disease, poisons and drugs, anoxia, congenital abnormalities, degenerative conditions and inborn or acquired errors of metabolism. The higher the threshold, the less likely that these conditions would cause epilepsy. Patients with the highest thresholds would be unlikely to develop epilepsy whatever the cerebral insult. This concept explains why some patients develop epilepsy and others with apparently similar conditions do not.

It is convenient to divide epilepsy in adults into two main groups, the generalised and the focal. This also applies to children, but there are many other factors to consider, partly because the maturing brain reacts differently to the adult brain and partly because children are subject to different diseases and hazards.

Focal or Symptomatic Epilepsy

The term implies that the attacks arise from a focal discharge. The attack may take any form from a brief focal event to a major convulsive seizure, and this is a continuum.

(a) *Aura.* A focal discharge may cause a brief focal disturbance usually called an aura, although it need not proceed any further. The nature of the attack depends on the location of the focus. Examples include a curious smell, usually unidentifiable and often unpleasant (uncinate attacks), a brief flash of light, a formed visual hallucination, auditory hallucination, *déjà vu* experiences, twitching of the thumb and index finger, abdominal sensations, feelings of fear and panic and numerous others. Nothing else develops and consciousness is preserved.

(b) *Epilepsia partialis continua.* Rarely a persisting focal discharge may cause a focal attack which continues for hours or days.

(c) *Aura with Jacksonian march.* A focal disturbance causing symptoms, such as twitching of the thumb and index finger, may spread across the cortex, causing twitching of the hand, face and arm in sequence. Consciousness need not be lost.

(d) *Aura with loss of consciousness.* If the disturbance becomes generalised, consciousness may be lost. This is often very brief and not associated with any convulsive features. Sudden loss of consciousness without a clinically identifiable aura does not exclude the presence of a focus, since the focal event may have been too brief to identify or have occurred in a part of the brain which is not symptomatically eloquent.

(e) *Aura, loss of consciousness and convulsive seizure.* The sequence outlined so far may finish with a major tonic–clonic seizure, often with tongue-biting and incontinence.

Treatment is effective in controlling the later stages of this progression, the initial focal event itself being the most refractory.

Generalised Epilepsy

In patients with a low epileptic threshold, the whole brain may discharge synchronously and the EEG shows a characteristic spike and wave pattern. This is not necessarily associated with loss of consciousness unless it lasts for several seconds. The clinical manifestations range from a brief absence to a major convulsive seizure. Many patients diagnosed as having *petit mal* suffer from a minor form of generalised epilepsy. The term *petit mal* should either be abandoned or reserved for the classical absence attacks of adolescents associated with three per second spike and wave in the EEG. The differentiation is important because true *petit mal* requires different medication.

Diagnosis. The diagnosis of epilepsy is made on the history alone. The account of a witness is often helpful since there are usually no abnormal signs. In developing focal lesions, such as a brain tumour, persisting signs may not appear for several years. Occasionally focal signs persist after the attack (Todd's paralysis), but this term should only be used when the signs resolve within twenty-four hours.

Investigation. In addition to a full clinical examination, all patients with epilepsy should have an EEG and, in the absence of any focal features, a lateral skull X-ray. When epilepsy develops later in life and in patients with focal features, either clinically or on the EEG further investigation may be necessary and a CT scan is the most appropriate. Serological tests for syphilis and a chest X-ray should also be done.

Treatment. The object of treatment is to control the attacks so that the patient may lead a normal life, and this can be achieved in the majority of patients.

Anticonvulsant Drugs

The biggest advance in recent years is the development of methods of measuring anticonvulsant blood levels, and this has profoundly affected the management of patients with epilepsy. The blood level cannot be predicted from the oral dose. Epilepsy can be controlled in over 80% of patients by the use of a single drug, provided the blood level is maintained in the upper part of the therapeutic range. The therapeutic range is arbitrarily derived; levels below the lower limit usually have little effect and levels above the upper limit are often associated with signs of toxicity; though it is, of course, the patient who requires treatment and not the blood level.

Drug treatment, however successful, is not a cure and patients may have to continue regular medication for many years. Since there may be no immediate consequence if a dose is missed, compliance is often poor. Medication given in one or two doses a day considerably improves compliance. Three doses a day necessitates taking tablets to school or work and is to be avoided. Dose frequency depends on the biological half-life of the drug. Drug interactions are particularly important for patients on long-term treatment and it may be necessary to advise patients accordingly. Drug combinations should not be used, since it is not possible to vary the doses independently.

Some basic data about the more commonly used drugs are given in Table 6.1.

Patients should be started on one drug in moderate dose (for example, the initial figure in Table 6.1 under 'usual daily dose range'). If the attacks are controlled, no further action is required. If attacks continue, the blood level should be measured and the dose adjusted, bearing in mind that it takes 2–3 weeks for most drug blood levels to stabilise. If attacks continue despite a blood level in the upper part of the therapeutic range, a different drug should be either substituted or added and the process repeated.

Phenytoin. Hydroxylation of phenytoin in the liver is a saturatable process, so that a small dose increment can result in a considerable rise in blood level. It is unwise, therefore, to increase the dose of phenytoin by more than 25 or 50 mg at a time when the daily dose exceeds 300 mg. In some patients, the addition of only 25 mg may convert a subtherapeutic blood level to a toxic level. The long half-life of phenytoin means that it need be given only once a day.

Valproate. This drug has a short half-life of about 8 hours but it is reasonable to give the drug twice a day since the anticonvulsant effect seems to last much longer. The short half-life also makes blood level measurements difficult to assess. 100 mg/l at peak and 50 mg/l at trough may also be used.

Table 6.1 Anticonvulsive drugs

Preparations	*Tablet or capsule size* (mg)	*Usual daily dose range* (mg)	*Therapeutic range* (mg/l)	*Approx half-life* (h)	*Usual dose frequency*	*Peak plasma level* (h)
Phenytoin	25 50 100	200–400	3–16	12–40	b.d. or daily	4–8
Carbamazepine	100 200 400	200–1200	4–14	9–15	b.d.	2–6
Valproate	200 500	600–2000	40–80	7–9	b.d.	7–9
Primidone	250	500–1500	< 14	5–15	b.d.	2–4
Phenobarbitone	15 30 60 100	30–90	9–25	75–108	daily	6–18

Primidone. A variable proportion of an oral dose of primidone is converted into phenobarbitone. There is, therefore, no reason to use a combination of primidone and phenobarbitone. Patients who are stabilised on primidone alone show a ratio of phenobarbitone to primidone which exceeds 2:1. If the primidone level exceeds the phenobarbitone level, it can be concluded that compliance is poor.

Phenobarbitone. Although still very widely used, phenobarbitone is no longer a treatment of first choice in adult patients with epilepsy. It may cause behavioural disturbance in children, the sedation is unacceptable to young adults and it may contribute to depression in the middle-aged. Blood levels should not normally exceed 25, especially in children, but many patients who have been stabilised on this drug for many years tolerate much higher levels without signs of toxicity. Withdrawal of the drug should be gradual owing to the risk of precipitating fits.

Status Epilepticus

Status epilepticus is a series of major attacks without full recovery between seizures. This is a dangerous condition with a high mortality and requires urgent treatment.

The priority is to stop the attack and this is best done with an IV injection of diazepam 10–20 mg or clonazepam 1–2 mg. It should not be given IM or diluted in IV infusion fluids. The diazepam injection may be repeated and is often all that is necessary.

Control must be maintained and if attacks recur less than an hour or two after more than two or three injections of diazepam, the patient must be transferred to an intensive care unit where methods of artificial ventilation are available. Chlormethiazole may be used by slow IV infusion and this may be combined with paralysis and ventilation. While paralysed and ventilated the patient's brain activity may be monitored by electroencephalography.

Epilepsy in Pregnancy

Phenytoin is a powerful liver enzyme inducer and when used in patients on the combined contraceptive pill it is necessary to prescribe a preparation containing at least 50 μg of oestrogen. There is about five-fold increase in the risk of cleft palate and cardiac abnormalities in children born to mothers with epilepsy on phenytoin; carbamazepine may be a safer drug to use in pregnancy. Phenobarbitone should be avoided. In the majority of patients with epilepsy it is important to maintain their anticonvulsant drugs during pregnancy but it is also important to ensure that the blood levels are not in the toxic range. As pregnancy advances the blood levels of most anticonvulsants falls; this is partly dilutional and partly due to more rapid clearance. It is, however, very rarely necessary to increase the dose during pregnancy, but if this is done, the dose must be reduced after delivery.

Most anticonvulsant drugs are excreted in small quantities in breast milk, but breast feeding is not contraindicated except for patients on phenobarbitone, which tends to cause drowsiness in the infant.

The risks of a child born to a patient with epilepsy of developing the same condition is only slightly greater than chance, provided that there is no history of epilepsy in the other parent's family, but in the latter case the risks then rise considerably.

Epilepsy and Driving

A single epileptic attack does not constitute epilepsy, which is by definition a liability to attacks. The law in the UK does not allow patients who have had more than one attack to drive until they have been attack-free for more than two years. If the attacks are nocturnal (i.e. while asleep) and continue to be solely nocturnal for more than three years, then a driving licence is allowed. The regulations are much stricter for HGV and PSV licences and any attack after the age of five permanently excludes these licences.

MIGRAINE

Migraine is a paroxysmal headache which may be clearly lateralised, but not necessarily always to the same side, or it may be generalised. The headache may be preceded by an 'aura' which can take many forms, the most common of which are a variety of visual disturbances such as fortification spectra, flashing lights or hemianopic defects. There may be numbness or tingling of the face and arms, weakness of one side of the body and, occasionally, dysphasia. These symptoms usually evolve over a few minutes and last for between 15 and 25 minutes. The headache starts towards the end of the aura and usually builds up to a maximum over an hour or so. It may remain severe for several hours and the whole attack is over in 6–12 hours; occasionally, attacks last a day or two. The headache is often accompanied by nausea and vomiting, photophobia and noise intolerance. The frequency of migraine is very variable, ranging from weekly to yearly but about once a month is common and attacks are often related to menstruation.

Pathophysiology. The aura stage of migraine is associated with cerebral vasoconstriction and it is likely that all patients go through this stage, even though it may not be clinically identifiable. The headache stage is associated with non-cerebral cranial vasodilatation. The cause of migraine is unknown, but there is probably a genetic factor because there is often a family history.

Treatment. The treatment of migraine falls into three parts:

(1) *Avoidance of Aggravating or Precipitating Factors.* Some patients are able to identify a major aggravating or precipitating factor and it is much easier to avoid this than to take medication. Only a few patients are sensitive to food substances and these are usually the tyramine-containing foods, but chocolate and citrus fruits are also potent aggravating factors in some patients. The contraceptive pill usually aggravates migraine and, though it may be reasonable to take simple treatment for the migraine, if severe attacks persist, then alternative methods of contraception should be used. The contraceptive pill is contraindicated in patients who repeatedly have the same aura. The commonest causes of an aggravation of migraine in middle age is the development of hypertension. The menopause is often associated with a change in the pattern of attacks. Other aggravating factors include stress and anxiety, alcohol, relaxation (weekend migraine) and the menstrual cycle.

(2) *Treatment of the Acute Attack.* The simplest treatment for an attack of migraine is a combination of soluble aspirin or an equivalent mild analgesic, taken together with metoclopramide 10 mg. The metoclopramide promotes the absorption of aspirin and is useful for its anti-emetic effect. Some patients benefit from the use of Migraleve. If these measures fail, an ergotamine preparation may be used and these are available either sublingually, to swallow, by inhalation or by suppository. Patients who have very occasional but very severe attacks may best be treated with a single large dose of a sedative and sleep the attack off.

(3) *Prophylaxis.* This is the most effective form of treatment for patients who have frequent attacks and may, of course, be combined with treatment for the acute attack; a number of drugs are effective:

On vascular smooth muscle—clonidine 0.025 mg t.d.s.
On vascular innervation—propranolol starting with 10 mg t.d.s.
By serotonin antagonism—pizotifen up to 3 mg a day.
On psychological factors—tricyclic antidepressants (amitriptyline 25–50 mg at night).

MIGRAINOUS NEURALGIA

This is a paroxysmal vascular headache but is otherwise different from migraine. It is much more frequent in men than in women and the attacks are not preceded by an aura. Attacks occur in clusters (hence 'cluster headache'), the patient usually having one or two attacks a day for several weeks before a remission, which may last for months. The attacks are sharply localised to one supra and retro-orbital region and it may spread to the cheek. The pain is very intense and lasts for less than an hour. The attack is associated with watering of the eye and blocking of the nose on the same side; subsequently the nose runs. In severe attacks there may be a Horner's syndrome (ptosis and a small pupil—see p. 333) and this occasionally persists between attacks. The attacks often occur at the same time every day and may waken the patient from sleep.

Treatment. The most effective treatment is an ergotamine suppository containing 2 mg either daily or twice a day for the duration of the cluster.

CEREBROVASCULAR DISEASE

INTRACRANIAL HAEMORRHAGE

Extradural Haemorrhage

This may occur after head injury and is due to the fracture line crossing a meningeal artery, usually the middle meningeal artery. The initial head injury is of sufficient severity to cause loss of consciousness, from which the patient often recovers. The bleeding is arterial, so that the haematoma forms over several hours, causing gradually increasing coma and in the later stages progressing hemiplegia with fixed dilated pupils. Removal of the haematoma is life-saving.

There may be no *lucid interval* if the initial injury is particularly severe. In suspected cases burr-holes should be made as a matter of urgency. The prognosis is related to the promptness of treatment, which should not be postponed until the patient is transferred to a neurosurgical unit if this is likely to result in undue delay. The haematoma can be demonstrated by a CT scan or by carotid angiography.

Subdural Haemorrhage

Subdural haematomas also follow head injuries but the injury may be quite slight and the history of trauma may be unobtainable. The haematoma is due to venous bleeding and it may take days or weeks to form. It usually occurs in the young and the elderly. The presenting feature may be headache or epilepsy. Later there are periods of fluctuating drowsiness leading to coma, and there may be clear lateralising signs or evidence of brain-stem compression. The haematoma may be demonstrated by a CT scan, though there is a stage at which the haematoma is isodense with brain. If unilateral, there will be displacement of the ventricles but, if bilateral, there may be no shift of midline structures. However, in such patients, the ventricles appear unusually small and the cerebral sulci are not very prominent. A gamma scan may be positive and the haematoma can be demonstrated by angiography.

Treatment. Small subdural collections, in the absence of any physical signs or symptoms or evolving clinical picture, may be left to resolve; otherwise the treatment is by surgical evacuation of the clot.

Subarachnoid Haemorrhage

This is usually due to the rupture of a berry aneurysm or bleeding from an arteriovenous malformation, and it most commonly occurs in middle life. The onset is usually abrupt with severe headache and often with loss of consciousness. Subsequently, the patient complains of severe occipital headache and this is often accompanied by vomiting. Examination may show subhyaloid haemorrhages and there is marked neck stiffness. Focal signs, such as aphasia, a visual field defect or hemiparesis may occur either because the bleeding is partly intracerebral and partly subarachnoid or because of associated spasm of major cerebral arteries. The clinical diagnosis can be confirmed by lumbar puncture. The CSF is often under pressure and the diagnostic feature is xanthochromia.

Cerebral Aneurysm. There are several different sorts of cerebral aneurysm, but the one most likely to cause subarachnoid haemorrhage is a berry aneurysm, which is due to a congenital defect of the arterial wall at major branches. Berry aneurysms are commonly found around the Circle of Willis, particularly on the internal carotid artery at the origin of the posterior communicating artery. Other common sites are on the anterior communicating artery and at the trifurcation of the middle cerebral artery. Aneurysms at either end of the posterior communicating artery may be associated with a third nerve palsy.

The fusiform aneurysms associated with degenerative vascular disease and hypertension and large saccular aneurysms seldom rupture and usually present with compression of nearby cranial nerves.

Cerebral Angioma. This is a congenital arteriovenous malformation which, although present from birth, may not give rise to symptoms until the second or third decade. Patients may complain of headache which is usually worse with exercise. It may present with subarachnoid haemorrhage, in which case the bleeding is usually less than occurs with the rupture of a berry aneurysm and often recurs. It may also present with epilepsy or with a very slowly progressive hemiparesis. A bruit may be heard over the mastoids or orbits and a venous hum may be heard in the neck.

Investigation of Subarachnoid Haemorrhage. If a patient survives the rupture of a berry aneurysm, investigations to find the source of the bleeding should be undertaken as soon as the patient has made a reasonable recovery. Patients are at risk from rebleeding at any time and there is no safe period. Bilateral carotid and vertebral angiography should, therefore, be undertaken as soon as possible with a view to a surgical approach to the aneurysm if such be found. After about 3–6 weeks the risk of rebleeding is about the same as the risks of surgery. No cause for the subarachnoid haemorrhage is found in about 20% of cases.

Intracerebral Haemorrhage

This is nearly always associated with systemic hypertension and the commonest cause is the rupture of a Charcot–Bouchard aneurysm. These micro-aneurysms occur on the short perforating arteries arising from the Circle of Willis and the lenticulostriate arteries. For this reason cerebral haemorrhage usually occurs in the internal capsule, corpus striatum, upper brain stem and thalamus. The onset is usually abrupt and the rapidly expanding lesion may cause loss of consciousness at or shortly after onset. The destruction of brain tissue and the site of the lesion usually results in severe deficit and recovery is often poor. It is not uncommon for the haemorrhage to rupture into the lateral ventricles. Surgical evacuation of the clot is usually disappointing.

CEREBRAL ISCHAEMIA

Cerebral ischaemia or infarction occurs when a cerebral artery is occluded by thrombus or embolus.

The important risk factors in cerebrovascular disease are hypertension, diabetes, hyperlipidaemia, syphilis, a haemoglobin above 15 g% or a PCV above 45 and the contraceptive pill. A cerebral thrombosis is unusual in young patients and in menstruating women. If a stroke occurs in these two groups, it is likely either to be an embolism from the heart or in association with one or more major risk factors. These risk factors need to be assessed in all patients with stroke and, if found, treated accordingly.

Cerebral Thrombosis

The onset is usually less abrupt than cerebral haemorrhage and the neurological defect may take several hours to evolve. This often occurs overnight and the patient wakes with a completed stroke. Occlusion is due to the formation of clot at a site where the artery is already narrowed by an atheromatous plaque. Occasionally a thrombus forms in a segment of inflamed artery (arteritis); causes include giant-cell arteritis, syphilis, polyarteritis nodosa and systemic lupus erythematosus.

Cerebral Embolism

Emboli to the brain may arise from any part of the vascular tree from the heart to the major cerebral vessels. The commonest sites are the heart and the carotid bifurcation.

Emboli from the Heart may arise from mural thrombi which form as the result of myocardial infarction or in the atria as a result of atrial fibrillation. In both cases the embolus consists of formed blood clot. In bacterial endocarditis, pieces of heart valve may break away to form emboli.

Emboli from the Carotid Arteries. The carotid bifurcation is a common site for atheromatous plaque formation. This may produce any degree of carotid stenosis to complete occlusion and at any stage in this process the surface of the plaque may ulcerate, giving rise to emboli of atheromatous debris, including cholesterol crystals. Platelets aggregate on the raw surface and may form platelet emboli. This process may also occur at the origin of the cerebral arteries from the aorta and in the carotid syphon.

Whatever the source of the embolus, the onset is abrupt, though the deficit may subsequently increase or repeated emboli may give rise to a 'shuttering hemiplegia' or 'stroke in evolution'. If an embolus impacts in a cerebral artery and subsequently fragments, the resulting transient neurological deficit is called a *'transient ischaemic attack'* (*TIA*) and is usually due to a platelet embolus. By international convention, TIAs resolve completely is less than 24 hours. Any attack which results in permanent neurological deficit is known as a *completed stroke*. If the deficit lasts longer than 24 hours but recovers completely, it is known as reversible ischaemic neurological deficit (RIND).

The clinical syndrome that results from cerebral embolism depends on which artery is involved, and for descriptive purposes the area of brain involved is identified by its feeding artery. Occlusion of the main trunk of the middle cerebral artery causes damage in its entire territory with motor and sensory deficit on one side of the body associated with aphasia if the dominant hemisphere is affected, and a homonymous hemianopia due to involvement of the optic radiation. Fragmentary forms of this syndrome occur with embolisation of more distant branches.

The Carotid Artery Syndrome. This consists of attacks of ipsilateral amblyopia and attacks with contralateral long tract signs, and is due to emboli from the carotid artery to the ophthalmic artery and middle cerebral artery. The emboli may be seen traversing the retinal circulation. If the eye and the brain are affected at the same time the cause is more likely to be a perfusion failure due to a tight carotid stenosis or occlusion.

About 30% of patients who have transient ischaemic attacks develop a completed stroke within three years and this may occur after only a few attacks. These patients should be investigated with a view to endarterectomy if a surgically treatable lesion is found. Vertebrobasilar transient ischaemic attacks should be managed conservatively since they have a better prognosis than those in carotid territory and since most of the vertebrobasilar system is not accessible for surgery. A bruit over the appropriate carotid bifurcation is a strong indication of stenosis of the artery at that site and considerably increases the chances of finding an operative lesion. Initial screening may be carried out with doppler ultrasonic angiology which can identify blood flow, turbulence and pressure drops and β mode scanning gives an image of the artery. Useful information may also be obtained from digital subtraction angiograms which produce images of the arteries following intravenous injection of contrast. The images are digitalised and subtracted in a computer. This technique is particularly useful in identifying occluded arteries and major stenoses. The definitive investigation is still by arteriography, usually performed by femoral catheterisation and subsequent selective catheterisation of the appropriate vessels.

If emboli are thought to arise in the heart, the patient should be anticoagulated. Emboli arising more distally in patients not suitable for surgery may be treated with antiplatelet drugs, such as aspirin 300 mg daily.

Any consideration of surgery must take account of the operative mortality and morbidity of carotid endarterectomy. It is doubtful if the operation should be performed if the combined mortality and morbidity exceeds 5%.

The Management of a Completed Stroke

About 50% of patients who have a hemiplegic stroke make a good recovery, about 25% die within the next month and the remainder are left severely disabled.

The immediate treatment consists of good nursing care with particular attention to the avoidance of chest infection and the management of urinary retention if it occurs. Although the blood pressure may be quite high in the hours after a stroke, it usually settles in a few days and treatment which causes a precipitous fall in pressure should be avoided. Dehydration must be prevented as it increases the tendency to thrombosis. Rehabilitation by physiotherapists and, if necessary, speech therapists should be commenced as soon as possible, as vigorous early treatment probably decreases subsequent disability.

VENOUS SINUS THROMBOSIS

This usually results from spread of infection from the middle ear, mastoid or air sinuses. It may be associated with cerebral abscess. Venous sinus thrombosis also occurs in association with pregnancy and may result from a head injury associated with skull fracture. Anticoagulants are contraindicated because of the risk of haemorrhage. Treatment is that of the cause and steroids may be helpful in reducing the associated cerebral oedema.

INTRACRANIAL TUMOUR

Any of the intracranial structures may give rise to tumour. The following list includes some of the common tumours.

meninges	—meningioma
brain parenchyma	—gliomas
cranial nerves	—optic nerve glioma, neurofibromas (acoustic and trigeminal)
endocrine	—pituitary and pineal
congenital	—craniopharyngioma, chordoma
blood vessels	—angioma, haemangioblastoma
granulomas	—TB, sarcoid and syphilis
metastatic tumours	—usually from lung or breast

In adults the most common neoplasms are supratentorial gliomas and metastatic tumours. In children, posterior fossa tumours are more common and they are usually medulloblastomas or astrocytomas.

Clinical Features. The presentation of an intracranial tumour depends very much on its location and speed of growth. About 5% of tumours present with fits or may initially be diagnosed as strokes. The majority of supratentorial tumours present with steadily progressive neurological deficit. A tumour in the frontal lobe may present with personality changes and dementia. If slightly more posterior, it may present with a slowly progressive hemiplegia and there may be speech involvement if it affects the dominant hemisphere. The earliest features of a temporal lobe tumour are facial weakness, slight drift of the outstretched arm and an upper quadrantic hemianopia. Parietal lesions often cause hemianopia and may be associated with receptive speech difficulty in the dominant hemisphere or difficulties with spatial orientation in the non-dominant hemisphere.

In a small proportion of patients epilepsy is the earliest symptom and this implies involvement of the cortex. In some very slowly growing tumours, such as meningiomas, the epilepsy may precede the development of other focal signs by many years.

Posterior fossa tumours usually present in a slightly different way. There is comparatively little space in the posterior fossa, so that a relatively small tumour quickly obstructs CSF pathways. Early symptoms are therefore often headache, vomiting and papilloedema which are much later features of supratentorial tumours. In addition, there may be signs of brain-stem compression.

Special Investigations. These should be carried out so that the presence of a tumour can be verified, its nature determined and appropriate treatment given.

(1) *Radiography.* Plain X-rays of the skull may show:

Erosion of the posterior clinoid processes,suggesting raised intracranial pressure; of the internal auditory meatus, indicating an acoustic neuroma; of the skull base in the region of the petrous apex and foramen ovale due to nasopharyngeal carcinoma.

Expansion of the sella turcica due to a chromaphobe adenoma or destruction of bone around the sella, perhaps with calcification, indicating a parasella tumour, such as a chordoma or an aneurysm.

Hyperostosis of the skull vault, sphenoid wings or olfactory grooves, indicating the site of a meningioma.

Shift of a calcified pineal gland, indicating the presence of an expanding lesion.

Abnormal calcification in the tumour itself; this may occur in very slowly growing gliomas, such as the oligodendroglioma and in about 50% of patients with craniopharyngioma.

The chest X-ray may show the presence of a bronchial carcinoma, the commonest primary associated with cerebral metastases.

(2) *Electroencephalography (EEG).* This is not the investigation of choice if a space-occupying lesion is suspected, but it may show a clearly focal disturbance in a patient presenting with epilepsy and this might indicate the need for further investigation. The EEG in cerebral abscess is very abnormal and shows high-voltage slow activity over the abscess.

(3) *The Isotope Brain Scan.* Gamma camera pictures are taken of the head from various angles following intravenous injection of Technetium-99^m. This is normally confined to the vascular system but may be extravasated and sequestrated in a number of abnormal conditions, including neoplasm, abscesses, haematomas and infarcts. Large vascular spaces may also be seen (angioma) and the venous sinuses are usually clearly visible.

(4) *Computerised Tomography (CT Scan).* The development of computerised axial tomography of the brain by EMI has been described as the greatest advance in the use of X-rays since their discovery by

Röntgen in 1895. A narrow pulsed beam of X-rays is passed through the brain and a detector records the amount that is transmitted. The X-ray source and its corresponding detector is rotated around the head and from the data obtained, the absorption coefficient or X-ray density of small volumes of brain can be computed. At present these volumes are 1.5 mm square in an 10 mm slice. The resulting composite picture clearly shows any structure whose X-ray density varies from that of calcium at one extreme to that of fat at the other. It is, therefore, possible to delineate tumours, abscesses, haematomas, infarcts and cerebral oedema. The ventricles are clearly seen, so that it is possible to say whether or not they are dilated or displaced and whether or not there is evidence of cortical atrophy. Tumours which are isodense with brain may not be seen but their presence inferred from distortion of normal structures. Many tumours are enhanced following the intravenous injection of an iodine-containing contrast material, since this makes the blood vessels appear denser than normal, and if it extravasates it may increase the apparent density of tumours. The CT scan is a rapid, accurate, reliable and atraumatic method of visualising the intracranial contents and it is associated with a low radiation dose. Early CT scanners were less reliable in the posterior fossa, particularly with small lesions lying close to the base of the skull. However, the latest generation of high definition machines provides very much better images. The use of these machines has considerably reduced the need for other diagnostic procedures, particularly pneumoencephalography.

(5) *Nuclear magnetic resonance (NMR).* This new imaging technique promises to provide very detailed images, comparable or better than X-ray CT scanning. The images are constructed by CT techniques from the radio frequency signal that is emitted as electron orbits return to normal, having been displaced by a powerful electromagnetic force applied to the patient by powerful magnets. In the brain, the difference between grey and white matter is particularly well shown and small lesions of white matter are easily seen. The widespread small lesions in multiple sclerosis can be well demonstrated. It is possible to reconstruct the image in any plane. It has the additional advantage of being entirely atraumatic and does not expose the patient to X-irradiation.

(6) *CSF Analysis.* Lumbar puncture for CSF analysis is contraindicated in the presence of an intracranial space-occupying lesion, because of the danger of herniation of the brain through the tentorial hiatus or foramen magnum (coning).

(7) *Cerebral Angiography.* The carotid and vertebral arterial system can be visualised by injection of a radio-opaque dye and rapid sequence X-rays show the arterial, capillary and venous stages. This is usually done by a femoral catheterisation and then by selective catheterisation of the artery concerned, but it can be carried out by direct arterial puncture. Angiography is indicated if the diagnosis on the CT scan is in doubt, if it appears to be a vascular lesion, particularly a cerebral

angioma, or if the detailed anatomy of the vascular tree is required by the surgeon planning operative intervention.

(8) *Pneumo-encephalography*. In this investigation air is used as the contrast medium and it displaces CSF in the ventricular system and cerebral subarachnoid space following lumbar injection. This investigation has almost completely been replaced by CT scanning, but may provide very useful information when used with tomography to outline small parasella and suprasella lesions and in some posterior fossa lesions, particularly by simultaneously outlining the aqueduct and fourth ventricle together with the basal cisterns.

(9) *Ventriculography*. Lumbar puncture is contraindicated in the presence of papilloedema and raised intracranial pressure. If visualisation of the ventricular system is required, air or a radio opaque medium can be introduced directly into the lateral ventricles through a brain needle. This is usually done immediately prior to operation and under the same anaesthetic.

Treatment. Treatment of intracranial tumours depends entirely on their nature and their situation. An attempt should be made to remove benign tumours, such as pituitary adenomas, acoustic neuromas and meningiomas, except where to do so would leave unacceptable deficit. Malignant gliomas are, on the whole, not removable, although if confined to the anterior part of the frontal lobe or the anterior part of the temporal lobe, it may be possible to carry out a radical resection. Otherwise, the nature of the tumour should be determined by biopsy and consideration given to the possibility of X-ray therapy. Metastatic tumours, if solitary and near the surface, can often be removed entirely. Chemotherapy has so far proved disappointing. Many cerebral tumours, particularly metastases and meningiomas, are associated with extensive white-matter oedema. This can be effectively treated with betamethasone (16 mg a day initially) and this treatment will often result in a dramatic improvement in the patient's condition.

DISSEMINATED SCLEROSIS (Multiple Sclerosis)

In this condition patches of demyelination occur at different times scattered throughout the central nervous system. These 'plaques' evolve and resolve to give the characteristic episodes of neurological dysfunction, from which there may be complete clinical recovery, although pathologically they leave small scars in the white matter.

Aetiology. The cause is unknown. There are features which suggest an immunological mechanism and some evidence to support the theory that it is an infection, perhaps with a slow virus, and these two possibilities are not mutually incompatible. In addition there is evidence that the composition of myelin in patients with multiple sclerosis is slightly different to normal subjects.

Epidemiology. The disease is much more common in temperate climates and is comparatively rare in equatorial countries. The prevalence in the Shetlands is twice that in Cornwall. Migration from a high-risk area to a low-risk area or vice versa only changes the risk for an individual if this migration takes place before adolescence. About 60% of patients have their first attack between the ages of 20 and 40 and a first attack below the age of 15 or over the age of 50 is rare. In the UK women are more affected than men in a ratio of 2:1.

Clinical Features. The signs and symptoms of disseminated sclerosis depend entirely on the site of the lesions but it is confined to the central nervous system. Although cranial nerve palsies occur, lower motor neurone signs in the limbs do not. Unilateral retrobulbar neuritis is often an early feature with the rapid progression of visual impairment, usually due to a central scotoma, associated with pain on eye movement. Vision may remain unchanged for days or a few weeks and then gradually improves. The disc may show swelling (papillitis) initially and later optic atrophy. Involvement of cerebellar pathways in the brain stem are common and result in nystagmus, internuclear ophthalmoplegia, dysarthria, ataxia and disequilibrium. Spinal cord involvement is also common with involvement of the pyramidal tracts and posterior columns. Sphincter disturbance is an early feature with spinal cord involvement.

These features usually evolve over a few days, last a few weeks and resolve over weeks or months. There may be complete remission of all signs and symptoms after the first episode and recurrence may not occur for many years. Often recovery is incomplete if the relapses are frequent, causing increasing permanent disability. It is not possible to predict the outcome of the disease in the early stages, but the state of the patient five years after the first attack is some guide to prognosis. In some patients, particularly the young, the disease shows wide fluctuations between exacerbations and remissions whereas others, particularly the older patients, may show a very slow progressive course over many years without obvious remissions.

Diagnosis. The diagnosis depends on the demonstration of multiple lesions within the nervous system and documented evidence of multiple lesions in time (definite multiple sclerosis). The demonstration of a single focal lesion for which no other cause can be found, with a history suggestive of other lesions, is usually designated 'probable multiple sclerosis', whereas a single lesion without any evidence of other lesions, but no alternative diagnosis, may be called 'possible multiple sclerosis'. It is, of course, necessary to exclude a focal lesion due to some other cause. This difficulty often occurs with a slow progressive spinal-cord lesion in middle age and no other features. A compressive lesion must be excluded by myelography.

Investigation. Analysis of the CSF may show a slightly raised CSF protein with a disproportionate increase in the amount of the immunoglobulin IgG. This is usually expressed as the IgG/albumin ratio. A more accurate test compares the relative amount of IgG to albumin in CSF to the same measurement in the blood and, by this means, it can be demonstrated that the immunoglobulin is produced on the brain side of the blood–brain barrier.

In patients with a single focal lesion both clinically and historically, additional focal lesions within the nervous system may be demonstrated by measurement of central conduction velocities:

Visual evoked responses. The patient is asked to look at a black and white checker-board pattern, which flashes black and white alternately. This produces a time-locked response in the visual cortex which can be recorded by surface electrodes. The amplitude is much less than that of the EEG so that an averager is required. Delayed conduction from one eye compared to the other or to normal values indicates a lesion of the optic nerve on that side. A similar technique can be used to measure central conduction velocities in the auditory system (auditory evoked responses and crossed acoustic response) and in the sensory system (somatosensory evoked responses).

Treatment. There is no specific treatment which influences the course of the disease. There is some evidence that a short course of high-dose steroids given during the acute attack induces a remission earlier and with less deficit than might otherwise have occurred. This is presumably by an effect on the oedema associated with an evolving plaque.

Neuromyelitis Optica (Devic's Disease).

This condition is closely related to disseminated sclerosis but it tends to develop at an earlier age, usually affecting adolescents. The clinical picture is that of bilateral retrobulbar neuritis occurring either simultaneously or consecutively and associated with a tranverse myelitis which results in a spastic paraplegia or quadriplegia. The pathological changes are similar to disseminated sclerosis. Recovery is often poor but relapses are rare. The treatment is with steroids.

THE HEREDITARY SPINOCEREBELLAR DEGENERATIONS

Any part of the neuraxis may be affected by genetically determined degenerative processes. The most common parts of the nervous system to be involved are the cerebellum, the spinal cord and the peripheral nerves. The extent to which these structures are involved varies from family to family but tends to breed true within a family. Although there is a continuum from a pure cerebellar degeneration to pure peripheral nerve involvement, some combinations of signs are much commoner than others and these were recognised early; an eponymous nomenclature has continued.

Friedreich's Ataxia

This is the commonest form of this group of degenerative disorders and is the result of degeneration in the cerebellum, posterior and lateral columns of the cord and less severe involvement of the optic nerves and peripheral nerves. The onset is usually in the first or second decade with unsteadiness of gait followed by clumsiness of the hands. The cerebellar degeneration results in nystagmus, dysarthria and ataxia. Spinal cord involvement results in pyramidal weakness of the legs with extensor plantar responses, but the knee and ankle reflexes are usually absent because of the associated peripheral neuropathy. The condition is associated with pes cavus, which may be found in unaffected members of the family, and there may be cardiac changes.

Peroneal Muscular Atrophy (Charcot–Marie–Tooth Disease)

This condition is characterised by pes cavus with wasting and weakness of the muscles which begins in the peronei and progresses proximally, later involving the hands. The wasting seldom progresses above mid-thigh to give an 'inverted champagne bottle' appearance to the legs. It is a degenerative disease predominantly of the peripheral nerves but there is evidence of anterior horn cell involvement and sometimes of cord involvement. There are two principal types, one presenting in the first decade (dominant and demyelinating) and the other in the fifth or sixth decade (dominant and axonal).

Hypertrophic Interstitial Neuropathy (Dejerine–Sottas Disease)

This condition is inherited as an autosomal dominant and affects peripheral nerves with marked thickening due to Schwann cell proliferation. There is marked slowing of peripheral conduction. The disease is slowly progressive, usually presenting in adolescence. If it starts in the first decade marked kyphoscoliotic deformities may develop. The CSF protein is always raised and, if greater than 10 g, there is likely to be obstruction of the CSF pathways due to hypertrophic roots.

NEUROFIBROMATOSIS (Von Recklinghausen's Disease)

This is a congenital ectodermal abnormality inherited as an autosomal dominant. Both the central and peripheral nervous system may be involved with multiple neurofibromas. The most striking feature is multiple tumours of the cutaneous nerves, which present as subcutaneous nodules of varying size, they may be pedunculated. Patchy cutaneous pigmentation is almost invariably present; these too may vary in size from a few millimetres to several centimetres. They are usually described as 'café au lait' spots and there should be more than five. Phacomas may be found in the retina and there are often congenital abnormalities of the skeleton.

Neurofibromas of the cranial nerves, particularly the V, VIII and IX, may occur in association or as an isolated occurrence. Similarly, isolated neurofibromas of spinal roots may occur and these give rise to wasting, weakness and pain in the myotome affected as well as causing a characteristic enlargement of the intervertebral foramen; the tumour assuming a dumbbell appearance on either side of the foramen, cord compression often occurs. Central nervous system neurofibromas are almost invariably associated with a markedly elevated CSF protein.

Complications. There is a high incidence of glioma, ependymoma and meningioma in association with neurofibromatosis. Occasionally, a neurofibroma may become sarcomatous.

DEFICIENCY STATES (See p. 599)

Thiamine Deficiency (Vitamin B_1)

Thiamine deficiency may present as a peripheral neuropathy (beri-beri) or as one of two forms of encephalopathy (Korsakoff's psychosis and Wernicke's encephalopathy).

(1) *Beri-beri.* Presents with pain and paraesthesia in the hands and feet, followed later by weakness. Examination shows wasting and weakness of the small hand muscles and the feet, absent reflexes and 'glove and stocking' cutaneous sensory loss. If there is associated cardiac failure with oedema, the condition is known as wet beri-beri.

(2) *Korsakoff's Psychosis.* This is often associated with polyneuritis. The syndrome is characterised by confusion, disorientation and striking loss of recent memory with a tendency to confabulate.

(3) *Wernicke's Encephalopathy.* This too may be associated with Korsakoff's psychosis and polyneuritis. The characteristic features are vertigo, nystagmus, ocular palsies, ataxia and drowsiness.

These clinical manifestations of thiamine deficiency are usually associated with chronic alcoholism but may be due to malnutrition. Wernicke's encephalopathy is a rare complication of hyperemesis gravidarum.

Treatment. The treatment is with large doses of thiamine, which may be given intravenously at first. Since thiamine deficiency is often associated with deficiency of other vitamins, it is usual to give a preparation containing other vitamins of the B complex and Vitamin C (Parentrovite Forte).

Vitamin B_{12} Deficiency (see p. 613)

Deficiency of Vitamin B_{12} may give rise to a macrocytic anaemia, subacute combined degeneration of the cord associated with a mild peripheral neuropathy, dementia, and optic atrophy.

The normal serum B_{12} level is above 400 ng/l. Macrocytosis may develop at levels below this but neurological complications are rare if the level exceeds 100. Neurological complications are virtually unknown in the presence of a normal blood picture.

Subacute combined degeneration of the cord is so called because of the combined involvement of the posterior and lateral columns of the cord. This gives rise to impairment of touch, vibration and joint position sense, together with pyramidal tract signs, which always involve the legs first. Patients complain of paraesthesia in the hands and feet, followed by increasing numbness and sensory ataxia. The knee and ankle jerks are absent because of the associated peripheral neuropathy but the plantar responses are extensor. Mental symptoms may accompany this condition but may rarely appear alone. Optic atrophy occurs in about 5% of cases.

Treatment. Treatment is by intramuscular injection of hydroxocobalamine 1000 μg given daily for the first week and then at increasing intervals to a maintenance dose of 1000 μg a month. This treatment must be continued for life.

NON-METASTATIC NEUROLOGICAL COMPLICATIONS OF CARCINOMA

Any part of the neuraxis may degenerate in the presence of a carcinoma elsewhere, usually an oat cell carcinoma of the lung. It is possible that the carcinoma produces a substance toxic to parts of the nervous system. The commonest manifestation is a mixed motor and sensory polyneuropathy but dementia, cerebellar atrophy and myelopathy may also occur. These conditions may occur in association with myeloma and the lymphomas.

FURTHER READING

Houston Merritt, H., *A Textbook of Neurology*, Lea and Febiger, Philadelphia, 1979.

M. R. C. Memorandum No. 45., *Aids to the Examination of the Peripheral Nervous System*, HMSO, London, 1980

Walton, J. N., *Brain's Diseases of the Nervous System*, 8th edition, Oxford University Press, Oxford, 1977.

Walton, J. N., *Disorders of Voluntary Muscle*, 4th edition, Churchill Livingstone, London, 1981.

CHAPTER 7

IMMUNOLOGICAL REACTIONS IN CLINICAL MEDICINE

Immunology has its roots in the observation that persons surviving certain infectious diseases seldom suffer from the same disease again. Apart from conferring specific resistance to various pathogens, it is now realised the immune system plays a fundamental role in other biological reactions of great clinical importance; the nature of these is outlined in this section.

NATURE OF IMMUNE RESPONSE

The immune response (Fig. 7.1) is initiated by a variety of substances referred to as antigens. These are classified according to their origin as (i) hetero-antigens which originate in a foreign species, e.g. pathogenic organisms or their products, (ii) iso-antigens which originate in a

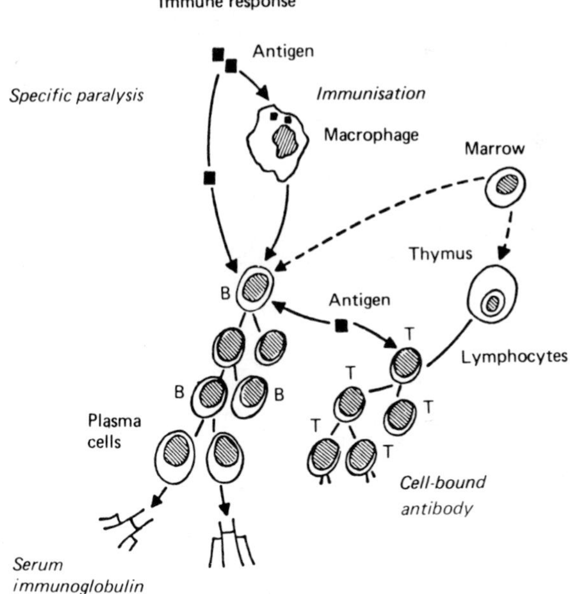

Fig. 7.1 Schematic representation of the immune response.

genetically dissimilar member of the same species, e.g. blood group substances, (iii) auto-antigens which originate in the sensitised host, e.g. thyroglobulin. Antigenic compounds may be complex proteins or carbohydrates of large molecular size. Many antigens which initiate a specific antibody response can be observed to undergo phagocytosis by tissue macrophages. These cells do not synthesise antibody but appear to participate in the immune response by concentrating antigen and presenting it to adjacent lymphocytes. The latter cells, which are derived from precursors in bone marrow, are widely distributed in lymph nodes, spleen, marrow and lymphoid tissues of the lung and gastrointestinal tract.

Adaptive immune responses are initiated by interaction of antigen with specific receptors on the surfaces of lymphoid cells. Two major classes of lymphocytes are recognised and these behave differently after reaction with antigen. T-lymphocytes undergo transformation and mitosis generating a population of cells specifically reactive with the inducing antigen; B-lymphocytes differentiate into plasma cells which secrete humoral antibody, but this process usually requires cooperation with T_H (T-helper) cells. Another subpopulation designated T_S (T-suppressor) cells interact with B cells to inhibit antibody synthesis. The immune reactions generated by these cellular responses therefore fall into two major categories. One is mediated by specific humoral antibody and the other by specifically sensitised T-lymphocytes (cell-mediated immunity). Antibody action may, in certain circumstances, be independent of cells, e.g. neutralisation of toxins, and certain specific cell-mediated reactions are independent of antibody, e.g. T_C (T-cytotoxic) killing of viral-infected or tumour cells. Several other specific immune mechanisms require the interaction of humoral antibody with cells. Such antibody-dependent cell reactions include macrophage endocytosis, mast-cell degranulation and ADCC (antibody-dependent cell-mediated cytotoxicity). In addition, the immune response generated by the interaction of antigen with lymphocytes may locally affect other cells which do not carry the specific antigen (non-specific immunity).

The Major Histocompatibility (HLA) System

The major histocompatibility (HLA) system includes a number of closely linked genetic loci which control cell surface antigens, certain complement components and immune responses. Three loci, HLA, A, B and C control Class I antigens present on all nucleated cells and responsible for graft rejection; HLA-D codes for a structurally distinct set of Class II antigens found only on lymphocytes and monocytes.

HLA genes	D	Complement Components	B	C	A	Chromosome 6
Class	II	III	I	I	I	

Experiments in mice indicate that histocompatibility antigens have a fundamental physiological role in the control of the cell interactions mentioned above. Thus, T-helper (T_H) or T-suppressor (T_S) cells and macrophages can interact functionally only if compatible at the mouse locus equivalent to HLA-D. Similarly, T_C (cytotoxic) cells can kill only target cells with corresponding specificities at the B, C and A loci. The association of several diseases such as ankylosing spondylitis, juvenile diabetes, Reiter's syndrome and gluten-sensitive enteropathy with certain MHC phenotypes, therefore, strongly suggests an immunological element in their pathogenesis.

The End Products of Immune Reactions

(i) *Serum Immunoglobulins.* Serum antibodies are confined to the γ-globulin fraction of serum proteins and are referred to as immunoglobulins (Ig). They are large proteins containing 2 heavy and 2 light polypeptide chains (Fig. 7.2). The different classes of immunoglobulin (IgG, IgA, IgM, IgD, IgE) are distinguished by the structure of their heavy chains. Each Ig chain is made up of repeating units of about 70 amino acids enclosed by a disulphide bond. This arrangement is of

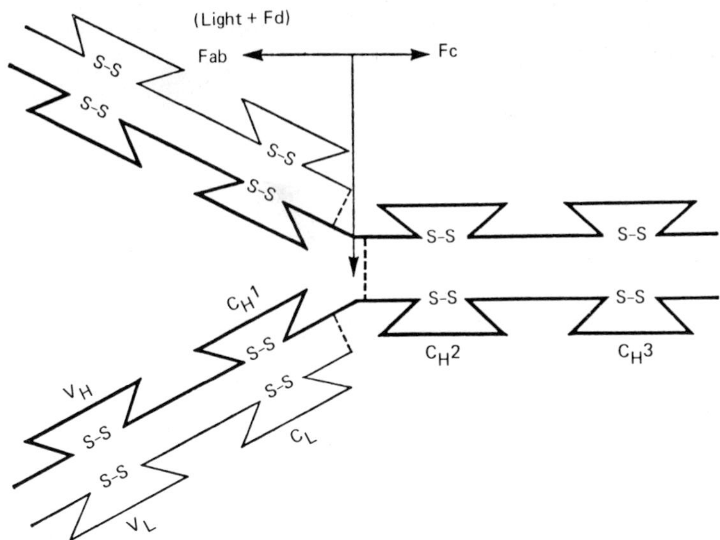

Fig. 7.2 Schematic representation of the antibody molecule showing 4-chain structure, site of cleavage by the enzyme papain (arrowed) and distribution of repeating units bounded by intra-chain disulphide bonds. The units labelled V_H and V_L contain the antigen binding sites while the C_H and C_L units carry sites for other activities such as complement fixation and membrane attachment.

interest since antibodies have evolved to perform two distinct functions which are separately localised in the molecule.

(a) Each antibody combines with a specific antigen. Every individual can probably make at least 10^6 antibodies with different specificities. The portions of the molecule which interact with antigen are called combining sites and there are two on each 4-chain molecule. These sites are generated by the interaction of the N-terminal units (V_H and V_L) of heavy and light chains, which show great variability of structure and are different in antibodies of distinct specificities. The V regions are common to all classes of immunoglobulins so that antibodies of a given specificity may be distributed in all the major Ig classes.

(b) Antibodies also carry out various effector functions which are consequent upon interaction with complement or with specific cells or membranes of the body. These effector sites are in C regions of the antibody molecule and given sites are present on some immunoglobulin classes but absent from others. Only IgG and IgM have sites for complement fixation, and only IgE has a site for attachment to mast cells, which is the basis for sensitisation of autologous tissues. Both IgG and IgM attach to the surface of macrophages and mediate endocytosis while IgG alone attaches to K (killer) cells to initiate antibody-dependent cell-mediated cytotoxicity (ADCC). These differences between the immunoglobulin classes account for the remarkable diversity of biological reactions mediated by serum antibody (Table 7.1).

(ii) *Monoclonal Antibodies Produced by Hybridomas.* Antigens carry several different antigenic sites each of which stimulates antibody production by several clones of B-cells. Antisera specific for a given antigen therefore contain a broad spectrum of polyclonal antibodies which have different combining specificities and may be of different classes. Individual B-cells and their clonal progeny, by contrast, produce a single antibody species, but such cells cannot be readily cultured in vitro. However, if B-cells are fused with myeloma cells the resulting hybridoma has the capacity to produce antibody and to proliferate in vitro. Such antibody comprises a single molecular species having defined specificity and class and can be produced in limitless amounts. The products of hybridomas therefore comprise standard immunological reagents previously unobtainable by conventional immunisation. Such antibodies have many increasingly important applications in clinical medicine which include:

Immunodiagnosis	Blood grouping; tissue typing; immunodiagnosis of infections and tumours.
Experimental analysis	Cell products e.g. interferon; Cell constituents e.g. for vaccine development; Cell subsets e.g. of lymphocytes and neurones.
Therapeutic agents	Drug targeting; immunotherapy.

Table 7.1 Properties of human immunoglobins

	IgG	*IgA*	*IgM*	*IgD*	*IgE*
Structural					
Molecular weight	150 000	160 000 (serum) 370 000 (secretory)	900 000	170 000	200 000
Heavy chain classes	γ	α	μ	δ	ε
Light chain types	κ, λ	κ, λ	κ, λ	κ, λ	κ, λ
Carbohydrate (%)	2.9	7.5	11.8	11.3	10.7
Biological					
Serum concentration g/l.	8–17	1.5–4.5	0.5–1.5	0.003–0.40	0.10–1.3 μg/l
Antibody activity	+	+	+	+	+
C fixation	+	0	+	0	0
Placental transfer	+	0	0	0	0
Seromucous secretion	0	+	0		+
Tissue sensitisation	0	0	0	0	+
Combination rheumatoid factor	+	0	0		
Attachment to macrophages	+	0	+		+
B-cell receptor	0	0	+ (monomer)	+	0
Attachment to K-cells (ADCC)	+	0	0	0	0

(iii) *Specific Cell-mediated Immunity*. In addition to the immunoglobulin response outlined above, antigenic stimulation leads to the proliferation of T-cells. These T-cells originate in bone marrow but are modified in some way by passage through the thymus gland (p. 391). Their surface receptors appear to have a structure related to the V regions of the serum immunoglobulins, but the identity of the receptor has not been established. T-cells comprise 80% of circulating lymphocytes. Functional subsets of T-cells include T_H (helper) cells which cooperate with B-cells in Ig synthesis, T_S (suppressor) cells which inhibit B-cells and T_C (cytotoxic) cells which can specifically kill virally infected target cells and tumour cells. Sensitised lymphocytes after combination with antigen can also exert widespread effects by producing factors which are called lymphokines and act upon other cell types (Table 7.2). Cell-mediated immune responses are directed predominantly against intracellular pathogens and organised tissue targets, and are associated with delayed hypersensitivity responses to specific antigen.

Table 7.2 Lymphokines

Cells affected	*Active lymphokine*
Macrophages and monocytes	Migration inhibition factor (MIF) Macrophage activating factor (MAF) Chemotactic factor for macrophages
Lymphocytes	Enhancement of antibody formation (helper factors) Suppression of antibody formation (suppressor factors) T-cell growth factors (Interleukin 2)
Polymorphonuclear leucocytes	Chemotactic factors
Other cell types	Lymphotoxin γ-interferon Collagen producing factor Osteoclast activating factor (OAF)

(iv) *Natural Killer (NK) cells*. These are a subpopulation of lymphoid cells comprising mainly large, granular lymphocytes. NK cells are able to kill some infected target cells and a range of tumour cells and do not require the presence of antibody. They are found in normal people and their activity does not depend upon previous sensitisation. NK cells possess an oxygen-dependent killing system which generates superoxide radicals and in this respect are akin to mononuclear phagocytes and granulocytes. NK cells are thought to be important in defence against tumour cells and their activity is augmented by interferons.

(v) *Immunological Paralysis.* Cells of the immunological system can respond in two alternative ways to the presence of antigen. On the one hand, antigenic stimulation, as outlined above, may induce the cycle of cell proliferation and differentiation which culminates in humoral or cell-mediated immunity. On the other hand, antigen may lead to specific immunological paralysis; this is not merely a failure to produce specific antibody, but is characterised by long-lasting loss of the capacity to synthesise antibodies specific for the paralysing antigen. Injection of antigens during foetal life tends to induce specific paralysis rather than antibody production, but specific paralysis can also be induced in adults by using the appropriate antigen dose or by modifying the physical character of the antigen. The mechanisms which determine whether an antigen will induce specific paralysis rather than antibody production are not fully understood. In some instances, the removal from antigen preparations of aggregated material liable to phagocytosis converts an immunising protein antigen into one inducing specific paralysis. This suggests that, at least in these instances, the immune response is initiated by antigen which has been modified by passage through macrophages while specific paralysis follows the direct interaction of antigen with lymphocytes.

(vi) *Non-specific Cell-mediated Immunity.* Sensitised T-lymphocytes reacting with antigen undergo blast transformation and may produce cytotoxic agents capable of damaging by-stander cells. In addition, other lymphocyte products may activate macrophages which become cytotoxic for a wide range of pathogens and cells.

DISORDERS OF ANTIBODY PRODUCTION

Clinical disorders may be associated with either diminished or increased production of antibody or lymphocytes. The most severe forms of antibody deficiency affect both cell-mediated and humoral immunity, but in other syndromes only one of these immune responses may be affected while the other remains intact. Unusual susceptibility to bacterial infections occurs with Ig deficiency and to viral infections where cell-mediated responses are defective. Patients with intact immune responses may rarely show increased susceptibility to infection associated with absence of complement components or defects of polymorph function.

Clinical immunodeficiency occurs in several rare congenital syndromes but more frequently is a complication of acquired disorders of the lymphoid system, e.g. Hodgkin's disease, myelomatosis, and lymphatic leukaemia.

AIDS (Acquired Immunodeficiency Syndrome) is an increasingly common disorder first observed in the UK in 1979. Over 1000 cases are known in the USA and the number is currently increasing by about 100 per month. The disease occurs predominantly in homosexual males and in drug addicts, but is seen also in haemophiliacs treated with antihaemophilic globulin isolated from donor blood. These facts suggest an infective origin for the disease, but no causative organism has been identified. AIDS is associated with repeated infections frequently involving opportunistic organisms e.g. pneumonia due to the protozoon *Pneumocystis carnii*, and with a high incidence of Kaposi's sarcoma. Humoral responses are normal in these patients, but cell-mediated immunity is very severely impaired. The disease runs a progressive course and the mortality is over 70%.

An excessive production of Ig leading to a diffuse increase of gammaglobulin detected on electrophoresis of serum is seen in many clinical disorders and results from proliferation of many different clones of lymphoid cells. The proliferation of a single clone, on the other hand, leads to production of monoclonal Ig which is homogeneous on electrophoresis and belongs to a single Ig class. This occurs in multiple myelomatosis and macroglobulinaemia, in association with various lymphomata and unrelated neoplasms and also, quite commonly, as an 'idiopathic' condition without detectable underlying pathology. Clonal proliferation of lymphocytes also occurs in acute and chronic lymphatic leukaemia, but these cells rarely produce immunoglobulin.

Disorders of Antibody Production

1. Deficient Production

(i) *Reduced cell-mediated and Ig responses*:
Combined Immunodeficiency
Combined Immunodeficiency (with thymoma)
Wiskott-Aldrich Syndrome (with thrombocytopenia and eczema)

(ii) *Reduced Ig response only*:
Transient hypogammaglobulinaemia of infancy
Congenital agammaglobulinaemia
Secondary hypogammaglobulinaemia (e.g. in Hodgkin's disease, nephrosis)

(iii) *Reduced cell-mediated response only*:
Thymic aplasia (di George's syndrome)
AIDS (acquired immunodeficiency syndrome)

2. Excessive Production

(i) *Diffuse hypergammaglobulinaemia*:
Chronic infections
Granulomata
Hepatic disease
'Connective tissue' disease

(ii) *'Monoclonal' Ig production*:
 Multiple myelomatosis (IgG, IgA, IgD, or IgE)
 Macroglobulinaemia (IgM)
 Lymphoma
 Idiopathic 'gammopathy'

(iii) *Clonal lymphocyte proliferation*
 Acute lymphatic leukaemia
 Chronic lymphatic leukaemia
 Burkitt's lymphoma

REACTIONS MEDIATED BY IMMUNE RESPONSES

Humoral antibodies and cell-mediated immunity are of fundamental clinical importance, not only in regard to protective immunity, but also in a wide range of pathological states involving immediate hypersensitivity reactions, auto-antibody formation or reactions to circulating immune complexes.

Protective Immunity

Immune reactions involve the primary interaction of antibody with the pathogen or its toxic products. Only in rare instances, however, e.g. some forms of viral immunity and toxin neutralisation, does this primary interaction constitute an effective immune response. Immunity is usually dependent on subsequent reactions of the bound antibody either with complement which leads to cell lysis, e.g. of Gram-negative bacteria, or with the surface of macrophages which promotes phagocytosis of the pathogen, e.g. pneumococci or with K-cells responsible for antibody-dependent cell-mediated cytotoxicity. It follows that protective immunity in systemic infections is mainly dependent upon IgG and IgM antibodies since only these can fix, complement and attach to effector cells. IgA is the predominant antibody of seromucous secretions and fulfils an important protective role at the epithelial surface of pulmonary and gastrointestinal tracts. Although IgA does not fix complement, it can act synergistically with lysozyme, present in seromucous secretions and activate complement by the alternative pathway to cause bacterial lysis. Cell-mediated immunity plays an important role in specific resistance to intracellular infections including tuberculosis, leishmaniasis, leprosy and some viral infections, and may be responsible for many of the papular and vesicular rashes which accompany common infectious diseases. The presence of cell-mediated immunity is indicated by the delayed hypersensitivity response, i.e. an inflammatory lesion appearing 24 hours after intradermal challenge with the antigen and characterised by local infiltration of the tissue with mononuclear cells.

Whether the immune response to infection is clinically effective or not depends mainly upon the serological character of the pathogen and its distribution in the body (Table 7.3). Lasting immunity occurs with organisms of uniform antigenicity widely distributed in the circulation, e.g. pertussis infection. Recurrent infections may be caused by serological variants of the original infecting pathogen, e.g. pneumococcal infections, or occur after localised infections which evoke a feeble immune response, e.g. diphtheria. Immunity may be totally ineffective where the organisms persists in modified form, e.g. the herpes virus as DNA or where the lethal dose of a toxic product, e.g. tetanus toxin, is less than the immunising dose.

The secretion of soluble cell surface antigens which combine with specific antibody or T-cells may effectively block immunity and promote survival of the pathogen, e.g. in schistosomiasis. Some intracellular pathogens are able to survive within phagocytic cells. Such survival may occur when a pathogen escapes from the ingested phagosome and lies free in the cytoplasm of the phagocyte, e.g. *Trypanosoma cruzi*; or when phagosomes fail to fuse with lysosomes and ingested organisms are therefore shielded from the potentially lethal lysosomal enzymes, e.g. *Toxoplasma*; or when fusion of phagosomes with lysosomes occurs, but the organisms are resistant to enzyme action, e.g. tubercle bacilli and *Leishmania*.

Immunity to tumours leading to involution of their growth may occur with virally-induced and chemically-induced tumours which carry recognisable foreign surface antigens. Unfortunately, tumours which arise spontaneously are not recognised as foreign and produce no effective immune response. The incidence of cancer is not increased in immunosuppressed subjects and the occurrence of lymphoid tumours in these patients could be related directly to the immunosuppressive agents used. NK cells (p. 396) are able to kill some tumour cell lines and interferon enhances their activity thus raising hopes for effective tumour therapy.

Immunopathology

In addition to specific protection, immune responses can cause tissue damage in several different ways (see Table 7.4):

Anaphylactic (*Type I reactions*). These reactions which include general and localised forms of anaphylaxis depend upon an immune response fundamentally similar to that responsible for protective immunity. There has long been speculation regarding the underlying mechanism producing such dramatically divergent reactions. It is now established that immediate hypersensitivity is mediated by one class of immunoglobulin, IgE (Table 7.1) and atopic individuals tend to produce this antibody in response to antigenic stimulation. The serum concentration of IgE is very low (p. 395) and most of this antibody is attached to

Table 7.3 Immune response to various infections

Clinical Immunity	*Serology*	*Distribution of Pathogen*	*Infections*			
			Bacterial	*Rickettsial*	*Viral*	*Protozoal*
Lasting	Uniform	Systemic or localised	Pertussis	Q-fever	Measles, Mumps, Rubella, Smallpox, Yellow-fever, Chickenpox	Cutaneous leishmaniasis
Strain-specific	Varied	Systemic or localised	Streptococcal Staphylococcal Pneumococcal	Typhus	Polio, Common-cold, Influenza	African trypanosomiasis
Poor	Uniform or varied	Localised (or intra-cellular)	Brucella		Common-cold, Influenza, Trachoma, Gonorrhoea	Malaria S. American trypanosomiasis
Ineffective			Tetanus		Herpes	Visceral leishmaniasis Schistosomiasis

Table 7.4 Immunopathology—mechanisms and clinical associations

Mechanism	*Antibody*	*Antigens*	*Clinical*
Anaphylactic (Type I)	IgE	Allergens e.g. drugs, pollen	Systemic anaphylaxis Bronchial asthma, Hay fever Urticaria
Cytotoxic (Type II)	IgG or IgM	Host tissue	Hyperthyroidism, Goodpasture's syndrome, Myasthenia gravis Auto-immune haemolytic anaemia
		Viral	Post-measles encephalitis
		Drugs	Haemolytic anaemia Thrombocytopenia
Immune Complex (Type III)	IgG or IgM	DNA	Lupus erythematosus nephritis
		Serum, Drugs	Serum sickness, Arthus reaction
		Viral	Serum hepatitis (arthritis, nephritis)
		Bacterial	Glomerulonephritis Lepromatous leprosy
		Protozoal	Malarial nephrosis
		Fungal	Farmer's lung
Cell-mediated (Type IV)	Cell-mediated	Host	Hashimoto's disease
		Chemical	Nickel sensitivity
		Viral	Herpes simplex
		Bacterial	Tuberculosis, Leprosy
		Protozoal	Cutaneous leishmaniasis
		Helminth	Schistosomiasis (cirrhosis)

tissue mast cells which are then said to be sensitised. On subsequent exposure, the antigen (allergen) reacts with tissue bound IgE and as a result the sensitised mast cells undergo degranulation, liberating various pharmacologically active compounds (Fig. 7.3) which cause the characteristic allergic symptoms (below). Desensitisation of atopic individuals can sometimes be achieved by injecting very small doses of the allergen. This stimulates the production of IgG antibody and on subsequent, natural exposure the allergen combines mainly with the predominant IgG (blocking) antibody so that reactions due to combination with IgE are prevented (Fig. 7.4). It is apparent that the biological consequences of antibody reactions depend fundamentally upon the relative proportions of the reacting Ig classes.

Auto-antibodies (*Cytotoxic Type II reaction*). The remarkable ability of the immunological system to distinguish 'self' from 'non-self' is

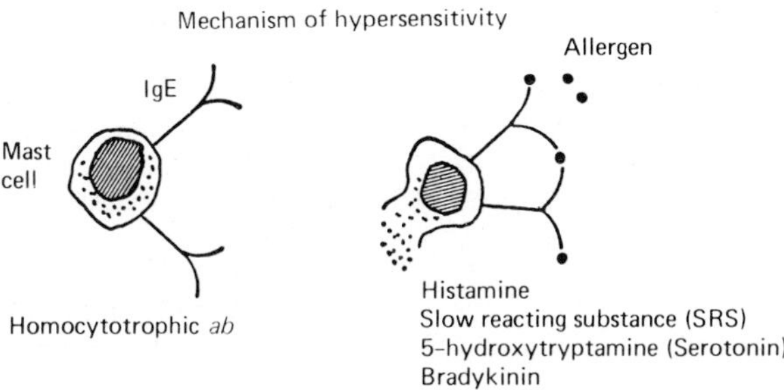

Fig. 7.3 Mechanism of local and generalised anaphylaxis. Antigenic stimulation of a susceptible subject leads to synthesis of IgE antibody which becomes attached to mast cells. A subsequent exposure to the same antigen leads to its combination with cell-bound IgE and consequent degranulation of mast cells and discharge of pharmacologically active compounds which cause anaphylaxis.

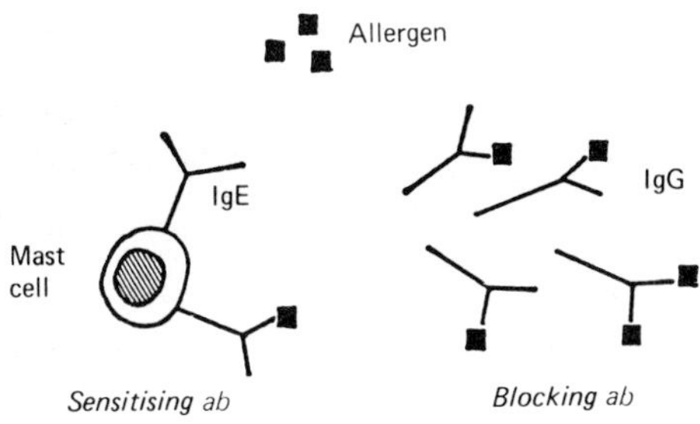

Fig. 7.4 Desensitisation of an atopic subject by injecting small amounts of the allergen may induce the formation of IgG antibody. By combining with this allergen after natural exposure the IgG acts as a 'blocking' antibody and prevents combination with IgE on sensitised mast cells.

thought to depend upon the development during foetal life of specific paralysis to auto-antigens. The appearance of auto-antibodies could, therefore, result from changes in the structure of auto-antigens (e.g. by drugs or infectious agents), entry into the circulation of antigens normally shielded from the immune system (e.g. spermatozoa, lens protein or thyroglobulin), the presence of cross-reacting heteroantigens (e.g. group A streptococci, which have antigens also present in human heart tissue) or loss of T_S (suppressor) activity (as in systemic lupus erythematosis). Viral infections which cause antigenic modification of cell surfaces may also induce antibody formation against the infected tissues (e.g. as probably occurs in post-measles encephalitis).

Table 7.5 Properties of some common auto-antibodies

Disease	*Antibody*	*Antigen*	*Test*	*Positive in*
Rheumatoid arthritis	Rheumatoid factor (IgM)	IgG	Rose-Waaler, Latex-particle } agglutination	Rheumatoid arthritis 70% SLE 20%, Normal 5% Sjøgren's syndrome 75%
Systemic lupus erythematosus	L.E. factor (IgG, IgA or IgM)	Deoxyribonucleohistose (nuclear protein)	LE cell phenomenon or immunofluorescence	SLE 90% Rheumatoid arthritis 50% Sjøgren's syndrome 75%
Thyroiditis	IgG or IgM	Thyroglobulin Thyroid microsomes	Precipitin reaction or Agglutination C^1 fixation	Hashimoto's disease 100% Thyrotoxicosis, Ca thyroid, non-toxic goitre 60% Normal females 15% Pernicious anaemia 40%
Thyrotoxicosis	LATS (IgG)		Release of labelled hormone from thyroid	Thyrotoxicosis 60%
Acquired haemolytic anaemia	IgG (non-agglutinating)	rH	Indirect haemagglutination (Coombs' test)	AHA 80%
Pernicious anaemia		Intrinsic factor Parietal cell	Binding of Radioactive Vitamin B_{12} Immunofluorescence	Pernicious anaemia 50% Thyroiditis 30%
Myasthenia gravis	IgG	Acetylcholine receptor of motor end plate	Immunofluorescence	Myasthenia gravis 85%

Auto-antibodies are being found in association with an increasing number of pathological states. In many instances these antibodies (Table 7.5) are directly responsible for the pathological lesions, e.g. in hyperthyroidism, myasthenia gravis and Goodpastures's syndrome. In other instances their presence is of diagnostic value, but several facts throw doubt upon the role of most of these antibodies in the *initiation* of pathological lesions. Many auto-antibodies occur in only a proportion of patients with the particular clinical syndrome and conversely, specific auto-antibodies are often found in the absence of the relevant disease (Table 7.5). In addition, their presence or level may show little correlation with the clinical state and autoimmune lesions are not usually induced by passive transfer of auto-antibodies. Thyroid stimulating antibody is an exception to this statement since thyrotoxicosis may occur in newborn offspring of thyrotoxic mothers who have circulating antibody. Muscle weakness may occur in babies born to mothers with myasthenia gravis associated with antibodies to acetylcholine receptors. These observations strongly support the idea that some forms of thyrotoxicosis and myasthenia gravis are caused by autoimmune reactions involving serum IgG antibody.

Immune Complex (*Type III reaction*). Antigen-antibody complexes present in the circulation may form microprecipitates in small blood vessels, fix complement and lead to accumulation of polymorphonuclear leucocytes, vascular occlusion and perivascular inflammation. Such lesions may occur in individuals injected with large doses of penicillin or horse serum (e.g. during passive immunisation for diphtheria or tetanus) who form antibodies which combine with the circulating antigen. The resulting syndrome, which is known as serum sickness, is characterised by glomerulonephritis, myocarditis, joint effusions, urticaria and pyrexia. Certain forms of pulmonary alveolitis which follow inhalation of fungal antigens, e.g. farmer's lung, also represent a reaction to circulating immune complexes. There is at present considerable interest in the possibility that various forms of renal disease, arthritis and periarteritis of obscure aetiology are caused by a similar immune mechanism.

Cell-mediated Immunity (*Type IV reaction*). Sensitised lymphocytes of thymic origin are involved especially in immunological reactions against organised tissues carrying foreign antigens. Such cell-mediated reactions are primarily responsible for rejection of foreign grafts, immunological responses to tumours and for certain forms of immunopathology, e.g. hepatic cirrhosis associated with schistosomiasis, granulomatous lesions in leprosy and sensitivity reactions to nickel, picryl chloride and poison ivy (p. 401). The presence of cell-mediated immunity is indicated by the delayed hypersensitivity response, i.e. an inflammatory lesion appearing 24 hours after intradermal challenge with the antigen and characterised by local infiltration of the tissue with round cells.

Conclusion

The immune system embodies an array of sensing cells which, through a wide repertoire of receptors, recognise antigens foreign to the host. This recognition event triggers a series of responses involving specific antibody formation and the production of a complex set of lymphokines which regulate the activities of many cell types. These reactions act individually and in concert to establish immunity to a variety of pathogens and to some tumours with recognisable antigenicity. Congenital and acquired disorders of the immune system may produce life-threatening susceptibility to microbial invaders. In addition, immune reactions can under circumstances outlined above cause damage to host tissue and generate a wide spectrum of pathological processes. Better understanding of factors which regulate immune responsiveness may permit more effective treatment of immunodeficiency and control of immunopathology.

CHAPTER 8

RHEUMATIC DISEASES

Rheumatic diseases constitute a heterogeneous group of conditions affecting joints, muscles, ligaments, and causing much suffering in the community through pain, stiffness and loss of mobility. Although acute episodes and life-threatening complications may be seen in certain of the conditions under consideration, the bulk of the problems encountered are less spectacular in their presentation and give rise to prolonged discomfort and disability without seriously impairing the general health of the patient. A wide spectrum of disease is seen in this group, including hereditary, inflammatory (both acute and chronic; infective and non-infective), metabolic, traumatic, degenerative, as well as neoplastic, neuropathic and psychogenic disorders. The aetiology and pathogenesis is in many cases unknown or poorly understood. Treatment is aimed at suppressing inflammation, reducing the disease activity and preserving and restoring the function of the locomotor system by physical therapy or surgical intervention or by adapting the environment to suit the patient's limited capabilities. Few of the diseases are amenable to eradication by medical means, but fortunately there is, in many cases, a strong tendency towards spontaneous recovery or remission. Twenty-three per cent of the work of a general practitioner involves rheumatic disorders. The importance of rheumatology in the medical curriculum is thus self-evident.

DEFINITIONS, ASSESSMENT AND DIAGNOSIS

The following terms are in common usage:

Arthralgia—pain in a joint
Arthritis—inflammation in a joint
Monarthritis—inflammation in a single joint
Oligoarthritis—inflammation in two, three or four joints
Polyarthritis—inflammation in five or more joints
Synovitis—inflammation of synovial membrane
Tenosynovitis—inflammation in a tendon sheath
Bursitis—inflammation in a bursa
Spondylitis—inflammation in the spinal joints
Spondarthritis—inflammation in the spine and peripheral joints
Osteoarthritis, osteoarthrosis—degeneration in a peripheral joint
Spondylosis—degeneration in the spinal joints
Effusion—presence of an excess of synovial fluid within a joint

Sciatica—pain in the distribution of the sciatic nerve
Cruralgia—pain in the distribution of the femoral nerve
Enthesopathy—inflammatory lesion at the point of insertion of a tendon or ligament in bone
Tendonitis—inflammation of a tendon
Arthropathy—any lesion affecting a joint
Myalgia—pain in a muscle
Myositis—inflammation in a muscle
Osteitis—inflammation in a bone
Chondritis—inflammation in cartilage.

The following terms have an imprecise meaning and are best avoided: *rheumatism*, *fibrositis* and *lumbago*.

The Assessment of the Arthritic Patient

Joint dysfunction from any cause gives rise to pain and reduction in the range of movement. In a mechanical disorder such as occurs when a fragment of bone or cartilage is impacted between the moving surfaces these may be the only abnormalities. In degenerative conditions crepitus may also be discerned, whilst in the presence of joint synovitis prolonged stiffness, warmth and joint swelling (often due to an effusion) are apparent. Important points in the history are the mode of onset, duration of symptoms, the subsequent progress, whether it follows a self-limiting, recurrent, acute or chronic course and the presence of relevant factors in the past, family and occupational history. Pathognomonic features such as rheumatoid nodules or tophi should be sought and deformities of the joints or spine considered not only from the diagnostic point of view but also for the effect on function.

Diagnostic Aids in Rheumatology

Many rheumatic diseases have characteristic clinical features so that clinical diagnosis is often not difficult.

The following diagnostic tests are helpful in difficult cases and as confirmation of the clinical diagnosis:

The ESR serves to distinguish inflammatory from degenerative and mechanical joint disease. The test for rheumatoid factor (latex fixation test and sheep cell agglutination test) are positive in two-thirds of patients with rheumatoid arthritis but also in a substantial number of patients with systemic lupus erythematosus (SLE) and in 5% of the normal population. Antinuclear factor is positive in most patients with SLE but in substantial numbers of patients with rheumatoid arthritis and scleroderma. The DNA binding test is more specific for SLE. Plasma urate is raised in primary and secondary gout. X-rays can provide diagnostic pointers to rheumatoid arthritis, osteoarthritis, ankylosing spondylitis and gout and pseudogout. Synovial fluid analysis should be undertaken whenever the diagnosis is uncertain and a joint effusion is detected. This is of paramount importance in patients suspected of infective arthritis and it can give positive evidence of gout and pseudogout by the recognition of crystals of sodium urate and calcium pyrophosphate respectively by polarising microscopy. Arthroscopy provides the opportunity (as yet only in the knee joint) of inspecting the inside of the joint and observing morbid anatomy, whilst synovial biopsy undertaken during arthroscopy or by closed needle biopsy can provide useful histological information on the underlying pathology.

No assessment of the chronic arthritic patient could be complete without a consideration of his capacity to undertake the basic tasks of daily living and his capacity for return to work.

RHEUMATOID ARTHRITIS (Rheumatoid Disease)

Rheumatoid arthritis is the most common form of chronic inflammatory disease affecting synovial joints. It should be seen, however, in a larger context as a multisystem disease of connective tissue which produces systemic manifestations in viscera as well as the locomotor system.

The precise aetiology is still unknown. There is a distinct familial tendency and an important recent discovery is a significant association between occurrence of the disease and an inherited tissue antigen, DRw4. The presence of an auto-antibody rheumatoid factor (which may be of the IgM or IgG class) in approximately 70 % of sufferers and the occasional identification of circulating immune complexes has led to the theory that the disease has an 'autoimmune' pathogenesis. The current prevailing view is that these features of autoimmunity are almost certainly epiphenomena triggered off by a virus yet to be isolated. The resultant synovial inflammatory response is characterised by hyperplasia, increased vascularity and a dense infiltration of lymphocytes and plasma cells, sometimes aggregated into follicles. This granulation tissue commonly known as pannus releases enzymes including collagenase, a neutral protease and lysosomal cathepsin D capable of destroying cartilage, ligament and bone. The process may result in destruction of the joint with subluxation and instability, ultimately leading to fibrous and, occasionally, bony ankylosis. A characteristic feature is the formation of the rheumatoid nodule over the ulnar aspect of the forearm and other points of pressure. Histologically, these are examples of a 'pallisading granuloma' with a central zone of connective tissue necrosis surrounded by radiating histiocytes and a peripheral zone with small round-cell infiltration.

The non-articular manifestations of the disease are explained on the basis of an arteritis occasioned by the deposition of immune complexes. This usually takes the form of a mild endarteritis but occasionally a more serious necrotising arteritis is seen. Secondary amyloid deposition may also occur in a small percentage (5–19%) of patients with rheumatoid arthritis which, with the falling prevalence of chronic sepsis, constitutes the major cause of secondary amyloid today.

Rheumatoid arthritis may affect all ethnic and geographical groups, but it is certainly more common and more severe in temperate than in tropical climates. In the UK the prevalence of adult rheumatoid disease is in the order of 1% with an annual incidence of new cases of approximately 0.02% per annum. The comparable figures for chronic juvenile arthritis are 0.06% and 0.006% per annum respectively. The adult disease is seen in between 3 and 8% of first-degree relatives of patients with the disease. There is evidence to suggest that life expectancy is reduced, particularly in those patients in whom the disease starts before the age of 45 years and those with more severe disease at the time of first diagnosis. Women are affected three times more often than men.

Clinical Features. The disease usually commences with articular symptoms, namely pain, swelling and stiffness in one or more synovial joints. The onset is usually insidious but may be acute, particularly in the aged. Classically, the joints favoured are the proximal interphalangeal joints, and metacarpophalangeal joints of the hands (the distal interphalangeal joints are usually not affected), the wrists, elbows, shoulders, hips, knees, ankles, tarsal joints and metatarsophalangeal joints. In the spine the cervical region is the only area commonly involved. Occasionally one encounters arthritis of the temporomandibular joints, the sternoclavicular joints, and even the crico-arytenoid joint may also may be affected. A typical feature of all inflammatory arthritides is the early-morning stiffness experienced by the patient on rising. The affected joints are tender, swollen and often warm and an effusion may be detected. In the hands the soft tissue swelling produces a spindling of the fingers with increased sweating of the skin and visible muscle atrophy. Involvement of weight-bearing joints causes difficulty in standing, walking and negotiating stairs. Occasionally, the disease commences in one solitary joint or two or three simultaneously, whence it may spread to become a widespread polyarthritis.

As the disease progresses unchecked, deformities commonly develop. These are seen as the characteristic ulnar deviation and flexion of the metacarpophalangeal joints, the 'swan-neck' or 'boutonnière' deformities of the fingers, fixed flexion deformities of the wrists, hip, knee and ankle, valgus deformity of the knee, hind foot and big toe and subluxation of the metatarsophalangeal joints. Subluxation of the cervical spine may occur in approximately 25% of the rheumatoid arthritis patients, either at the atlanto-axial joint (C1/C2) or lower down. This may cause compression of the cervical cord, but fortunately tetraparesis from this is surprisingly uncommon. Crico-arytenoid involvement when present may give rise to hoarseness, laryngeal discomfort or even stridor.

A common feature of knee involvement is the development of a Baker's cyst. This arises when synovial fluid under pressure is forced from the knee joint into a communicating bursa which enlarges to produce a palpable and often painful swelling in the popliteal fossa or upper calf. While often asymptomatic a Baker's cyst may rupture its contents into the tissues of the calf to produce a painful, oedematous lower extremity with a positive Homans' sign, thereby mimicking a deep vein thrombosis. Rheumatoid synovitis also commonly affects tendon sheaths and bursae, producing soft tissue swelling seen over the dorsum of the hand, the flexor aspect of the fingers, the olecranon, the deltoid region and the malleoli. Synovial swelling may give rise to compression of peripheral nerves, in particular, the median nerve of the wrist, causing a carpal tunnel syndrome. Rheumatoid arthritis may be complicated by pyogenic infection, either blood-borne or introduced at the time of an intra-articular injection through faulty technique. Suspicion of this is aroused when a single joint appears to be more actively inflamed than the remainder.

Extra-articular Manifestations. Weight loss, lethargy, anorexia, pyrexia and symptoms of anaemia may be seen in varying degrees of severity and exemplify the systemic nature of the conditions. Reactive depression not infrequently results from the pain, disability and frustration that ensues.

Subcutaneous rheumatoid nodules, most commonly seen over the ulnar border of the forearm and olecranon, over the sacrum, the fingers and in large tendons, notably the achilles, occur in one third of patients. Although unsightly and occasionally liable to infection, these are painless and cause little trouble. Their presence, however, is of diagnostic and prognostic significance, in that it helps to establish the precise diagnosis and implies a liability to more destructive joint disease and vasculitis. Patients with nodules are invariably seropositive with a high titre of rheumatoid factor. Visceral involvement may occur as a result of nodule formation, arteritis or amyloid deposition as follows:

(1) Rheumatoid nodules may form in the lung parenchyma or pleura, pericardium, myocardium or endocardium and occasionally in the meninges. Pleural and pericardial effusions are not uncommon. The latter may be complicated by cardiac tamponade or constrictive pericarditis. Nodule formation in the sclera may lead to perforation of the eye.
(2) Endarteritis of small-calibre vessels (of the order of 15 μm diameter) may develop in seropositive patients and present as an asymmetrically distributed Raynaud's phenomenon, 'nail-fold lesions' (micro-infarcts) around the margin of the fingernails, sensory neuropathy of the fingers and/or foot and episcleritis. All of these manifestations are of minor significance and tend to remit spontaneously.
(3) Necrotising arteritis is by contrast a life-threatening complication,

fortunately rare, which causes a severe sensori-motor neuropathy of the limbs, large necrotic skin ulcers of the legs, occlusion or rupture of major mesenteric or other visceral arteries.

(4) Amyloid deposition occurs in the bowel, liver, kidneys and spleen. Clinically it presents as persistent proteinuria. This progresses to nephrotic syndrome and later irreversible renal failure. The prevalence of amyloid in rheumatoid arthritis studies is approximately 5% in clinical studies and some three to four times that number on autopsy studies.

(5) 'Rheumatoid lung'. In addition to nodules and pleurisy mentioned above, fibrosing alveolitis is seen in association with rheumatoid arthritis; as is *Caplan's syndrome*, a severe form of pneumoconiosis seen in coalminers with rheumatoid arthritis.

(6) Eye involvement. In addition to the episcleritis and scleral nodule mentioned above, kerato-conjunctivitis sicca is frequently seen in association with dryness of the mouth (xerostomia) in rheumatoid arthritis, as one form of *Sjögren's syndrome*.

(7) Haemopoietic system. A normochromic normocytic anaemia as seen in other chronic inflammatory diseases is commonly present. It responds more to improvement in the disease rather than to haematinics. Hypersplenism with splenomegaly is not uncommon and may manifest as leucopenia or thrombocytopenia. This is the so-called *Felty's syndrome*, which may confer a liability to infection and the possibility of thrombocytopenic purpura.

Diagnosis. The erythrocyte sedimentation rate is raised whilst the disease remains active. Recently, it has been suggested that measurement of acute-phase proteins e.g. C-reactive protein, may be a more reliable index of disease activity. As mentioned, normochromic normocytic anaemia is a feature of the active disease, but a superimposed iron deficiency pattern should raise the suspicion of gastrointestinal blood loss, possibly the result of drug treatment.

As previously mentioned, the antiglobulin *rheumatoid factor* is present in approximately 60% of patients with established rheumatoid disease. The tests commonly in use include the *Rose–Waaler test* in which sheep red cells coated with gamma-globulin agglutinate in the presence of a patient's serum, or the *latex fixation test* in which similarly coated polystyrene particles are used. The latter tends to be more sensitive but is less specific, being positive in a variety of other conditions including bacterial endocarditis, tuberculosis and cirrhosis. The titre of rheumatoid factor tends to parallel the activity of the disease, rising with exacerbations and falling with remissions. In some patients the test is negative at the onset, later becoming positive as the condition progresses. Subsequently, when the disease becomes totally inactive, it may return to a negative state. A high titre is associated with the possible development of nodules and arteritic manifestations. Rheumatoid factor is invariably negative in the so-called seronegative arthropathies (see below), but may be positive in SLE, scleroderma and Sjögren's syndrome. A positive antinuclear factor and a positive LE cell preparation may be seen in up to 20% of patients with rheumatoid arthritis, and this occasionally causes diagnostic confusion. Such patients, however, follow the pattern of rheumatoid disease rather than SLE. Plasma electrophoresis frequently reveals an increase in the alpha-2 and gamma-globulin fractions during the active phase of the disease.

Radiography is helpful in monitoring the progress of the disease. Early features include juxta-articular osteoporosis, later leading to erosion of the articular surface and loss of joint space. Finally, total destruction of a joint may be seen with or without bony ankylosis.

Synovial fluid analysis generally reveals a loss of the normal viscosity, a cellular exudate (predominantly polymorphonuclear leucocytes) containing anything between 5000 and 60 000 cells/dl. Synovial biopsy, performed when the diagnosis is in doubt, may reveal the characteristic synovial reaction referred to above.

Treatment. Since the aetiological agent is unknown, it is not yet possible to eradicate the disease by chemotherapeutic means. Much, however, can be done to mitigate the effects of the disease. The principal aims of treatment are:

(a) to control the synovitis, thereby relieving symptoms and reducing the likelihood of erosions. This is achieved by rest, anti-inflammatory drugs, disease-modifying drugs and, where single joints are involved, by surgical or radio-isotope synovectomy.
(b) To prevent deformities by splinting inflamed joints, which would otherwise develop serious flexion contractures, e.g. hand, wrist, knee, ankle.
(c) Where irreversible damage has occurred to a joint to improve joint and muscle function by physiotherapeutic means—exercises, appropriate surgical appliances (splints, collar, caliper, corset, etc.)—and surgical means where necessary (prosthetic joint replacement).

Acute exacerbations respond to a short period of joint immobilisation by splinting in the case of a single joint, or by a short period (one week) of bed rest in the presence of a polyarthritis. The latter must be carefully supervised since bed rest carries certain risks (bed sores, deep-vein thrombosis, contractures, muscle atrophy and pneumonia) especially in the elderly or debilitated. Light resting splints are essential when joints of the hand, wrist, knee or ankle are involved if serious deformity is to be avoided. A cervical collar is helpful if the cervical spine is affected. Isometric exercises at this stage help to prevent muscle atrophy. The most actively inflamed joints may be aspirated and injected with corticosteroid, e.g. hydrocortisone acetate 25–50 mg, methylprednisolone acetate 20–40 mg or triamcinolone hexacetonide 5–20 mg, the dose depending on the size of the joint. The effect of these injections is often dramatic. The duration of benefit varies and is often prolonged, particularly with the longer-acting preparations.

Non-steroidal Anti-inflammatory Drugs (NSAIDs)

These drugs are also administered at this stage, and will continue to be required as long as the synovitis remains active, in most cases over a period of several years or even decades. It is essential, therefore, to choose the best drug for each individual patient—a process of trial and error. Many NSAIDs are now currently available. They consist of:

(1) *Aspirin*—potent, still widely used, liable to cause tinnitus, deafness and overt or occult gastrointestinal bleeding in therapeutic doses, 4–6 g in divided doses. These side-effects and the large numbers of tablets required reduces its acceptability and thereby patient compliance. Alternative formulations include enteric-coated and micro-encapsulated aloxiprin, choline magnesium trisalicylate, diflunisal, salsalate, and benorylate (an ester of aspirin with paracetamol) have proved more acceptable than soluble aspirin.
(2) *Indomethacin*—potent, but liable to cause headaches and dizziness in many patients. Long-term use may give rise to prepyloric gastric ulceration. Dose: 25–50 mg 3 times daily. A suppository (100 mg) is available for night use and helps to control morning stiffness. Sulindac is a chemically related preparation which has fewer side-effects.
(3) *Phenylbutazone*. This is pyrazole which may cause fluid retention, gastric ulceration and bone-marrow depression, particularly with long-term use. It is, therefore, suitable only for short-term use for acute exacerbation. In the UK this drug is only available for hospital-treated patients with ankylosing spondylitis. The chemically related preparation azapropazone is less toxic.
(4) The *propionic acid derivatives*—ibuprofen (400–600 mg t.d.s.), naproxen (250 mg in the morning, 500 mg at night), ketoprofen (50 mg t.d.s.), fenoprofen (300–600 mg t.d.s.), flurbiprofen (50 mg q.d.s.), indoprofen (200 mg t.d.s.) and fenbufen (600–900 mg once daily).
(5) The *aryl–acetic acid derivatives*—fenclofenac, diclofenac and tiaprofenic acid.
(6) *Miscellaneous*—tolmetin, a pyrrole derivative, and piroxicam (20 mg once daily), an oxicam derivative.

By and large, all the drugs listed in groups 4–6 have been shown in clinical trials to be comparable in terms of efficacy with the older drugs (groups 1–3). They are undoubtedly better tolerated, although rashes occur. Gastric intolerance is common and occasionally gastric haemorrhage may be seen. They should be used with extreme caution in the elderly, patients suffering from known peptic ulceration, those on anticoagulants, and should all be avoided in pregnancy. All the newer preparations are more expensive than the earlier ones. With few exceptions their mode of action is believed to be by inhibition of prostaglandin synthetase. Their use is applicable in other forms of inflammatory joint disease, including acute gout. They may also be helpful in degenerative joint disease and soft tissue lesions when symptoms merit their use.

Disease Modifying Agents in Rheumatoid Disease (DMARDs)

These drugs are introduced as second line drugs where NSAIDs have failed to control joint inflammation and/or where erosions have developed on X-ray. They include gold salts, d-penicillamine, chloroquine, immunosuppressive and immunopotentiating drugs and corticosteroids.

(a) *Gold.* Injections of sodium aurothiomalate are given by weekly IM injections of 50 mg (after a test dose of 10 mg) until a total of 1 g has been given. If by the end of that time a favourable response is seen, treatment is continued indefinitely on a monthly basis, providing that side-effects are not forthcoming. Skin reactions are common and may be severe. Temporary suspension of the injections is recommended. Many patients, however, are subsequently able to resume the course. Proteinuria should be looked for at each attendance and injections are not given if it is present. Gold nephropathy is a rare complication which may lead to nephrotic syndrome. Gold should be withdrawn, but even so, it may take a year before the kidney recovers. Of greatest importance is the liability to bone-marrow depression which may lead to serious (even fatal) aplastic anaemia. Fortunately, this is rare but thrombocytopenia alone is more common. These haematological complications can only be prevented by careful and regular monitoring of blood and platelet counts preferably before each injection. With these precautions gold salts have proved themselves over a half century to be a useful and effective means of suppressing rheumatoid synovitis. Gold-induced remissions are accompanied by an improvement in systemic features. Its mode of action is still uncertain.

(b) *D-penicillamine.* This drug has been introduced for the treatment of rheumatoid arthritis in the past decade and has been shown in trials to be equivalent to gold in its efficacy, though similar and serious side-effects do occur. These include rashes, proteinuria (with nephrotic syndrome), loss of taste (which is transient), abdominal symptoms and thrombocytopenia (rarely aplastic anaemia). Like gold its effect does not become apparent until 3–6 months after starting treatment. It has the advantage of being administered orally. Experience has shown that a 'go low, go slow' policy of dosage is safer—125 mg daily as the starting dose rising by 125 mg per day at monthly intervals until a satisfactory remission has occurred. It is rarely necessary (or advisable) to exceed 750 mg daily.

(c) *Chloroquine.* This antimalarial drug was introduced in the 1950s for rheumatoid arthritis. It has somewhat fallen out of favour owing to its propensity for causing retinal damage. It should only be used if facilities are available for an ophthalmological examination at 6-monthly intervals.

(d) *Immunosuppressive drugs*, which include azathioprine, chlorambucil and cyclophosphamide are mainly used to treat the serious arteritic complications. This is because of their tendency to serious side-effects including bone-marrow depression. The immunopotentiating drug levamisole, which is an antihelminthic agent has recently been shown to be effective in rheumatoid arthritis. However, it too poses problems of serious adverse effects and has largely been abandoned.

(e) *Corticosteroids*. Oral corticosteroids are now rarely used in the treatment of rheumatoid arthritis owing to the cumulative side-effects—osteoporosis, skin atrophy, peptic ulceration, steroid myopathy, steroid cataracts and suppression of the hypophyseal–pituitary–adrenal axis. If they are to be used at all, it should be a very minimal dose, e.g. 5–7.5 mg prednisolone daily. It has been shown that alternate day therapy is less harmful, particularly in children where suppression of growth is an additional hazard.

Synovectomy

Persistent refractory inflammation in a single joint may be treated by synovectomy—removal of the synovial membrane—by either medical or surgical means. In either case, relief of pain and stiffness and restoration of movement is achieved, although relapse may occur subsequently. Medical synovectomy is obtained by the intra-articular injection of a radio-isotope, e.g. $Yttrium^{90}$ in colloidal form. The isotope is taken up by the synovial cells and the membrane is thereby ablated by the ionising radiation (beta particles). This form of treatment is reserved for patients over the age of 45, on account of the (theoretical) risk of oncogenesis.

Surgical synovectomy is the surgical excision of the synovial membrane as far as this is possible, and it is most widely used in the knee and small finger joints. Postoperative stiffness of the joint is a hazard, which usually responds to manipulation under anaesthetic and vigorous physiotherapy.

Other Surgical Measures

Total joint destruction may be treated either by arthrodesis (still widely practised in the wrist, big toe and thumb joints), or total joint replacement in those joints where a satisfactory prosthesis is available. This is most successful in the hip joint where the Charnley type of low-friction arthroplasty (metal on plastic) is the most widely used. Many total knee prostheses are now available and prostheses are available for the shoulder, elbow, ankle and the MCP and PIP joints of the hands. In other joints attempts at joint replacement have been less successful. The main problems of joint replacement are inadequate facilities for carrying out all the operations that need to be undertaken, and the complications of infection and/or loosening of the prosthesis which may require it to be removed. Subluxation of the cervical spine which causes cord compression requires cervical fusion.

Rehabilitation

Total management of the patient with rheumatoid arthritis requires a team approach in which specialist medical and nursing skills are supplemented by those of the trained physiotherapist, occupational therapist and medical social worker. Careful assessment of the patient's ability to cope with daily living, together with monitoring of progress, enables realistic goals to be set for the patient to return to as full and active a life as possible. Skills lost as a result of the ravages of the disease may be restored partly by retraining and partly by adapting the environment to the needs of the handicapped patient. Both home and work environments need to be considered and it is essential that both the patient and his family and employer be put into the picture in order to achieve an optimal result.

THE SERONEGATIVE SPONDARTHRITIDES

This group of chronic arthritic conditions is characterised by the absence of rheumatoid factor in the serum, the absence of nodules, a largely asymmetrical distribution of peripheral joint involvement and a tendency towards bilateral sacro-iliitis progressing, in some cases, to a picture of ankylosing spondylitis. The presence of spinal disease is commonly associated with the tissue antigen HLA B27. Despite this important hereditary factor the precise aetiological agent responsible for these diseases is as yet unknown.

ANKYLOSING SPONDYLITIS

This disease predominantly affects young men and has a prevalence of approximately 1 per 1000 of the population. Recent epidemiological studies suggest that it may be considerably more common than this. This condition has a predilection for synovial joints of the vertebral column, commencing in the sacro-iliac joints and spreading cranially. Larger peripheral joints may also be affected. HLA B27 is present in 90–95 % of cases compared with 5–10 % in the normal population. Recent evidence suggests that *Klebsiella pneumoniae* may be an important pathogen in this disease, but this is as yet unconfirmed. Although the synovial histopathological reaction is similar to that seen in rheumatoid arthritis, the tendency is for bony ankylosis to occur. Syndesmophytes or bony bridges form between adjacent vertebrae and ultimately the facet joints, intervertebral discs and ligaments ossify, giving rise to the classical radiological appearance of the 'bamboo spine'.

Clinical Features. Persistent low back pain with morning stiffness in the young adult male is the classical presentation. Imperceptibly progressive loss of spinal movement occurs with flattening of the lumbar spine, dorsal kyphosis and a compensatory cervical hyperlordosis. Loss of chest expansion results from costovertebral joint involvement. As the spinal deformity develops the patient tends to adopt a hyperextension of the hips in order to maintain his centre of gravity. Symptoms may be so mild that the condition remains undiagnosed until advanced or it may be ascribed in error to intervertebral disc disease or psychogenic backache. On occasion, the pain may be severe, particularly at night, waking the patient in the early hours. Pain and limitation of movement in the hip joints and shoulders and/or effusions in the knees indicate peripheral joint involvement which adds to the disability imposed by an increasingly rigid spine. Enthesopathies (tender lesions at the site of tendinous insertions, e.g. plantar fasciitis) are common, and alternating sciatic pain may occur as well as discomfort around the thoracic cage.

A tendency to recurrent, acute iritis occurs in 20% of cases. A normochromic normocytic anaemia is common during active phases of the disease, which may be aggravated by gastrointestinal blood loss caused by NSAIDs. Amyloid deposition (see above) is said to occur in 6% of patients coming to necropsy. Rarely, cardiac involvement with conduction defects (e.g. complete heart block) and/or aortic incompetence occur from aortitis. A bilateral upper lobe fibrosis of the lungs has been reported in this condition.

Diagnosis. The diagnosis is based on the clinical history and examination and is confirmed by the radiological appearance of the spine, notably the sacro-iliac joints (blurring of the joint margins, sclerosis, erosion and ultimately ankylosis) and the vertebral bodies (formation of syndesmophytes, squaring of the vertebrae and ultimately the appearance of the 'bamboo spine'). The sedimentation rate and C-reactive protein is raised while the disease remains active.

Treatment. The aim is to relieve pain and stiffness by the application of non-steroidal anti-inflammatory drugs, which permit the patient to take part in vigorous physiotherapy necessary to restore and maintain the spinal mobility and to prevent flexion deformity of the spine. The patient is encouraged to lie prone as much as possible and to practise mobilising exercises daily for the rest of his life. The DMARDs are ineffective, corticosteroids are contraindicated owing to the risk of osteoporosis, and deep X-ray therapy (formerly used widely to relieve pain and stiffness) is now no longer used owing to the increased risk of leukaemia. Total hip replacement is indicated in the presence of advanced hip-joint destruction and spinal osteotomy is occasionally used in the presence of severe spinal deformity. Acute iritis is treated along conventional lines by local corticosteroid drops and mydriatics.

PSORIATIC ARTHRITIS

Arthritis associated with psoriasis may take one of the following forms:

(a) A widespread polyarthritis typically involving the distal interphalangeal joints, the interphalangeal joints of the thumb and great toe as well as larger joints.
(b) A severe mutilating arthritis affecting the hands causing widespread osteolysis as well as total destruction of the small finger joints.
(c) A polyarthritis which from the point of view of distribution is indistinguishable from rheumatoid arthritis. This is the most common variety. It does, however, pursue a more benign course, though erosions do occur. Rheumatoid nodules and rheumatoid factor are, of course, absent.
(d) Sacro-iliitis progressing in many cases to a picture of ankylosing spondylitis.

Treatment. The general principles are similar to those adopted for rheumatoid arthritis. Because of the more benign nature of the condition, drug treatment is usually limited to the NSAIDs. In more severe cases gold injections, methotrexate and razoxane may be effective, but D-penicillamine is ineffective and oral corticosteroids are rarely indicated.

REACTIVE ARTHRITIS

This term denotes the development of arthritis in a patient suffering from an infective process elsewhere in the body (usually in the gastrointestinal or genital tracts), but without evidence of infection in the joint itself. It occurs almost exclusively in patients showing the tissue antigen HLA B27 who develop enteric infection with *Salmonella, Shigella, Yersinia* or *Campylobacter* organisms. It may also occur as sexually acquired reactive arthritis (SARA), and there is evidence to suggest that the offending organism here may be *Chlamydia trachomatis*, though this remains to be confirmed.

Reiter's Syndrome, originally described as a triad of urethritis, conjunctivitis and arthritis, but often presenting additional features including balanitis circinate or sicca, keratoderma blennorrhagica, uveitis, aortitis, sacro-iliitis and ankylosing spondylitis. It has long been known that Reiter's syndrome may complicate sexually acquired nonspecific urethritis or dysentery, but living micro-organisms have never been isolated from the affected joints. For this reason Reiter's syndrome is now classified as a form of reactive arthritis.

Acute rheumatic fever can be considered as a reactive arthritis and is considered on p. 171.

ARTHRITIS ASSOCIATED WITH BOWEL DISEASE

An inflammatory polyarthritis may occur in patients suffering from ulcerative colitis, Crohn's disease and Whipple's disease. This tends to be a recurrent, acute or persistent affection of large, predominantly lower limb joints. By and large, the activity of the arthritis mirrors that of the underlying intestinal disease.

In addition some 18% of patients suffering from inflammatory bowel disease will develop sacro-iliitis, approximately one half of whom proceed to the full picture of ankylosing spondylitis. In these circumstances the activity and progression of the spinal disease appears to bear no temporal relationship to the activity of the underlying bowel condition.

BEHÇET'S SYNDROME

A subacute or chronic arthritis with a predilection for knee joint involvement, but with occasional involvement of the axial skeleton, is seen in association with buccal and genital ulceration and uveitis in Behçet's syndrome.

INFLAMMATORY DISORDERS OF CONNECTIVE TISSUE

The group of diseases included under this heading (formerly referred to as the collagen diseases) include systemic lupus erythematosus (SLE), polyarteritis nodosa, dermatomyositis and polymyositis and scleroderma (systemic sclerosis). The members of this group have a number of features in common, namely, abnormal immunological reactivity, multi-system involvement, a (variable) therapeutic response to corticosteroids and a usually unremittent course. Overlap syndromes do occur.

SYSTEMIC LUPUS ERYTHEMATOSUS (SLE)

This is a multi-system disease with protean manifestations. It is nine times more common in women than in men, with an onset during the child-bearing years, though occasional onset during childhood or advanced age occurs. It appears to be much more common in negroes than caucasians and a familial tendency is seen.

Pathology. Widespread fibrinoid deposition (containing gammaglobulin and fibrin, together with complement) is seen throughout the body, notably in relation to small arterioles and capillaries, in connective tissue and in serous membranes. These changes are almost certainly due to the deposition of immune complexes which, particularly in the kidney, is an important pathogenetic mechanism. A wide variety of humoral antibodies is encountered in the serum. These include antinuclear antibodies, directed against a variety of nuclear constituents native and single-stranded DNA, DNA-histone (detected in the LE cell preparation), double-stranded ribonucleoprotein (RNP) and Sm antigen. In addition, both IgG and IgM rheumatoid factors and a biological false positive test for syphilis (BFP) are found in approximately one third of patients. Serum complement levels (C3, C4 and total haemolytic complement) are lowered, particularly in the presence of renal involvement, and cryoglobulins and antibodies directed against erythrocytes (detected by the Coombs test), leucocytes, lymphocytes and platelets are widely seen. Circulating anticoagulants are found in up to 10% of patients. In addition, there is also evidence of impaired cellular immunity in SLE, resulting from an impairment of suppressor T-lymphocyte activity. A possible viral aetiology responsible for the immunological abnormalities is likely, but as yet no viral agent has been identified. An SLE-like illness occurs in some patients treated with hydralazine, penicillamine, procainamide, practolol, isoniazid and anticonvulsant drugs. In patients so afflicted renal involvement is absent and complete recovery is seen on withdrawal of the offending drug.

Clinical Features. These are considered under the following headings:

(a) *General.* Fever, malaise, anorexia and weight loss are common.

(b) *Skin.* The classical rash of SLE is the erythema seen typically in the 'butterfly' region of the cheeks and bridge of the nose but also elsewhere, particularly areas exposed to ultraviolet light to which the skin in this condition is particularly sensitive. Other skin lesions include urticaria, peri-ungual erythema and cutaneous vasculitis. Alopecia is a frequent feature limited to SLE within this group of conditions.

(c) *Joints.* A symmetrical peripheral polyarthritis affecting predominantly small finger joints and reminiscent of rheumatoid arthritis is a common finding. Ulnar deviation of the hands may occur but erosions are characteristically absent. Subcutaneous nodules are uncommon.

(d) *Tenosynovitis.* Tenosynovitis may occur in the hands and *aseptic necrosis* of the femoral head (osteonecrosis) is a common finding even in the absence of corticosteroid treatment.

(e) *Respiratory System.* Pleurisy with effusion is common, and parenchymal pulmonary involvement (pneumonitis) may be seen. Diffuse pulmonary fibrosis is less common.

(f) *Cardiovascular System.* Raynaud's phenomenon may be a presenting symptom. Pericarditis with effusion, myocarditis and verrucose (Libman–Sacks) endocarditis may all occur.

(g) *Kidney.* Renal involvement occurs in most patients, although in only half is it clinically significant. It may take the form of thickening of the glomerular basement membrane, a proliferative glomerulitis and fibrinoid change. Presentation is with proteinuria which may be heavy and lead to nephrotic syndrome and be associated with hypertension and renal failure. Clues to the ultimate prognosis may be gleaned from renal biopsy, examined by immunofluorescence, light and electron microscopy.

(h) *Haemopoietic and Reticuloendothelial Systems.* Anaemia (often haemolytic), neutropenia and thrombocytopenia are common events and may be severe. Hepatosplenomegaly and lymphadenopathy are commonly seen.

(i) *Gastrointestinal Tract.* Sjögren's syndrome may be present and abdominal pain and diarrhoea occasionally occur due to intestinal arteritis, pancreatitis or peritonism. Significant involvement of the liver does not occur and the formally styled 'lupoid hepatitis' formerly thought to be a feature of SLE is now termed 'chronic active hepatitis' and considered to be a separate entity (see p. 111).

(j) *Central Nervous System.* Brain involvement is now known to be one of the most common features, presenting as a neuropsychiatric disorder, convulsions, hemiplegia, cranial nerve lesions, cerebellar disorder or aseptic meningitis. Transverse myelitis may also occur. Conventional neurological investigations (angiography, brain and CT scanning) are generally unhelpful. EEG may show a non-specific diffuse abnormality. By contrast, oxygen^{15} scanning appears to be a promising marker.

(k) *Eye.* Retinal haemorrhages and exudates are common but major ocular disturbances are rare.

Diagnosis is based on the above-mentioned clinical features. The LE cell preparation has been largely replaced by the antinuclear antibody immunofluorescent test, which is present in virtually all cases, though it is not specific for the disease (see above). The DNA binding test for double-stranded (native) DNA is a more specific indicator of SLE though it may be negative during inactive phases of the disease. It may therefore be used as an index of disease activity, and in this context is a more reliable pointer than the sedimentation rate which is often markedly elevated in this condition.

Prognosis. There has been a remarkable improvement in the prognosis of this disease in recent years, due in part to the wider (and earlier) recognition of this condition and part due to the greater restraint in the use of corticosteroids for treatment. The five-year survival has virtually doubled in the last twenty-five years and is now over 90%.

Treatment. NSAIDs are valuable in the treatment of the articular complaints, while antimalarials are also capable of suppressing the disease, particularly in those patients with skin and joint involvement. Severe manifestations are treated by oral corticosteroids, sometimes supplemented by immunosuppressive drugs, e.g. azathioprine or cyclophosphamide. These drugs undoubtedly carry a morbidity and mortality in their own right and should be used with extreme caution and prudence. Recent evidence suggests that low-dose prednisolone (7.5 mg daily) is a more satisfactory treatment than high dose (over 30 mg daily) even for mild renal and brain involvement.

POLYARTERITIS NODOSA (PAN)

This disorder is characterised by a necrotising arteritis of small and medium-sized vessels, thought to be due to the deposition of as yet unidentified immune complexes. Hepatitis-associated antigen has been found in the serum and in the lesions of patients with polyarteritis, which suggests that serum hepatitis virus may be participating in the pathogenesis. The arteritic lesions are widely disseminated throughout the body and may lead to aneurysm formation, rupture and haemorrhage, thrombosis and, ultimately, recanalisation. A rare variant of PAN is Wegener's granulomatosis—a locally destructive granuloma affecting the nasal passages and upper and lower respiratory tract which may be associated with glomerulonephritis.

Clinical Features. Males predominate with an incidence rising with age. Features include fever, weight loss, hypertension, tachycardia, gangrene on the extremities, asthma, pneumonitis, an acute abdomen (due to mesenteric arteritis), proteinuria and renal failure, arthralgia and myalgia, cutaneous vasculitis and peripheral neuropathy of the mononeuritis multiplex type. In addition, focal brain and spinal-cord involvement and ocular vascular accidents complete the truly protean nature of the disease.

Diagnosis. There are no specific laboratory tests for PAN. Serological tests such as the ANA and the rheumatoid factor are usually negative. Confirmation is usually obtained histologically by muscle, skin, kidney or nerve biopsy. Hepatic or renal arteriography may reveal multiple small aneurysms which are said to be diagnostic of this condition.

Prognosis. Depends on the distribution of organ involvement.

Treatment. High-dose corticosteroids (prednisolone 40–80 mg daily) is generally recommended initially with a view to slowly reducing and eventually withdrawing the drug in the light of the subsequent progress. Use of the immunosuppressive drugs may be helpful.

GIANT CELL (TEMPORAL) ARTERITIS

Pathology and Aetiology. This is a granulomatous form of arteritis affecting predominantly the branches of the external carotid artery, notably the temporal and facial arteries, and certain branches, notably the ophthalmic, of the internal carotid artery. Only occasionally are arteries emanating from the aorta, e.g. coronary arteries, involved. A possible immunological mechanism has been suggested by the finding of increased cellular immune responses by lymphocytes from patients with this condition to constituents of the arterial wall. The condition is predominantly seen in middle and old age.

Clinical Features. The common presentation is with pain in the head and face due to ischaemia and intermittent claudication of the muscles of mastication has been reported. The temporal arteries are characteristically thickened, tender and pulseless and the overlying scalp may be reddened and occasionally frankly gangrenous. Other modes of presentation include sudden visual failure due to ophthalmic artery thrombosis and polymyalgia rheumatica (see p. 433).

Diagnosis. The sedimentation rate is invariably elevated, often markedly so. Since the arteritis may be distributed patchily, the temporal arteries may be normal on palpation, and where doubt exists it is prudent to perform a temporal artery biopsy. The characteristic features are thickening of the media with infiltration by inflammatory cells including giant cells and intimal proliferation leading to gross narrowing of the lumen. The condition should be suspected in particular in elderly patients suffering from (often vague) headaches or rheumatic symptoms in the presence of a raised ESR.

Treatment. Oral corticosteroid treatment is indicated as soon as the diagnosis is made in order to prevent blindness, since this is irreversible. Prednisolone 40–60 mg a day may be required to bring the condition under control, the dose being tapered in response to the fall in the sedimentation rate. Long-term surveillance is essential if relapse is to be avoided. The condition may remain active for months or years.

Pulseless Disease

Brief mention is made of *Takayasu's disease* which is an arteritis affecting branches of the aorta near their origin. It is seen chiefly in young women and is also associated with a raised sedimentation rate. It is also responsive to corticosteroid treatment.

SCLERODERMA (Systemic Sclerosis, SS)

This uncommon condition is characterised by an excessive deposition of collagen in the dermis and in the viscera, notably, the gastrointestinal tract, together with a small-vessel arteritis involving, in particular, the extremities.

The cause is unknown, but it is relatively more common among miners. The finding of antinuclear antibodies and other features of altered immunity in approximately one half of patients suggests a possible immunological pathogenetic mechanism.

Clinical Features. It is three times more common in women than in men. The onset is often insidious and Raynaud's phenomenon may antedate other symptoms by several years. Pain and stiffness in the small joints and tendon sheaths is a common early symptom. Gradually the skin of the distal extremities becomes thickened, tethered and rigid, inhibiting movement. This progress gradually extends proximally and may envelop the whole body. Puckering of the mouth leads to a characteristic appearance. Calcinotic nodules appear over the fingertips and pressure areas. Telangiectasia are seen on the skin of the extremities, face and on the tongue. Joint and tendon-sheath involvement causes pain and additional stiffness and flexion deformities of the fingers. A palpable crepitus is a feature of tenosynovitis of the wrist. Tapering of the fingers is due to osteolysis occasioned by ischaemia. Muscle involvement also commonly occurs, although this may be mild.

Gastrointestinal involvement occurs in 70% of patients. The most common manifestation is in the oesophagus, where a loss of peristalsis results in dysphagia which may be severe. Small-bowel involvement may give rise to malabsorption, which may be aggravated by bacterial overgrowth. A rare complication is the presence of collections of gas in the intestinal wall (pneumatosis intestinalis). Co-existent primary biliary sclerosis or chronic active hepatitis may be seen. Colonic involvement is common but usually asymptomatic. Occasionally distension or perforation may occur.

Pulmonary fibrosis occasionally progressing to 'honeycomb lung' is common, though it may be asymptomatic in the initial stages. In the heart, pericarditis and myocardial fibrosis may be present. A variety of ECG changes is seen including arrhythmias and heart block. Frank renal involvement tends to lead to a rapidly progressive spiral of hypertension and renal failure. Central nervous system involvement does not occur but trigeminal neuropathy has been described. Sjögren's syndrome may occur in association with scleroderma.

Diagnosis. The ESR is raised in two thirds of patients while one third give a positive test for rheumatoid factor. Antinuclear antibody is present in over 50%. Characteristic changes in the skin biopsy include increased dermal collagen, a thinning of the epidermis and a loss of the normal appendages.

Prognosis. In the absence of major organ involvement scleroderma may pursue a relatively benign though progressive course. Over 70% survive five years. In the presence of lung but no heart or kidney involvement, or heart but no kidney involvement, the corresponding figures are 50 and 30%. Renal involvement imposes usually a less than one-year survival. 'Diffuse scleroderma', i.e. widespread skin involvement including the trunk, is usually associated with major organ involvement and a poorer prognosis whereas the CREST syndrome (calcinosis, Raynaud's, oesophageal, sclerodactyly and telangiectasia) carries a more favourable outlook. It has recently been shown that anticentromere antibodies are common in this subgroup.

Treatment. There is no really effective treatment for this disorder. D-penicillamine has been used and is helpful with regard to the skin condition if instituted early. Corticosteroids are of little benefit except in relieving the rheumatic symptoms which are probably better treated by NSAIDs. Raynaud's phenomenon and digital ischaemia have been treated by intra-arterial reserpine and a variety of other vaso-active drugs, but with limited success. Cervical sympathectomy, plasmapheresis and hyperbaric oxygen give only limited and transient relief. Cardiac pulmonary, renal and gastrointestinal symptoms are treated on their own merits along conventional lines.

DERMATOMYOSITIS AND POLYMYOSITIS

This is an inflammatory disorder of striated muscle of unknown aetiology, which presents with weakness of the limbs and trunk, respiratory difficulties, dysphagia and diplopia. The term dermatomyositis denotes an additional skin involvement, notably the heliotrope eruption around the eyelids, peri-ungual erythema, an inflammatory oedema of the skin causing induration and later atrophy, collodion patches and subcutaneous calcinosis. Other features include Raynaud's phenomenon, arthralgia and arthritis, cardiac failure and occasionally, pulmonary fibrosis.

An association between malignancy and both dermatomyositis and polymyositis is generally accepted. Carcinoma of the lung, prostate, uterus, ovary, breast and large bowel are the most common tumours.

Diagnosis is confirmed by typical EMG changes, histological evidence of degeneration of muscle fibres, regeneration and chronic inflammatory infiltration on muscle biopsy. The serum creatine phosphokinase is elevated. The ESR may be mildly elevated or normal in the presence of active disease and serological tests are unhelpful.

Treatment. Oral corticosteroids [dose prednisolone 40–60 mg (occasionally more) daily initially] are used to suppress the disease and are usually effective. The addition of methotrexate, azathioprine, or cyclophosphamide may be helpful in resistant cases. During acute phases the patient is treated with bed rest with appropriate splinting to avoid contractures and deformities. Even in the absence of an associated malignancy the prognosis may be poor, particularly in older subjects with heart or lung complications.

Overlap Syndromes

Not infrequently clinical features of two or more of the inflammatory disorders of connective tissue are seen in the same patient, causing diagnostic difficulty. A particular subset, called 'mixed connective tissue disease' has been identified by the presence in the serum of antibodies to extractable nuclear antigen (ribonucleoprotein (RNP) component).

METABOLIC ARTHRITIS, GOUT, PSEUDOGOUT AND OCHRONOSIS

Acute synovitis may be provoked by the liberation into the joint cavity of microcrystals—monosodium urate monohydrate in the case of gout and calcium pyrophosphate dihydrate in pseudogout.

GOUT (p. 505)

The concentration of urate in plasma and body fluids represents a fine balance between production and excretion. Owing to the limited solubility of urate, its accumulation (recognised as hyperuricaemia—plasma urate in excess of 0.5 mmol/l) leads to precipitation of crystals, particularly in joints, subcutaneous tissues and in the renal collecting system. This may arise as a result of increased de novo purine synthesis, from excessive intake of high purine foods or from excessive catabolism of nucleoproteins as occurs in the myeloproliferative disorders, leukaemia, myeloma and polycythaemia rubra vera (secondary hyperuricaemia), particularly when these conditions are treated by cytotoxic agents. Failure of the kidney to excrete urate, as in renal failure, or tubular retention of urate, as occurs with certain drugs, e.g. oral diuretics and pyrazinamide, also results in accumulation.

Gout occurs in approximately one third of patients with hyperuricaemia, the risk increasing with the height of the urate level. Gouty subjects tend to be obese, hypertensive and regular drinkers of alcohol. There is also an association with hyperlipidaemia and coronary artery disease. There is a strong familial tendency; the pattern of inheritance suggests a multifactorial aetiology. Other conditions in which hyperuricaemia is seen include chronic lead poisoning, toxaemia of pregnancy, starvation, hyperparathyroidism, hypothyroidism, mongolism and glycogen storage disease. Urate deposits are seen as tophi in and around joints and bursae, in cartilage such as the pinnae, over bony prominences and (rarely) in the kidney. Renal changes are those of hypertension with nephrosclerosis and interstitial nephritis. Urate calculi may be seen in a proportion of patients.

Clinical Features. Acute self-limiting attacks of arthritis favouring the first metatarsophalangeal joints, but occurring in others too, is the classical presentation of gout. These may be associated with pyrexia, leucocytosis and an elevated sedimentation rate. Spontaneous remission (if the attack has not been aborted by medical treatment) occurs within a week in most patients, though a migratory polyarthritis is sometimes seen. The natural history is for recurrent acute attacks to occur with increasing frequency, and eventually, a chronic deforming arthropathy may result from tophus formation. These may discharge releasing a chalky material, composed of urate crystals, and readily identified as such by microscopic examination or chemical analysis. Despite hypertension, proteinuria and mild renal impairment gout does not usually reduce longevity.

Diagnosis. Clinical diagnosis is confirmed by the finding of hyperuricaemia and the identification of urate crystals seen on polarising microscopy as negatively birefringent needles within synovial fluid polymorphs. X-rays are normal in the early stages, but eventually punched-out areas caused by the tophi are seen in relation to the chronically affected joints.

Treatment. Acute gouty episodes respond to oral colchicine (0.5 mg 4-hourly until relief or diarrhoea ensues!) or full doses of indomethacin. The newer NSAIDs constitute a promising and better tolerated alternative. An intra-articular steroid injection often aborts an attack. Systemic steroids are reserved only for the most intractable cases.

In the face of recurrent acute attacks it is justified to institute hypouricaemic drugs—probenecid or sulphinpyrazone which are uricosuric agents promoting the excretion of urate, or allopurinol, which is a xanthine-oxidase inhibitor which curtails urate synthesis by blocking the last stage of the pathway. All these drugs require to be taken indefinitely and patient compliance may be a problem. Their institution may result in a temporary exacerbation of acute attacks during the first few months and it is wise, therefore, to cover this period by the concurrent administration of an anti-inflammatory drug. Allopurinol is the drug of choice in the presence of renal failure, renal stones or overproduction of uric acid, particularly when cytotoxic drugs are used to treat malignant disease. The usual daily dose is 300 mg. It is adjusted by monitoring the serum urate level. Smaller doses are required in patients with renal failure.

PSEUDOGOUT

This a disorder principally seen in elderly subjects and is rarely encountered in early life. It occurs as a result of calcium pyrophosphate deposition in cartilage (chondrocalcinosis) which in most patients appears to be a feature of ageing of cartilage. In a few patients it is a manifestation of a metabolic disorder, e.g. hyperparathyroidism or haemochromatosis. A familial variety has been recorded.

Clinical Features. Recurrent acute episodes of arthritis occur predominantly in the larger joints, knee, wrist, etc. resembling urate gout, and following a similar self-limiting course. Occasionally polyarticular involvement occurs and a destructive arthropathy may be seen.

Diagnosis. The sedimentation rate may be elevated during an attack, but other blood investigations are normal (except when there is an associated metabolic disorder). X-ray examination will reveal fine stippling of chondrocalcinosis seen in the fibrocartilage—menisci of the knee or wrist joints—or as a fine line within the articular cartilage of involved joints. Chondrocalcinosis is a common finding in elderly subjects, only a small percentage of whom suffer from pseudogout. It should not be assumed, therefore, that the presence of chondrocalcinosis is pathognomonic of pseudogout. Confirmation of this diagnosis can only be made satisfactorily by identifying the intraleucocytic crystals of calcium pyrophosphate on polarising microscopic examination of synovial fluid aspirated from an affected joint. These crystals (unlike those of gout) are oblong in shape and are weakly positively birefringent.

Treatment. Acute attacks are treated by resting the affected joint and the administration of NSAIDs. An intra-articular steroid injection is helpful in aborting an attack. There is no known means whereby the deposited articular calcification can be removed. Even treatment of an associated metabolic disorder, e.g. removing a parathyroid adenoma in hyperparathyroidism or venesection in haemochromatosis, fails to halt the progression of the chondrocalcinosis.

OCHRONOSIS

This inborn error of metabolism is due to an absence of the enzyme homogentisic acid oxidase which results in deposition in connective tissues, notably cartilage, of polymerised homogentisic acid. The resultant premature degeneration of cartilage results in destructive changes in the intervertebral discs and larger peripheral joints. The disc spaces become extremely narrowed with sclerosis of vertebral plates. The result is a severe loss of spinal movement. In the peripheral joints, the features are those of severe osteoarthritis. The condition is diagnosed by the detection of homogentisic acid in the urine, which classically turns black on standing or when alkali is added.

INFECTIVE ARTHRITIS

Invasion of a synovial joint by pathogenic micro-organisms occurs in a wide variety of infections caused by viruses, bacteria and fungi. For practical purposes, the most important infections are those due to pyogenic bacteria, including the *Staphylococcus, Streptococcus, Gonococcus, Meningococcus, Pneumococcus, coliform bacillus, Salmonella,*

Haemophilus, *Brucella* and *M. tuberculosis*. Spread to the joint is usually via the blood stream, though direct invasion may occur from adjacent osteomyelitis, or when organisms are inadvertently introduced into the joint during aspiration procedures or surgical operations.

VIRUS INFECTIONS

A symmetrical self-limiting polyarthritis occurs in *rubella* about the time that the rash develops, and it is particularly common in young, adult female subjects suffering from this condition. A similar complication is seen after rubella immunisation with live attenuated virus. Arthritis is occasionally seen in other virus conditions including mumps, chickenpox, smallpox, infectious mononucleosis and infective hepatitis. In some of these conditions the arthritis is due to the presence of live virus within the joint, in others it appears to be due to the deposition of immune complexes.

BACTERIAL ARTHRITIS

Involvement of one or more joints may arise in the presence of bacteraemia in the course of an infection from a wide variety of bacteria (see above). A focus of infection elsewhere in the body would be an important clue to this diagnosis. However, any patient with an acute monarthritis should be suspected of suffering from bacterial arthritis, particularly in the presence of unexplained fever, until proved otherwise. Bacterial endocarditis may present with this manifestation. Rheumatoid arthritis sufferers are particularly prone to secondary bacterial joint infection.

The only way to confirm (or exclude) this diagnosis with certainty is to obtain a sample of synovial fluid by aspiration of the affected joint and submit it to full bacteriological examination including Gram staining of the smear and culture. This procedure has the added advantage of permitting antibiotic sensitivities to be undertaken and correct therapy to be instituted.

Undiagnosed (and therefore untreated) bacterial arthritis may rapidly lead to total destruction of the joint—a sad affair in a condition so readily amenable to treatment.

In *gonococcal arthritis* a febrile illness is seen, particularly in female subjects presenting with fever and oligoarthritis, or migratory polyarthritis, and tenosynovitis in association with a widespread skin eruption composed of macules, petechiae, vesicles or pustules.

Though arthralgia is a common event in *brucellosis*, attention is drawn to a true arthritis, usually monarticular, and favouring the hip or knee joint. Spondylitis may also occur.

Tuberculous infection frequently occurs in bone, notably the spine, where it may give rise to serious destructive changes and compression of the spinal cord. Peripheral joint involvement may also occur, particularly in the knee or hip with pain and gradual loss of mobility. Severe destructive changes are seen on X-ray. Other manifestations include tenosynovitis, particularly involving the flexor tendon sheaths at the wrist, and tuberculous dactylitis which presents as a painless swelling in relation to a metatarsal or metacarpal bone.

Treatment of Infective Arthritis. Rational treatment will depend on identifying the precise aetiological agent involved, and no amount of effort should be spared to this end. It is important to emphasise that where bacteriological culture is concerned appropriate examinations should be carried out expeditiously and before antibiotic treatment is instituted, otherwise negative cultures will result, confusing the issue. For reasons already stated, bacterial arthritis is a medical emergency and needs to be handled as such. Antibiotic therapy with broad-spectrum drugs is instituted as soon as synovial fluid has been sent to the laboratory pending the outcome of sensitivity testing. The affected joint should be treated by splinting and anti-inflammatory analgesic drugs prescribed as appropriate. Full parenteral antibiotic therapy obviates the need for intra-articular installation of antibiotics, though daily aspiration of the joint should be performed to remove accumulated purulent exudate. As the bacterial inflammation subsides the joint may be gently mobilised, though antibiotic therapy should be continued for between 6 and 12 weeks depending on the severity of the condition. Surgical drainage is performed for bacterial arthritis only when medical treatment fails.

Tuberculous infection in bone and joint (which can only be confirmed by histological and bacteriological examination biopsy material) is treated by antituberculous drugs in combination for a period of not less than eighteen months.

DEGENERATIVE JOINT DISEASES
(Osteoarthritis, Spondylosis)

These common conditions result from degeneration of cartilage, both articular cartilage in synovial joints and fibro-cartilage in the intervertebral discs. The prevalence sharply increases with advancing age but other factors, notably previous fracture in relation to a joint, recurrent dislocation, occupational over-use, previous joint or spinal disease whether congenital or acquired are important. Hereditary factors may also play an important aetiological role. Where five or more joints are involved the term 'generalised osteoarthrosis (GOA)' is used. One particular variety, 'nodal GOA', in which Heberden's nodes are a common feature, shows a strong hereditary tendency, tending to present chiefly in females at around the time of the menopause.

Clinical Features. Osteoarthritis is suspected in any middle aged or elderly patient who presents with pain, stiffness and deformity of one or more joints in the absence of symptoms and signs of inflammation. Commonly involved joints are the distal interphalangeal and proximal interphalangeal joints of the hands (with bony deformities known as the Heberden and Bouchard node respectively), the first carpometacarpal joint at the base of the thumb as well as the weight-bearing joints—hip, knee, ankle and metatarsophalangeal joint of the great toe. Hip involvement causes a limp and difficulty in climbing stairs, and examination reveals limitation of passive movement—notably, rotation. Knee involvement gives rise to pain on walking and difficulty with stairs and may be recognised by crepitus on passive movement, deformity,—genu varum and loss of joint range, both flexion and extension. Quadriceps wasting is usually evident and an effusion may be present though this is usually small. A Baker's cyst may be seen.

Cervical spondylosis may cause local pain and restriction of movement of the neck; pain, parasthaesiae and weakness in the upper limb due to cervical nerve-root compression by osteophytes; (rarely) cord compression known as cervical myelopathy; or brain-stem ischaemia due to vertebral artery compression.

Dorsal spine involvement is usually asymptomatic but may give rise to local pain or referred pain radiating around the side of the chest.

The lumbar spine is particularly vulnerable to acute and chronic trauma occasioned by lifting, bending, etc. Prolapse of a lumbar intervertebral disc is a common disorder affecting adults of both sexes. Herniation of the nucleus pulposus through a rent in the annulus fibrosus may compress one or more nerve roots constituting the cauda equina. The clinical picture is one of acute lumbar pain after strenuous activity, inability to move the spine followed by pain down the leg in the distribution of either the femoral (cruralgia) or sciatic (sciatica) nerve. Signs of femoral or sciatic nerve tension (femoral nerve stretch test and reduced straight leg raising test respectively) and an associated neurological deficit may be present and cauda equina compression may occur. Causes of acute lumbar pain in the absence of evidence of nerve-root compression include a central disc prolapse; facet joint dysfunction; muscle and ligamentous injury; vertebral fracture due to trauma or secondary to infective metabolic or neoplastic disease of the bones; spondylolysis or spondylolisthesis as well as visceral causes.

Chronic low back pain is a serious problem both in human and economic terms. Any of the above-mentioned causes may participate and there may be a strong psychogenic element. The syndrome of intermittent claudication of the cauda equina' in which symptoms of lumbar nerve-root compression are brought on by exercise has now been accepted as being due to further reduction in the capacity of the vertebral canal of those with a congenitally small canal by acquired pathology (spinal stenosis).

Diagnosis of DJD. This is usually made on clinical grounds. Evidence of systemic disease is absent and blood tests are usually normal. Radiological appearances are characteristic and include narrowing of the joint space and loss of the normal joint contour and the presence of osteophytes. Such changes, may, however, be present in asymptomatic individuals, and undue importance should not be placed on their finding in the absence of appropriate clinical features.

In spondylosis confirmatory evidence of cord and/or nerve-root compression may be found using contrast radiculography or myelography.

Treatment. There is no known way of halting the progress of this condition. Fortunately, it is often asymptomatic and patients may be tided over painful episodes by short courses of NSAIDs coupled with physiotherapy in the form of heat and exercises, hydrotherapy or gentle manipulation. Intra-articular injections of corticosteroids are generally not indicated except in the presence of a joint effusion. Compression of nerve roots should be treated by immobilisation—with a collar in the case of the cervical spine or with bed rest in an acute lumbar intervertebral disc prolapse. In the latter case failure to respond may be treated by epidural corticosteroid injections or failing that, discectomy. Acute cauda equina compression is a surgical emergency requiring urgent decompression.

Advanced osteoarthritis affecting the hip or knee joint may be satisfactorily treated by total joint replacement.

NON-ARTICULAR RHEUMATIC DISORDERS

POLYMYALGIA RHEUMATICA

This condition of elderly patients presents with muscle pain and stiffness predominantly affecting the muscles of the shoulder and the pelvic girdle and the proximal limb muscles. Muscle weakness and tenderness are not seen, though occasionally synovitis of central joints, e.g. sternoclavicular joint, may be present. Some patients also experience malaise, weight loss and anaemia and a proportion show features of temporal (cranial) arteritis (see p. 423). Tests for rheumatoid and antinuclear factor are usually absent, though increase in the gamma globulins may be present and the immunoglobulin levels may be raised. The ESR is strikingly elevated, which is a hallmark of the condition. Another characteristic feature is the dramatic response to oral corticosteroid medication, the response being evident within hours of starting. The usual dose is between 10 and 20 mg of prednisolone daily until such time as the ESR falls to within normal limits, whereupon the dose may be tapered accordingly. Because of the close relationship between this condition and temporal arteritis (with the attendant risk of retinal artery occlusion) it is important that this condition be recognised and adequately treated without delay and careful follow-up instituted. Because of the rather non-specific nature of the symptoms alternative diagnoses including myeloma, carcinomatosis and polymyositis should be borne in mind. A temporal artery biopsy, a muscle biopsy, a creatine phosphokinase estimation and an EMG are helpful in this regard.

SOFT TISSUE LESIONS

Under this heading are included a group of common, benign, though troublesome conditions seen in clinical practice that may mimic arthritis and cause diagnostic difficulties in the unwary. For convenience they may be divided up into five main categories:

(a) **Enthesopathies.** These may be either acute traumatic episodes or chronic over-use injuries affecting sites of attachment of ligaments, tendons or fascial bands. Common examples include *lateral epicondylitis* (*'tennis elbow'*), *medial epicondylitis* (*'golfer's elbow'*), and *plantar fasciitis*.

(b) **Periarthritis** (including capsulitis and periarticular tendonitis). These lesions affect predominantly the shoulder joint which, being a shallow ball and socket, depends to a considerable extent for its stability to the complex of muscles, tendons and joint capsules known collectively as the rotator cuff. Four syndromes are commonly described within this entity—*tendonitis of supraspinatus, infraspinatus, subscapularis or long head of biceps*—identified by a painful arc of movement when the affected muscle is moved; *subacromial bursitis* with tenderness over the site of the bursa; *acute calcific tendonitis* associated with a brisk inflammatory reaction due to crystals of hydroxyapatite reminiscent in its ferocity of acute gout and distinguished by the presence of calcific material seen on X-ray; *adhesive capsulitis* (*'frozen shoulder'*) in which gross restriction of movement in the shoulder joint is apparent in all directions though pain is variable. Adhesive capsulitis is commonly seen after pleurisy, myocardial infarction, hemiplegia and certain operations in the region, notably mastectomy. An extension of this condition is known as the *shoulder/hand syndrome* in which the hand becomes diffusely swollen and tender followed by progressive atrophy of muscle, bone and skin with severe contractures and deformities. It is believed to be due to a reflex neurovascular dystrophy (algodystrophy).

(c) **Entrapment neuropathy** of which *carpal tunnel syndrome* (p. 359) is the most commonly seen variety.

(d) **Bursitis.** Excessive friction between bone and overlying moving soft tissues may give rise to bursitis. Commonly affected sites include *olecranon bursitis*, *prepatella bursitis* and *pre-achilles bursitis*.

(e) **Tenosynovitis.** Inflammation of synovium of the tendon sheaths occurs in a wide variety of conditions of over-use, particularly involving the long flexor tendons of the fingers or the extensor and abductor tendons of the thumb. Blocking of the movement of the tendon within the sheath may result in 'triggering'. This condition is known as *stenosing tenosynovitis* or *de Quervain's disease*.

For a more detailed description of the conditions mentioned in this section the reader is referred to standard rheumatological and orthopaedic texts. The majority of the conditions listed are amenable to treatment which may be on the basis of local corticosteroid injections, physiotherapeutic techniques or minor surgical procedures. Drug treatment has little part to play in the management of these conditions.

PSYCHOGENIC RHEUMATISM

This term is used to denote a condition whereby rheumatic-type symptoms manifest an underlying psychological disorder such as depression, hysteria, anxiety or compensation neurosis. Arthralgia and low back pain in the absence of clinical signs of organic disease are characteristic features of this condition.

TIETZE'S SYNDROME (Costal Chondritis)

In this obscure condition pain and tenderness are observed in the costochondral junctions. It is usually selflimiting but occasionally local infiltrations of corticosteroids are required which may be helpful.

HERITABLE DISORDERS OF CONNECTIVE TISSUE

These are multi-system disorders resulting from the inheritance of abnormalities in either the fibrous proteins (collagen and elastin) or the ground substance (glycosaminoglycans).

The disorders of fibrous proteins share a common feature, namely, generalised laxity of ligaments resulting in hypermobility of joints, which may result in articular symptoms. They include *Marfan's syndrome* (long, slender extremities, arachnoidactyly, high arched palate, dislocation of the lens and dilatation of the ascending aorta: *homocystinuria* (due to a deficiency of the enzyme cystathionine synthetase and similar to Marfan's syndrome with the additional features of thrombosis in medium-size arteries, osteoporosis and mental handicap); *Ehlers–Danlos syndrome* (characterised by hyper-extensible and fragile skin, a tendency to bruising and rupture of arteries); and *osteogenesis imperfecta* (*fragilitas ossium*,) in which a marked tendency to fracture of bone and a blue appearance of the sclerotic of the eye are the most characteristic features.

With the exception of homocystinuria which is inherited as a recessive, all these conditions are inherited as a dominant gene. The term 'hypermobility syndrome' denotes generalised laxity of ligaments in otherwise healthy subjects. It, too, may be an hereditary disorder (albeit mild) of connective tissue. Hypermobility, irrespective of the cause, may result in synovitis of the joints, recurrent dislocation and possibly premature osteoarthritis.

The disorders of ground substance comprise the mucopolysaccharidoses, a group of eleven diseases with differing manifestations (including the Hurler, Hunter, Scheie, Sanfilippo, Morquio and Maroteaux–Lamy syndromes). Patients manifest a variety of features including dwarfism, stiff joints, clouding of the cornea, aortic regurgitation, hepatosplenomegaly and mental handicap. Excessive quantities of mucopolysaccharides are found in the urine. In a number of these conditions the underlying enzyme defect has been identified.

MISCELLANEOUS RHEUMATIC CONDITIONS

(1) **Erythema Nodosum.** A self-limiting symmetrical arthritis notably affecting the knees and ankles is seen in this condition. Treatment is with NSAIDs. Occasionally short courses of steroids are required.

(2) **Sarcoidosis.** In early sarcoid the arthropathy of erythema nodosum may be seen. Later in the disease sarcoid granulomata may appear in the synovial membrane or bone causing synovitis and destructive arthropathy respectively.

(3) **Henoch–Schönlein Purpura.** A transient, non-migratory arthritis affecting predominantly the ankles, knees and hips, wrists and elbows with effusions, is seen in this condition.

(4) **Familial Mediterranean Fever.** Episodic arthritis of short duration with spontaneous remission is common and a chronic, destructive arthritis has also been reported. The episodes of arthritis respond to colchicine.

(5) **Hyperlipoproteinaemias.** A migratory polyarthritis is seen in Type II hyperlipoproteinaemia whilst in Type IV an episodic arthropathy is reported.

(6) **Hypogammaglobulinaemia.** An arthropathy similar to rheumatoid arthritis is seen, although destructive changes are rare.

(7) **Haemophilia and Christmas Disease.** In these bleeding diatheses recurrent haemarthroses give rise to acute episodes of joint pain and swelling and eventually to severe destructive changes, deformity and fibrous ankylosis.

(8) **Leukaemia.** Arthralgia, arthritis and bone pain are frequent symptoms in acute leukaemia, whilst in chronic leukaemia symmetrical

arthritis of larger joints results from infiltration of articular structures. Secondary gout may also occur in these conditions.

(9) **Sickle-cell Disease.** In this condition bone infarction, arthralgia or synovitis may occur during crises.

(10) **Pigmented Villonodular Synovitis.** This granulomatous condition of synovium may affect joint tendon sheath or bursa. It presents as a painless swelling of a single joint, usually of the knee, leading to erosion and cyst formation. Treatment is by synovectomy.

(11) **Hypertrophic (Pulmonary) Osteoarthropathy.** This is the combination of finger clubbing with painful, tender swelling of ankles and wrists with characteristic periosteal new bone formation seen radiologically. Joint effusions may occur. It is associated with intrathoracic or intra-abdominal pathology, usually infective or neoplastic.

(12) **Avascular Necrosis of Bone (Osteonecrosis).** The femoral head is the most commonly affected site though the humeral head and femoral condyles may be affected. It is seen in trauma, sickle-cell disease, caisson disease, high-dose corticosteroid therapy, SLE and alcoholism.

(13) **Neuropathic (Charcot's) Joints.** A severe form of destructive arthropathy seen in certain neurological diseases with loss of pain sensation. The common causes are tabes dorsalis, syringomyelia, diabetes mellitus with peripheral neuropathy and congenital indifference to pain.

JUVENILE CHRONIC ARTHRITIS

Many patients carry their chronic rheumatic disease into adult life from childhood. It is for this reason that a note on juvenile chronic arthritis is not out of place in a volume devoted to adult medicine. It is now known that several clinical and pathological entities fall within this broad title and the use of the term 'Still's Disease' to cover them all is no longer tenable. Rheumatic fever is not included and is dealt with separately (p. 171).

The following entities have been delineated:

(1) **Seropositive** (adult-like) **juvenile rheumatoid arthritis.** This variety is very similar to the adult one with IgM rheumatoid factor, nodules and erosive disease.

(2) **Juvenile ankylosing spondylitis.** This presents in childhood as a peripheral arthropathy and only in the late teens do the classical features of ankylosing spondylitis develop with spinal involvement. These patients are almost exclusively HLA B27 positive and have a tendency to recurrent acute iritis.

(3) **Juvenile chronic arthritis** (Still's disease) comprises three entities.

(i) Systemic onset, with fever, lymphadenopathy, splenomegaly and pericarditis which may all precede the polyarthritis and cause diagnostic confusion.

(ii) Pauci-articular disease. As its name implies it commences in a small number of joints (1–4). Although the articular disease may not be very severe there is a real danger of severe eye problems following chronic iritis which may be insidious in its onset and pass undetected. The antinuclear factor is commonly positive.

(iii) Polyarticular disease. The arthritis develops in 5 or more joints, particularly in the knees and wrists. Small finger joints may also be involved including the distal IP joints. The cervical spine may also be involved.

(4) Juvenile scleroderma
(5) Juvenile dermatomyositis
(6) Juvenile systemic lupus erythematosus
(7) Juvenile psoriatic arthritis
(8) Polyarthritis associated with ulcerative colitis and regional enteritis

These are uncommon childhood ailments and their clinical presentation follows the general pattern of adult disease (see above).

FURTHER READING

Scott, J. T., (ed.), *Copeman's Textbook of the Rheumatic Diseases*, 6th Edition, Churchill Livingstone, Edinburgh, 1983.

Reports on Rheumatic Diseases, Collected Reports, The Arthritis and Rheumatism Council for Research, London, 1983.

CHAPTER 9

DISEASES OF CALCIUM METABOLISM AND BONE

INTRODUCTION

Bone

Bone consists of connective tissue made rigid by the orderly deposition of mineral. The connective tissue of bone consists of collagen fibres lying in a polysaccharide ground substance. In this connective tissue framework are deposited crystalline bone salts which consist of calcium, phosphate and carbonate; the proportion of these ions may vary but dahlite ($CaCO_3 . 2Ca_3(PO_4)_2$) is probably the commonest combination. In addition to calcium bone contains about one third of the total body sodium.

Calcification depends on the concentration of calcium and phosphate at the bone face and on other variables such as pH. The exact mechanism is not known but it is clear that phosphatase plays a part, perhaps by raising the local concentration of phosphate; a rise in plasma alkaline phosphatase therefore indicates an increased rate of breakdown and renewal of bone. *Calcitonin* a hormone which is secreted by the thyroid, parathyroid and thymus causes deposition of calcium and phosphate in bone. It is produced in large amounts by medullary carcinoma of the thyroid.

Vitamin D (cholecalciferol) is manufactured as a result of the action of sunlight on the skin or is obtained from the diet. It is then metabolised to more active forms. In the liver it is converted to 25-hydroxy-cholecalciferol and then further hydroxylated in the kidneys to the active hormone 1,25-hydroxycholecalciferol, which is concerned with calcium absorption and bone mineralisation. When Vitamin D is deficient the osteoid tissue of growing bone fails to calcify. The salts of bone are not metabolically inactive; rapid exchange can occur between the minerals in bone and those in the tissue fluids. Furthermore bone is not a static structure but is constantly being remodelled by a process of breakdown and renewal. Osteoclasts are concerned with bone resorption and osteoblasts with calcification.

Vitamin D Analogues

In addition to the 25-hydroxy and 1,25-hydroxy analogues of cholecalciferol there are a number of similar compounds produced in vivo by metabolic processes. The physiological importance of these substances is not yet known. Some analogues have been synthesised and

1,α-hydroxycholecalciferol (alfacalcidol) is available for clinical use. It has the advantage that unlike Vitamin D (cholecalciferol) its action is relatively short, so if overdosage with resultant hypercalcaemia occurs it can be rapidly reversed by stopping the drug.

Metabolism of Calcium

Calcium is absorbed from the small intestine and this requires the presence of 1,25-hydroxycholecalciferol. The average daily diet contains about 25–50 mmol of calcium and of this about 2.5–5.0 mmol is absorbed, the exact amount being regulated by the needs of the body. In health about 2.5–7.5 mmol are excreted daily in the urine. Most of the body calcium is in bone. This is undergoing continuous absorption and excretion with a turnover of about 10 mmol daily and here again calcium release equals calcium uptake.

If the calcium in the diet is increased, balance is maintained largely by a decrease in the proportion absorbed and urinary excretion rises little. Conversely, if the diet is deficient in calcium, absorption is increased and urinary excretion decreases. Vitamin D is essential for the absorption of calcium from the gut and if it is deficient calcium loss exceeds intake with subsequent decalcification of bones. Excessive urinary loss, however, is balanced by an increase in uptake and decalcification is unusual.

The plasma normally contains between 2.10–2.60 mmol calcium/litre. A little over half of this is ionised, most of the remainder is bound to protein (chiefly albumin) and a small fraction is diffusible but un-ionised. The ionised fraction plays the most important part in the clinical states hypo- and hypercalcaemia, although its concentration is rarely measured. Because of the binding of calcium to protein, total calcium levels are influenced by plasma protein concentration and corrections may be required. The binding of calcium and plasma albumin is also affected by pH; acidosis decreases protein-binding and thus increases the ionised fraction. The level of plasma calcium is controlled by the *parathyroid* glands and by 1,25-hydroxycholecalciferol (see above). A fall in plasma calcium increases parathormone secretion and vice versa. The actions of parathormone are:

(1) To mobilise calcium from bone and thus increase the plasma calcium concentration.
(2) To increase the renal excretion of phosphate and thus to lower plasma phosphate concentration and to increase the reabsorption of calcium by the renal tubules and thus elevate the plasma calcium levels.
(3) To stimulate production of 1,25-dihydroxycholecalciferol by the kidney (see above) and thus increase the intestinal absorption of calcium.

The non-protein-bound calcium and phosphate pass freely through the glomerulus. About 95 % of the filtered calcium is reabsorbed, probably by the distal tubule. The urinary excretion of calcium is only slightly dependent on dietary intake. In health it should not exceed 7.5 mmol/24 h. Phosphate is both reabsorbed and excreted by the renal tubules. In addition small amounts of calcium are excreted by the intestine.

HYPOCALCAEMIA

Introduction

The commonest cause of a sustained fall in plasma calcium is parathyroid hormone deficiency, for under normal circumstances any lowering of plasma calcium leads to increased secretion of parathormone with mobilisation of calcium from bone and return of the blood level to normal. Hypocalcaemia also occurs rarely in Vitamin D or calcium deficiency (i.e. malabsorption, rickets or during lactation) or in renal osteodystrophy.

Long-standing hypocalcaemia produces striking structural changes in the body. Reduction in the level of ionised calcium in the blood causes increased neuromuscular excitability, and the clinical syndrome of tetany. This usually appears when the total plasma calcium level has fallen to about 1.8 mmol/litre. It is also seen in alkalosis where, although the total plasma calcium concentration is normal, the ionised fraction is reduced. It is probable too that magnesium and potassium can play a part in the genesis of tetany.

Clinical Features of Tetany

Symptoms

(1) Paraesthesia in lips, nose, and fingers which is worse before breakfast.
(2) Spontaneous muscle cramps.
(3) Epileptic fits.
(4) Laryngeal spasm in children.
(5) Rarely arteriolar spasm, with pallor and raised blood pressure.
(6) Psychoses may develop.

Signs

The diagnostic point is the demonstration of increased neuromuscular excitability. *Chvostek's sign* is elicited by tapping over the facial nerve as it emerges from the parotid gland beneath the zygoma. A hemifacial twitch constitutes a positive response. Minor contractions confined to the angle of the lips should be ignored. The combination of twitching of the eyelids and the lips is usually significant but for certainty there should be movement of the whole side of the face. *Trousseau's sign* is elicited by the application of a sphygmomanometer cuff to the arm and raising the pressure to above the patient's systolic blood pressure for three minutes, by which time the hands should have adopted the classical 'main d'accoucheur' position—wrist and metacarpophalangeal joints flexed and fingers extended.

Signs of Long-standing Hypocalcaemia

Long-standing hypocalcaemia is associated with well-marked ectodermal defects. There may be coincident tetany.

(1) Dry, scaly skin.
(2) Loss of eyelashes, sparse eyebrows, patchy alopecia, and scanty axillary and pubic hair.
(3) Wrinkling and brittleness of nails.
(4) If present before they are fully formed, hypoplasia or aplasia of teeth.
(5) Changes in nervous system; cataracts are common and so is calcification in the basal ganglia and dentate nuclei. Papilloedema occurs rarely.
(6) Susceptibility to moniliasis probably due to immune deficiency.

Differential Diagnosis of Hypocalcaemia and Tetany

(1) **Alkalosis** usually results from hyperventilation; this is commonly hysterical but may be an epileptic phenomenon. It produces a fall in the concentration of ionised calcium in the plasma, partly by raising the pH of the blood and partly by increasing the level of plasma citrate which combines with free calcium. Hyperventilation produces transient attacks of tetany. A history of overbreathing is diagnostic but subjects vary considerably in the amount of hyperventilation required to produce tetany. Typical findings in the blood are a reduced $P\text{CO}_2$, with a normal or slightly reduced bicarbonate and a normal total calcium concentration. *Treatment* consists of re-breathing from a paper bag and suitable sedation.

Tetany may also occur with alkalosis due to acid loss from prolonged vomiting or gastric aspiration or rarely after ingestion of too much alkali.

(2) **Hypoparathyroidism** is usually the result of too radical thyroidectomy (secondary hypoparathyroidism). Transient tetany may develop soon after operation and in a few patients symptoms persist. In others the onset of symptoms may be delayed for several years. Occasionally the parathyroids are absent or non-functioning (primary hypoparathyroidism).

Clinical Features. The typical findings in parathormone deficiency are due to hypocalcaemia. They consist of tetany and sometimes epilepsy combined with widespread ectodermal defects (see above). Patients with primary hypoparathyroidism frequently develop chronic monilia infection of the skin. The plasma calcium level is low and the phosphate is high. The 24-hour urinary calcium output is usually low and the plasma parathormone level is unmeasurable.

Pseudohypoparathyroidism is a rare condition in which the parathyroid functions normally but the tissues are incompletely responsive to parathormone. In addition to showing the features of hypocalcaemia these patients are short of stature and have thickset bodies, round faces, and short hands and fingers. The plasma parathormone level is raised.

(3) **Osteomalacia and Rickets.** In these disorders (p. 448) there is a decrease in calcium absorption. However, a lowered plasma calcium level is unusual, presumably because the parathyroid glands maintain it at a normal level by mobilising calcium from bone, although the evidence for this is scanty. Occasionally, however, hypocalcaemia with attendant symptoms is found.

(4) The **malabsorption syndrome** may be associated with hypocalcaemia due to poor absorption of calcium and perhaps also of Vitamin D.

(5) **Renal disease** can cause hypocalcaemia which may complicate chronic renal failure (see p. 486). It can also result from excessive loss of calcium in the urine due to renal tubular acidosis (see p. 500).

(6) Occasionally patients are seen with recurrent tetany where there is no apparent biochemical abnormality.

Treatment of Hypocalcaemia

(1) *Tetany* can be abolished by injecting calcium gluconate (10 ml of a 10 % solution) slowly intravenously.

(2) The diet should be of adequate calorie value and have a high protein and calcium content. This latter is achieved by giving calcium lactate 5.0–10.0 g daily.

(3) Patients with hypoparathyroidism are best treated with 1,α-hydroxycholecalciferol (alfacalcidol) 1–2 μg daily by mouth. This increases calcium and phosphate absorption from the gut.

The dose must be controlled by estimation of plasma calcium and phosphate levels.

HYPERCALCAEMIA

Hypercalcaemia may result from increased calcium absorption (Vitamin D poisoning, sarcoidosis or milk poisoning) or from increased calcium mobilisation from bone as in hyperparathyroidism, or primary bone disease.

Clinical Features. Several systems are affected by hypercalcaemia:

(a) *Kidneys.* Hypercalcaemia interferes with reabsorption of water by the renal tubules producing polyuria and causing thirst. Eventually calcium may be deposited in the renal tubules producing nephrocalcinosis and renal stones.

(b) *Voluntary Muscle.* There is decreased neuromuscular excitability, which may lead to general muscular weakness.
(c) *Gastrointestinal Tract.* Decreased excitability also affects smooth muscle causing constipation. Anorexia and vomiting are also common. Abdominal pain of a vague but persistent nature may occur in hyperparathyroidism (see below).
(d) Patients with hypercalcaemia may feel generally ill and depressed and may indeed be diagnosed as having some psychological disorder.
(e) *Deposits of calcium* may occur at the junction of the cornea and sclera. The deposits have a granular gritty appearance and are associated with increased vascularity.
(f) If bone is affected by the primary disease there may be pain and weakness perhaps with fractures.
(g) *Marked hypercalcaemia* produces confusion, coma, anuria and death. Such symptoms develop at a blood level between 3.5–4.0 mmol/litre.

Differential Diagnosis of Hypercalcaemia

(1) **Primary Hyperparathyroidism.** This usually results from one or more parathyroid adenomas; less commonly all four glands show diffuse hypertrophy. Carcinoma of the parathyroids occurs in less than 1 % of patients with this condition but the tumour is always hormone-secreting. About 70 % of the patients are women. The disease exists in two clinical forms, with and without involvement of bone. Whether these represent two distinct disorders is not known but it seems more probable that bone changes are merely due to more severe disease, the basic cause of both types being overproduction of parathormone. Sometimes parathyroid adenomas are associated with hormone secreting adenomas in other endocrine glands, particularly the pancreas, the anterior pituitary and the adrenal cortex.

Clinical Features

(a) *Without bone disease* (90 %); presents with symptoms of hypercalcaemia (see above) or of renal stones. About 10 % of patients with recurrent renal stones have hyperparathyroidism and it must be emphasised that renal stones may be the only signs of the disorder. If hypercalcaemia persists over long periods there is progressive renal destruction with stones and finally fibrosis with hypertension and renal failure. There is an association between hyperparathyroidism and several other disorders including duodenal ulcer, pancreatitis and hypertension.
(b) *With bone disease* (only about 10 % of patients have clinical bone disease although a higher proportion have biochemical evidence of bone involvement with raised plasma alkaline phosphatase or urinary hydroxyproline). Bone disease is often associated with

Vitamin D deficiency, either dietary or associated with renal failure. Symptoms may be either generalised with skeletal pain, waddling gait, loss of height, pseudoclubbing and bony tenderness; or localised, when tender bony lumps occur. These are the *brown tumours* of hyperparathyroidism; they contain osteoclasts, but unlike the osteoclastomas they are not locally malignant. They usually arise in the jaw or tibia, though no bone is immune. These localised and generalised forms of skeletal involvement are not mutually exclusive.

Special Investigations

Biochemistry

(1) In primary hyperparathyroidism the plasma calcium level is usually persistently above normal, though occasionally it may be only intermittently raised so that several estimations are advisable if the condition is suspected clinically. Changes in the plasma protein concentration affect the level of bound calcium and thus of total calcium and a correction for these fluctuations may have to be made. It is important to avoid prolonged compression of the arm when taking blood as this may concentrate plasma protein and thus give falsely high figures for calcium. It should be remembered that if renal failure develops the plasma calcium level may fall and thus obscure the diagnosis. The daily urinary excretion of calcium is nearly always increased.

The plasma phosphate level may be reduced but this is not constant particularly when there is concomitant renal damage. The plasma chloride level is raised. If there is bone involvement there is elevation of the plasma alkaline phosphatase and of the urinary hydroxyproline.

(2) If there is difficulty in the differential diagnosis, cortisone 100 mg daily can be given for 10 days and will cause a fall in the plasma calcium level in sarcoidosis and in most patients with malignant disease, but will not alter the level in hyperparathyroidism.

(3) It is now possible to measure the plasma parathyroid hormone concentration, but in mild hyperparathyroidism levels are apt to be in the upper end of the normal range; therefore in these cases the estimation is not useful diagnostically.

Radiology. Early radiological changes occur in the phalanges which show subperiosteal and phalangeal tuft erosion and the laminae durae surrounding the roots of the teeth disappear. Later changes consist of fuzziness of trabeculae and in long-standing cases widespread patchy erosions and cystic changes occur with bowing and sometimes fractures of pelvis and long bones. 'Brown tumours' may be present. Calcification appears in soft tissues.

Treatment. The treatment of primary hyperparathyroidism is surgical and prognosis is good provided renal damage is not too extensive. Occasionally it is necessary to treat severe hypercalcaemia (see below) before operation. Patients with bone disease may require Vitamin D after operation, and this can be given as 1,α-hydroxycholecalciferol 1.0 μg daily.

Secondary hyperparathyroidism with hypertrophy of the parathyroid glands occurs secondary to chronic renal failure (see renal osteodystrophy) and with long-standing steatorrhoea. In secondary hyperparathyroidism the plasma calcium level is only very rarely higher than normal.

(2) **Sarcoidosis** (p. 305). About 20% of patients have raised serum calcium level; this bears no relationship to increase in plasma globulin or to involvement of bones. It appears to be due to hypersensitivity to Vitamin D leading to increased absorption of calcium. It is accompanied by hypercalciuria which may lead to nephrocalcinosis or stone formation.

(3) **Myelomatosis.** The bone changes and raised plasma and urinary calcium levels closely resemble those of hyperparathyroidism. Bence Jones proteinuria and abnormal plasma proteins are strongly in favour of myelomatosis. Marrow biopsy is diagnostic.

(4) **Carcinomatosis.** With or without osteolytic secondary deposits may be associated with hypercalcaemia. The reason is obscure but there may be some substance produced by the tumour which resembles parathormone and releases calcium from bone.

(5) **Paget's Disease of Bone** (p. 452). If these patients are immobilised, e.g. in a plaster spica for a fractured femur or kept in bed for a long period, the plasma calcium (otherwise normal) may rise to very high levels.

(6) Overdosage with **Vitamin D** or undue sensitivity to its actions cause hypercalcaemia.

(7) **Milk Alkali Syndrome.** Patients with peptic ulcers who have taken very large quantities of milk and alkalis may develop hypercalcaemia, hypercalciuria and tissue calcification.

(8) Mild hypercalcaemia may occur in **thyrotoxicosis**. The plasma calcium returns to normal when the thyroid disease is controlled.

Treatment of Acute Hypercalcaemia

A plasma calcium level of about 4.0 mmol/litre may cause cardiac arrest. This occurs most commonly as a complication of malignant disease and require immediate treatment. This consists of:

(a) Intravenous infusion of normal saline to correct dehydration which is frequently present and also to increase the excretion of calcium in the urine. Loop diuretics such as frusemide 60 mg 4-hourly also increase urinary calcium excretion and can be used in combination with saline infusions.

(b) Hydrocortisone 100 mg IV and repeated 6-hourly will often lower the plasma calcium due to malignant disease, sarcoid and Vitamin D excess.

(c) Mithramycin 15 μg/kg body weight is effective in patients with malignant disease.

For long-term treatment a solution containing phosphate or phosphate effervescent tablets (Phosphate Sandoz) given orally is very effective in reducing plasma calcium levels by preventing calcium absorption.

Asymptomatic Hypercalcaemia

Since the introduction of biochemical screening a number of subjects have been found with persistent elevation of plasma calcium levels, but who have no symptoms. Full investigation of these patients may reveal no cause for the abnormality although it is presumed that they have mild hyperparathyroidism. Follow-up of such patients suggests that about one third of them will develop symptoms or further evidence of disease in the ensuing five years.

In these circumstances it would seem reasonable to observe and repeat the estimation at regular intervals if the patient is elderly and the plasma calcium is only slightly raised. In younger patients or in those with more than minimal elevation of the plasma calcium the neck should be explored surgically if no cause is apparent after investigation.

HYPERCALCIURIA

Hypercalciuria is important because it may lead to nephrocalcinosis and renal stone formation. The main causes are:

(1) Hypercalcaemia (see above).
(2) Increased absorption of calcium as in Vitamin D excess or sarcoidosis.
(3) Increased bone breakdown as in immobilisation and Paget's disease.
(4) Renal tubular disorders.
(5) Idiopathic hypercalciuria.

Idiopathic hypercalciuria is now thought to be a disorder of calcium absorption, although a few of these patients are believed to be suffering from mild hyperparathyroidism with a normal calcium concentration in the plasma. On a low calcium diet absorption and excretion are normal, but as the amount of calcium in the diet is increased so a larger fraction than normal is absorbed and the urinary calcium rises often to figures of 10–20 mmol/litre calcium excreted in 24 hours.

Hypercalciuria can be controlled by a low calcium diet but this may prove irksome. Calcium absorption can also be decreased by giving sodium cellulose phosphate (5.0 g three times daily with meals).

RICKETS AND OSTEOMALACIA

The essential feature of both osteomalacia and rickets is a failure to calcify bone resulting in an excess of osteoid which is uncalcified bone matrix. In children the syndrome is known as rickets and in adults as osteomalacia.

Vitamin D is essential for bone calcification. It is obtained from certain foods including butter, vitaminised margarine and fish liver oils. It is also formed by the action of sunlight on the skin. Coloured people living in Britain are therefore particularly susceptible if their diet is deficient in the vitamin.

Lack of Vitamin D leads to decreased absorption of calcium from the gut. This is associated with a fall in extracellular calcium concentration and it is believed (although the evidence is incomplete) that this in turn stimulates the production of parathormone. The plasma calcium is thus usually kept at normal levels, but there is an increased urinary excretion of phosphorus and the plasma phosphorus concentration is lowered. The calcification of osteoid depends in part on the solubility product of calcium and phosphorus $(Ca)^3 + (P)^2$ in the plasma and tissue fluids. When this is decreased as in Vitamin D deficiency there is a failure to calcify *osteoid*. In rickets the main changes are seen where new bone is being formed from the epiphyseal cartilage. In the adult there is no new bone formation at the epiphysis but remodelling of bone continues throughout life and in osteomalacia too there is a failure to calcify new bone.

Vitamin D deficiency may be due to several causes:

(a) Dietary deficiency.
(b) Failure to absorb Vitamin D—this may occur after gastrectomy or in the malabsorption syndrome.
(c) Failure of hydroxylation of Vitamin D (cholecalciferol). This may occur as a result of chronic liver disease. It can also occur in renal disease and plays a part in the clinical picture of renal osteodystrophy (see p. 450).
(d) Induction of liver enzymes may lead to rapid breakdown of Vitamin D; this has been reported in patients with epilepsy who have been taking phenytoin, which is a powerful enzyme inducer, over long periods.
(e) Resistance to the action of Vitamin D is also found in some renal tubular disorders (see below).

Clinical Features

Rickets. The earliest clinical symptoms are tiredness and muscular weakness. There is bone pain and pain on movement. Dentition is delayed and the teeth may be deformed and quickly become carious. Swelling and tenderness of the distal ends of the radius and ulna are common, and so is the rickety rosary (costochondral swellings). Frontal and parietal bossing of the skull occurs and occipitoparietal flattening may result from the softness of the skull (craniotabes).

If the child can stand or walk, bowing of the legs may result from weight bearing, and kyphoscoliosis may appear.

Radiographs show widening and decreased density of the line of calcification next to the metaphysis, with irregularity and concavity of the metaphysis itself. In severe cases there may be rarefaction with deformities in the shaft of the bone.

Osteomalacia. Early symptoms are fatigue, stiffness and skeletal pains followed by muscular weakness and hyporeflexia. The gait is waddling and there is marked adductor spasm. Climbing up stairs may be particularly difficult. Costochondral swelling is common, and there is striking spinal curvature and the pelvic outlet is narrowed. Pathological fractures may appear in the pelvis and long bones, and may be exquisitely painful. Occasionally the plasma calcium level is low enough to produce tetany.

Radiology. Pseudo-fractures (Milkman, Looser) are the most frequent defect. These are lines of increased translucency running in from the surface of the bone, commonly found in the upper ends of the humerus and femur and in the pubic rami. They are strips of decalcification occurring in relationship to arteries or in areas of stress. In severe cases the bones show generalised decalcification with deformity and fractures.

The biochemical changes are similar in rickets and osteomalacia. The plasma calcium is usually a little low and occasionally considerably reduced. The plasma phosphate level is low but the alkaline phosphatase is frequently increased.

Treatment. Depends on the cause. For simple dietary deficiency, Vitamin D 0.05 mg (2000 units) or liq calciferol (BP) 1.0 ml (3000 units) are sufficient. In malabsorption doses of Vitamin D up to 50 000 units daily by mouth may be required, or 20 000 units can be injected weekly. Treatment should be continued until healing occurs and a watch kept for Vitamin D poisoning. In coeliac disease a gluten-free diet will frequently decrease the oral Vitamin D requirements.

Calcium is also required and effervescent calcium tablets (Sando-Cal) 2.0 g daily for an adult is satisfactory.

Vitamin D Resistant Rickets. This small group have the symptoms of rickets but do not respond to small doses of Vitamin D. The onset is usually late and there may be a family history. They are associated with disorders or renal tubular function.

(a) *Phosphaturic rickets* is probably due to a failure of the renal tubules to reabsorb phosphorus. The plasma calcium concentration is normal and the phosphate low. The bony lesions respond to 1,α-hydroxycholecalciferol (alfacalcidol) 1.0 μg daily and modified as required, and a supply of phosphorus in the form of sodium phosphates should be added to the diet.

(b) *Renal tubular acidosis* (p. 500) and *Fanconi's syndrome* (p. 500) may both be associated with rickets.

RENAL OSTEODYSTROPHY

Renal or uraemic osteodystrophy is a disease of calcium metabolism associated with chronic renal failure. The bones show a number of changes including osteomalacia, osteitis fibrosa, and new bone formation elsewhere. In the blood there is a normal or lowered calcium level, a normal or raised phosphorus level and frequently evidence of acidosis. The blood urea is always raised.

There are probably several factors responsible for the clinical picture of osteodystrophy. They include:

(1) Failure to form 1,25-hydroxycholecalciferol by the diseased kidney, leading to impaired absorption of calcium and bone changes of osteomalacia.
(2) Increased parathyroid activity with enlargement of the glands and typical changes in the bones (secondary hyperparathyroidism) (see below). Rarely the parathyroids become autonomous and this leads to hypercalcaemia (tertiary hyperparathyroidism).
(3) Phosphate retention. A rise in plasma phosphate is usual in renal failure and would tend to depress plasma calcium levels. This may be particularly associated with ectopic calcification.
(4) Acidosis may play a small part.

Clinical Features. In children dwarfism with bone deformities similar to those found in rickets are the most prominent features. In adults the symptoms of chronic renal failure usually overshadow the bone lesions although bone pain and fractures occasionally occur. The other feature is metastatic calcification which is occasionally palpable but is more frequently seen in radiographs. The *radiological* changes in the bones are complex and may be divided into:

(1) Changes similar to rickets.
(2) Changes similar to hyperparathyroidism, with subperiosteal absorption of bone often most marked in the phalanges.
(3) Patchy osteosclerosis most marked in the skull. The vertebrae may show alternating bands of sclerosis and decalcification producing the 'rugger jersey' spine.
(4) Metastatic calcification may be widespread, both muscles and particularly blood vessels being affected.

Treatment. Bone symptoms can be controlled by giving 1,α-hydroxycholecalciferol (alfacalcidol) 1–2 μg daily together with calcium gluconate 5.0 g b.d. The plasma calcium level must be estimated at least once a month and the dose modified accordingly.

Long-term management is less successful and the bone changes may progress in spite of continued treatment.

If metastatic calcification is a problem and the blood phosphate level is raised, phosphate absorption can be decreased by giving aluminium hydroxide orally.

Early treatment of this condition in the asymptomatic stage is now recommended using a Vitamin D analogue, phosphate binding drugs and calcium supplements.

OSTEOPOROSIS

This may be defined as an atrophy of bone; although the volume of the bone remains the same, its content of bone tissue decreases. It affects both bone matrix and calcium and is most evident in the axial skeleton.

Aetiology

(1) *Idiopathic (senile) osteoporosis* is a common disorder. Atrophy of the skeleton is part of the general process of ageing, and starts at about the age of twenty. In certain people atrophy progresses fast enough to produce symptoms which usually appear in late life. This occurs more commonly in women than in men. There are probably several aetiological factors including androgen or oestrogen deficiency, Vitamin D and calcium deficiency (particularly in the elderly), and physical and circulatory factors.

(2) In *Cushing's syndrome* and *steroid administration* a negative nitrogen balance and failure to form bone matrix are important.

(3) *Hyperthyroidism* and *acromegaly* may be complicated by osteoporosis and are associated with increased loss of calcium in the urine.

(4) *Immobilisation* leads to osteoporosis and increased excretion of calcium in the urine, sometimes complicated by stone formation.

(5) In *intestinal malabsorption* osteoporosis may co-exist with osteomalacia.

(6) *Rheumatoid arthritis* is frequently associated with osteoporosis especially in those treated with steroids.

Clinical Features. The disease may be symptomless, or there may be pains in the back, round the trunk, or down the limbs. They are made worse by jarring or flexing the spine, but rarely have the characteristics of root pain. Sudden severe back pain suggests the collapse of a vertebra. On examination, the spine is shortened so that height is lost and the distance from the ground to the iliac spine exceeds that from the iliac spine to the crown. Gross kyphosis is the rule and may decrease the vital capacity, but compression of the spinal cord is almost unknown. The consequent buckling of the trunk causes a characteristic transverse skin crease across the upper abdomen above the umbilicus. The infolded skin is keratinised, emphasising that the changes are of long standing. Radiographs show rarefaction of the spine and biconcave (cod fish) vertebrae. No typical biochemical changes are recognised and the alkaline phosphatase is normal.

Treatment consists of mobilising the patient and the administration of hormones and calcium. Oestrogens will reduce the severity of the osteoporosis after the menopause. Their use is probably best restricted to patients who have been given an early menopause or those with symptoms. An oral contraceptive containing 30 μg of ethinyloestradiol for three weeks out of four is satisfactory but the patient may object to withdrawal bleeding. In men norandrostenolone (Durabolin) 25 mg intramuscularly once weekly or norethandrolone (Nilevar) 10 mg three times daily have been used but are of doubtful value. A reasonably high protein diet and calcium 1.0 g daily (Sando-Cal three tablets daily is a useful preparation) are necessary to replace deficiencies. In older patients it is important to ensure that they are not Vitamin D deficient. Relief of pain often occurs within a month or so, though it is rare for radiological improvement ever to be seen.

PAGET'S DISEASE OF BONE (Osteitis Deformans)

Paget's disease usually affects a number of bones to greater or lesser degree, but some bones are completely spared. This is in distinction from osteomalacia and osteoporosis where the whole skeleton is affected, albeit unequally. Sometimes Paget's disease affects just one bone, particularly the tibia, femur, a clavicle, or a vertebra. It is rare before forty and affects men more than women in the proportion of 3:2. Occasionally it is familial. No disorder of metabolism has been identified, nor is there any indication that it is an inflammatory process. Two clues to its cause are the association with Hashimoto's disease and the occurrence of a similar disease in horses fed on a diet low in calcium and high in phosphorus (*big head disease*). It is said to be rare in oriental countries, where the phosphorus content of the diet is low.

The bones in order of affection are the sacrum, pelvis, spinal column (from below upwards), femur, tibia, skull, fibula, clavicle, humerus, rib. The hands and feet are almost always spared. Clearly the distribution is to some extent governed by stress and strain; the part of the skull which is particularly affected is at the sites of origin of the temporal muscles.

Clinical Features. The earliest symptom is pain, usually in the lower back, and often worse at night. Headaches are common, and there may be an unpleasant feeling of hotness from circulatory derangements. Deafness, often of nerve type, is common and the patient may have noticed increase in the size of his head. The picture may be complicated by platybasia and pathological fractures are common.

Examination of advanced cases shows enlargement of the head, kyphosis, shortening of the spine and bowing of the long bones, especially in the legs. The bones are highly vascular and act as an arteriovenous shunt. This causes tachycardia, wide pulse pressure with a collapsing pulse, and dilatation of the heart. The limbs and extremities are hot, and often a murmur can be heard over affected bones. *Congestive cardiac failure* of 'high output' type may supervene. In the earliest cases these signs are absent, but there is limitation of hip movement, especially rotation, by pain.

The serum alkaline phosphatase level is always raised, often to great heights (350–1000 u/litre). No other biochemical abnormality is found in the blood unless the patient is immobilised, when the serum calcium level rises. The changes in the bones are essentially the result of increased resorption, and are characterised by cystic fibrosis, in this respect resembling hyperparathyroidism. Radiography shows a typical picture; there is increase in total diameter of affected bones, with thickening and broadening of the cortex, and abnormal architecture of the cortex and cancellous bone. In some cases only the proximal part of a long bone is affected, and the area immediately beyond its distal extent is rarefied (*osteoporosis circumscripta*). The disease spreads distally, progressing about 1 cm every two years.

Complications are frequent. *Pathological fractures* are common, and generally heal well. *Deafness*, either from auditory nerve compression or otosclerosis, is ultimately the rule, and the optic nerve too may be compressed, causing *blindness*. Vertebrae may collapse and cause *spinal cord compression* and the effects of platybasia may be extreme. As more bone is involved so the tendency to *cardiac failure* increases. It is claimed that both hypertension and atheroma are more common than usual in Paget's disease. But the most serious (and least common) complication is the occurrence of *sarcomatous change* in the affected bone.

There are several drugs which can be used to relieve bone pain and neurological complications by slowing down the pathological processes in Paget's disease. They are not indicated in asymptomatic patients.

(a) Calcitonin 100 i.u. given subcutaneously daily for 6 months will usually relieve bone pain. It can also be used to control developing neurological lesions and promote healing of fractures.

(b) The phosphonate disodium etidronate stabilises calcium phosphate crystals. The usual dose is 5–10 mg/kg daily orally. It may be successful when calcitonin fails and should relieve symptoms within six weeks.

OSTEOPETROSIS (Albers–Schönberg's Disease)

The outstanding feature is a great increase in bone density so that radiographically they warrant the description of 'marble bones'. It exists in three forms foetal, juvenile and adult. The foetal form may be diagnosed radiographically *in utero*, and death always occurs shortly after birth. It is sporadic, whereas the juvenile and adult forms are familial and have Mendelian recessive characters.

Clinical Features. The *juvenile form* is severe, and death before puberty is the rule. Effects are produced by increase in size of bones, so as either to compress nerves (auditory, optic) or to encroach on the medullary cavity and to interfere with blood formation. This causes anaemia initially, later leuco-erythroblastic anaemia, ultimately marrow aplasia. Attempts at extramedullary haematopoiesis cause hepatoplenomegaly and generalised lymphadenopathy. *In adults* the disease is relatively benign. About one third of all cases sustain pathological fractures which heal badly; otherwise there are no symptoms or signs, and the diagnosis is made by chance radiography.

There is no special change in blood chemistry, but *radiography* shows a typically symmetrical increase in bone density. Characteristic appearances in individual bones are described, e.g. 'celery stick' in long bones, 'sandwich' vertebrae, and 'bone within bone' in the carpal and tarsal bones.

CONGENITAL ABNORMALITIES OF BONE

(a) **Osteopsathyrosis** (Osteogenesis imperfecta) exists in two forms, *intra-uterine* and *infantile*. The intra-uterine form causes multiple fractures *in utero* and death either before or shortly after birth. The infantile form presents as pathological bone fragility, resulting in frequent fractures. The bone changes are due to a defect in the connective tissue scaffolding of bone. Other evidence of connective tissue abnormality is found in the characteristic blue sclerotics which may however be absent in the most severe cases.

Clinically these children suffer many fractures from trivial injury. With increasing age fractures often becomes less frequent, probably due to greater care. Otosclerosis may develop in adult life.

(b) **Achondroplasia.** This disease appears in foetal life, and is hereditary. In most instances the pattern of occurrence is of Mendelian dominance, but sometimes recessive characters appear. There is defective ossification of bones formed in cartilage. For this reason the skull vault and spinal bones are normal, but the arms and legs are abnormally short, like those of a dachshund.

These are the typical circus dwarfs. The average height is about 4 feet; the trunk is normal but the arms and legs are short and the head misshapen. The vault appears large and the face is small with a sunken bridge to the nose. Musculature is well developed, and the hands rather small; the fingers are almost equal in length.

Many achondroplasics are stillborn, or die soon after birth. In those who survive the expectation of life is normal. No treatment is useful.

Table 9.1 Biochemical changes in some metabolic bone diseases

Normal	Ca^{2+} *2.10–2.60 mmol/l*	PO_4^{3-} *0.60–1.40 mmol/l*	*Renal function*	*Alk. phos. 7–106 u/l*	*Urinary* Ca^{2+} ***Men < 10 mmol/24 h Women < 8.5 mmol/24 h***
Rickets/osteomalacia	N or ↓	N or ↓	N	↑ or N*	↓
Primary hyperparathyroidism	↑	↓	N or ↓	N	↑ or N
" " with bone disease	↑	↓	N or ↓	↑	↑ or N
Secondary hyperparathyroidism	N or ↓	N or ↑	↓	N or ↑	↓
Hypoparathyroidism	↓	↑	N	N	↓
Osteoporosis	N	N	N	N	N
Paget's disease of bone	N or ↑ †	N	N	↑	N or ↑†

* Rarely if complicating malabsorption
† If immobilised
N Normal
↑ Raised
↓ Decreased

MARFAN'S SYNDROME

Marfan's syndrome is a hereditary disorder of connective tissue. There is no particular sex incidence and it can appear in incomplete forms.

The main manifestations are:

(1) *Skeleton.* The bones are elongated and thin and the span exceeds the height. The palate is high arched and the hands show arachnodactyly.
(2) *Cardiovascular System.* There is necrosis of the elastic tissue of the aortic wall leading to aneurysm formation, dissecting aneurysm or aortic incompetence, sometimes with superimposed infective endocarditis.
(3) *The lens of the eye* may be dislocated.
(4) *The urine* may show increased excretion of hydroxyproline, a constituent of collagen.

There is no treatment.

FURTHER READING

Paterson, C. R., *Metabolic Disorders of Bone*, Blackwell Scientific Publications, Oxford, 1975.

Resnick, D. and Niwayama, G., *Diagnosis of Bone and Joint Disorders*, W. B. Saunders, Philadelphia, 1981.

CHAPTER 10

DISEASES OF THE KIDNEY

INTRODUCTION

The kidney has three main functions:

(1) The *excretion* of the end products of metabolism and of foreign substances and their metabolites. These include such substances as urea, uric acid and creatinine, and a large number of drugs or their breakdown products.
(2) The *maintenance* of the tissue fluids at a constant composition. The kidney is concerned not only with the concentration of various substances in the tissue fluids, but also helps to maintain the pH and volume of the latter within physiological limits.
(3) The *secretion* of hormones and hormone-like substances. These include renin, erythropoietin, the active form of Vitamin D (1,25-dihydroxycholecalciferol) and several prostaglandins.

There is a continual tendency for the composition of the tissue fluids to change. This results from wide variation in the intake of fluid and electrolytes and from the changes in the rate of metabolism which occur from hour to hour, resulting in uneven production of the end products of metabolism. The kidney must respond to these changes by excreting varying quantities of fluids and electrolytes; and as many of the end products of metabolism are acid it is continuously excreting hydrogen ions.

THE STRUCTURE OF THE KIDNEY

The functional unit of the kidney is the *nephron*. This consists of a glomerular tuft, situated in the cortex, and a tubule. The tuft leads into the proximal convoluted tubule which in turn leads to the loop of Henle which dips into the medulla, turns back on itself and ends in the distal convoluted tubule, which drains into a collecting tubule. There are two types of nephron: those in the outer part of the cortex which have short loops of Henle and are largely concerned with filtration and reabsorption, and those in the inner cortex which have long loops and play an important part in the countercurrent concentrating mechanism (p. 459). There are about one million nephrons in each kidney.

The *blood supply* to the glomerulus is directly from the renal artery. Efferent vessels leaving the glomerular tuft form a capillary network around the convoluted tubules, ending in a branch of the renal vein.

The cells lining the convoluted tubules and part of the ascending limb of the loop of Henle are columnar epithelium whereas those lining the rest of the loop are much flatter.

RENAL FUNCTION

THE GLOMERULUS

The glomeruli receive blood almost direct from the renal arteries at a considerable pressure. It seems probable that glomerular filtration is a passive process and that glomerular fluid is an ultrafiltrate, the formation of which depends on the balance between the capillary hydrostatic pressure forcing water and solutes through the glomerular membrane and the osmotic pressure of the plasma proteins keeping it within the vessel. Provided that the concentration of plasma proteins is constant, the rate of glomerular filtration depends therefore on the intraglomerular pressure and stresses the need for an adequate blood pressure and flow to maintain glomerular filtration.

The *glomerular filtrate* contains water with glucose, sodium, chloride, potassium, urea, uric acid, creatinine, and a number of other substances. It contains a little protein, which is reabsorbed in the proximal tubule. The volume of the glomerular filtrate is enormous, probably about 180 litres/24 hours.

The *glomerular filtration rate* (GFR) can be measured. This is done by giving a substance which passes freely through the glomerular membrane and is not reabsorbed by the renal tubules. The rate of excretion of this substance is therefore the same as its rate of filtration.

TUBULAR FUNCTION

The tubules selectively reabsorb the various constituents of the glomerular filtrate so as to maintain the composition of the body fluids constant and at the same time allow the excess of electrolytes, products of metabolism, and water to pass to the collecting tubules and be excreted as urine.

Table 10.1 shows the approximate composition of the glomerular filtrate and urine in 24 hours.

Reabsorption of Water

(a) *Diuresis.* About 85 % of the water filtered by the glomerulus is reabsorbed by the proximal tubule. It is believed that this is a passive process and follows the active reabsorption of sodium. The remaining water, greatly diminished in volume but with the concentration of

Table 10.1 Composition of glomerular filtrate and urine in 24 hours

Substance	*Amount in glomerular filtrate*	*Amount excreted in the urine*
Sodium	15 mol	150 mmol
Calcium	127 mmol	5.0 mmol
Glucose	11 mol	—
Urea	10 mol	5.8 mol
Water	180 litres	1.51

(After Robinson.)

sodium unaltered, then passes to the distal tubules and collecting ducts where further reabsorption occurs. This distal reabsorption is under control of the antidiuretic hormone (ADH) from the posterior pituitary. Osmoreceptors in the paraventricular and supra-optic nuclei respond to changes in plasma osmolarity. Dilution of the plasma decreases the release of ADH so that less water is reabsorbed in the distal tubules and collecting ducts and diuresis results.

When an osmotic diuretic is given reabsorption by the proximal tubule is decreased and the volume arriving at the distal tubule is so great that only a fraction can be reabsorbed. This is why in chronic renal failure there is a failure to concentrate urine. The increased amount of filtered urea which is not reabsorbed acts as an osmotic diuretic.

(b) *Urine Concentration.* When the osmolarity of the plasma increases, there is an increased release of ADH which leads to concentration of the urine. The mechanism of this action has now been clarified. The loops of Henle as they dip into the renal medulla act as a *countercurrent multiplier*; sodium passes across from the ascending to the descending limbs so that as the urine descends into the loops it becomes more and more concentrated and as it ascends it becomes more dilute. The osmotic concentration which develops in the lowest part of the loops is reflected in the interstitial tissue of the medulla and renal papillae.

The action of ADH is to render the cells lining the collecting ducts more permeable to water, so that when urine passes down these ducts and through the area of high osmotic concentration in the renal papillae, water is absorbed from the ducts and the urine becomes concentrated.

Reabsorption of Sodium and Excretion of Acid

One of the important functions of the kidneys is to conserve sodium which is the chief extracellular cation, and to excrete hydrogen ions produced by the body's metabolic processes. Under normal conditions about 80% of sodium reabsorption occurs in the proximal tubule, largely in association with chloride and with an osmotically equivalent volume of water. The remainder occurs in the ascending limb of the loop of Henle and in the distal tubule where it is under hormonal regulation.

Sodium reabsorption is adjusted so that the total body sodium remains constant. One of the important controlling mechanisms is the hormone *aldosterone* which is secreted by the adrenal cortex. Aldosterone causes increased tubular reabsorption of sodium and excretion of potassium and is produced in response to a fall in blood volume or a decrease in renal blood flow.

The metabolic processes of the body lead to the production of various acids. The chief one is carbonic acid, the end result of oxidisation of foodstuffs, and this is eliminated in the form of its anhydride carbon dioxide, which is excreted through the lungs. The other important acid products of metabolism are phosphoric, sulphuric and organic acids, whose anhydrides are not volatile and must be excreted in solution through the kidneys. Although this forms only 0.2% of the total H^+ production, its importance is disproportionately large. The excess hydrogen ions of these acids are absorbed by the buffer systems of the blood, mainly the sodium bicarbonate system, with the release of CO_2 which is excreted by the lungs.

The bulk of secreted hydrogen ion combines with filtered bicarbonate (see below); this normally results in removal of bicarbonate so that none

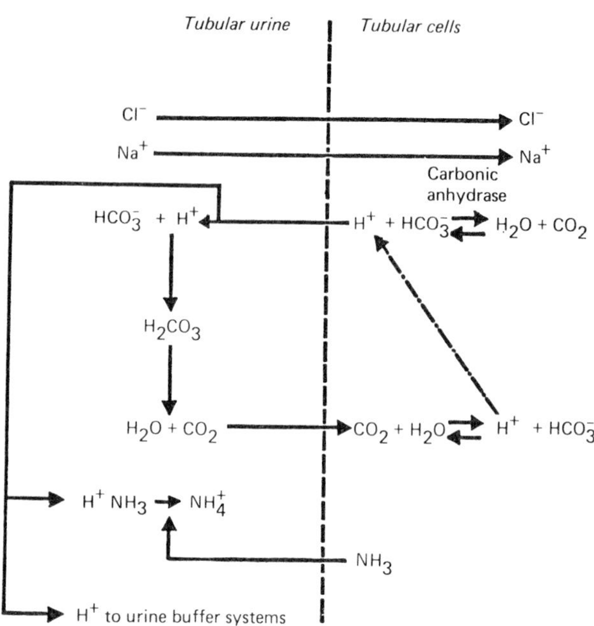

Fig. 10.1 Tubular mechanism for excretion of acid and conservation of sodium.

is lost in the urine. Hydrogen ions are secreted in the distal tubule, and without the ability to establish a gradient of hydrogen ion from blood to tubule at this site acidosis will result. Equally, failure to reabsorb bicarbonate in the proximal tubule will overwhelm the distal H^+ excretion.

Because the kidney cannot establish a pH gradient of urine: blood greater than 4.6:7.3 it is necessary to reduce the number of free hydrogen ions in the urine. This is done in three ways.

(1) In acidosis, urine hydrogen ions combine with ammonia in the tubular cell:

$$NH_3 + H^+ \rightarrow NH_4^+$$

(2) The buffer systems of the urine (largely phosphate) absorb hydrogen ions without producing too great a change in pH of the urine.
(3) Hydrogen ions combine with filtered bicarbonate (see below).

These mechanisms are important for without them the kidney could only excrete a small amount of acid (i.e. hydrogen ions).

Excretion of Bicarbonate

When hydrogen ions are excreted into the renal tubules they combine with bicarbonate:

$$H^+ + HCO_3^- \rightleftharpoons H_2CO_3 \rightleftharpoons H_2O + CO_2$$

The carbon dioxide thus produced diffuses back into the tubular cells to reform bicarbonate. This is one possible method of bicarbonate reabsorption, although bicarbonate ions are absorbed as such. The urine is normally bicarbonate-free on a mixed diet.

If, however, plasma bicarbonate is raised, less hydrogen ions are exchanged for sodium bicarbonate being excreted and the urine becoming alkaline. Again, if the proximal tubules are damaged or defective, bicarbonate will reach the distal tubular mechanism in excess and the urine will be alkaline with production of systemic acidosis.

Excretion of Potassium

It appears probable that all the filtered potassium is absorbed by the proximal tubules and that further potassium is excreted by the distal tubules. The pathway of tubular potassium excretion competes with that for hydrogen ion excretion, so that increased hydrogen ion excretion decreases potassium excretion and vice versa. Potassium is also exchanged for sodium by the renal tubules, so that if little sodium is available potassium excretion is decreased. Finally certain drugs, particularly diuretics and the adrenal steroids, increase renal excretion of potassium.

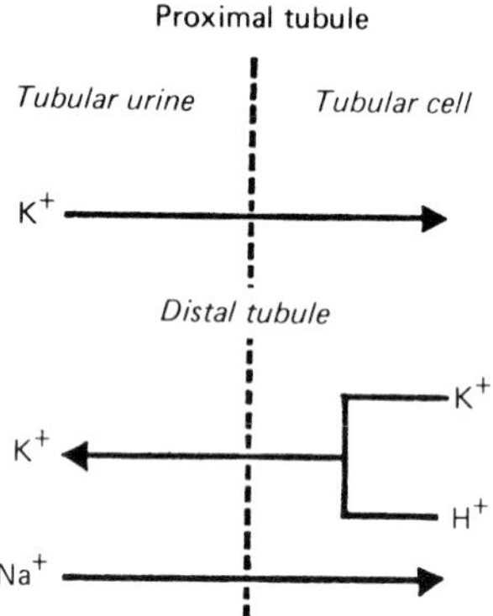

Fig. 10.2 Tubular mechanism for excretion of potassium.

Reabsorption of Glucose and Amino Acids

This occurs in the proximal tubule. If the plasma level of glucose rises as in diabetes mellitus the reabsorbing system can no longer deal with the increased load and glucose is passed in the urine.

HORMONES PRODUCED BY THE KIDNEY

Renin is an enzyme which splits off a polypeptide *angiotensin* from plasma protein. Angiotensin is important in the control of blood pressure and blood volume. It has a direct constricting action on the arterioles and also promotes salt and water retention by stimulating the release of *aldosterone* by the adrenal cortex. Renin is released from the kidney by reduced renal circulation, usually following hypovolaemia or rarely narrowing of a renal artery or by a fall in sodium concentration in the fluid of the distal tubule.

Erythropoietin stimulates the production of erythrocytes. Overproduction may be responsible for the polycythaemia seen in some renal diseases, particularly renal tumours.

The kidney is also important in activating cholecalcifierol (Vitamin D) by further hydroxylating 25-hydroxycholecalciferol to *1,25-hydroxycholecalciferol* which is very active in promoting the absorption of calcium. Failure of this step in chronic renal failure may play a part in the development of renal osteodystrophy (see p. 450). The renal medulla produces several prostaglandins, one of which may be important in regulating blood pressure by lowering vascular tone.

THE URINE

Volume. The volume of urine passed in 24 hours in health usually lies between 700 and 3000 ml. The urinary output of normal people is modified by fluid intake and by loss of fluid in sweat and the stools.

Appearance. The colour of normal urine varies from deep yellow to almost colourless. The colour is due to the presence of urochrome.

The osmolality of the urine depends on the weight of substances in solution. Generally speaking, a high osmolality indicates that the kidney is capable of concentrating the urine. It may also however be raised by such substances as glucose, mannitol and contrast media which have been excreted by the kidney. In health under the appropriate stimulus the kidney should be able to achieve an urine osmolality of 800 mOsmol/kg. The hydrometer provides a rough method of estimating the osmolality of the urine and the specific gravity (SG) varies between 1002 and 1032.

Proteinuria. Normal adults excrete about 100 mg/m^2 of protein in 24 hours. The amount is increased in the upright posture or after exercise. Protein is now usually detected by 'Labstix' which is a colorimetric method depending on the presence of an indicator. By this method it is possible to detect 150 mg of protein per litre of urine which is at the top of the normal range. If therefore a faint trace of protein is found in the urine of an apparently normal person and if there is no suspicion of renal disease on other grounds this finding should be disregarded.

Excess protein in the urine, provided that there is no lesion of the urinary tract, indicates that protein has leaked from the blood to the urine across the glomerular membrane. Being the smallest molecule, completely retained, albumin leaks the most easily, but if the glomerular leak is severe all fractions of the plasma proteins may appear in the urine. Proteinuria is found in almost every variety of renal disease and generally speaking its presence is evidence of disease of the renal parenchyma. The amount of protein in the urine is no indication of the severity of the renal damage and it is a common experience to find only a small amount of protein in the urine of some patients with advanced renal disease (notably advanced pyelonephritis).

Symptomless Proteinuria

In patients with significant proteinuria who are otherwise symptom-free it is important to avoid over-investigation, but it is necessary to exclude treatable lesions and form an idea of the seriousness of the underlying disease if present and of the prognosis. The first step is to decide whether the proteinuria is intermittent or persistent.

Intermittent Proteinuria. In some patients proteinuria is intermittent and may be related to posture, exercise and other factors. It may occur in a wide variety of renal diseases but in young people is frequently due to **orthostatic proteinuria.** In this condition protein is found in the urine secreted when the subject is up and about, but is absent from urine secreted when he is recumbent. Urine passed on rising therefore contains no protein. It is unusual for these patients to pass more than 1.0 g protein in 24 hours.

About half the patients with orthostatic proteinuria have minor glomerular changes but follow-up studies have shown that they do not develop progressive renal disease and the condition is harmless. However, before orthostatic proteinuria is diagnosed as harmless, renal disease must be excluded and investigations should include renal function tests, examination of the urinary deposit and an intravenous pyelogram.

Persistent proteinuria is most commonly due to glomerulonephritis either with minimal glomerular change, mesangial proliferation or membranous change. It may also be due to pyelonephritis or surgical renal disease. If no abnormality is found on clinical examination and renal function studies and the pyelogram are normal and the urine contains no red cells, the patient should be observed. Provided there is no deterioration in renal function over a year or two further investigation such as renal biopsy is unnecessary and the prognosis is usually good. The presence of hypertension, impaired renal function or red cells in the urine suggests progressive renal disease, may carry a worse prognosis and the diagnosis should therefore be clarified by renal biopsy.

Haematuria. Blood in the urine may arise from the kidney or from the renal tract. If it arises from the kidney it is intimately mixed with the urine; if from the lower renal tract it may appear only at certain phases of micturition. Large amounts of blood in the urine are obvious; smaller amounts give it a smoky appearance and minimal haematuria can only be detected by centrifuging the urine and examining the deposit under the microscope for red cells or by using 'Labstix' which detects free haemoglobin. Haematuria must be distinguished from haemoglobinuria and various drugs which may colour the urine red, notably phenindione.

Important causes of haematuria are:

From the Kidney	*From the Renal Tract*
Glomerulonephritis (various)	Papilloma of the urinary tract
Infarct of the kidney	Acute pyelitis or cystitis
Subacute infective endocarditis	Carcinoma of the bladder
Renal carcinoma	Prostatic infection
Overdosage with anticoagulant drugs	Tuberculosis of the renal tract
Bleeding diseases	Renal stone
Injury to the kidney	

Urinary Deposit

Fresh urine can be examined under the microscope for cells and casts. It can either be looked at uncentrifuged or can be centrifuged at 3000 r.p.m. for 5 minutes and the deposit studied.

White Cells in the Urine. White cells may be found in any inflammatory disease of the urinary tract, including glomerulonephritis, cystitis, and prostatitis. In infective conditions they may be present in such quantities as to warrant the term 'pyuria'. Pyuria may be severe enough to cloud the urine. The uncentrifuged sample should contain no more than 5 white cells/μl in men and 10 white cells/μl in women.

Casts in the Urine. Casts are composed of Tamm Horsfall protein, a normal constituent of urine which has solidified in the renal tubules, together with filtered plasma protein, particularly albumin. If they contain cells, either epithelial cells from the renal tubules or leucocytes or red cells, they are called *cellular casts*. If these cells have undergone cloudy swelling the casts are called *granular casts*. Casts which do not contain cells are called *hyaline casts*.

A few hyaline casts are often found in the urine of normal people and

Table 10.2 Usual urine abnormalities in renal disease

Disease	*Appearance*	*Volume*	*Specific gravity*	*Protein*	*Deposit*
Acute Nephritis	Smoky or red	Decreased	High	Present	Red cells, white cells and casts
Nephrotic syndrome	Normal or pale	Normal	Normal range at first, low and fixed later	Present in large amounts	Casts and sometimes red cells
Chronic renal failure	Pale	Increased	Low and fixed	Trace	Casts and few red cells
Essential Hypertension	Normal	Normal or increased	Normal range or low and fixed	0 to small amounts	Normal or excess casts
Acute renal infection	Cloudy 'fishy' odour	Often decreased	Normal range unless previous renal damage	Trace	White cells and bacteria

may be present in large quantities after exercise. Cellular and granular casts are found only in renal disease.

Crystals are rarely of importance and are common in old specimens of urine.

RENAL FUNCTION TESTS

Renal function resolves itself broadly speaking into filtration and reabsorption. A number of tests have been devised which assess one or other of these aspects of renal function. It must be realised that renal function tests merely indicate the degree of impairment of one aspect of renal function; they rarely indicate the nature of the underlying disease. Moreover, they are relatively insensitive and there may be considerable renal damage before these tests show evidence of impaired renal function.

The Blood Urea and Blood Creatinine

The blood urea should always be estimated in patients with suspected renal disease. Although it is a rough-and-ready test of renal function it is simple to perform and often gives as much information as more elaborate investigations.

The normal blood urea level lies between 2.5–7.1 mmol/litre. Persistent elevation indicates considerable interference with glomerular function; this may be due to primary renal disease, or be secondary to a failure of the renal circulation. Unfortunately, although the estimation of the blood urea level is easy it is not a very sensitive test of glomerular function; on a normal protein intake glomerular filtration must be reduced to about 30% before there is any rise in blood urea level. The blood urea level also varies consistently with dietary protein intake and the degree of protein catabolisms, the variations becoming greater with decreasing renal function. Blood creatinine levels can be used in the same way (normal range 50–130 μmol/litre, varying with age and muscle mass) and are less susceptible to changes in diet. There is however a group of patients with seriously impaired renal function who are able to excrete creatinine via the renal tubules and thus have a misleadingly low figure for plasma creatinine. The relationship between the plasma creatinine and the GFR is not linear, so that as the GFR falls there is at first only a small rise in plasma creatinine. With further decline in the GFR the plasma creatinine rises more rapidly so a false impression is given of an accelerating deterioration in renal function. A better correlation is obtained if 1/(plasma creatinine) is related to the GFR. The plasma *β,2-microglobulin* behaves in a similar way to creatinine and can be used as an alternative.

TESTS OF GLOMERULAR FILTRATION RATE (GFR)

The GFR can be measured by giving a substance which is completely filtered by the glomerulus and is neither absorbed nor excreted by the tubules. Such a substance is the polysaccharide inulin. Under these circumstances the excretion of inulin in the urine (in mg/min) divided by the plasma level of inulin (in mg/ml) gives the number of ml of plasma filtered per minute. The general calculation is given by the formula:

$$\text{GFR/per min} = \frac{\text{urine vol per min} \times \text{urine concentration of inulin}}{\text{plasma concentration of inulin}}$$

In practice inulin clearance studies are rather complicated to perform so that creatinine (a substance which occurs naturally in the blood) is often used.

Creatinine Clearance Tests

The rate of clearance of creatinine from the blood almost exactly parallels glomerular filtration although in man there is slight tubular excretion of creatinine balanced by some binding to plasma proteins. In a few patients with massive proteinuria the creatinine clearance may give an erroneously high figure for glomerular filtration. The blood creatinine levels are very constant and a 24-hour collection of urine can be used with a single plasma sample taken at some point during the collection. Generally speaking, creatinine clearance provides the most practical method of estimating GFR.

'Single Shot' Clearance

Substances such as ^{51}Cr EDTA or ^{125}I iothalamate which are not metabolised and are excreted only by glomerular filtration can be injected intravenously. The rate of their disappearance from the blood, which is measured by timed blood samples, is proportional to the glomerular filtration. This avoids urine collection, the least accurate step of the clearance measurement. These substances can also be used as substitutes for inulin in formal GFR measurements.

TESTS OF TUBULAR FUNCTION

Urine Concentration

The kidney will fail to concentrate the urine in the face of dehydration if there is:

(1) Inadequate release of ADH.
(2) An osmotic diuresis as in diabetes mellitus or chronic renal failure.

(3) Nephrogenic diabetes insipidus—a failure of the kidney to respond to ADH.
(4) Hypercalcaemia.

Conversely poor renal perfusion prevents the kidney producing a dilute urine.

The concentration of the urine can be measured by:

(a) The specific gravity which usually varies between 1002 and 1032.
(b) Osmolarity which represents the total solute content of the urine and is measured by the depression of the freezing point. It varies between 100 and 1200 mOsmol/kg.

The most widely used test for the concentrating ability of the kidney is:

Concentration Test

Method 1: Many people achieve a concentrated urine on their usual fluid intake. All urine passed over a 24 hour period is collected and at least one sample should reach a concentration of 800 mOsmol/kg (SG 1022) or above. If this is not achieved Method 2 should be used.

Method 2: The discomforts of dehydration can be avoided by injecting intramuscularly 4.0 μg of desmopressin in the morning. Urine samples are taken over the next 9 hours. The osmolality of one specimen should exceed 800 mOsmol/kg (SG 1022). Excessive fluid intake should be avoided during this period.

Patients with many forms of renal disease are unable to concentrate the urine which is then found to have fixed osmolality (SG about 1010).

The Ability to Produce an Acid Urine

This is an important aspect of tubular function, for if the kidney cannot secrete an acid urine it is failing in one of its most important functions, the excretion of the acid products of metabolism.

A simple test of the kidney's ability to produce an acid urine is by giving ammonium chloride by mouth in a dose of 0.1 g/kg body weight. The urine should then become acid (pH 5.3 or less) within five hours. Failure to produce an acid urine under these circumstances indicates a derangement of tubular function.

In chronic renal failure even with a systemic acidosis, the kidney can still usually produce an acid urine but in various tubular disorders particularly renal tubular acidosis, it cannot produce a pH of less than 6.0.

RADIOGRAPHY OF THE KIDNEY

The outline of the kidney can usually be seen on a straight X-ray but to obtain a clearer picture and to outline the renal pelvis and collecting system requires pyelography. This entails intravenous injection of contrast material which is filtered by the glomerulus and concentrated in the tubules before being excreted by the kidney.

In renal failure the amount of contrast medium filtered per unit of time is diminished and the outline of the collecting system is less vivid. It is possible by special techniques, however, to obtain a reasonable picture up to a blood urea level of 20 mmol/litre.

Fluid intake is usually restricted before pyelography to increase the density of the shadow; but it must be remembered that with impaired renal function this may precipitate renal failure, particularly in myelomatosis.

DISORDERS OF THE KIDNEY

ACUTE RENAL FAILURE

Acute renal failure from any cause is a serious condition with a mortality which remains about 50% overall. This relates mostly to the precipitating circumstances and complications, many of them grave; no patient should die of the uraemia itself with proper management. Acute renal failure, clinically, comprises any condition in which, temporarily, the kidneys are unable to carry on their excretory and regulatory functions. There are therefore a variety of circumstances and outcomes to consider.

The *first* and most important group is reversible acute renal failure from renal hypoperfusion, usually coupled with renal intravascular coagulation (DIC), endothelial swelling within vessels and sometimes *tubular necrosis*. The factors which may lead to this are:

(1) Loss of circulating volume haemorrhage, saline depletion, protein loss (e.g. burns, gut losses and massive proteinuria).
(2) Septicaemia or endotoxaemia, especially but not exclusively with Gram-negative organisms.
(3) Circulating nephrotoxins. (a) exogenous, e.g. poisons and drugs especially some antibiotics. (b) endogenous, e.g. bile salts, haemoglobin from mismatched transfusions, myoglobin from crush injuries.
(4) Concealed accidental haemorrhage in toxaemia of pregnancy, probably because of DIC and renal vasoconstriction.
(5) Hypoxaemia from lung disease, heart failure, etc.
(6) Acute pancreatitis.

In most patients more than one factor is involved and in many most of these circumstances are present. This state of affairs may pass through three phases of increasing severity and irreversibility:

(1) A phase of *reversible renal hypoperfusion* when restoring the circulation and treatment of precipitating factors leads to immediate restoration of renal function.
(2) A phase of *established acute renal failure*, when, despite these measures, a period of days or weeks must be passed before renal function returns spontaneously. The reasons for this delay are obscure.
(3) A phase of *cortical necrosis* which may be patchy or complete; if the latter then renal function will not return.

The *second* important group is acute failure from *post renal obstruction of the urinary tract*. This may occur in the renal tubules themselves, from precipitated substances such as myeloma protein or insoluble compounds such as uric acid or sulphadiazine. More commonly, the obstruction is extra-renal from things within the ureter (e.g. stones), within the wall (e.g. tumours), or without the ureter (e.g. retroperitoneal fibrosis or tumours).

The *third* group consists of a variety of intrinsic renal diseases such as acute glomerulonephritis, severe acute pyelonephritis or amyloidosis, where filtration ceases.

The *fourth* and final group is that in which pre-existing renal damage or obstruction was present and the acute episode represents acute renal failure of any of the above varieties superimposed on this, or worsening of the primary condition.

Diagnosis of which group the patient may fall into begins alongside the management of the acute uraemia (see below). The *urine composition* is of help in distinguishing immediately reversible from established renal failure and a spot urine sample should be analysed:

Urine	*Incipient Reversible*	*Established*
Osmolality	more than 1.3 × the plasma osmolality	equal to or less than plasma
Urea concentration	above 350 mmol/litre	less than 175 mmol/litre
Specific gravity	above 1020	1010 or less
Sodium concentration	below 20 mmol/l	30 mmol/l or more

The next most valuable investigation is a *high dose* (2 ml/kg of meglumine iothalamate) *pyelography* preceded by a straight X-ray of the abdomen. This will establish the presence of renal blood flow, show the size of the kidneys and demonstrate obstruction if it is present. Finally, as a diagnostic and therapeutic measure the response to a high dose (500–1000 mg) of frusemide intravenously over 4 hours may be tested; in a proportion of patients a brisk diuresis will be obtained.

Clinical Features. In the first (*oliguric*) stage of acute renal failure the urinary output drops below 700 ml/24 hours (30 ml/hour). Complete anuria is unusual except in obstruction of the urinary tract. During this period urea and potassium released from cell breakdown accumulate with ever rising plasma levels. The failure to excrete hydrogen ions causes an acidosis with a fall in plasma bicarbonate. The patient becomes sleepy and stuporose; nausea and vomiting are frequent. The chief danger is cardiac arrest due to hyperkalaemia.

The *oliguric* phase usually lasts from one to twenty-one days and is followed by a *diuretic* phase. The urinary output rises sharply until the patient is passing several litres of dilute urine which is largely glomerular filtrate as the renal tubules are not yet working. The danger now is excess loss of water, sodium and potassium. Slowly the urine volume and composition return to normal as tubular function recovers.

Throughout both phases many patients have a bleeding tendency and all are highly susceptible to intercurrent infection if this has not been present from the outset.

Treatment is aimed at keeping the patient alive until spontaneous recovery of renal function occurs. The management of the precipitating circumstances may dominate the clinical picture.

Proper management requires daily measurement of the fluid and electrolyte state of the patient.

Infection should be investigated and treated promptly with the appropriate antibiotic, bearing in mind that most antibiotics are excreted in the urine. Among those which are particularly suitable are the penicillins, erythromycin and fucidin.

In the stage of *reversible renal hypoperfusion* correction of precipitating factors such as fluid and/or sodium depletion, raising cardiac output or treating infection and giving intravenous frusemide may well restore renal function rapidly. However it is important to guard against fluid overload.

In the phase of *established acute renal failure*, the aim is to *replace the small fluid and electrolyte losses* in urine, sweat and gastrointestinal secretions to avoid over-hydration and to *feed the patient a high* 3000 cal (12.54 kJ) diet containing 1 g/kg of protein and low in electrolytes (less than 20 mmols of Na^+ and of K^+ per day). In milder forms of renal failure, where oliguria is brief and the patient not catabolic, it is possible to do this by 'conservative' management, especially if oliguria is not profound. However, better management of patients following surgery, better ante natal care, and better management of incipient shock has resulted in many parts of the world in the virtual elimination of such cases of acute renal failure, leaving only the much more severe varieties who cannot be managed without the aid of dialysis. In managing the patient conservatively, the patient should be weighed daily, and should maintain constant weight or lose weight slowly.

(i) The fluid intake may be calculated from the urinary output, loss of fluid from other causes (i.e. diarrhoea, fistulae, etc.) together with the insensible loss (500 ml daily) corrected for fever (if any).

(ii) Calories can be given orally as artificial carbohydrates such as Caloreen (Milner Scientific) made up as a 4:1 concentration in water, or Hycal (Beecham's) which is rather nauseating to many patients unless diluted. Oral fat emulsions are also used but may cause diarrhoea.

Many patients will require intravenous feeding because of nausea and vomiting. A central venous catheter is useful as there is a tendency to thrombosis in peripheral veins when 50% or 33% glucose solutions are infused. Fat emulsions suitable for intravenous use (Intralipid, Lipiphysan) can supply up to 2000 cal (8.36 kJ)/litre; they are invaluable and relatively free from side effects.

One advantage of dialysis in these circumstances is that 60 g of protein either by mouth or as a casein hydrolysate such as Aminosol which can be given intravenously.

(iii) Electrolytes. Sodium balance is not usually a problem unless excess sodium has been given or there is excessive loss. Plasma sodium estimations are only a rough guide to sodium balance in the patients and must be combined with the history, previous balance (if any) and general clinical picture (i.e. hypotension, loss of elasticity of the skin). Replacements should be given if required.

Hyperkalaemia is a more common problem, particularly in the hypercatabolic patient. It can be temporarily controlled by giving glucose and insulin (1 unit of insulin to 4.0 g of glucose) or 10% calcium gluconate 10–20 ml slowly intravenously.

With this regime some patients can be maintained until diuresis occurs. Dialysis is required if:

(a) Clinical condition deteriorates, with drowsiness, twitching, etc.
(b) Blood urea rises above 35 mmol/litre particularly if it is rising rapidly (more than 8 mmol/litre in 24 hours).
(c) Plasma potassium rises above 7.5 mmol/litre.
(d) Plasma bicarbonate falls below 15 mmol/litre.
(e) Dialysis may be required for gross overhydration.

In general patients are dialysed earlier than formerly, so that they can be maintained in better health with a more reasonable diet. In general dialysis is best performed in an experienced unit, but peritoneal dialysis can be used if the abdomen is intact to tide the patient over for transfer.

In the *diuretic* phase, which may develop very quickly, the aim of treatment is to replace the large amounts of water, sodium and potassium which are lost in the urine.

Acute on Chronic Renal Failure

Patients already suffering some form of chronic renal disease are more liable to develop acute renal failure from all the causes listed above. The clinical features are similar to those in uncomplicated renal failure but the diagnosis may be suggested by finding small kidneys on the radiograph or by the presence of renal osteodystrophy.

The management is as given above but if the chronic renal disease is very advanced the patient may never recover adequate renal function and will require long-term dialysis.

GLOMERULONEPHRITIS

Classification

Glomerulonephritis may be defined as bilateral, non-suppurative diffuse disease of the kidneys, affecting primarily the glomerulus. There is no entirely satisfactory classification of glomerulonephritis, which can be on a basis of aetiology, pathogenesis, histology or clinical presentation. At the bedside, glomerulonephritis presents as one of a number of syndromes each of which is associated with several different pathologies, i.e.:

acute nephritic syndrome;
recurrent haematuria;
hypertension with microscopic haematuria;
nephrotic syndrome;
chronic glomerulonephritis.

Table 10.3 relates the clinical condition to pathological changes. It is to some degree a simplification as patients do not always fit neatly into one category or another and there is often an overlap. Histology is more important in determining prognosis and response to treatment by steroids than it is in deciding the aetiology of the glomerulonephritis.

Immunological Basis

It is now believed that many types of nephritis are due to circulating soluble immune complexes. These will develop when there is an excess of antigen present. Among the antigens which have been implicated are streptococcal DNA (in lupus erythematosus), Australia antigen, tumour antigens and *Plasmodium malariae*. There are almost certainly other antigens yet to be discovered.

The *immune complexes* are filtered out at the glomeruli together with *complement*. The subsequent activation of the complement cascade leads to a combination of inflammation and coagulation which damages the glomeruli. This may resolve entirely as usually happens in post-streptococcal glomerulonephritis or may lead to progressive scarring and obliteration of the glomeruli.

Table 10.3 Relationship between clinical syndromes and pathological changes in glomerulonephritis

	Glomerular inflammation	*Mesangial proliferation*	*Focal lesions*	*Minimal changes*	*Focal glomerulo-sclerosis*	*Proliferative with crescents*	*Membranous*
Acute nephritic syndrome	+					+	
Recurrent macroscopic haematuria		+	+				
Microscopic haematuria/proteinuria		+	+				(+)
Nephrotic syndrome				+	+	+	+
SLE			+			+	+
Henoch's purpura		+	+				

ACUTE NEPHRITIC SYNDROMES

The syndrome of acute glomerulonephritis usually presents as oedema which affects the face as much as the rest of the body, a decreased output of urine which contains blood and albumin, and usually some rise in blood pressure.

The syndrome of acute glomerulonephritis may occur:

(1) following an acute streptococcal infection;
(2) occasionally after other bacterial or virus infections;
(3) without any clear previous cause;
(4) as a complication of:
 polyarteritis nodosa;
 anaphylactoid purpura;
 systemic lupus erythematosus;
 Goodpasture's syndrome;

Much the most common is *acute post-streptococcal glomerulonephritis*, which is probably an atypical reaction to infection with β-haemolytic streptococci of the *Lancefield Group 12* in the throat, or types 49 or 55 in infected skin lesions. It is due to the formation of soluble antigen–antibody complexes in the blood which are trapped in the kidney and fix complement. They damage the glomerular membrane and attract polymorphonuclear leucocytes.

ACUTE POST-STREPTOCOCCAL GLOMERULONEPHRITIS

Pathology. Macroscopically, the kidneys appear hyperaemic. On microscopy the glomeruli show inflammatory changes with increased numbers and swelling of the capsular cells, and sometimes polymorph infiltration. Electronmicroscopy shows 'humpy' deposits on the glomerular membrane which contain immunoglobins and complement. In a proportion of cases the tubular cells show some damage. Later in the evolution the glomeruli show only proliferation of the mesangial stalk.

Many of the clinical features can be explained by the morbid anatomical findings. The widespread damage to the glomeruli is responsible for blood and protein leaking into the urine. The oedema is due to a marked reabsorption of salt and water in the presence of reduced filtration by the relatively undamaged tubular cells with subsequent overloading of the circulation.

Clinical Features. Acute glomerulonephritis occurs most commonly in children and adolescents. There is usually a history of a streptococcal throat infection one to three weeks previously. The onset is fairly sudden with malaise, shivering, and fever and some patients complain of a pain in the loins or abdomen. Vomiting in children is common.

Examination shows oedema, particularly around the eyes and giving the face a characteristically puffy appearance. The blood pressure is usually moderately raised, the jugular venous pressure is often elevated, and examination of the lungs often reveals fine râles from oedema. *The urine* is decreased in volume during the early stages of the disease; it is of high specific gravity but low in sodium and contains protein and red cells. The amount of blood is usually sufficient to produce a smoky appearance in an acid urine. The ESR is raised. The blood urea, provided there is no previous renal damage, may be within normal limits; frequently, however, it is raised. Renal biopsy is only rarely required unless the disease persists or is in some way unusual.

About 85–95 % of children with acute nephritis make a complete and permanent recovery. A diuresis occurs after a few days, following which the temperature settles, the oedema subsides, the blood pressure falls and the blood and protein disappear from the urine. Proteinuria, then microscopic haematuria, are generally the last of the abnormal signs to go and may take several months or even a year or more to disappear completely. In the remaining 10 % or so of patients the disease takes one of the following courses:

(1) A few patients develop *rapidly progressive nephritis*. The symptoms and signs persist with increasing evidence of renal failure and death occurs, usually within a year, from uraemia and hypertension. In this group early epithelial crescent formation round the glomeruli is common.

(2) A further small group of patients develop complete anuria, this is a very serious complication and most of them die unless treated with dialysis.

(3) Some patients apparently make a good recovery, but continue to pass protein in the urine and although they may feel perfectly well for many months or even years they eventually develop either the nephrotic syndrome or chronic renal failure.

There is some difference of opinion as to the prognosis in adults, but it seems that ultimately the majority of patients make a complete recovery although complete resolution may be delayed for some years.

Treatment is designed to maintain water and electrolyte balance and to provide adequate calories until spontaneous recovery of renal function occurs. In the early stages the patient is kept in bed but is usually allowed up when his general condition improves even if there are still red cells and protein in the urine. There is no evidence that prolonged bed rest improves the prognosis.

The diet should contain at least 1000 cal (4.18 kJ), largely in the form of carbohydrate and fat to prevent endogenous protein breakdown, but only 20–30 g of protein daily. It is particularly important to restrict the salt intake as the retention of salt is responsible for the oedema and raised blood pressure. Such a diet consists of bread and butter (salt free), jam, honey, cereals, and fruit. Potatoes baked in their jackets or mashed with salt-free butter are a good source of calories. The most useful fluids are barley water, fruit drinks containing glucose, or weak tea with very little milk. At the beginning of treatment fluids should be restricted to 750 ml in 24 hours; as the urinary output increases the fluid intake is increased. The usual method of calculation is 500 ml plus a volume equal to the amount of urine passed in the previous 24 hours.

On this regime a diuresis usually develops within a few days; when this occurs the patient can resume a normal diet.

Procaine penicillin 600 000 units daily should be given for a few days at the beginning of treatment to clear streptococci from the throat. Otherwise there is no evidence that any drug influences the course of acute glomerulonephritis.

Complications include fits and cardiac failure. Fits can be controlled by giving diazepam 2.5–10.0 mg intravenously. If pulmonary oedema is particularly troublesome large doses of frusemide (up to 1.0 g daily for an adult) will induce a diuresis. The control of a hypertensive crisis is considered on p. 171.

A very small proportion of patients develop anuria which may require dialysis. This complication carries a serious prognosis and biopsy is essential at this stage.

Convalescence. As the clinical state improves the patient should make a gradual return to full activity. Proteinuria may persist for up to a year and there is nothing to be gained by prolonging convalescence until it has entirely disappeared. A gradual return to full activity should be made. On returning to normal life, chills and throat infections should be avoided as much as possible and streptococcal throat infections must be treated vigorously with antibiotics if they occur. Wholesale removal of tonsils should not be practised, but if they are grossly diseased they should be taken out at a later date.

Glomerulonephritis Complicating Systemic Disease

Systemic Lupus Erythematosus (SLE)

The kidney is involved in about 60 % of patients with systemic lupus erthematosus. The glomerular lesion is probably due to circulating immune complexes, the antibodies being directed against DNA. The histological lesions are variable and include thickening of the basement membrane (wire loop appearance) and cell proliferation or membranous change which is indistinguishable from other forms of glomerulonephritis.

Clinical Features. General features of SLE are usually, but not always, present. The common renal presentation is isolated proteinuria or the nephrotic syndrome (see p. 480) which progresses with exacerbations and remissions to renal failure. Rarely it may present as a progressive acute nephritis. The diagnosis depends on finding a high level of antinuclear factor in the blood combined with kidney changes (seen on biopsy) which are compatible with SLE.

Treatment. The disease process can be suppressed by high doses of steroids and/or cytotoxic drugs. If treatment is started before too much renal damage has occurred, a majority of patients will survive five years and some considerably longer.

Anaphylactoid Purpura

About half the patients with anaphylactoid purpura have haematuria and proteinuria or more rarely the nephrotic syndrome. Biopsy usually shows mesangial proliferation with deposits of IgA or focal crescentic lesions. In children the prognosis is good, although recovery may be slow. In adults renal failure develops occasionally. There is no clear evidence that steroids or cytotoxic drugs influence the course of the disease.

Polyarteritis Nodosa

Renal involvement is common in this disease. The lesion may be either a thrombosis in a small artery causing an infarct, or a glomerulitis. The patient may present as acute nephritis, which is often progressive, or as recurrent haematuria often combined with hypertension. The disease process can be controlled by treatment with steroids which may be combined with cytotoxics.

Subacute Infective Endocarditis

The presence of red cells in the urine has long been known as a useful diagnostic feature of infective endocarditis. The kidney may show either a focal nephritis or diffuse glomerulonephritis; these lesions are believed to have an immunological basis. In addition, emboli may cause frank renal infarcts. The severity of the renal involvement varies, but deterioration in renal function with proteinuria and haematuria may progress unless the infection is controlled.

Goodpasture's Syndrome

This is a rare disease involving the lungs and kidneys. It is thought to be due to an antibody directed against the basement membrane of the glomerulus and pulmonary capillaries. The nature of the antigen is unknown.

Clinical Features. Young adults are most commonly affected. Early symptoms are cough, dyspnoea and haemoptysis together with anaemia. After a variable period these are followed by haematuria and progressive renal failure. Death usually ensues within a few weeks or months.

Treatment. The disease process can be partly suppressed by steroids or azathioprine.

RECURRENT MACROSCOPIC/MICROSCOPIC HAEMATURIA

Recurrent Haematuria

Recurrent haematuria is a syndrome in which haematuria occurs at the height of an infection and not after the lapse of some days as in patients with the more serious acute diffuse lesion. The disorder occurs most commonly in children or young adults and most patients give a long history of repeated attacks of haematuria without oedema and without developing any evidence of impaired renal function or hypertension. Biopsy of the kidney usually shows focal proliferative glomerular lesions or mesangial proliferation often with deposits of IgA in the stalk.

Treatment should be directed to treating the infection and persuading the patient (or parents) to lead a normal life. The disorder does not respond to steroids. In the majority of patients the prognosis is good, occasionally chronic renal failure develops. Warning signs are persistent proteinuria, hypertension and deteriorating renal function.

Microscopic Haematuria with/without Hypertension

Various combinations of these symptoms are not uncommon. Renal biopsy usually shows mesangial proliferation or focal proliferative lesions. In general the progress of this group of disorders is slow and many patients retain reasonable renal function over many years. It is important to control hypertension which otherwise will accelerate the process.

Focal Nephritis and Mesangial Proliferative Nephritis

These are histological descriptions and not clinical entities. The essential feature of mesangial proliferative nephritis is an increase in mesangial cells which may be associated with deposits of IgA in the glomerulus when it is sometimes called *IgA nephropathy*. It is a common pathological finding and may be associated with recurrent haematuria, proteinuria and hypertension with microscopic haematuria. The cause of this type of nephritis is not known. The clinical course is relatively benign and there is no specific treatment.

In focal nephritis the glomerular change which may be proliferative or sclerotic is confined to part of the glomerular tuft; clinically it is associated with a number of syndromes including recurrent haematuria, symptomless proteinuria, SLE and Henoch's purpura. The management and prognosis depend on the underlying disease.

THE NEPHROTIC SYNDROME

The nephrotic syndrome is characterised by heavy proteinuria, low plasma proteins and oedema. There are a number of causes of this state:

(1) Glomerulonephritis. This accounts for 80 % of nephrotic syndrome in the adult. The disorder is of unknown cause. It most commonly arises *de novo*, but sometimes follows an episode of acute glomerulonephritis. It has also been called nephrotic nephritis or Type II nephritis.
(2) Diabetic nephropathy.
(3) Systemic lupus erythematosus.
(4) Amyloid disease.
(5) Anaphylactoid purpura.
(6) Complicating Hodgkin's disease.
(7) Complicating malaria.
(8) Thrombosis of renal veins or inferior vena cava.
(9) Poisoning by mercury, troxidone or other substances.

Pathology and Natural History of the Nephrotic Syndrome. The nephrotic syndrome is the result of excessive loss of plasma proteins in the urine. This is due to glomerular damage of differing aetiology. The smaller albumin molecules pass more easily through the damaged glomerular membrane than the larger globulin molecules and there is therefore a disproportionately large loss of albumin. With increasing glomerular disease the leak of the larger-molecular-weight proteins increases and it is possible to measure the profile of the protein leak by measuring the clearance of protein of differing molecular weights. The fall in plasma proteins, particularly albumin, leads to a low plasma osmotic pressure and diffusion of fluid into the tissue spaces, forming oedema and causing a fall in blood volume. It seems probable that the fall in blood volume stimulates the release from the adrenal cortex of excess aldosterone which in turn is responsible for the retention of more salt and water (see Fig. 10.3).

In parallel with the fall in plasma albumin there is a rise in plasma cholesterol and triglycerides; the significance of this is unknown but it does not appear to be associated with an increased incidence of atheromatous diseases. The plasma-protein-bound iodine may be reduced with subsequent depression of the basal metabolic rate. The loss of gammaglobulin which contains the circulating antibodies makes patients with this condition highly susceptible to intercurrent infections. In the early stages this protein leak may be the only disorder of renal function, but if the disease progresses there is obliteration of the nephrons and picture of chronic renal failure develops.

The nature of the glomerular lesion varies. In glomerulonephritis four types of change may be found:

(1) *Minimal Change*. In this type little abnormality can be seen in the

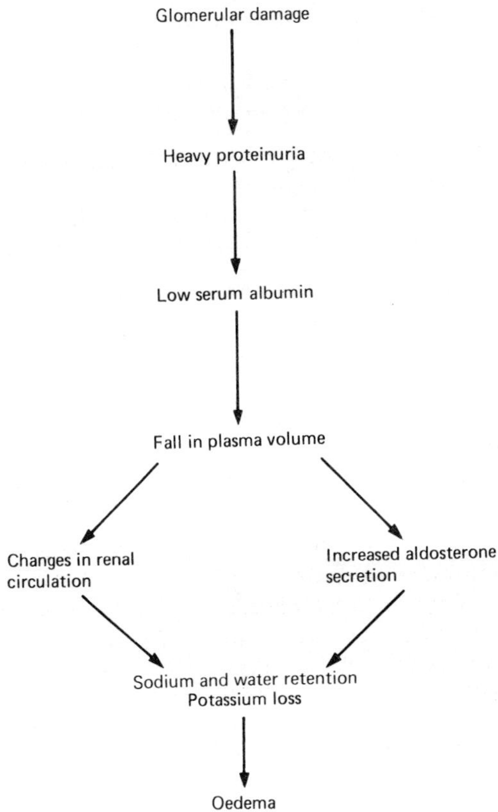

Fig. 10.3 Development of oedema in the nephrotic syndrome.

glomerulus on light microscopy. It is believed to be due to an allergy and occasionally the allergen can be identified. It accounts for 85% of childhood nephrotics and only 25% in adults. Patients with minimal change usually respond well to steroids; if these are ineffective or produce excessive cushingoid changes a cytotoxic immunosuppressive agent may be tried. The ultimate prognosis is good and renal failure rarely develops.

(2) *Focal glomerulosclerosis* is usually associated with a slowly progressive deterioriation in renal function, but many patients live for ten years or more.

(3) *Proliferative changes* are variable. The less severe lesions include subvarieties of mesangial proliferation and focal proliferation (the latter being also associated with recurrent haematuria). These changes carry a good prognosis with little if any deterioration in renal function. Severe

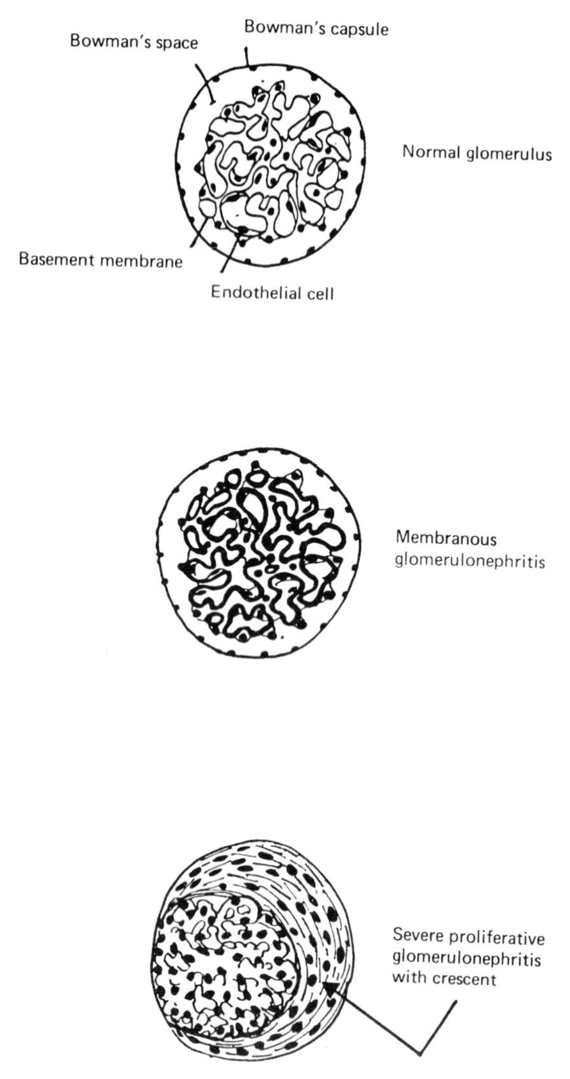

Fig. 10.4 Glomerular changes found in the nephrotic syndrome.

degrees include endo- and extracapillary sclerosis and extracapillary proliferation with crescent formation. Here the disease is progressive with developing hypertension, haematuria and ultimately renal failure, and the course is unaltered by treatment.

(4) *Membranous Change.* The wall of the glomerulus is thickened by the deposition of soluble complexes of antigen/antibody/complement.

Membranous changes as well as occurring with glomerulonephritis are also seen in systemic lupus erythematosus, complicating various neoplasms, associated with some infections (malaria and hepatitis B) and with certain drugs (gold, tridione and penicillamine). The course is usually slowly downhill and is unaffected by treatment (see prognosis below).

The various other causes of the nephrotic syndrome listed above may produce characteristic changes in the glomerulus (ie, amyloid or diabetes mellitus). Confusion can arise however, for example, systemic lupus erythematosus can cause membranous, proliferative or 'wire loop' appearances. Renal vein thrombosis, where presumably mechanical factors are involved, can be confused with membranous nephritis.

Clinical Features. The onset of the nephrotic syndrome is usually insidious. The appearance of oedema is preceded by a period of proteinuria; when the plasma albumin drop below a critical level (20 g/litre) oedema begins to appear. At first this may be confined to the ankles and be fleeting, but as the disease progresses it extends until finally it may affect the whole body, so that the face is pale and puffy, the legs show particularly severe distension and fluid may accumulate also in the peritoneal cavity, the pleural cavities and the pericardium. In the early stages of the disease, the blood pressure is not usually raised and the blood urea level may be normal or even low. The urine contains large amounts of protein, usually more than 5.0 g in 24 hours; in addition it may contain red cells, the persistence of which usually indicates a severe lesion and a poor prognosis. Renal tract infection is quite a common complication and the urine may contain pus cells and organisms.

The continued protein loss leads to considerable muscle wasting and this becomes obvious when the oedema disappears. Owing to increases in blood clotting factors (V, VII and fibrinogen) spontaneous venous thrombosis may occur, particularly if the patient is kept at rest.

The prognosis of the disease is variable and depends on the underlying lesion. Those with minimal changes respond to treatment and those with minor proliferative lesions carry a good prognosis. In more severe lesions, whether due to glomerulonephritis, systemic lupus or amyloidosis, the ultimate prognosis is poor. About 50% of patients with membranous changes survive ten years, although some survive much longer, and in about 20% of patients the disease appears to become quiescent. In those with membranoproliferative lesions, renal failure develops in about five years and with severe proliferative lesions survival may be considerably shorter. In such patients the oedema may persist, often fluctuating in severity. The blood pressure and blood urea levels begin to rise, the proteinuria and oedema often diminish at this stage and death ultimately ensues from renal failure. Before the introduction of antibiotics many of these patients died of intercurrent infection, but such infections can now usually be controlled.

Because of the variable nature of the glomerular lesion and its bearing on prognosis and treatment, *renal biopsy is nearly always necessary*.

Treatment. When the cause of the nephrotic syndrome has been determined it is occasionally possible to remove or treat that cause, for example drug-induced renal damage or secondary amyloid disease. In most patients, however, the only treatment possible is that of the renal disease itself.

Treatment of the nephrotic syndrome is aimed at reducing proteinuria and oedema, restoring the plasma proteins to normal and combating intercurrent infection as it arises. In the majority of adult cases all these objectives cannot be achieved, but temporary remission of symptoms is usually possible.

Symptomatic Treatment

Bed rest should be avoided if possible as it does not influence the course of the disease and may precipitate venous thrombosis. If it is essential the patient should receive 5000 units of heparin subcutaneously twice daily.

Diet. Although low plasma proteins are a cardinal feature of the nephrotic syndrome it is doubtful whether very high protein diets are beneficial as the limiting factor is the ability of the liver to manufacture albumin. The diet should therefore contain 80–90 g of protein daily. Salt restriction is rarely necessary as salt balance can be controlled by the use of diuretics which is easier and more pleasant for the patient. If oedema is persistent it is possible to reduce sodium intake to 40–50 mmol daily by excluding salt from the table and cooking, but further reduction of salt intake requires specially prepared diets.

Diuretics. Frusemide in doses up to 240 mg daily or bumetanide 20 mg daily are very effective in controlling oedema; supplementary potassium will usually be needed. Sometimes the addition of spironolactone to counteract the action of aldosterone increases the diuresis and reduces potassium loss in the urine.

Resistant oedema can be treated with a combination of an intravenous diuretic and salt free albumin or dextran. This combination not only produces an effective diuresis but prevents the development of acute hypovolaemia, which is always a danger when large doses of diuretics are used.

Specific Treatment

Steroid. Nearly all patients with minimal change lesions (usually children) respond to steroids within one month of starting treatment, but the mode of action is not known. Longer treatment, or treatment of most other varieties of nephrotic syndrome, is inadvisable and may be dangerous. The nephrotic syndrome due to systemic lupus may respond but high doses of steroid are usually required.

There are many schemes of dosage and the most suitable has not yet been settled. In children aged ten years and upwards, 60 mg of prednisolone are given daily for 14 days. The dose is then reduced by

10 mg every five days, until a daily dose of 10 mg is reached. If the urine is now protein-free this dose is continued for 8 weeks and then tailed off. If proteinuria persists the histology should be reconsidered and cytotoxic treatment considered. After this regime about 50 % of patients will have a permanent remission; the remainder will relapse, often following intercurrent infection, and will require some form of maintenance of intermittent steroid treatment.

If patients fail to respond to steroids, or develop steroid toxicity, *immunosuppressive drugs* may produce a remission. *Cyclophosphamide* in doses of 3.0 mg/kg/day is the most satisfactory and is given for 8 weeks. Weekly blood counts must be done, but leucopenia and hair loss are rare. The long-term effects of treatment on the testes or ovaries is not known, but longer courses are certainly toxic.

Renal Vein Thrombosis

This can complicate the nephrotic syndrome, particularly renal amyloidosis. It may be due to tumour growth from a hypernephroma spreading along the renal veins or it may occur for no apparent reason.

Clinical Features. A rapidly progressive thrombosis produces a clinical picture of acute renal failure, sometimes combined with haematuria. With a more slowly developing obstruction the appearance is that of the nephrotic syndrome. Diagnosis may well require venography of the inferior vena cava and renal veins.

Treatment is with anticoagulants and the prognosis is variable.

CHRONIC GLOMERULONEPHRITIS

Clinical Features. Chronic glomerulonephritis may follow an attack of acute glomerulonephritis or the nephrotic syndrome or it may occur without any history of renal disease. It may develop immediately after the attack of acute glomerulonephritis, or there may be a latent period of many years in which albuminuria is the only symptom of the underlying and progressive renal damage.

Sooner or later chronic renal failure develops, often complicated by severe hypertension. When this occurs the progress is usually steadily downhill and most patients are dead within two years unless treated by dialysis or transplant.

CHRONIC INTERSTITIAL NEPHRITIS

The kidneys appear contracted and scarred. There is a mixture of fibrosis and infiltration with lymphocytes and plasma cells. The tubules are dilated and the glomeruli become sclerosed. These changes have several causes and thus represent a pathological appearance rather than a specific disease. They occur in:

Chronic pyelonephritis (p. 497)
Analgesic abuse (p. 506)
Gouty nephropathy (p. 505)
Infiltration of the kidney with lymphoma
Lead poisoning
Balkan nephropathy.

There are also a number of patients in whom the aetiology is unknown.

CHRONIC RENAL FAILURE

Chronic renal failure may be the result of a number of pathological processes, but in the end the clinical picture is remarkably constant whatever the original cause.

The most important causes of chronic renal failure are:

Chronic glomerulonephritis
Chronic pyelonephritis
Malignant hypertension
Amyloid disease
Analgesic abuse
Systemic lupus erythematosus
Various types of urinary tract obstruction
Polyarteritis nodosa
Diabetic nephropathy
Myelomatosis
Renal stones
Polycystic kidneys
Renal tuberculosis.

Sometimes it is difficult to decide precisely the original cause of the renal disease.

The glomerular filtration has to fall to 30 ml/minute before there is any obvious effect on renal function. As renal function deteriorates further a condition of *renal insufficiency* develops with a moderately raised blood urea but minimal symptoms. When the glomerular filtration rate reaches about 5.0 ml/minute the symptoms and signs of *terminal* (*end stage*) *renal failure* develop, and the fully developed clinical picture of uraemia emerges.

Renal Function in Chronic Renal Failure

In chronic renal failure there is a considerable decrease in the number of functioning nephrons and thus in the glomerular filtration rate. Those nephrons which remain appear to function normally so that disturbances of function are probably due to overloading of the remaining nephrons, rather than to any abnormality of the nephrons themselves. This has been called the *intact nephron hypothesis*. However, sometimes there is evidence of specific tubular defects, e.g. in pyelonephritis and polycystic kidneys there may be early and disproportionate failure to concentrate and acidify the urine. The result is a loss of flexibility of renal function *with an inability to regulate water and electrolyte balance.*

(1) **Urea and Metabolite Retention.** The excretion of urea depends on the GFR; when this drops to about 30% of normal, retention of urea occurs. The raised concentration of urea in the plasma increases the concentration of urea in the filtered fraction and by this means an adequate excretion is maintained. In addition to urea, sulphate and phosphate are retained together with potentially toxic substances such as phenols, guanidine compounds and aromatic amines.

(2) **Polyuria and Hyposthenuria.** The passing of large volumes of urine of a specific gravity around 1010 (300 mOsmol/kg) is characteristic of chronic renal failure, this is associated with the loss of the normal diurnal rhythm of urine production so that nocturia is a common feature. This is largely an osmotic diuresis due to the increased filtered load of urea, although occasionally (particularly in pyelonephritis) damage to the tubular concentrating mechanism is contributory.

(3) **Acidosis.** Acidosis is a common feature of chronic renal failure. With the falling GFR, there is a decreased filtration of hydrogen ions. In addition although the kidneys are still capable of secreting an acid urine, there is a reduced production of ammonia and a reduced excretion of phosphate which are not therefore available to combine with hydrogen ions, so that total acid elimination is diminished. Also the tubules are less efficient at reabsorbing bicarbonate.

(4) **Electrolyte Disturbances.** The fall in glomerular filtration may lead to some retention of sodium and water with subsequent oedema particularly of the lungs. Hyperkalaemia may also occur and can be very dangerous. It may be due to potassium retention, but also to the acidosis in which potassium ions pass from the intra- to the extracellular space and are replaced by hydrogen ions. Sodium and sometimes potassium depletion may also occur, and is particularly common when there is loss of these ions from elsewhere, for instance in diarrhoea. The prolonged osmotic diuresis interferes with tubular function so that the kidney cannot respond by reducing sodium excretion.

(5) **Calcium.** The disorders of calcium metabolism are considered on p. 450.

(6) **Anaemia.** The anaemia of chronic renal failure is largely due to a failure of production of *erythropoietin* by the damaged kidneys, though decreased red-cell survival is certainly present, and haemostatic disturbances may lead to increased losses.

The Early Clinical Features of Chronic Renal Failure

Renal Insufficiency

The onset of renal failure is usually insidious. Symptoms may be minimal, but may include some polyuria, nocturia, and perhaps some loss of energy. On examination the blood pressure is usually raised and the urine contains a little protein together with a few red cells and granular casts. The blood urea level is a little raised, but in the early stages of renal failure this can often be restored to normal by a diet low in protein. This stage may persist for a considerable period, sometimes years, before the classical terminal picture develops and it is in this stage that judicious management of diet, fluid intake, and electrolyte balance can keep the patient in moderately good health.

The Terminal Clinical Features of Chronic Renal Failure

For convenience these may be considered systematically:

Central Nervous System. The patient is at first *tired* and *listless* and *headaches* are common. As the disease progresses, he becomes drowsy and may finally lapse into coma. Muscular twitching and sometimes *epileptiform convulsions* may occur.

The biochemical abnormality underlying the symptoms arising in the nervous system is not clear, but it seems probable that they are due to an upset in balance of the blood electrolytes. The muscular twitching can sometimes be relieved by intravenous calcium salts.

Alimentary System. The tongue is dry and coated with a dirty brown fur, the breath has an uriniferous smell and hiccoughs, *nausea*, and *vomiting* are often distressing symptoms. Sometimes bleeding from the gastrointestinal tract occurs leading to haematemesis or bloodstained *diarrhoea*. These symptoms are caused by the excretion of urea into the gut, where it breaks down and releases ammonia. This is highly irritant.

Respiratory System and Acid/Base Balance. Acidosis causes a typical gasping form of respiration known as Kussmaul breathing; Cheyne-Stokes respiration may also occur in the terminal stages.

Pulmonary oedema may occur and *dyspnoea* is a common symptom. Pulmonary infection is not uncommon and may be due to unusual bacteria such as *E. coli* or to fungi.

Cardiovascular System. *Hypertension* is frequently found in association with chronic renal failure and is probably due to several factors: increased cardiac output, sodium and water retention, and in the more severe cases, an increased production of *renin* (see p. 462). It may produce no symptoms, but more commonly the *vascular system* is severely affected. This is most easily seen in the retinae which show:

(1) Papilloedema.
(2) Soft exudates which often take the form of a star at the macula. They are caused by oedema of the retina.
(3) Haemorrhages into the retina.
(4) Thickening of the arteries with variations in calibre and tortuosity, increased light reflex, and nipping at the arteriovenous crossings.

Pericarditis frequently appears in the late stages of renal failure. It may cause chest pain and usually a loud rub. Effusions are uncommon and usually bloody. The cause is unknown.

A small proportion of patients die from heart failure or cerebrovascular accidents, although the majority die of renal failure itself.

Skin. The skin is dry and becomes yellowish or brownish in colour and since the sweat glands excrete urea or other substances normally excreted by the kidney, *pruritus* is common. Occasionally there is so much urea in the sweat that it crystallises on the skin to give a 'urea frost'.

Blood. Microcytic normochromic *anaemia* which is resistant to iron treatment is very common in uraemia. It is due to decreased production of red cells with some haemolysis and can only be relieved by blood transfusion.

The Skeleton. A small proportion of cases of chronic renal failure shows widespread disorder of the bone which is called *renal osteodystrophy* (renal rickets, p. 450). *Pseudogout* due to high blood phosphate level can occur.

Endocrine System. Apart from the secondary *hyperparathyroidism* there is failure of gonadal function, *infertility*, loss of libido and *amenorrhea*, being common. Uraemia mimics *hypothyroidism* but sometimes true thyroid failure is present.

The Urine. The urine volume per 24 hours is increased and there is nocturia. It is usually of fixed specific gravity (between 1010 and 1012) and contains protein, although often in quite small amounts. Microscopy shows increased numbers of red cells and granular casts.

Treatment of Chronic Renal Failure. There is unfortunately no way of preventing the progress of renal damage in most patients with chronic renal failure. All that can be done is to help the kidney to function as well as possible under the circumstances. Patients can frequently be kept alive and in moderately good health for years. The important points in management are:

(a) *Fluid intake* should be at least 3 litres daily. In chronic renal failure the excretion of urea and other waste products is proportional to the urinary flow, so a high urine output is essential. It is important, however, not to overhydrate these patients since this results in oedema. They should be weighed regularly and the fluid intake adjusted to keep their weight steady. Sodium intake will have to be adjusted to the needs of the patient as sodium loss in the urine is variable but is usually in the region of 40–70 mmol/day. Evidence of hypernatraemia with venous congestion and rising blood pressure call for a reduced intake and frusemide in large doses (500 mg daily) orally may be required in a crisis. Some patients lose a lot of sodium in the urine and if this is complemented by loss from vomiting or diarrhoea depletion develops with hypovolaemia and deteriorating renal function. In these circumstances sodium can be given orally or intravenously in the form of sodium bicarbonate.

Hyperkalaemia can be prevented by reducing the intake if necessary, and the use of an ion-exchange resin (Resonium A 15 g three times daily) sometimes helps. In the terminal stages hyperkalaemia may be impossible to control.

(b) Severe *dietary restrictions* are irksome and it is doubtful if they are useful. When the blood urea rises above 15 mmol/litre (plasma creatinine 375 μmol/litre) the daily intake of protein should be reduced to 40 g and the diet should be largely composed of carbohydrates and fat, producing 3000 calories. As failure becomes more severe the protein intake may be reduced to 20 g daily, or the Giovenetti diet may be used. This diet provides the minimal necessary quantity of first class protein. This extreme type of diet requires very close supervision, since if not strictly adhered to, especially with regard to calorie intake, it results in increased catabolism weight loss and actual deterioration. For the treatment of disturbed calcium metabolism see p. 450.

(c) The *anaemia* of renal failure does not respond to haematinics. It may be treated by transfusion but the benefit is very transitory. It is fruitless to try and maintain a normal PCV by repeated transfusions and carries with it the risk of immunising the patient against transplantation antigens, or of turning the patient into a hepatitis carrier. Many of these patients get along very well with a PCV of 25% or even lower.

(d) *Hypertension* which accompanies the renal failure may be very severe, and accelerates the progression of the renal damage. It is usually worth while trying to lower the blood pressure to safer levels by means of drugs (p. 168), but the control of blood pressure in these patients is difficult. A loop diuretic such as frusemide is needed to reduce sodium retention and this may be combined with a β blocker which is not excreted by the kidney, such as metoprolol. A direct vasodilator may be added to the regime if necessary.

(e) Eventually a stage is reached at which only symptomatic treatment can be given. Chlorpromazine often prevents the nausea and vomiting and morphine may relieve discomfort and alleviate anxiety and fears.

(f) *Drugs in Renal Failure.* Renal failure may modify the action of drugs. This is most often due to alteration of the drug's kinetics although receptor sensitivity is occasionally affected. Changes may occur in distribution of the drugs and alteration in plasma protein levels may influence their protein binding. Renal failure may also affect the metabolism of drugs. These changes are usually quite small quantitatively and the most important effect of renal failure on drug elimination is concerned with those drugs which are excreted by the kidney.

The excretion of a drug by the kidney is related to the creatinine clearance however the drug is handled by the kidney, and normograms are available which allow the reduction of dosage to be calculated to avoid accumulation. Drugs which should be avoided or reduced in renal failure include:

Aminoglycosides	Digoxin
Co-trimoxazole	β Blockers excreted by the kidney
Cephaloridine	Allopurinol
Nitrofurantoin	Chlorpropamide
Nalidixic acid	Cyclophosphamide
Isoniazid	Methotrexate
Tetracyclines	Azathioprine

Maintenance Haemodialysis and Renal Transplant

When the glomerular filtration rate falls below about 3 ml/min in patients without hypertension and 5 ml/min in the presence of this complication, terminal renal failure has been reached and the patient will die. It is possible to maintain such patients in fair health by haemodialysis.

The patient is given a permanent external arteriovenous shunt or subcutaneous arteriovenous fistula and through this is attached to a dialysis machine for about 10 hours three times a week. The choice of patients for such treatment is not always easy, as a certain amount of mental resilience is required, and they should not be suffering from any progressive systemic disease outside the kidneys. Hypertension, however, is no bar and is usually considerably improved after dialysis has been started.

An alternative is continuous ambulatory peritoneal dialysis in which the patient retains intraperitoneal dialysis fluid for 4–6 hours four times daily. It is cheap and allows the patient more scope but is often complicated by recurrent bouts of peritonitis. Nevertheless it is useful where haemodialysis is impracticable.

Renal transplant with either a cadaver or live donor offers an alternative method of rescuing patients with terminal renal failure. The main problem of transplantation is rejection of the donor kidney by an immune response involving both cellular and humoral mechanisms. Although this can possibly be minimised by matching donor and recipient in terms of both ABO and HLA antigens as closely as possible, prolonged immunosuppression is required. About half the transplanted cadaveric kidneys survive four years and the survival rate is rather better with live donors. Transplantation does however allow the patient to lead a more normal life than dialysis.

Immunosuppression and Cancer

When renal transplant is followed by immunosuppressive treatment there is an increased incidence of malignant disease. These are largely reticulum cell sarcomas or microgliomas and brain involvement is common. There is also some increase in skin cancers and mesenchymal tumours.

RENAL FAILURE DUE TO OBSTRUCTION
(Obstructive Uropathy)

Although this type of renal failure is often treated surgically it forms an important part of the differential diagnosis of both acute and chronic renal failure. Among the causes are:

Stones in the renal tract
Neoplasms of the urinary tract
Prostatic enlargement
Retroperitoneal fibrosis
Lymphomas causing ureteric obstruction.

Clinical Features. Obstructive uropathy may present as acute or chronic renal failure. Other symptoms such as pain and haematuria may give some clue as to the diagnosis. Intravenous pyelography is usually essential to clarify the situation. Subsequent management depends on the cause of the obstruction.

Retroperitoneal Fibrosis

In this unusual condition there is fibrosis of the posterior abdominal wall with involvement of the ureters which can ultimately become obstructed. The cause of the fibrosis is unknown but the following groups are recognised:

(a) idiopathic;
(b) associated with prolonged use of methysergide;
(c) associated with neoplastic infiltration of the posterior abdominal wall usually by carcinoma of the breast or a lymphoma.

Clinical Features. The picture is one of slowly developing renal failure. Often there are no other specific symptoms, although low back ache may occur sometimes. The pyelograph shows dilation of the renal pelvis on one or both sides with variable dilation of the ureters which may be displaced medially. Sometimes the disorder appears to be unilateral at first.

Treatment. This is essentially surgical to release the trapped ureters. Steroids will often produce temporary relief of the obstruction.

URINARY TRACT INFECTION

Three clinical syndromes of urinary tract infection will be described:

(1) frequency and dysuria syndromes;
(2) acute bacterial pyelonephritis;
(3) chronic pyelonephritis.

The relationship between these three syndromes has long been the subject of debate. There is little doubt that lower urinary tract infection can be followed by acute pyelonephritis. The connection between acute urinary tract infection and the contracted kidneys of chronic pyelonephritis is important. In adult women, provided there is no obstruction in the urinary tract, it is very rare for acute infection to progress to chronic pyelonephritis. In adult men, where urinary infection is rare, an underlying cause should always be suspected. Children, however, are a different matter. Infection in this age group frequently means some structural abnormality of the renal tract, usually causing vesico-ureteric reflux. If the infection is not corrected there is real danger of progressive kidney damage. Finally, the clinical and pathological condition known as *chronic pyelonephritis* probably arises from several causes, of which infection is only one.

The Significance of Bacteriuria

E. coli is the common infecting organism; others include *Staphylococcus albus* or *aureus, Proteus vulgaris* (frequently associated with stones), *Pseudomonas pyocyanea, Klebsiella* and *Streptococcus faecalis.*

The culture of a *fresh* specimen of urine (a midstream or catch specimen is satisfactory) is essential in the investigation of urinary tract infection. The work of Kass has shown that the urine of normal individuals does not contain more than 10 000 organisms per ml of urine. In urinary tract infection, even if it is latent, it is usual to find more than 100 000 organisms/ml.

The clinical importance of symptomless bacteriuria depends largely on the circumstances in which it is found. In women who are not pregnant it is of little significance, it is only rarely associated with subsequent renal tract infection, and does not usually need treatment. It is particularly common in elderly women. Bacteriuria in pregnancy is discussed on p. 496. In children bacteriuria is more liable to be associated with structural disease of the urinary tract and requires treatment.

Acute Infections

Frequency and Dysuria Syndrome (Cystitis)

This is a disease of women and there are several aetiological factors. Using routine methods it is possible to culture bacteria from the urine of about 50 % of these patients, though with refined techniques a variety of organisms including lactobacilli and corynebacteria can be grown in a high proportion of urines. In this group of patients the disorder is thought to be due to infection of the posterior urethral glands and trigone of the bladder and it is sometimes termed *bacterial cystitis.*

In the remaining patients no evidence of infection can be found and causative factors include minor injury to the urethra during coitus and local reaction to soaps, deodorants, etc. This disorder is called the *urethral syndrome.*

Clinical Features. This is a very common complaint. It may be precipitated by sexual intercourse or complicate prolapse. Often attacks occur for no obvious reason. The usual symptoms are frequency and dysuria; fever or general malaise are not common. The attacks are usually self-limiting and only last a few days. The main problems are:

(1) Attacks frequently recur and even if they are not medically serious they are socially distressing.
(2) In a small proportion of patients the infection may spread to the kidneys and cause a pyelonephritis.

Acute Pyelonephritis

The term pyelonephritis is used to emphasise that with inflammation of the ureters and renal pelvis there is also infection of the renal parenchyma. The renal medulla is particularly involved, the high osmolality in this area interfering with the normal immune mechanism and making it especially vulnerable. It seems probable that infection reaches the kidney via the ureter, but the exact mechanism is not clear except where there is vesicoureteric reflux.

Colonisation of the bladder, ureters and renal pelvis by bacteria is normally prevented by the urinary flow which washes out any organisms from the lower urinary tract and is perhaps combined with a local antibacterial action of immunoglobin and bladder epithelial cells. Anything which interferes with the free flow of urine will therefore predispose to infection, and causes of such interference are:

(a) pregnancy;
(b) prolapse;
(c) bladder neck obstruction, renal stones etc.;
(d) neurological disorders which interfere with bladder emptying.

In addition the short female urethra predisposes to ascending infection.

In children, outflow tract obstruction, particularly in the posterior urethra, may be combined with reflux of urine from the bladder into the ureters, leading to pyelonephritis. This is probably due to some congenital defect and can be demonstrated by a micturating cystogram; its recognition is important since it can cause progressive renal damage if infection is not controlled. It usually recovers as the child grows older.

In men pyelonephritis is nearly always secondary to some abnormality in the urinary tract.

Clinical Features. The onset is usually sudden, although there may be a short history of lower urinary tract infection. Symptoms include fever, shivering and rigors, general malaise, aching in one or both loins and sometimes in the suprapubic region, frequency and dysuria. On examination there is usually tenderness over one or both kidneys. There is a leucocytosis and a large number of pus cells are found in the urine.

Treatment of Acute Infection

(a) *Frequency and Dysuria Syndrome.* Symptoms nearly always disappear within a few days but it is usual to give a short course of antibiotics (co-trimoxazole, one tablet twice daily for 5 days). Recurrence is the real problem and will require pyelography and cystoscopy to exclude a local cause although this is rarely found. Sometimes cystoscopy is combined with urethral dilation, although there is little evidence of its therapeutic effectiveness. To prevent recurrent attacks simple measures such as a reasonable fluid intake, micturition after sexual intercourse and personal cleanliness may be helpful.

(b) *Acute Pyelonephritis.* The patient is nursed in bed and given a fluid intake of at least 3 litres daily. A urine sample should be sent for culture and to determine sensitivity of the organism to antibiotics. Since the infecting organism is usually *E. coli*, treatment can be started with a suitable antibacterial drug without waiting for the result of urine culture. A list of drugs is given below and the most useful is co-trimoxazole one or two tablets twice daily, trimethoprim 200 mg twice daily or amoxycillin 250 mg 3 times daily. Symptoms usually subside rapidly but treatment should be continued for 5 days. If the patient fails to respond a resistant organism is probably responsible and the result of urinary culture will reveal its nature. Sensitivity tests will now show the most effective antibiotic to use.

It is important to ensure that the infection has been eradicated and patients should have their urine cultured one month after completion of treatment to ascertain that it is sterile.

Recurrence of bacterial infection, even in women with an apparently normal urinary tract, is common. If they do not occur too frequently each attack can be treated as above. For a few patients it is necessary to continue treatment over long periods to control symptoms. Co-trimoxazole one tablet at night or nitrofurantoin 100 mg once or twice daily are satisfactory.

Any patient who has had a bacterial kidney infection must have an intravenous pyelogram to exclude underlying disease and with recurrent infections more extensive investigation may be required.

Renal Infection in Pregnancy

Routine urine tests show that about 5% of pregnant women have a significant bacteriuria (more than 100 000 organisms per ml), although they may be symptomless at the time, and about 40% of these bacteriuric women develop overt urinary infection as pregnancy progresses. About 2–3% of all pregnant women develop clinical renal tract infection. This is believed to be due to dilatation of the ureters and interference with urinary flow by the foetus. Urinary infection may be associated with an increased incidence of toxaemia, foetal abnormality and prematurity.

Clinical infection should be treated (see above) and a sulphonamide or amoxycillin is usually satisfactory. Patients with asymptomatic bacteriuria should be given a week's course of antibiotic treatment and thereafter be observed throughout the pregnancy. A few patients whose kidneys have already been damaged by previous infection may require treatment throughout pregnancy. Sulphadimidine 0.5 g t.d.s. is usually satisfactory (provided the organism is sensitive). However, sulphonamides must be stopped four days before delivery as they interfere with binding of bile pigments by the infant's plasma proteins, and thus increase the risk of kernicterus. Other chemotherapeutic agents have not been fully evaluated in pregnancy, and co-trimoxazole, which is a folate antagonist, should be avoided.

Renal Infection in Childhood

Although diseases of childhood are outside the scope of this book it is impossible to consider renal tract infection in adults in isolation as it may have started very early in the lives of these adult patients.

It is now believed that chronic pyelonephritis starts in childhood. It is due to infection in the renal tract combined with a structural abnormality which is usually vesico-ureteric reflux. Most damage probably occurs before 2 years of age.

When a child presents with dysuria and frequency it is first necessary to confirm the presence of infection by urinary culture, as only about 20% of children with symptoms of this type actually have bacterial infection. If infection is proved the child should have a pyelogram and about half of them will be found to have ureteric reflux. In children under two years and in special cases they should also have a micturating cystogram.

If the urinary tract is anatomically normal infection should be treated with an appropriate antibiotic and follow-up urinary cultures. If reflux is present the child should be given trimethoprim 2.5 mg/kg as a single dose at night. Vesico-ureteric reflux is a self-limiting condition and antibacterial treatment should be continued until the reflux disappears.

Surgical correction of reflux is only required if:

(a) there is gross reflux;
(b) infection is not controlled;
(c) there is progressive renal scarring.

Chronic Pyelonephritis

Chronic pyelitis is responsible for about 15% of end-stage renal failure in this country. In the majority of patients the disease arises in early childhood and is due to a combination of ureteric reflux and infection but it may not present clinically until adult life. It is considerably more common in women than in men.

Table 10.4 Drugs used in renal infection

Drug	*Dose*	*Comment*
Sulphamethizole	100–200 mg	Use only outside hospital where chance of resistance is lower. Can be used in pregnancy up to 1 week before delivery.
Co-trimoxazole	1–2 tabs b.d. Prophylactic 1 tablet at night	Very effective. Preferred drug in uncomplicated infections. Do not use with severely impaired renal function.
Trimethoprim	200 mg b.d.	As for co-trimoxazole.
Nalidixic Acid	1.0 g q.i.d.	Wide antibacterial range. Side-effects: nausea, light sensitivity and neurological disorders.
Nitrofurantoin	100 mg t.d.s. Prophylactic 100 mg at night	Should be avoided in pregnancy and with impaired renal function. Not effective against proteus.
Amoxycillin	250 mg t.d.s. or 3.0 g repeated once after 12 hours	Can be used in pregnancy. Resistant strains appearing.
Gentamicin	80 mg 8-hourly IV or IM	For severe infections. Reduced dose in renal failure. Monitor blood levels.

One or both kidneys may be affected. In the late stages the changes are those of chronic interstitial nephritis. The kidneys are contracted and irregularly scarred, there are areas of round cell infiltration and periglomerular fibrosis. Some patients have a long history of recurrent urinary infections, others have none and even at post-mortem it may be impossible to culture bacteria from the kidneys. It may therefore be difficult to decide whether the changes of chronic interstitial nephritis are due to infection or some other cause (see p. 485).

Chronic pyelonephritis may complicate renal stones and structural abnormalities of the renal tract and a number of patients, even in adult life, show persistent ureteric reflux.

Clinical Features. Chronic pyelonephritis may present as a chronic or recurrent infection with fever, shivering attacks, aching in the loins and perhaps some frequency. It is then easy to diagnose.

Often, however, it presents as chronic renal failure (see p. 486) with no history of infection, and may be difficult to distinguish from other causes of this syndrome. Renal failure may be preceded by a symptomless proteinuria of many years' duration.

Features suggesting chronic pyelonephritis:

(1) The presence of pathogenic organisms in the urine (see bacteriuria above).
(2) As chronic pyelonephritis attacks mainly the renal medulla, abnormalities of tubular function are more prominent than in chronic glomerulonephritis. Inability to concentrate the urine appears early and some patients lose excessive amounts of sodium through the kidney.
(3) Straight radiography may show irregularity in the outline of the kidneys due to coarse scarring, and they may be unequal in size. The cortex may be thinned and the calyces may show clubbing (Fig 10.5).
(4) Vesico-ureteric reflux of urine may be detected on micturating cystography.

The diagnosis may be confirmed by renal biopsy.

All patients with suspected chronic pyelonephritis should have an intravenous pyelogram and usually cystoscopy and micturating cystogram or retrograde pyelogram to exclude any structural disorder which requires surgical treatment.

Prognosis. Unilateral disease usually runs a prolonged and benign course. In bilateral disease, particularly if it is complicated by hypertension, renal function may deteriorate progressively. Infection *per se* does not appear to accelerate the development of renal damage.

Treatment. Symptomatic renal infection should be treated with the appropriate antibiotic (see p. 497) but there is little evidence that long and complicated courses of antibiotics eradicate the infection or alter the progress of the disease. Amoxycillin and co-trimoxazole (provided

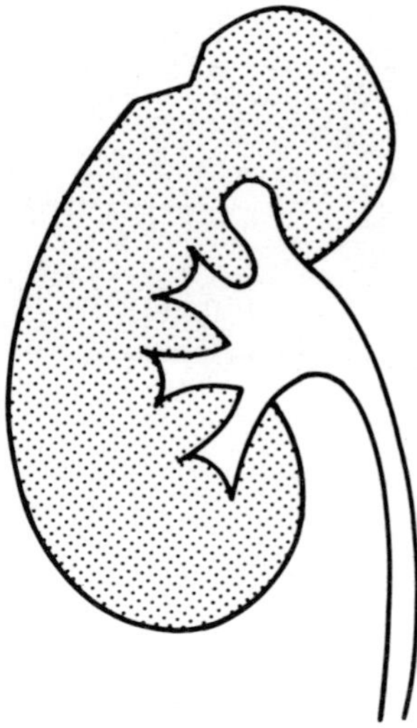

Fig. 10.5 The kidney, showing pyelonephritic scarring and a clubbed calyx.

the GFR is not below 30 ml/min) are useful. Hypertension, if present, should be controlled.

If a patient with chronic pyelonephritis develops renal failure he should be treated as already described (p. 489). The following points, however, should be remembered:

(1) Renal failure in these patients may be precipitated by an acute exacerbation of renal infection and antibiotic treatment may induce a remission.
(2) Patients with chronic pyelonephritis are particularly prone to electrolyte disturbance, correction of which may produce considerable improvement in renal function.

DISORDERS OF TUBULAR FUNCTION

A small number of patients will be encountered who appear to have disorders of tubular function without much evidence of glomerular disease. In many of these patients the disorder is congenital but in others it is the result of various forms of renal disease, particularly chronic pyelonephritis. These disorders may be simple or multiple and may affect nearly every aspect of tubular function. Three such disorders are considered here:

Fanconi's Syndromes

There are two Fanconi syndromes.

(a) *Lignac–Fanconi Syndrome (Cystinosis)* is an inherited metabolic disorder of childhood. There are widespread deposits of cystine throughout the body together with tubular renal defects. Death is usually due to renal failure which may be associated with renal rickets.

(b) *Adult Fanconi Syndrome* is a disorder of both the proximal and distal tubules. It may occur as an idiopathic inherited disorder or be secondary to poisoning by heavy metals or some antibiotics.

There is a failure by the tubules to reabsorb phosphate, amino acids, glucose, bicarbonate and uric acid which are excreted in the urine. This form of Fanconi's syndrome usually presents in adult life as renal osteodystrophy and carries a relatively good prognosis.

Renal Tubular Acidosis

In this condition there is a failure by the kidneys to produce an acid urine (below pH 6.0). Normally the tubular cells excrete hydrogen ions which combine with ammonia or are absorbed by the buffer system of the urine (see p. 459). For this system to work efficiently the tubular cells must be able to produce a pH in the urine of about 5.4. In renal tubular acidosis the failure to achieve a urinary pH of less than 6.0, even in the face of systemic acidosis, makes the excretion of hydrogen ions much less efficient. The main metabolic results are:

(a) systemic acidosis;
(b) low plasma phosphate;
(c) hypokalaemia (if distal tubule is involved);
(d) hypercalcuria.

Several varieties are described.

Type I (Distal tubular) where the defect is in the distal tubular secretion of the hydrogen ions. It can occur as a self-limiting disorder of infancy or be found in adults due to an inherited defect or secondary to renal disease such as pyelonephritis.

Type II (Proximal tubular) may be an isolated phenomenon, usually developing in childhood or it may be part of multiple proximal tubular defects as in the adult Fanconi's syndrome when acidosis is caused by bicarbonate loss.

Clinical Features

(1) *In infants* renal tubular acidosis is characterised by failure to thrive, dehydration, and vomiting. The urine is never more than slightly acid. If the child survives, renal function tends to become normal and the disease does not progress into adult life. Rickets may need treating, either with thiazides (which increases the bicarbonate reabsorption) or with carefully controlled doses of Vitamin D. If phosphate loss is also present, this should be supplemented.

(2) *In adults* the main symptoms are osteomalacia of the skeleton and calcification of the kidney which may ultimately lead to chronic renal failure. Sometimes in addition there are symptoms of potassium deficiency.

Treatment is to try and correct the acidosis by giving bicarbonate and citrates and to replace the calcium deficiency if present.

Amino-acidurias

Amino acids are normally almost completely reabsorbed in the proximal renal tubule. They appear in the urine in two circumstances; *overflow amino-aciduria*, when because of an abnormality of amino acid metabolism some amino acid (or amino acids) is produced in excess; and amino-aciduria due to *failure of reabsorption*. This occurs in the multiple proximal tubular defect referred to as the Fanconi syndrome and discussed above, when all amino acids are present in the urine (*generalised amino-aciduria*). However, there are a number of rare conditions in which specific renal tubular transport mechanisms for amino acids are defective. The only clinically important condition is *cystinuria*. This disorder is due to failure by the proximal tubule to reabsorb a group of four dibasic amino acids. This is associated with a similar transport defect in the jejunum. The only important amino acid is cystine since it is insoluble in all but very alkaline urine and in about 5% of cystinurics this leads to recurrent renal stone formation, and symptoms usually develop in early adult life. It is important to remember that these stones are only faintly opaque on X-ray.

Treatment consists of maintaining a high fluid intake (3.0 litres in 24 hours) combined with alkalisation of the urine with bicarbonate, when stones may even dissolve and further formation be inhibited. Penicillamine which forms a soluble complex with cystine may be used occasionally, but it has troublesome side-effects and is very expensive.

Medullary Sponge Kidney

Medullary sponge kidney (cystic disease of the renal pyramids) is not uncommon. Cysts of varying size are found in the pyramids and they communicate with the collecting tubules, which are dilated. The cysts often contain stones. The condition may be generalised, or affect one kidney, or part of one kidney. It is only found in adults and there is no preponderant sex incidence. It is not progressive and is thought to be congenital in origin. Renal function is not affected except secondarily by infection or stones.

Clinical Features. The symptoms are not specific, patients presenting with urinary infection, haematuria and stones. The diagnosis is radiological and is best shown on pyelography. The pyramids are widened, and the cysts show with the dye. The dilated collecting tubules often opacify in a fan-like fashion in the pyramids. Stones grouped like clusters of flowers are present in the medulla of the kidneys.

Management is conservative and is confined to the treatment of urinary infection or renal colic and stones. Rarely, nephrectomy for unilateral disease is indicated. When the condition is confined to one pole of one kidney partial nephrectomy can be done.

RENAL LESIONS IN SYSTEMIC DISEASE

The Kidney in Hypertension

Although hypertension causes some changes in the renal arterioles, this is not usually enough to interfere seriously with renal function and renal failure occurs very ràrely in essential hypertension. In the small group of hypertensives in whom there is a very high diastolic blood pressure associated with marked arteriolar changes and severe retinopathy, often called *malignant or accelerated hypertension*, severe renal damage can, however, rapidly develop. Sometimes this is associated with fibrin thrombi in the arterioles and capillaries of the kidney, a fall in the platelet count, and red cell fragmentation seen in the blood film (*microangiopathic anaemia*). The arterioles become thickened and the afferent arterioles of the glomerulus undergo hyaline necrosis with subsequent ischaemic lesions of the glomerulus.

Clinical Features of Malignant Hypertension. In addition to the usual symptoms of severe hypertension (p. 165), the patient develops evidence of renal damage: protein, casts, and red cells appear in the urine and the blood urea rises. Nearly all untreated patients are dead within two years.

Treatment. The blood pressure must be reduced (p. 168) and there is now good evidence that with control of blood pressure, the prognosis is considerably improved if treatment is started before renal function is seriously impaired.

Unilateral Renal Disease and Hypertension

The experiments of Goldblatt showed that ischaemia of one kidney in the dog produced hypertension, and a small proportion of patients with hypertension have demonstrable unilateral renal disease. Hitherto, however, removal of the abnormal kidney, although occasionally dramatically successful, has seldom cured the hypertension.

The unilateral renal disease may be pyelonephritis, hydronephrosis, or stenosis of the renal artery. This last type exactly mimics Goldblatt's experiment and it is in this group that nephrectomy or relief of the stenosis should be successful, for it is renal ischaemia resulting in excess renin production with activation of the renin-angiotensin system which is responsible for the rise in blood pressure. The stenosis is usually due to fibrous hyperplasia when it occurs in young patients and to atheroma in the older group.

Clinical Features. Suspicion should be aroused if the patient is young (under 40) with severe hypertension of rapid onset and with a negative family history. Physical examination is unhelpful except that a murmur may be heard over the affected renal artery.

Unilateral renal ischaemia as a cause of hypertension is very rare and the most useful screening test is an intravenous pyelogram which will show:

(a) A smaller kidney on the affected side;
(b) Delayed appearance of the contrast medium in the ischaemic kidney. This will require X-rays taken minutes after the injection of the contrast medium;
(c) Ultimately a denser shadow on the affected side because the contrast medium is more concentrated by the ischaemic kidney.

If pyelography suggests unilateral renal disease which might be ischaemic the next step is to confirm the presence of stenosis by aortography which outlines the renal arterial tree. Even the presence of a stenosis, however, does not necessarily imply that the kidney is ischaemic. *Divided renal function studies*, for which under standard conditions the urine is collected from each kidney separately, are rarely required.

When the kidney is ischaemic the pattern of tubular function changes. Essentially the tubules reabsorb more of the filtered load of water and proportionally even more of sodium. This means that the urine from the ischaemic kidney is:

(a) Decreased in volume;
(b) Higher in PAH concentration;
(c) Lower in sodium concentration;
(d) The inulin and PAH clearances are often decreased on the ischaemic side (but this is not characteristic of ischaemia and may occur with any type of renal damage).

Treatment. The correct management is very difficult, for no test shows without doubt which patient will derive benefit from operation. Renal vein renin levels from the affected abnormal kidneys, when compared with the level in the peripheral blood, provide the best prediction of successful relief. If there is unequivocal evidence of unilateral renal artery stenosis and the other kidney is normal there is about a 50% chance of relieving the hypertension by nephrectomy or by some plastic operation on the stenosed renal artery. Most patients with hypertension and renal artery stenosis can be controlled with drugs, and if possible, this course is preferable even in those patients in whom it is likely surgery will be of benefit. In general, these patients are being managed more conservatively than in the recent past.

Diabetes Mellitus

Proteinuria is common in patients with diabetes. Sometimes in addition there may be other evidence of renal involvement such as a nephrotic syndrome or chronic renal failure. The various renal diseases associated with diabetes are classified thus:

(1) *Pyelonephritis*. This is probably the commonest lesion and accounts for the majority of diabetes who develop chronic renal failure. Some diabetes have autonomic neuropathy affecting the bladder, and many are catheterised in acute episodes.

(2) *Glomerular Lesions*. There are two types:

   (a) The Kimmelstiel–Wilson acellular lesion, which is characterised by nodules of eosinophilic material in the glomerular tuft and is entirely confined to diabetics.

   (b) A generalised thickening with sclerosis of the basement membrane of the glomerular capillary. This change may be found in other types of renal disease.

   The relationship between these changes and clinical evidence of renal disease is not clear but it would seem that the nodular lesions are not necessarily associated with clinical renal disease, which correlates much more closely with the generalised sclerosis. Glomerular lesions in diabetes are frequently associated with diabetic retinopathy.

(3) *Arterial Changes*. The smaller arteries of the kidney may show generalised sclerosis.

(4) *Papillary Necrosis*. In this condition the papilla may slough and it is frequently associated with acute renal infection. It may also be found in analgesic nephropathy.

Treatment is directed to controlling the diabetes as well as possible, although there is no evidence that this prevents the development of renal disease. It is very important to recognise chronic pyelonephritis, as in this group it may be possible to control the infection with antibiotics and thus halt or slow down the progress of the disease.

Amyloid Disease

Amyloid disease may occur as a primary phenomenon or may complicate various systemic disorders (see p. 555). It usually produces a nephrotic syndrome and now that more accurate diagnosis is available by means of renal biopsy it does not appear to be as rare as was formerly considered. Rapid deterioration in renal function suggests renal vein thrombosis.

The prognosis is variable. The primary disease is usually progressive, but if the underlying cause can be removed secondary amyloidosis can be arrested, although it is very doubtful that it will actually reverse.

Myelomatosis

Myelomatosis can damage the kidney in a number of ways. Proteinuria is common and the urine also contains immunoglobin fragments. These may gel in the renal tubules producing an obstructive nephropathy and ultimately renal failure. In addition a small number of patients develop amyloidosis. The rapid proliferation of cells in the bone marrow can lead to hypercalcaemia which also damages the kidney and reduces renal function.

Gout

Gout may damage the kidney in three ways:

(a) Urate crystals may be precipitated around the tubules causing an interstitial nephritis. This may lead ultimately to hypertension and renal failure.
(b) The sudden rise in the plasma uric acid concentration which follows the treatment of leukaemias or lymphomas by cytotoxic drugs can cause precipitation of uric acid in the tubules and acute renal failure. Allopurinol should therefore be given before patients start taking these drugs.
(c) Uric acid stones may complicate hyperuricaemia but can also occur when uric acid levels in the blood and urine are normal. The reasons for this are not clear but many patients excrete a continuously acid urine in which uric acid is poorly soluble.

Treatment is with allopurinol 300 mg daily which decreases uric acid formation and excretion. It may be combined with a high fluid intake and alkalinisation of the urine with sodium bicarbonate.

Decreased doses are required with impaired renal function.

DRUG-INDUCED RENAL DISEASE

A large number of drugs may occasionally cause renal damage. The lesions produced vary and sometimes the same drug may be associated with differing pathologies. The following clinical syndromes are listed together with some of the drugs believed to have been incriminated.

Acute renal failure caused by a number of mechanisms including tubular necrosis and glomerulonephritis.

Aminoglycosides	Amphotericin B
Some cephalosporins	Penicillin
Heavy metals	Sulphonamides
Carbon tetrachloride	Phenylbutazone

Concurrent use of loop diuretics will increase the toxicity of cephalosporins and aminoglycosides.

Nephrotic Syndrome

Gold Penicillamine Troxidone	probably due to immune complex formation

Systemic Lupus Syndrome

Hydralazine	Penicillin
Isoniazid	Phenytoin
Procainamide	

Retroperitoneal Fibrosis. This produces extra renal obstruction. Classically it occurs with methysergide but has been reported with other drugs.

Analgesic Nephropathy

The prolonged use of analgesics is associated with the development of renal damage, the usual pathological picture being that of renal fibrosis with papillary necrosis and sometimes even detachment of the papillae. It seems that *phenacetin* is the most important analgesic involved. However, analgesics are quite often given as mixtures and it is difficult to completely exonerate other mild analgesics such as aspirin and paracetamol.

Clinical Features. The patient may present with chronic renal failure, hypertension, recurrent renal infection or haematuria. Straight X-ray may show calcification of the papillae which may outline the papilla if they are lying free in the renal pelvis. Pyelography may show small irregular kidneys similar to chronic pyelonephritis. The dye may show detachment of the papillae and may outline the spaces found by the disappearance of the pyramids.

Treatment. There is no specific treatment, but if the analgesic is stopped renal function should not deteriorate further and may actually improve. If further analgesia is required for chronic pain, the safest analgesics to give are indomethacin, ibuprofen or the fenemates, none of which have yet been shown to produce or exacerbate analgesic nephropathy.

NORMAL VALUES

Venous Plasma Concentrations

Bicarbonate	25–29 mmol/litre
Potassium	4–5.5 mmol/litre
Sodium	138–145 mmol/litre
Total calcium	2.12–2.62 mmol/litre
Inorganic phosphate	0.8–1.4 mmol/litre

Creatinine	50–130 μmol/litre
Urea	2.5–7.1 mmol/litre
Urate Male	0.15–0.42 mmol/litre
Female	0.12–0.40 mmol/litre
Osmolality	280–295 mOsmol/kg

24-hour Urine Output

Calcium	1.20–8.8 mmol
Creatinine	9–18 mmol
Potassium } Sodium }	Depends on intake Usually 50–200 mmol
Urea	250–600 mmol
Protein	Less than 150 mg
Cystine	0.04–0.42 mmol

Renal Function (corrected to 1.73 m^2 surface area)

Renal plasma flow	400–750 ml/min
Glomerular filtration rate*	100–160 ml/min
Maximum concentrating capacity	800 mOsmol/kg
Maximum acidifying capacity	pH 4.6–5.1

* Decreases with age.

FURTHER READING

Black, D. A. K. and Jones, N. F., (eds.), *Renal Disease*, 4th edition, Blackwell Scientific Publications, Oxford, 1979.
Cameron, J. S., Russell, A. M. E. and Sale, D., *Nephrology for Nurses*, 2nd edition, Heinemann, London, 1976.
Gabriel, R., *Renal Medicine*, Baillière, London, 1981.
Wardener, H. E. de, *The Kidney*, 4th edition, Churchill, London, 1973.

CHAPTER 11

DISORDERS OF WATER AND ELECTROLYTE METABOLISM AND OF ACID/BASE BALANCE

INTRODUCTION

A normal man with a body weight of 70 kg contains about 42 litres of water. The proportion of the body which is accounted for by water varies with sex and age.

Adult man: 65 % of weight is water.

Adult woman: 55 % of weight is water.

Infant: 50 % of weight is water.

Fat, which contains no water, also influences these figures and in very obese subjects the proportion of body weight due to water may be significantly lower.

In considering disturbances of water and electrolyte balance the body water is divided into the *intra- and extracellular* spaces or compartments. The intracellular space contains about 70 % (approx 30 litres) and the extracellular space about 30 % (approx 12 litres) of the body water.

The extracellular space can be further subdivided into the intravascular space and the interstitial fluid. Ions and water pass freely between these compartments and although the capillaries are largely impermeable to protein so that the concentration of protein is much higher in the plasma than in the interstitial fluid, the interstitial and plasma spaces may be regarded as a single compartment. The maintenance of an adequate volume in the intravascular compartment is however essential or circulation will fail.

The most important ions are:

		Plasma (mmol/litre)	*Intracellular Fluid (mmol/litre)*
Cations	Na^+	136–142	11
	K^+	4.0–5.5	164
	Ca^{2+}	2.5	1.0
	Mg^{2+}	1.0	1.4
Anions	Cl^-	95–105	0
	HCO_3^-	25–28	10
	HPO_4^{2-}	2	110
	SO_4^{2-}	1	18
	Protein	16	66
	Organic Acids	6	5

Extracellular Osmolality 285 mOsmol/litre.

The intra- and extracellular spaces are separated by the cell membrane which is freely permeable to water but in health is largely impermeable to sodium and potassium. In health the cell water and the extracellular fluid are iso-osmotic.

It can be seen that the main extracellular cation is sodium and the main intracellular cation is potassium. The maintenance of the high concentration gradient of these ions across the cell membrane is dependent on energy-producing metabolic activity within the cell.

Changes in the concentration of these ions in either the intra- or extracellular spaces result in the passage of water from the low concentration to the high concentration space until the osmolalities of the two spaces are again equal. The shift of water results in the shrinkage and expansion of the respective spaces.

In general, therefore, it can be stated that provided there is adequate hydration the amount of sodium in the body determines the volume of the extracellular fluid and the amount of potassium in the body the volume of the intracellular fluid.

Assessment of Volume Changes

(a) *Vascular Compartment.* A fall in the plasma volume is followed by vasoconstriction and a rise in pulse rate in an effort to maintain the circulation. This causes cold extremities, a fall in blood pressure which is more marked on standing and a fall in central venous pressure. Alternatively a rise in plasma volume is associated with a rise of blood pressure and of central venous pressure.

(b) *Tissue Fluid Compartment.* This is difficult to assess. Loss of skin elasticity when pinched is a classical but late sign of deficiency of tissue fluid. Excess will produce oedema.

(c) There is no satisfactory way of assessing the volume of intracellular water.

The sum of the anions and cations of the plasma should of necessity balance. Clinical measurements usually show a small difference between cations and anions which is called the *anion gap*. An increase in this gap may be evidence of a metabolic acidosis due to accumulation of acids such as salicylic or lactic acid.

CLINICAL DISORDERS

The diagnosis of clinical disorders of salt and water metabolism requires an awareness of the circumstances in which these disorders may occur; if these are remembered diagnosis is not usually difficult. However, it is usually much harder to assess the extent of the disorder.

The management of these conditions is made more precise by daily measurement of intake and output of water and electrolytes and

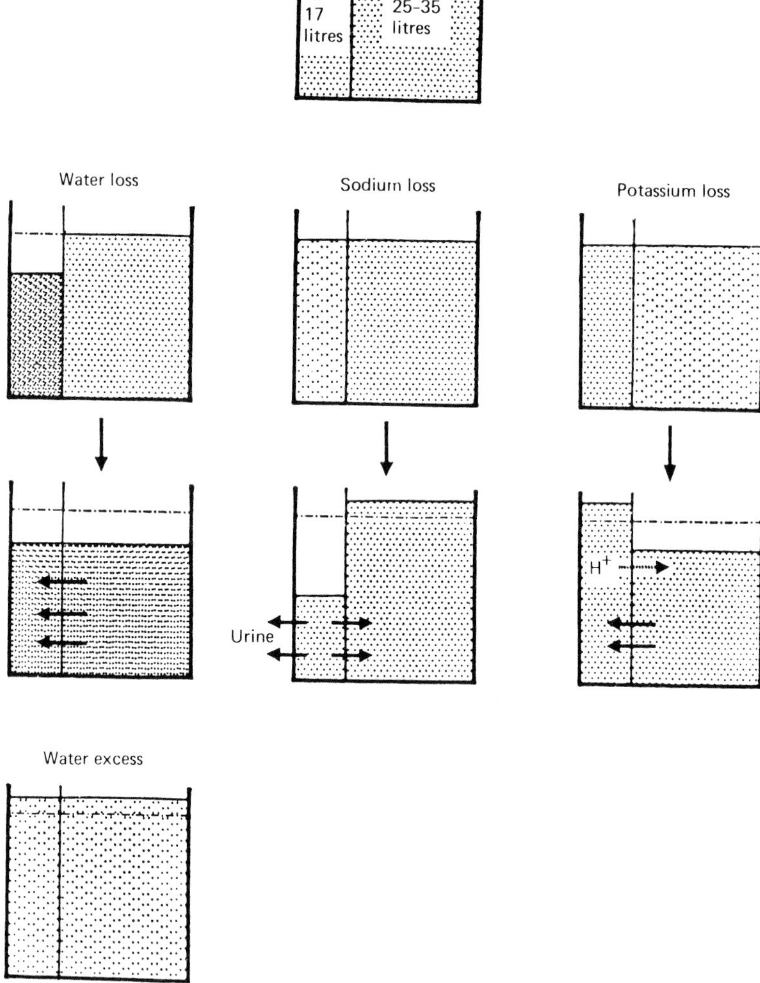

Fig. 11.1 Disorders of water and electrolyte balance.

estimation of plasma levels of electrolytes. The main measurements required are careful records of the volume and electrolyte content of oral and intravenous fluids, the levels of sodium, potassium, bicarbonate and chloride in the plasma, and the volume of urine passed in each 24 hours. In more complicated disorders measurements of sodium and potassium concentrations in the urine may be necessary. In special cases the volume and electrolyte content of other excreta (vomit, aspirate and faeces) may be needed. Regular weighing is a most useful guide to net fluid balance.

Losses which may be expected are given below:

Aspirate / Vomit	Water H^+ K^+ Na^+
Fistulae	Water Na^+ K^+ HCO_3^-
Diarrhoea	Water Na^+ K^+
Osmotic diuresis (as in uncontrolled diabetes)	Water Na^+ K^+

Some assessment of renal function is very useful and measurement of blood urea or creatinine is usually sufficient for this purpose. Good renal function is a great help in returning the patient to normal fluid balance provided ions and water are supplied in adequate quantities. The problem is much harder when renal function is impaired.

If intake and output records are available from the start of the patient's illness the nature and degree of the disorder of electrolyte and water balance can easily be calculated. However, for most patients records are either incomplete or non-existent. Diagnosis must usually be made on clinical grounds and confirmed by plasma concentrations of electrolytes, although as will be seen below these may only give a very rough idea of the extent of the disorder. There are now methods of measuring the total body sodium and potassium, but they are not generally available for routine use and are slow and clumsy.

Finally it must be remembered that it is unusual for a single disorder to exist alone. Any change in the total body electrolytes affects the amount of water in the body, and loss of more than one electrolyte occurs frequently. Although for simplicity individual disorders are examined separately, in practice combinations are the rule.

WATER

The volume of body water depends on the amount ingested and produced by metabolic processes and the output in the urine; in addition about 900 ml/24 h are lost through the lungs and skin. Diarrhoea or excessive vomiting are also factors in some patients; in addition, feverish patients may lose more water by sweating. It is important to remember that although the volume of water in the stools is normally small (less than 300 ml/24 h), a large volume passes in and out of the gut and any disturbance of this exchange can produce rapid dehydration. Healthy kidneys require to excrete at least 700 ml/24 h to get rid of waste

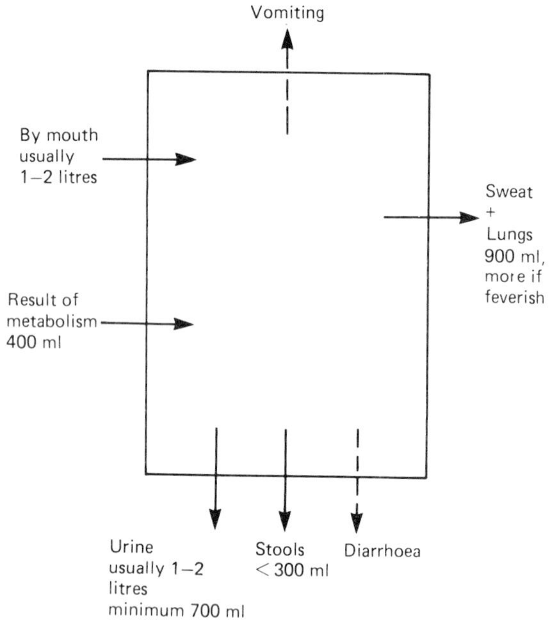

Fig. 11.2 Water intake and water loss over 24 hours.

products. Many patients do not have healthy kidneys and the urine output may have to be considerably higher to prevent uraemia.

Dehydration. Isolated dehydration is not common in this country and usually results from decreased intake. Comatose or debilitated patients may not be given sufficient water. Excessive loss of water from the intestinal tract or through the kidneys is much more common, but, except in diabetes insipidus, there is a concomitant loss of electrolytes and thus a complicated picture.

In pure water deficiency shrinkage of both the intra- and extracellular spaces occurs (see p. 508). The main symptoms are thirst due to rise in the osmolality of the extracellular fluid and in severe cases confusion or coma. Signs are not prominent except for a dry mouth. The volume of urine is low and the urine is concentrated. The plasma proteins, sodium and haemoglobin are raised. Assessment of water deficiency is not easy and will depend on the history, fluid balance charts (if available), and the clinical state of the patient. The best way to follow changes in body water is by regular weighing.

Treatment. Water should be given by mouth or intravenously as 5% dextrose solution. The amount required may be difficult to assess, but the plasma sodium level or osmolality may be used as a guide.

Over-hydration. This occurs when excessive water intake is combined with failure of water excretion. The common causes are acute renal failure or excessive production of antidiuretic hormone. Inappropriate ADH secretion may complicate certain malignant tumours particularly oat cell carcinoma of the bronchus. It may also occur following head injury, in the first 48 hours after major surgery, in acute porphyria and in acute alcoholism. Other causes of over-hydration are excessive intake as the result of overinfusion of dextrose solution or compulsive water drinking. Occasionally it may complicate treatment with chlorpropamide. The excess water is distributed evenly through the intra- and extracellular spaces. Subcutaneous oedema may be present and pulmonary oedema detected by râles at the lung bases. Cerebral oedema also develops and is responsible for much of the clinical picture. Clinical features are confusion, convulsions and ultimately coma. The plasma electrolytes and osmolality are low although the blood urea may be raised if there is associated oliguria. The urine is of low osmolality.

Treatment. In mild cases it is sufficient to restrict water intake. If overhydration is severe it will be necessary to give hypertonic saline (1.8% or 4.5%) to raise the plasma sodium level (and thus osmolality) of the body water. If there is acute renal failure some form of dialysis may be needed to remove excess water.

SODIUM

The freely exchangeable sodium in the body (about 2500 mmol) is almost entirely confined to the extracellular space. There is in addition a considerable amount of sodium in bone but it is not readily available for exchange.

In health the amount of exchangeable sodium in the body depends on intake and loss in the urine. Normal kidneys are very effective in regulating excretion to keep the body sodium steady. If there is severe loss or excessive intake, particularly if renal function is temporarily or permanently disturbed, upsets in sodium balance occur.

Sodium Depletion. This can be caused by excessive loss, usually from the *gastrointestinal* tract or through the *kidneys*. Gastrointestinal loss results from vomiting, diarrhoea, and fistulae. Renal loss is usually the result of prolonged diuretic therapy, although it may also occur in uncontrolled diabetes (p. 541) or with renal tubular lesions. It is also a feature of adrenal failure.

Vomiting causes sodium deficiency, not only from loss in the vomit but also by producing an alkalosis, and thus an obligatory excretion of sodium in an alkaline urine. Decreased intake is not common in this country, but in the tropics excessive sweating plus a low salt intake can be important.

As the sodium concentration (and thus the osmolality) in the extracellular space falls, water is lost both in the urine and into the intracellular space (p. 508) so that the volume of extracellular space including the blood volume decreases. Finally, this adjustment fails and the sodium concentration in the extracellular space falls. This means that by the time the plasma sodium is significantly reduced, considerable depletion has occurred.

It will be noted that in many instances the loss of sodium is combined with loss of water so that the picture is one of combined water and sodium depletion.

Clinical features are weakness, vomiting and cramps. The shrinkage of the extracellular space causes hypotension (particularly postural), tachycardia, lax skin and sunken facies. The plasma sodium concentration is reduced with severe depletion but owing to the fall in extracellular volume the plasma sodium concentration underestimates the extent of sodium deficit. The urine volume is usually normal in the early stages with a low sodium concentration. Ultimately a fall in renal perfusion due to the low blood volume leads to a decreased urine volume and a rising blood urea.

Treatment. If charts are available, the degree of sodium depletion can be calculated, but this is unusual. There is no ideal way of establishing sodium deficiency which is suitable for routine use. A rough approximation may be obtained by multiplying the number of milliequivalents the plasma sodium is below normal by the extracellular volume.
Deficiency in mmols of Na =

$$140 - \text{observed Na conc.} \times \frac{25}{100} \times \text{body weight in kg.}$$

This formula does not allow for the shrinkage in extracellular volume which occurs in sodium depletion and which tends to keep up the plasma sodium concentration. The calculated deficiency should therefore be multiplied by a factor of 2 to give a truer estimate of deficiency.

It is usual to spread the repletion of sodium over 24–48 hours although with severe deficiency it is reasonable to give 1 litre of isotonic saline in the first hour. It should also be remembered that the day to day loss of sodium may be continuing, and sodium depletion is frequently associated with water depletion so that correction of dehydration may also be required. A patient with severe sodium depletion may easily need as much as 10 litres of water and 1000 mmol of sodium. Sodium is usually given as 0.9 % (isotonic) sodium chloride solution, though if the plasma sodium concentration is below 120 mmol/litre, 1.8 % sodium chloride can be used. If sodium depletion is associated with acidosis, due perhaps to uncontrolled diabetes or excessive intestinal loss, it is usually sufficient to infuse isotonic sodium chloride solution and the kidneys will correct the acidosis by secreting an acid urine. With very severe acidosis (plasma pH < 7.1) or with impaired renal function isotonic sodium bicarbonate (1.4%) can be used instead of sodium chloride. During the repletion period, continued observation of the clinical and biochemical state of the patient is necessary.

In patients in whom it is suspected that cardiac function is impaired a careful watch must be kept on the central venous pressure and the bases of the lungs as over-rapid infusion can precipitate heart failure and pulmonary oedema.

Sodium replacement can also be achieved by giving oral isotonic sodium chloride solution provided it contains 2% glucose or 4% sucrose. The absorption of glucose enhances the absorption of electrolytes. This form of replacement has proved invaluable in the treatment of cholera.

Hyponatraemia

It is not uncommon for patients to have reduced levels of plasma sodium. This may be due to *sodium depletion* (see above), or it may be due to *water retention* following inappropriate secretion of ADH or an ADH-like substance (see p. 597).

Sodium Excess

This may occur in two different contexts with different clinical pictures:

(a) Uncomplicated sodium excess is commonly due to heart failure, acute glomerulonephritis or over-infusion with saline solutions. There is concommittent retention of water with expansion of the extracellular space including the blood volume. This leads to oedema and if cardiac function is not impaired to hypertension.

(b) Hypoalbuminaemia is usually due to the nephrotic syndrome, cirrhosis of the liver or malabsorption from protein losing enteropathy. The initial change is loss of salt and water into the tissue spaces causing a reduction of circulatory volume. This induces retention of sodium and water in the kidneys and thus sodium excess. The clinical picture is one of oedema which may be associated with hypovolaemia, postural hypotension and poor peripheral circulation.

Treatment is aimed at relieving the primary condition if this is possible. Diuretics are useful for relieving oedema but may exacerbate hypovolaemia if used too vigorously in hypoalbuminaemic states. Spironolactone can be used if excessive production of aldosterone is believed to be a factor in sodium retention. Although albumin infusions can be used in an acute situation they are not particularly helpful for long-term treatment.

POTASSIUM

Potassium is the major intracellular cation. It plays an important part in cell membrane activity and in the concentration of muscle. In health the adult male body contains about 3000 mmol of potassium, the amount being regulated by renal excretion, although the conservation of potassium by the kidneys is not as effective as that of sodium.

Potassium is also excreted into the gut in the bile and intestinal fluid, but is reabsorbed. If, however, there is excessive loss of intestinal fluid, depletion can occur.

The intracellular distribution of potassium makes the measurement of total body potassium very difficult. Unfortunately the plasma potassium concentration (normal 3.5–5.0 mmol/litre), though usually giving some indication of the situation, may be misleading, especially as considerable depletion (up to 200 mmol K) can occur with no fall in the plasma level and without development of symptoms. Further if potassium is passing from the cells to the circulation, plasma levels may be normal even with progressive intracellular depletion. More accurate methods of measuring total body potassium are available but are not suitable for routine use.

Potassium Depletion

Excessive loss of potassium can occur from the *gastrointestinal tract*, due to vomiting, fistulae, or prolonged diarrhoea. Excessive use of purgatives is an occasional cause. Severe *renal loss* occurs in uncontrolled diabetes mellitus (p. 541) or the recovery phase of acute renal failure and in renal tubular acidosis. Steroids also cause increased renal potassium loss, and it is a feature of primary aldosteronism and Cushing's syndrome (p. 571). Long-term use of diuretics can also cause potassium depletion. If used in low doses as in the treatment of hypertension depletion is rarely severe (plasma potassium is usually above 3.0 mmol/litre) and supplements are not often required. With larger doses, particularly if there are complicating factors such as secondary hyperaldosteronism, supplements are usually necessary.

Loss of potassium from the cell causes a fall in intracellular osmolality, and thus loss of water from the cell. There is some shift of hydrogen and sodium ions into the cell. In addition the urine becomes acid because hydrogen ions are exchanged for potassium ions in the distal tubule and excreted in the urine. This loss of hydrogen ions from the plasma results in a *hypokalaemic alkalosis* with a raised plasma bicarbonate concentration.

Clinical features are muscle weakness and fatigue, and in severe depletion actual paralysis may occur. The muscle of the intestine may lose tone, causing ileus. Potassium depletion can also damage the cells of the renal tubule producing polyuria and a failure to acidify the urine.

Potassium depletion can cause cardiac arrhythmias and sensitise the heart to the toxic effects of digitalis. The plasma potassium is usually low in severe depletion and the ECG shows typical changes (Fig. 11.3) and various arrhythmias.

Treatment. The extent of potassium depletion is impossible to assess and estimations based on plasma levels will usually be misleading. In general it can be said that depletion severe enough to produce symptoms means a deficit of at least 500 mmol and with severe symptoms it may be considerably higher.

Whenever possible potassium should be given by mouth. Potassium chloride is most satisfactory in doses of 30–100 mmol of potassium daily. Prolonged use of potassium chloride sometimes produces intestinal ulceration with stricture formation. Potassium chloride effervescent tablets (Sando-K), (12 mmol K and 8 mmol Cl per tablet), or tablets of Slow K (8 mmol/tablet) which contain potassium chloride in a slow release form, seem to be free from side-effects. Satisfactory natural sources of potassium are fresh orange juice (5.0 mmol/100 ml) and tomato juice (6.0 mmol/100 ml).

If intravenous replacement is necessary a potassium chloride solution containing 1.5 g KCl (20 mmol) in 10 ml can be added to 500 ml of infusion fluid. In general, potassium should not be infused at a greater rate than 20 mmol of potassium every hour and plasma levels should be monitored. Great care is required if renal function is impaired as there may be a sudden swing to hyperkalaemia.

Potassium Excess

The symptoms of potassium excess develop when the extracellular potassium concentration is raised and most commonly occurs when the kidney fails to excrete potassium. This is found in acute renal failure when oliguria is frequently associated with widespread muscle injury, infection and fever, all of which tend to release potassium from the tissues into the extracellular space. In chronic renal failure the kidneys usually excrete potassium normally or even in excess until the terminal stages. In conditions of circulatory failure a combination of low partial pressure of oxygen and reduced renal blood flow leads to migration of potassium from the cell and raised plasma levels. A mild hyperkalaemia may also be seen in Addison's disease, and is due to aldosterone deficiency.

Hyperkalaemia can also be iatrogenic either due to rapid infusion of potassium (particularly if renal function is impaired) or to the combination of potassium-sparing diuretics such as amiloride with potassium supplements or their use in patients with impaired renal function.

Clinical Features. The main effect is on muscle. The patient becomes increasingly weak and may eventually become paralysed with hypotonia and absent reflexes. The heart's action becomes irregular and heart block

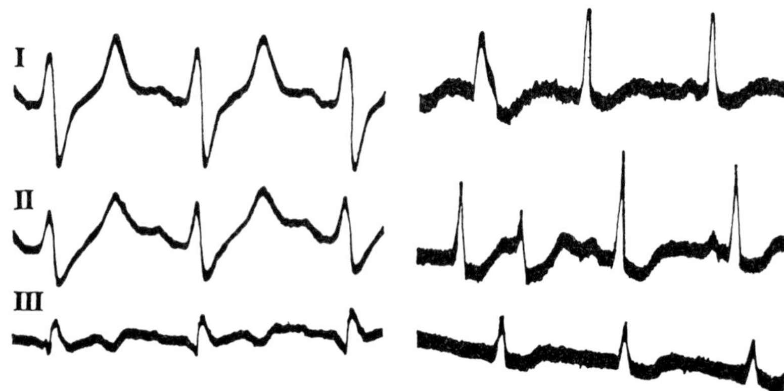

Fig. 11.3 ECG from patient with a raised serum potassium level (9 mmol/l): note wide QRS and tall T waves.

ECG from patient with low serum potassium (2.7 mmol/l): note extrasystole, wide QRS and S-T depression.

and asystole may ensue. The ECG shows typical changes (Fig. 11.3). The diagnosis is confirmed by estimating the plasma potassium level, and a concentration of over 7.0 mmol/litre can be dangerous but the rate of rise is also important.

Treatment

(a) *Preventive*

(1) High calorie diet, low in potassium.
(2) An ion exchange resin calcium polystyrenate 15 g four times daily by mouth or 3.0 g rectally.
(3) Dialysis.
(4) If possible correct the underlying cause.

(b) *Emergency*

(1) Infusion of 20% glucose with 25 units of insulin per 500 ml.
(2) 10 ml of calcium gluconate (10 g/100 ml) slowly IV.

MAGNESIUM

Magnesium is mainly an intracellular ion, the normal plasma range is 0.7–1.2 mmol/litre.

Deficiency can arise from excessive loss from the gut due to vomiting or malabsorption, or in the urine from excessive use of diuretics.

Clinical features include tetany, muscular weakness, cardiac arrhythmias and confusional states.

Treatment. Intravenous magnesium chloride is be given at a rate of 0.5 mmol/min or magnesium hydroxide can be given orally.

ACID/BASE BALANCE

Physiology

The intracellular pH is believed to be about 7.0. The end products of non-nitrogenous metabolism are carbon dioxide and small amounts of organic and inorganic acids. These substances are temporarily buffered by the intracellular buffers but ultimately pass from the cells and are carried in the blood to their sites of elimination (the lungs and the kidneys) with a minimal change in plasma pH. Carbon dioxide being a gas is excreted via the lungs and the organic and inorganic acids are excreted by the kidneys.

Excretion of Carbon Dioxide. On entering the blood carbon dioxide is converted to carbonic acid by the enzyme carbonic anhydrase in the red cells. This reaction is so rapid that dissolved CO_2 may be considered as an effective acid. Measurements are usually given in terms of partial pressure of carbon dioxide ($P\text{CO}_2$) rather than concentration of carbonic acid. Some 90% of the hydrogen ions released by the dissociation of this carbonic acid combine with haemoglobin, thus preventing a large fall in blood pH. In the tissues the release of oxygen from haemoglobin allows the uptake of hydrogen ions by the imidazolyl groups on the haemoglobin molecule.

$$HbO_2 + CO_2 + H_2O \xrightarrow{\text{carbonic anhydrase}} H^+Hb + HCO_3^- + O_2$$

Oxygen in the lungs similarly causes a release of hydrogen ions which combine with bicarbonate with the formation of carbon dioxide which is excreted. In addition some carbon dioxide is carried on the amine groups of haemoglobin and plasma proteins and released in the lungs.

$$H^+Hb + O_2 \rightarrow HbO_2 + H_2O + CO_2\uparrow$$

Maintenance of pH and Excretion of Hydrogen Ions. The stable pH of the blood is preserved by a number of buffer systems. These consist of strong bases which on the addition of hydrogen ions (acid) form weak acids. The bases and weak acids which act as buffers in this context are frequently called buffer bases and buffer acids.

The pH of the blood depends on the ratio buffer base to buffer acid. It can be derived from the equation propounded by Henderson and Hasselbalch in 1908.

$$pH = pK + \log\left(\frac{\text{buffer base}}{\text{buffer acid}}\right)$$

The buffer systems of the blood with their approximate relative buffering capacity are:

	Percentage of Total Capacity		*Percentage of Total Capacity*
HCO_3^-/H_2CO_3	37	Hb/HbH	34
HPO_4^{2-}/H_2PO_4	5	Protein/PrH	24

If hydrogen ions are added to these buffer systems, they combine with the buffer bases to form weak buffer acids. The fall in pH resulting from the addition of acid is therefore minimised.

In the plasma the compensation is almost entirely due to HCO_3/H_2CO_3 system because CO_2 can be excreted immediately.

$$HCO_3^- + H^+ \rightarrow H_2CO_3 \rightarrow H_2O + CO_2\uparrow$$

and the ratio log HCO_3/H_2CO_3 (i.e. pH) maintained at near normal levels.

Similarly if hydrogen ions are removed from the system and the pH rises, buffer acid is changed into buffer base with the release of hydrogen ions and the increase in pH is minimised.

The *total buffer base* is the sum of all the buffers (bicarbonate + protein + Hb + phosphate). If ventilation is normal then the plasma bicarbonate level reflects the total buffer base. If however there is an abnormality of ventilation then this is no longer true. This is because retention or deficit of carbon dioxide (and thus carbonic acid) will influence bicarbonate levels without altering the total buffer base, i.e.

$$\begin{array}{c} H_2CO_3 \rightarrow H^+ + HCO_3^- \\ \downarrow \\ \text{Buffer base} \end{array}$$

The hydrogen ion released thus reduces the buffer base, but at the same time bicarbonate is added. The net result being no change in total buffer base, but an increase in bicarbonate. The terms 'base excess' or 'base deficit' are used to indicate abnormalities of total buffer base.

The role of haemoglobin in the excretion of carbon dioxide has already been considered. In addition small amounts of hydrogen ions (about 75 mmol/24 h) are produced as organic and inorganic acids (sulphuric and lactic). They are accommodated in the buffer systems of the blood and excreted in the urine. Provided the influx from the cells equals efflux through the kidneys, the pH of the blood remains constant.

Clinical Applications

Introduction. Acid/base disturbances can be divided into those which are primarily due to disorders of carbon dioxide excretion (respiratory) and those due to inequality of acid or base production or excretion (metabolic or non-respiratory). The symptoms due to acid/base disturbances are ill-defined and are often overshadowed by the primary disease. Once the possibility is recognised the diagnosis is usually not difficult.

Investigation. The bicarbonate buffer system of the blood is usually studied as it is the easiest to measure. Bicarbonate is usually estimated by the autoanalyser using venous blood. Provided that respiratory function is normal this estimation usually gives an adequate approximation of the buffer base situation in the blood. If however there is CO_2 retention it will underestimate the deficiency in base and vice versa, so that where there is a respiratory disorder or where the situation is complicated, it is usual to measure the plasma CO_2 and pH using arterial blood, the bicarbonate concentration can then be computed. Mixed venous blood can also be used but gives a figure about 6 mm higher than arterial blood for $P\text{CO}_2$.

Acid/base disorders are often associated with electrolyte deficiencies, so that the plasma and often urinary concentrations of sodium and potassium should be measured. Estimation of blood urea levels gives an indication of overall renal function.

Normal Values

$$\text{Plasma pH} = 7.35-7.45$$
$$\text{Plasma bicarbonate} = 24-28 \text{ mmol/litre}$$
$$P\text{CO}_2 = 4.5-6.0 \text{ kPa } (35\text{–}45 \text{ mmHg})$$

Disorders of Carbon Dioxide Excretion

1. Impaired Excretion (Respiratory Acidosis)

The carriage of carbon dioxide from the tissues to the lungs is described above. In health, ventilation is physiologically maintained so that the partial pressure of carbon dioxide in the alveoli is about 5.5 kPa, the concentration of dissolved carbon dioxide in arterial blood being that which is in equilibrium with this partial pressure.

If there is inadequate alveolar ventilation, the partial pressure of carbon dioxide rises leading to an increase in the dissolved carbon dioxide (hypercarbia).

This causes a fall in the ratio $HCO_3^- / P\text{CO}_2$ (increased) and therefore a fall in pH.

The decrease is minimised by the other buffer bases combining with carbon dioxide and being converted to buffer acids with the release of bicarbonate.

$$\text{Buffer base} + CO_2 + H_2O \rightarrow \text{Buffer acid} + HCO_3^-$$

Following carbon dioxide retention the excess hydrogen ions are excreted by the kidney, producing an acid urine and reabsorption of bicarbonate by the tubules is increased.

Impaired carbon dioxide excretion occurs:

(1) Most commonly in chronic bronchitis, emphysema and asthma. It may occur acutely in bronchial obstruction with collapse.
(2) More rarely with depression of respiration in morphia or barbiturate poisoning, or from weakness of the respiratory muscles in poliomyelitis, polyneuritis, myopathy or myasthenia gravis.
(3) Head injuries.

Clinical Features. Symptoms usually appear when the $P\text{CO}_2$ rises to

60 mmHg. The patient is dyspnoeic and cyanosed (due to the concomitant hypoxia) with a full pulse and warm extremities from peripheral vasodilation. The blood pressure is frequently raised in acute hypercapnia. Further increase in $P\text{CO}_2$ brings about confusion with twitching and finally coma. Papilloedema may develop due to cerebral vasodilation. The treatment is directed towards increasing alveolar ventilation and relieving hypoxia.

Treatment. This is directed towards increasing alveolar ventilation and relieving hypoxia, and the method of treatment depends upon the cause. In bronchial infection antibiotics, antispasmodics and physiotherapy are important. In opiate overdose the appropriate antagonist should be used. When there is muscular weakness various forms of assisted respiration may be necessary. Respiratory stimulants are rarely helpful.

2. Excessive Excretion (Respiratory Alkalosis)

This is due to hyperventilation which leads to excessive loss of carbon dioxide and to a rise in the ratio $HCO_3^-/P\text{CO}_2$ (decreased) and a rise in plasma pH.

This is minimised by the other buffer acids converting to buffer bases with the release of hydrogen ions which combine with bicarbonate.

$$\text{Buffer acid} + HCO_3^- \rightarrow \text{Buffer base} + H_2O + CO_2$$

Renal conservation of hydrogen ions results in an alkaline urine.

Excessive excretion to carbon dioxide is often due to over-breathing as a result of hysteria, fear or pain. It is a constant feature of salicylate poisoning; rarely it is found in subjects with alveolar block causing hypoxia but not affecting carbon dioxide excretion and it may also complicate various forms of cerebral damage.

Clinical features are increased neuromuscular excitability with twitching, paraesthiae, and tetany. Patients with fear or anxiety should be given the appropriate analgesic or sedative but it is important to ensure that respiratory depression (i.e. with opiates) does not lead to hypoxia. In hysteria the easiest treatment is to raise the $P\text{CO}_2$ in the alveoli by rebreathing from a bag. In those with cerebral damage careful depression of respiration with morphia is sometimes useful.

Disorders of Hydrogen Ion Excretion

1. Gain of Acid or Loss of Bicarbonate (Metabolic Acidosis)

When the rate of production of hydrogen ions exceeds the rate of excretion either because of increased ingestion of acid substances, undue metabolic production of acids or impaired excretion by the kidneys, the condition of metabolic acidosis develops.

The rise in pH is minimised by the acid combining with buffer bases,

$$\text{Buffer base} + H^+ \rightarrow \text{Buffer acid}$$

resulting in a fall in the ratio buffer base/buffer acid.

A similar state can result from the loss of bicarbonate ions.

An excessive influx of acid into the blood can arise from the following causes.

(a) Ingestion of substances which produce acid, the commonest being ammonium chloride and aspirin.
(b) Increased production of acid occurs with severe exercise, in uncontrolled diabetes mellitus and sometimes after major surgery.
(c) Tissue hypoxia as may occur in cardiac arrest or septicaemic shock leads to rapid production of lactic acid with resulting acidosis. Overproduction of lactic acid is also seen with the use of biguanides (see p. 537) and in methanol poisoning.
(d) In both acute and chronic renal failure the kidneys fail to excrete enough acid.

Bicarbonate deficiency follows loss of intestinal secretions due to diarrhoea or fistulae. There is often an associated sodium and potassium deficiency. Failure of the renal tubules to reabsorb bicarbonate (with subsequent deficiency) also occurs in renal tubular acidosis.

Anion Gap. Normally the gap between $Na^+ + K^+ - HCO_3^- + Cl^-$ is 10–15 mmol. If acidosis is due to excess acid production (i.e. lactic acid, etc.) the gap will be increased. If however it is due to bicarbonate loss it will be unaltered, bicarbonate being replaced by chloride.

Clinical Features. Hyperventilation is a cardinal sign. This is initially due to stimulation of the carotid chemoreceptors. Later the CSF bicarbonate and pH fall and this further increases ventilation. Central signs are increasing drowsiness and finally coma.

Acidosis also depresses cardiac function and increases the tendency to arrhythmias. Other clinical features will depend on the underlying cause.

Treatment

(1) Relief of the primary cause if possible.

(2) Re-establishment of optimal renal function by correcting dehydration and electrolyte deficiencies.

(3) It is often sufficient to restore circulation by infusion of isotonic sodium chloride solution and allow the kidneys to excrete the excess acid. In severe acidosis (pH < 7.1) the depleted buffer base can be restored by the infusion of isotonic sodium bicarbonate solution (1.4%–163 mmol/litre). As a rough guide, the total base deficiency can be calculated:

$$25 - \text{plasma bicarbonate (mmol/litre)} \times 0.3 \text{ body weight in kg} = \text{deficiency in mmol.}$$

This will almost certainly underestimate the deficit and further base will be required, the amount depending on the levels of plasma bicarbonate. Too rapid correction of base deficit can cause disequilibrium across the cell membranes. Bicarbonate only diffuses slowly into the cells and CSF so that although extracellular acidosis may be corrected rapidly, intracellular and CSF acidosis persists for 24 hours or more.

2. Loss of Acid or Gain of Bicarbonate (Metabolic Alkalosis)

Gain of bicarbonate is due to its excessive ingestion in the treatment of peptic ulcer. Healthy kidneys can cope with almost unlimited amounts of bicarbonate but if there is renal disease, base excess may develop. Loss of acid is usually due to vomiting or gastric aspiration. Metabolic alkalosis can also complicate potassium deficiency (p. 516).

The rise in pH results in buffer acid being changed to buffer base.

$$\text{Buffer acid} \rightarrow \text{Buffer base} + H^+$$

and a rise in the ratio buffer acid/buffer base.

The kidneys secrete an alkaline urine containing large amounts of sodium and bicarbonate.

Clinical features include clouding of consciousness and in addition there may be paraesthesiae, tetany and convulsions.

Acid loss from vomiting or aspiration is often coupled with sodium and potassium deficiency. This is due partially to loss in gastric secretion and to increased excretion in the urine.

Treatment. It is usually sufficient to correct dehydration and electrolyte deficiencies and the kidneys will excrete the excess base.

Definitions

Acid. A substance which donates hydrogen ions. Strong acids are those which are highly dissociated in solution, and weak acids are those poorly associated in solution.

Base. A substance which accepts hydrogen ions. A strong base accepts hydrogen ions more readily than a weak base. Important physiological bases are bicarbonate, dibasic phosphate and some amino acids.

Buffer Base. A base which takes part in the buffer systems of the body.

Acidosis and Alkalosis. These terms cannot be precisely defined. They are generally used to indicate the primary direction of the change of plasma pH, acidosis indicating a fall and alkalosis a rise in pH.

	Partial Pressure CO_2	*Plasma pH*	*Plasma Bicarbonate*
Impaired excretion CO_2 (respiratory acidosis)	Increased	Decreased	Increased
Excessive excretion CO_2 (respiratory alkalosis)	Decreased	Increased	Decreased
Retention of acid or loss of base (metabolic acidosis)	Normal or Decreased	Decreased	Decreased
Loss of acid or retention of base (metabolic alkalosis)	Normal	Increased	Increased

Plasma changes in acid/base disorders.

FURTHER READING

Cameron, J. S., in *Medical Treatment* (Vol. III). Edited by K. S. Maclean and G. W. Scott, Churchill, London, 1970.
Tweedle, D. E. F., *Metabolic Care*, Churchill Livingstone, Edinburgh, 1982.

CHAPTER 12

DISEASES OF METABOLISM

DISORDERS OF CARBOHYDRATE METABOLISM

Introduction—Metabolism of Carbohydrate

Glucose is absorbed from the small intestine and passes through the portal vein to the liver. Here it is phosphorylated and some is stored as glycogen, some broken down to pyruvate and some dephosphorylated and passed into the plasma. These changes are effected by enzyme systems.

The normal fasting level of glucose in venous blood is less than 6.0 mmol/litre. Glucose passes freely through the glomerular filter and is totally reabsorbed by the cells of the proximal tubule. If the plasma glucose level (and hence the level in the glomerular filtrate) is above 11 mmol/litre, then the tubule's power of reabsorption is exceeded and sugar appears in the urine.

Glucose passes from the plasma into the interstitial fluid and then into the cell. Inside the cell it is again phosphorylated and either stored as glycogen, or broken down to pyruvate, then to CO_2 and water, with consequent release of energy; or converted to fatty acids and ultimately to fat. It has been estimated from tracer studies in animals that of the total glucose which is metabolised daily 67 % is oxidised to CO_2 and water, 30 % is converted to fatty acids and only 3 % is stored as glycogen. 65 % of this glucose is dietary in origin, 30 % arises from gluconeogenesis and only 3 % from glycogen.

A number of hormones serve to regulate carbohydrate metabolism, the most important being insulin, which is synthesised as a long polypeptide chain in the beta cells of the islets of Langerhans. This chain folds over on itself and through the establishment of disulphide links forms the pro-insulin molecule. Removal of the 'connecting peptide' results in the 'A' and 'B' chained insulin molecule, which usually polymerises in the resting state and forms the insulin granules visible by electron and light microscopy. Insulin is released, and synthesised in response to a rise in plasma glucose levels; release is possibly initiated by gastrointestinal polypeptide hormones. The plasma insulin level as determined by radio-immune assay lies between 5 and 30 microunits/ml. It circulates both in a free form and bound to the albumin and alpha-2 globulin of the plasma. At the same time as insulin is released from the pancreas the remaining part of pro-insulin (the C peptide chain) also enters the circulation and the C peptide can therefore be used as an index of insulin release.

The action of insulin is mediated by insulin receptors on the cell membrane. It varies in different tissues but in general it increases the uptake of glucose and suppresses the release of non-esterified fatty acids by adipose tissue.

Thyroxine is mildly hypoglycaemic in effect but pituitary and adrenal hormones and the secretion of the alpha cells in the islets of Langerhans, glucagon, are all hyperglycaemic. The importance of hormones other than insulin in clinical diabetes is uncertain.

Carbohydrate metabolism may be deranged so that there is too much or too little sugar in the blood. The first is commoner and by far the most important; it causes the syndrome of diabetes mellitus.

DIABETES MELLITUS

This syndrome is characterised clinically by polyuria and polydipsia, and biochemically by hyperglycaemia and glycosuria.

Incidence of Diabetes. This varies widely in different populations; it is generally low in areas of low nutrition and high where food is plentiful. Best estimates suggest that up to 15% of the population of Western Europe is affected.

Studies of incidence related to age show that there is a small peak in the second decade which falls again and then rises steadily with increasing age to reach a plateau at about 60.

Diagnosis. Diabetes may be suspected from the clinical picture but can only be proved biochemically. The presence of glycosuria is not sufficient, for this may result from a low renal threshold (p. 528) or a 'lag' curve. Normal values of blood glucose are taken as less than 5.0 mmol/litre fasting and less than 10 mmol/litre two hours after food. *Diagnostic levels* for diabetes mellitus are shown in Table 12.1.

Table 12.1 Diagnostic blood sugar levels in diabetes mellitus (mmol/l)

	Venous blood	*Capillary blood*
Fasting	> 7.0	> 7.0
2 hours after meal	> 10.0	> 11.0

In doubtful cases and to establish the level of the renal threshold (Fig. 12.1) a glucose tolerance test (GTT) should be carried out. A loading dose of glucose (75 g) is given and blood glucose levels measured every half hour for 2 hours (Fig. 12.1). The diagnosis of diabetes mellitus (DM) is certain if three criteria are fulfilled:

(a) The fasting level exceeds 7.0 mmol/l
(b) The maximum level achieved exceeds 10.0 mmol/l
(c) The value 2 hours after the loading dose is above 10 mmol/l venous blood or 11 mmol/l capillary blood.

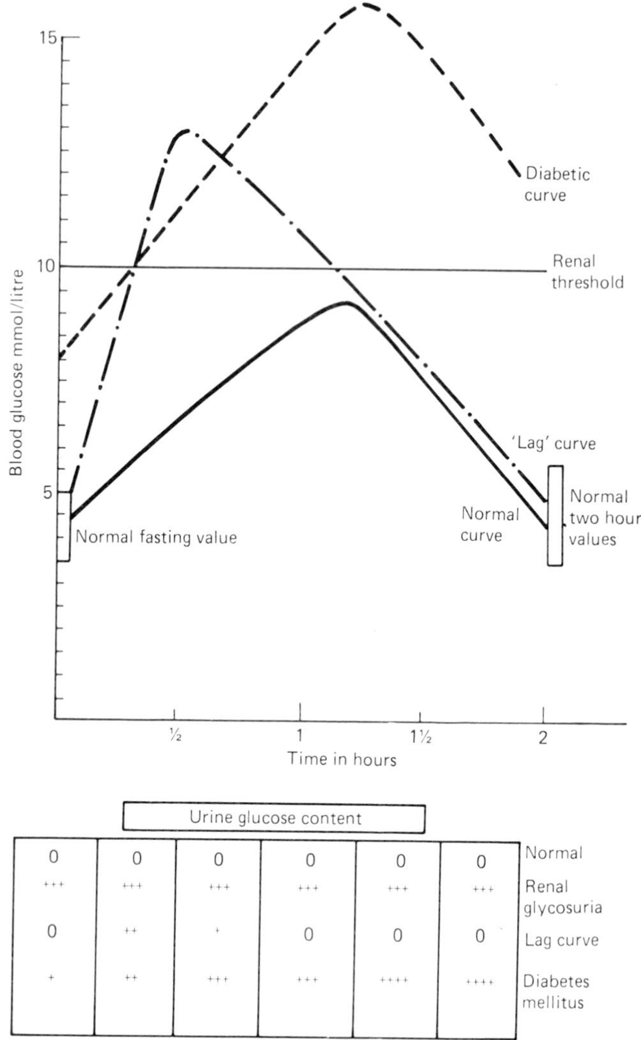

Fig. 12.1 Glucose tolerance test showing various types of curves.

If only two of these criteria are present the diagnosis is less certain and the patient should not be labelled diabetic. He should be regarded as showing *impaired glucose tolerance (IGT)* and suggested criteria for this diagnosis are as given in Table 12.2.

No significant excess mortality has been demonstrated in men with IGT but it is a warrant for continued surveillance. Women with IGT do

Table 12.2 Diagnostic blood sugar levels in impaired glucose tolerance

	Venous blood	*Capillary blood*
Fasting	< 7.0	< 7.0
2 hours after glucose	> 7.0	> 8.0
but	< 10.0	< 11.0

Table 12.3* Crude mortality at 10 years in DM and IGT compared with controls (Bedford Survey)

	Men		*Women*	
	Numbers	*All deaths*	*Numbers*	*All deaths*
Controls	102	20 (19.2%)	85	9 (10.6%)
Diabetics	51	19 (37.2%)	63	25 (39.2%)
IGT	130	29 (22.3%)	119	35 (29.4%)

* (Modified from Keen *et al.* (1979), *Diabetologia* **16**, 283)

show a slight excess mortality but both sexes with diabetic curves show a greater and more significant excess mortality than controls.

Other abnormal but non-diabetic results may be obtained from glucose tolerance tests:

(a) *Renal Threshold.* Glucose is normally filtered by the glomerulus and completely reabsorbed by the proximal renal tubules. Above a plasma glucose level of 11 mmol/l (the renal threshold) the reabsorptive capacity of the tubules is exceeded and glucose appears in the urine. With increasing age the renal threshold rises (Fig. 12.2) and this is of some importance in the control of diabetes by urine testing. In some apparently normal people the tubular reabsorption of glucose is defective so that although they have a normal glucose tolerance test, glucose appears in all urine specimens including the first morning specimen after an overnight fast. This is an hereditary condition, known as *renal glycosuria*. It is not connected with diabetes mellitus and is of no importance. There are no complications and treatment is unnecessary. It may also occur as a transient phenomenon in pregnancy.

(b) *Lag Curves.* There is an implied lag in insulin production so that high blood glucose levels and possibly glycosuria are found in the early samples during a GTT. It may occur after gastroenterostomy or in association with hyperthyroidism or during steroid therapy; sometimes there is no apparent explanation. It is more commonly seen in the elderly. Usually it is of no significance but it is a warrant for annual observation in those patients with a family history of diabetes.

(c) *Flat curves* are seen in myxoedema, hypopituitarism and the malabsorption syndrome.

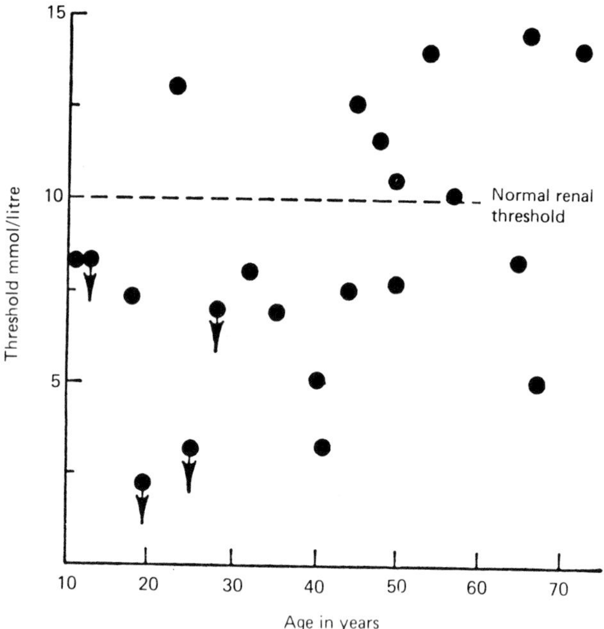

Fig. 12.2 Renal glucose threshold in 22 diabetic patients. Note the high thresholds which may be found in the older age group.

Clinical Features. Depending upon the severity and rapidity of the metabolic decompensation hyperglycaemic patients may present in four ways irrespective of the possible precipitating factors.

(1) *Acute Onset.* The patient suffers acute polyuria, polydipsia, rapid loss of weight, becomes ketoacidotic and unless treated usually passes into coma within a few days or weeks. Less frequent symptoms include irritability, vomiting, abdominal pain, muscle cramps and peripheral tingling. This onset is usual (but not universal) among children and adolescent diabetics, but may also occur among the elderly.

(2) *Gradual Onset.* The thirst and polyuria are less intense although nocturia may be noted. The obese may lose 1–2 stones over a period of months, or may have gained weight lately. Pruritus vulvae or crops of boils may occur, lassitude is common and middle-aged males may complain of loss of libido and impotence. This onset is common in middle life but may be observed among younger and older patients.

(3) *Symptoms of Complications.* Many older diabetics present with symptoms from the complication of diabetes; in the eye (cataract, retinopathy); peripheral nerves (neuropathy); kidneys (nephrotic syndrome); blood vessels (coronary artery disease, intermittent claudication and gangrene).

(c) *Iritis Rubeosa.* Reddening of the iris at the margin of the cornea due to new vessel formation obstructing the canal of Schlemm and so blocking the drainage of the anterior chamber of the eye which may lead to glaucoma.

(2) In the Blood Vessels

Evidence of impaired circulation to the feet (cold toes or feet, atrophic skin, poor hair or nail growth) should be sought, as gangrene is severely incapacitating and should be prevented whenever possible. Particularly significant are small ischaemic areas which seem to be related to the obstruction of endarteries with glycoproteins.

(a) All peripheral pulses should be palpated; absent ankle pulses may occur with ageing but are more common among diabetics.
(b) The main vessels should be auscultated, especially the abdominal aorta, renal arteries, iliac and femoral vessels, and the findings recorded. Hyperlipidaemia must be suspected and if present treated.
(c) An electrocardiogram should be recorded.

(3) In the Nervous System

Diabetic Neuropathy:

(a) Peripheral neuritis in diabetics is of three varieties:
   (i) Chronic peripheral neuritis (p. 362) affecting only the legs and associated with gross weakness and extensive anaesthesia. Frequently complicated by perforating ulcers, sometimes by Charcot's joints (p. 369) and osteomyelitis. The occurrence of lightning pains may heighten the resemblance to tabes dorsalis. The peripheral nerves may be thickened and the protein in the CSF is usually raised.
   (ii) Acute peripheral neuritis affecting the hands and feet in young acutely uncontrolled diabetics, causing tingling and numbness of fingers and toes with pain on use of muscles and on squeezing them. This is rapidly relieved by control of the disease.
   (iii) Mononeuritis multiplex (p. 359).
(b) Diabetic amyotrophy is characterised by symmetrical pain and weakness in the buttocks and thighs with muscular wasting and areflexia. The CSF protein is usually raised and the electromyogram shows the typical pattern of lower motor neurone disease. It is believed to be a motor radiculopathy.
(c) Damage to the autonomic nervous system causes impotence in males and loss of orgasm in females, nocturnal diarrhoea, postural hypotension and loss of sweating over the lower limbs. The Valsalva response may be impaired.
(d) Optic atrophy is an occasional occurrence.

(4) In the Renal Tract (p. 504).

(5) In the Skin

(a) At blood sugar levels over 13mmol/litre glucose appears in the sweat. Skin infections, particularly boils and monilial infections of the vulva are common in diabetics.

(b) Hypercholesterolaemia and hyperlipaemia occasionally lead to the formation of xanthomata in the skin, small hard yellowish nodules up to a few millimetres in diameter.

(6) Infection

Severe vulvo-vaginitis or balanitis are common and present with intense itching. Less commonly there may be generalised pruritus. Recurrent urinary infections and acute pyelonephritis are frequent and may be fulminating. Infection in the skin creases is common in the obese and carbuncles still occur although less frequently nowadays. The incidence of pulmonary tuberculosis is increased and all diabetics should have a chest radiograph. Delayed healing of any infection should always arouse suspicion of diabetes.

Treatment of Diabetes Mellitus

Introduction. In the past there have been two schools of thought, those who advocated strict control and those who felt that provided the patient was neither hypoglycaemic nor ketotic, little need be done. Longer experience suggests that only by the most careful control can complications be postponed and life prolonged. Unfortunately even the strictest control by present methods will not prevent complications developing ultimately in some cases; nevertheless, the incidence of some complications—cataracts, skin infections—is less and expectation of life is far greater in those diabetics who have always been carefully controlled.

Control may be assessed by the urinary glucose provided that the renal threshold is normal and renal function is not impaired. It should be checked by blood-sugar estimations every three months. The patient should be 'lean and spry', neither gaining nor losing weight, eating an adequate and enjoyable diet, taking exercise reasonable for his age, free from all diabetic complications and subject to neither hyperglycaemia nor hypoglycaemia at any time during the 24 hours. Assuming a normal renal threshold the metabolic management should keep the urine as nearly sugar-free as possible. Glycosuria should not exceed 5–10 g a day, and although this is compatible with a single 2 % glycosuric sample, wherever possible urine samples should not contain more than 0.5 % glucose.

Treatment of Type II Diabetes

When diabetes is diagnosed the patient should be fully examined clinically and any complications noted. A chest radiograph should be taken and his urine tested for sugar, acetone bodies, protein and casts. A midstream specimen of urine should be cultured and any existing infection treated. A diet suitable to his age and occupation should be prescribed and if he is obese his weight reduced. The majority—about 85%—of diabetics present with obesity and mild diabetes in the second half of life, and they represent Type II of those previously described. Nearly all of them can be treated by diet alone provided they will cooperate. It is essential to reduce their weight to near their ideal and this can only be done by dieting. In effect this means taking less food than the patient requires so that the body is forced to draw on fat depots as a source of energy. When the weight is sufficiently reduced for the age, height and sex then a diet supplying adequate calories should be prescribed with limitation of carbohydrate.

In general, patients are offered too much to eat. Only the heaviest labourers require more than 3000 calories daily; most patients need between 1800 and 2500 calories, and women rather less than men. Few patients are adequately controlled on diets containing much more than 150 g of carbohydrate in 24 hours. It is important to realise that some diabetics may take up to four weeks to respond fully to dietary restriction.

Oral Hypoglycaemic Agents

There are many advantages in the use of oral agents to control diabetes. They save the necessity for injections which may indeed be impossible for the aged, handicapped or partially sighted patient.

If it could be shown that these preparations prevent the development of complications as effectively as they control blood sugar levels there would be little reservation for their use. Unfortunately this is far from certain and there is some evidence that suggests that the tendency to vascular disease may be increased in patients whose hyperglycaemia is controlled by tablets but whose dietary restrictions are neglected. It is therefore wise to restrict the use of oral hypoglycaemic agents to patients for whom diet has manifestly failed in spite of conscientious efforts by patient and doctor. They should always be regarded as an adjunct to diet and not a substitute.

Sulphonylureas. These drugs probably act by stimulating the release of endogenous insulin from the remaining active β cells. They should not be used in the undieted patient, in pregnancy or in patients who are ketotic.

A number of sulphonylureas are now available and the main features are given in the Table 12.5. Tolbutamide has a short action and is the weakest of the group, therefore it is safer for old people. Glipizide and glibenclamide are short-acting but rather more powerful. Chlorpropamide is long-acting so that one daily dose is sufficient; however it may cause hypoglycaemia as the full effect of once daily dosage develops slowly over 1–2 weeks. In addition, doses above 250 mg are rarely more effective but increase the incidence of side-effects.

Table 12.5 Details of sulphonylureas in current use

Approved name	*Proprietary name*	*Dose range (mg)*	*Dose frequency (24 h)*	*Tablet size (mg)*	*Duration of action (hours—approx)*
Tolbutamide	Rastinon	500–3000	1–3	500	8
Chlorpropamide	Diabinese	50–500	1	100 250	24
Glibenclamide	Euglucon Daonil	2.5–20	1–2	2.5 5.0	12
Glipizide	Minodiab	2.5–20	1–3	5.0	6

The sulphonylureas interact with a number of drugs including sulphonamides, salicylates, anticoagulants, monoamine oxidase inhibitors and β blockers.

Biguanides lower the blood sugar in diabetics but paradoxically not in normal subjects. They reduce hepatic glucose release, increase peripheral insulin action and in high doses reduce intestinal absorption. Their main use is in overweight diabetics and as an adjunct to the sulphonylureas in patients resistant to treatment. Nausea and diarrhoea can be a problem and it is usual to start with a small dose of metformin 500 mg b.d. with meals and to increase it every 3–4 days.

Biguanides must not be used in patients with impaired liver or renal function or in alcoholics. It is usual for a slight rise in plasma lactic acid to occur with these drugs but some of the above patients may develop *acute lactic acidosis*. This presents with general malaise, clouding of consciousness and ultimately coma. Serum lactate, which is normally below 1.0 mmol/litre, is considerably raised. The prognosis is poor. Treatment consists of stopping the biguanides and infusing bicarbonate to combat the acidosis.

Treatment of Type I Diabetes

All young thin diabetics require both insulin and diet, and these should be matched to the amount of exercise they take. A heavy worker needs more calories than a clerk. For adequate control a regular amount of activity and regular meals are essential, and occupations such as commercial travelling involving irregular hours are unsuitable careers for young diabetics to choose. Variations in diet and activity are a major problem during school years, but with patience and persistence most juvenile diabetics remain reasonably well controlled whilst being educated. In general these children are less suitable for boarding school. A useful guide to diet is to prescribe at least 70–80 g of protein per day, not more than 150–200 g of carbohydrate and the balance of calories needed as fat.

Insulin. Insulin became available therapeutically in 1922 and until 1930 only directly prepared short-acting insulins were available. Between 1930 and the early 1950s long-acting insulins were introduced. This was first achieved by attaching the insulin molecule to a protein (isophane, protamine zinc, globulin) and later by modifying its physical state so that a suspension of crystals, amorphous (semilente) or crystalline (ultralente) or a mixture (30 % amorphous, 70 % crystalline) known as lente was injected. These insulins were not always satisfactory and their prolonged use occasionally resulted in damage to the subcutaneous tissues (insulin fat atrophy or hypertrophy).

This led to attempts at further purification of commercial insulin and finally to the separation of three fractions:

(i) (MW *ca.* 20 000) This fraction is strongly antigenic and contains various non-insulin pancreatic proteins. It is believed to be the chief cause of tissue damage.

(ii) (MW *ca.* 9 000) The major component is pro-insulin and it is highly antigenic.

(iii) (MW *ca.* 6 000) Non-antigenic and biologically the most powerful. Highly purified insulins derived from the 'C' fraction are now available and are known as monocomponent (MC) insulins.

Insulin with the exact structure of human insulin is now available. It is prepared either by genetic modification of E. coli so that the bacteria produce insulin or by changing enzymatically the structure of animal insulin. The resultant product is less antigenic than animal insulin. On changing from animal insulin to human insulin, some dosage reduction may be required.

Some of the insulins used today are shown in Table 12.6.

Precise measurements of the duration and degree of activity of the different insulin preparations may be made in animals (Table 12.6), but should not be uncritically extended to patients. Variations in absorption from repeatedly used sites, in the activity of the individual and in the carbohydrate load all serve to modify exact timing of the biological activity of injected insulin. In clinical practice it is enough to regard some insulins as acting chiefly through the day, and others principally in the late afternoon and evening and through the night, but with the increasing realisation of the importance of control throughout the 24 hours many physicians now advise their patients to take two or even

Table 12.6 Details of source and activity of insulins in common use

Type of Insulin	*Peak Activity*	*Source*	*Monocomponent*
Short-Acting			
Insulin injection (BP)	2–4 h	Beef	No
Actrapid MC	2–4 h	Pork	Yes
Long-Acting			
Insulin zinc suspensions (mixture 30% amorphous, 70% crystalline)			
Lente	3–8 h	Beef	No
Lentard MC	3–8 h	Beef/pork	Yes
Monotard MC	3–8 h	Pork	Yes
Biphasic insulin (mixture of rapid and long-acting insulins)			
Rapitard MC	4–10 h	Beef/pork	Yes
Protamine zinc (BP)	5–14 h	Beef	Now available
Human insulins			
Neutral insulin	1–2 h	—	—
Isophane insulin	4–6 h	—	—

three injections of short-acting insulins rather than risk indifferent control by one injection of a retard insulin.

Insulin preparations were presented in varying concentrations, 20, 40 or 80 units/ml. This led to confusion in prescribing, dispensing and measuring, and now one standard strength of 100 units per ml (U100) is being introduced with a standard insulin syringe graduated in 100 divisions per ml.

Insulin is a polypeptide and if taken by mouth is digested to its constituent amino acids. It must therefore be injected subcutaneously at least once daily. A standard insulin syringe should be used with needles of adequate size. The site of injection should be varied and the front of the thigh, over the deltoid muscle and the lower abdomen are the most convenient sites for self-injection. Insulin absorption may be marginally faster in warm weather, especially in lean subjects.

Controlling Diabetes with Insulin

Assuming a normal renal threshold, the urine may be used as a rough index of control. The patient is taught to test the overnight urine, then after breakfast, lunch and tea, and immediately before bed, and to record the results. An initial dose of 20 units of soluble insulin just before or just after breakfast and 10 units just before or just after the evening meal are prescribed and the effect on the urinary glucose observed. Changes should not be made at less than three-day intervals unless hypoglycaemia occurs. Appropriate adjustments are made until the patient is sugar-free and not hypoglycaemic; this is much better done as an outpatient under normal life conditions. One caveat—all diabetics on soluble insulin in the morning must take a small mid-morning carbohydrate snack, especially if their overnight urine is sugar-free.

Once control is achieved the urine need be tested only once daily, but at a different time each day, so that in five days tests are made at all critical times. Hospital attendance can also become infrequent; well-controlled cases should be reviewed quarterly when blood-sugar estimation and urine tests for sugar, ketones and protein should be done. Careful records of weight must be kept, and chest radiographs taken annually. Care of the feet should be emphasised, especially in the elderly, and chiropody arranged when necessary.

In view of the outstanding success of laser beam treatment in diabetic retinopathy, it is imperative to diagnose retinal lesions at an early stage. For this reason annual examination of the fundus with the pupil dilated is mandatory, and if suspicious lesions are observed then a fluoroscein retinogram should be ordered. If these lesions are then confirmed the patient should be referred to an ophthalmologist for appropriate laser beam therapy.

The Control of Diabetes

It is generally conceded that the stricter the control of the blood glucose level, the less the chances of developing complications of diabetes. There are two ways in which stricter control can be implemented and whether one or other method comes into general use remains to be seen.

(a) *Self-monitoring.* This implies regular estimation of blood glucose levels by the patient. The present method is to use dextrosticks or some similar colour reaction combined with a reflection spectrometer which enables him to obtain accurate measurements. These tests should be done four times daily and also at 3.00 a.m. once a week. In this way it is possible to obtain a much tighter control of diabetes than by the usual estimation of urinary sugar.

(b) *Haemoglobin A1c.* Glucose becomes incorporated in a number of protein molecules including those of haemoglobin with which it forms Hb A1c. The concentration of Hb A1c in the blood gives an estimation of the overall plasma glucose levels over the preceding three weeks or so and this is an indication of the control of the diabetes. This estimation is useful in picking up poorly controlled diabetics but is not so good at distinguishing patients who are having periods of hypoglycaemia.

Indications for a Change to Monocomponent Insulins

Most diabetics are satisfactorily controlled by the older insulins. There are, however, several indications for switching patients to monocomponent insulins:

(a) The development of generalised allergies to unpurified insulins.
(b) The development of fat atrophy at the injection sites.
(c) Severe local reactions at the site of injection.
(d) When very large doses of insulin are required, suggesting that antibodies are interfering with the action of insulin.
(e) In pregnancy when antibodies produced by impure insulins can cross the placental barrier and damage the foetal islet cells.
(f) Newly diagnosed insulin dependent diabetes.

Complications of Insulin Treatment

(1) Repeated use of the same site for insulin injections may lead to gross thickening of subcutaneous tissues, chiefly fat, called lipohypertrophy. It is often due to insulin being injected too deeply, directly into the subcutaneous adipose tissue. In other patients the subcutaneous fat rapidly disappears at the site of injections (lipoatrophy), due to insulin injections being too shallow. It usually occurs early in the treatment and cannot be avoided by varying the site. It is usually self-limiting, and is less likely to occur with monocomponent insulins.

(2) Hypoglycaemia may result from an overdose of insulin. This may be caused by mis-measurement, by unwittingly using insulin of increased strength, by the too rapid action of insulin either from increased physical activity or from failing to take an expected meal, or from careless change to a preparation using insulin of a different species. For treatment, see p. 546.

Difficulties in Diabetic Control

Insulin resistance in diabetics who require insulin is rare. The diagnosis is usually made when insulin is either incorrectly prescribed (for 'elderly' diabetics) or incorrectly given. The common causes of failure of control if insulin is correctly prescribed and injected are:

(1) Failure to diet. It is difficult to persuade patients with only minor symptoms to accept dietary restriction, but failure to comply is soon revealed by serial observation of body weight. Alcoholics, narcotic addicts and psychopathic patients are unable to accept restrictions and suffer accordingly.

(2) Cryptic infection. Pulmonary tuberculosis is the most serious of these, chronic pyelonephritis the commonest. Septic teeth, tonsils and adenoids especially in children may be important. Cholecystitis should be excluded.

(3) Marked variation in physical activity. This applies particularly to schoolchildren and great ingenuity must be used to balance diet, activity and insulin. Some adult occupations are also too irregular to be suitable.

(4) Genuine insulin resistance rarely exists. It occurs when there is failure to absorb insulin from a frequently used site at which severe lipoatrophy or hypertrophy has occurred, when there are antibodies to insulin present in the plasma, and when there are abnormalities of intracellular glucose metabolism which are not wholly corrected by insulin. These cases may present as unstable or brittle diabetics who pass easily and rapidly from hypo- to hyperglycaemia and ketosis.

Diabetic Crisis

This may occur in any diabetic at any age, and comes on over 24–48 hours. If there is insufficient circulating insulin to allow glucose to be used as a source of energy by the cells two things occur. Glucose accumulates in the blood in large quantities and the cells are forced to use fat as an alternative fuel with resulting ketosis. The first causes an osmotic diuresis with the loss of water, glucose, potassium, sodium, magnesium, phosphate and sulphate in excessive quantities. The second leads to accumulation of acetone (acetoacetic acid and β hydroxybutyric acid) bodies in the blood resulting in acidosis (ketosis). Ketone bodies also act directly on the brain to cause drowsiness and on the respiratory centre to stimulate excessively rapid and deep respiration (Kussmaul's respiration, Lufthunger).

Eventually these metabolic derangements lead to coma, but short of coma there is still a medical emergency. The occurrence of glycosuria of 2% or more with ketonuria and ketonaemia in a drowsy patient who appears ill should be regarded as a diabetic crisis. It must be appreciated that all degrees of crisis exist and the severity is proportional to the ketosis, not to the level of the blood sugar. In the presence of renal disease urinary ketones are not an adequate index of ketosis, and blood ketones of plasma bicarbonates should be estimated.

Clinical Features. There are signs of dehydration and sodium depletion (p. 513), the pulse is weak and rapid, and the blood pressure low. The tongue is dry and coated, and the breathing is forced and noisy, the breath smells of acetone. The abdomen is scaphoid and there may be abdominal pain, tenderness and guarding.

Treatment. Before starting treatment a careful examination must be made to try to discover the initiating cause of the crisis, infection, cardiac infarction, trauma or neglect being the commonest. But treatment is a matter of urgency, and should not be unduly delayed by a prolonged search for causes. Two other words of warning—the patient should be disturbed as little as possible, routine nursing procedures may be omitted until he is fully conscious. Better a dirty diabetic than a clean corpse. Second—with ketosis there will be resistance to the action of insulin. As the ketosis subsides, sensitivity to the action of insulin increases sharply and it is possible to precipitate hypoglycaemia by too vigorous therapy.

The regime below is suitable for a diabetic who is deeply in coma. It should be discreetly interpreted for minor stages of crisis.

(i) *Fluid and salt replacement* starts with intravenous 0.9% saline. The first litre should be given as fast as possible, in ½–1 hour; thereafter, one litre per hour for 2 hours and then one litre every 2–3 hours.

(ii) As the blood glucose falls, *potassium passes into the cells and the plasma potassium level decreases.* To prevent serious hypokalaemia, 20 mmol of potassium (1.5 g KCl) should be added to the infusion and given hourly. Regular measurements of plasma potassium are made and the rate of infusion of potassium adjusted to keep the plasma level between 4 and 5 mmol/litre.

(iii) Although *acidosis* is a consistent finding in diabetic coma it is better if possible to restore salt and water deficiency and allow the kidneys to correct the acidosis by secreting an acid urine, thus avoiding too rapid acid/base shifts between the intra- and extracellular compartments.

Very severe acidosis (plasma pH 7.0 or less) should however be corrected by giving 200–400 ml (65–130 mmol) of a 2.74% solution of sodium bicarbonate over one hour. The plasma pH should then be estimated again and further infusion adjusted accordingly. If necessary it should be alternated with 500 ml of 0.9% saline containing 20 mmol K.

(iv) *A broad-spectrum antibiotic* should be given.

(v) *Low-dose heparin* (5000 units twice daily subcutaneously) should be given to prevent venous thrombosis.

(vi) The stomach should be emptied via Ryle's tube.

(vii) Catheterisation should only be carried out if the bladder is palpable and no urine has been passed in the first 4 hours.

(viii) *Insulin* should be given using either soluble insulin or Actrapid. For adults the dose is:
Initial dose—20 units IM.
Subsequent dose—6.0 units IM hourly or 4–6 units/hour by continuous intravenous infusion. This will require an infusion pump.

When the blood glucose level reaches about 14 mmol/litre the infusion should be changed to 5% dextrose and the insulin continued as either, 6.0 units IM every 2 hours or 10 units by continuous infusion over 4 hours. Potassium replacement should continue.

Oral feeding is resumed as soon as possible and potassium given in the form of Slow-K and potassium-rich foods such as orange or tomato juice.

Success depends on *close clinical and biochemical attention.* Initially, *hourly blood estimations for glucose, potassium, bicarbonate, pH, urea and PCV are required*, then at longer intervals as the patient improves.

A chest radiograph should always be taken and an ECG recorded. Leucocytosis is the rule and does not necessarily indicate infection.

Recovery is slow and with the best treatment severe cases take 48–72 hours.

Diabetics in Special Circumstances

(a) *During Surgical Operations.* If the patient is having elective surgery and is already being treated with insulin, he should be controlled by soluble insulin or its monocomponent analogue given three times daily. Very mild diabetics who are well controlled by diet or small doses of hypoglycaemic agents do not usually require any change of management but the blood sugar must be estimated regularly. Poorly controlled diabetics on hypoglycaemic agents should be temporarily switched to soluble insulin.

On the day of the operation a 5% dextrose infusion should be started giving 1.0 litre every 8 hours and soluble insulin should be infused by pump at the rate of 3 units per hour. This regime will usually prevent hyperglycaemia and ketosis which often develop as a result of surgery. Blood sugar should be estimated regularly particularly in the postoperative period and the urine tested for ketones. The infusions of dextrose and insulin can be adjusted as necessary. For emergency operations a similar regime can be used.

As the patient recovers and starts oral feeding again the infusion can be stopped and a return made to infections of soluble insulin 3 times daily.

(b) *Pregnancy.* Diabetic women are less fertile, more prone to miscarry and to toxaemia of pregnancy and hydramnios than their healthy sisters.

Their babies are more likely to die *in utero*, to be born grossly overweight, to suffer congenital malformations or to perish shortly before or after birth. Whereas the maternal mortality rate has improved markedly in the last twenty-five years, the foetal mortality in babies born to diabetic mothers remains over 10%.

Diabetes almost always becomes more severe during pregnancy; indeed, it may be precipitated or unmasked by it. Insulin requirements usually increase sharply for the first trimester, remain steady for the second, and usually increase but occasionally decrease during the third. They decline very sharply after parturition and close observation is necessary to avoid hypoglycaemia. Breast feeding almost always fails, and many obstetricians artificially suppress lactation immediately after birth. Because the power of the cells in the proximal renal tubule to reabsorb glucose is impaired in pregnancy the renal threshold falls, and therefore the urinary glucose is not an adequate index of control and blood glucose levels must be estimated.

Because of the dangers of intra-uterine death, termination of pregnancy either by induction of labour or elective caesarian section is indicated at 36 weeks. Some of the fatalities in the infants can be traced to a hyaline membrane lining the alveoli, a few to hypoglycaemia, but many remain unexplained.

(c) *During Infection.* Insulin requirements increase with infection, and this is true of gastroenteritis with vomiting and anorexia. The prescribed insulin dose should always be given, and if glycosuria or ketonuria perists it should be increased. Even minor infections in diabetes should be treated seriously.

DIABETES INSIPIDUS

Introduction. This is a rare disease, characterised by the excretion of a large (10–20 litres/24 hours) urinary volume and consequent great thirst. It is caused either by an absence of antidiuretic hormone from the posterior pituitary gland, or by an inability of the distal renal tubule to respond to its action. Failure of secretion may occur when disease processes affect the region of the pituitary, for example tumours (*ca.* 50%), inflammatory disease (*ca.* 25%), vascular changes (*ca.* 10%), trauma (*ca.* 10%) and Hand–Schüller–Christian disease (*ca.* 2–3%).

Clinical Features. The effect of the diuresis is to cause intense thirst, and if fluids are withheld dehydration is rapid, and the signs and symptoms of water deficiency (p. 512), soon appear. The urinary osmolality is always low. The condition should be suspected in all patients secreting over 4 litres of urine per 24 hours and drinking more than 5 litres per 24 hours. It must be differentiated from diabetes mellitus (glycosuria), terminal renal failure (proteinuria, uraemia) and hysterical over-drinking. Only the last is difficult to separate. The most useful confirmatory test is to deprive the patient of water for 8 hours. Normal subjects will achieve a urine concentration of at least 600 mOsmol/kg whereas those with diabetes insipidus will achieve only a small rise in osmolality. This test requires care as it is possible to dehydrate the patient seriously and it should not be performed if the plasma osmolality is above 300 mOsmol/kg.

Symptomatic treatment is by means of the pitressin analogue desmopressin. The dose is 10–20 μg intranasally once or twice daily or 2.0 μg IM daily. Some patients are helped by thiazide diuretics and chlorpropamide is sometimes of value. Cure can only be achieved by treating the cause.

Nephrogenic diabetes insipidus is almost always congenital, very rarely the result of destruction of the distal renal tubule in pyelonephritis. The congenital form is easily recognised by the family history, its early onset, male predominance, and failure to respond to desmopressin. Low sodium diets are recommended as treatment, but prognosis is poor.

Inappropriate Secretion of Antidiuretic Hormone

In some patients with malignant disease, almost always carcinoma of the bronchus, antidiuretic hormone may be secreted by the tumour cells and cause water retention with progressive dilution of the plasma electrolytes and urea. This usually presents clinically as a 'low sodium syndrome' (pp. 515, 597). Treatment is by water restriction, aldosterone, and the treatment of the underlying condition.

HYPOGLYCAEMIA

Introduction. Symptoms usually appear when the blood glucose has fallen to between 2.2–2.8 mmol/litre. They seem more related to the rate of fall than to the actual level reached, and commonly occur when patients are hungry. Sometimes they can be averted by eating carbohydrate, e.g. chocolate.

Symptoms are of rapid onset and begin with slight unsteadiness, tremulousness, difficulty in concentration, and often headache. They proceed to irrational behaviour, stupor, and coma. Urine may be voided.

Signs. The patient becomes pale, sweats, and the pulse is initially rapid and jerky. When coma is complete the pulse and blood pressure are normal. Severe and prolonged hypoglycaemia may produce irreversible cerebral changes. Epileptic fits may occur and coma may proceed to death.

Cause of Hypoglycaemia

(1) *Insulin overdose*; mismeasured doses, failure to take an expected meal, overexertion.
(2) *Reactive*.
(3) *Liver disease*. Cirrhosis, subacute necrosis.
(4) *Gastrointestinal disease*—post gastrectomy syndrome; steatorrhoea; after alcoholic excess.
(5) *Endocrine*. Hypopituitarism, hypothyroidism, adrenal insufficiency, as a premonitory occurrence in diabetes mellitus, and in insulin-secreting tumours of the pancreas.
(6) *Sarcomas, secondary carcinomatosis*.
(7) Use of *chlorpropamide*, and other *hypoglycaemic drugs*, especially in non-diabetics.
(8) Side-effects of salicylates, antihistamines or monoamine-oxidase inhibitors.

Careful history and clinical examination will make nearly all these conditions sufficiently obvious. It is only when it is reactive or when it is due to an insulin secreting tumour that further investigation is usually necessary for diagnosis.

A five hour glucose tolerance test is useful in establishing a diagnosis of reactive hypoglycaemia (Fig. 12.4).

In hypoglycaemia due to an insulin producing tumour a prolonged fast (14 hours at least) will lead to a progressive fall in blood glucose (Fig. 12.5). The presence of a low plasma glucose together with an inappropriately high plasma insulin is characteristic of an insulinoma.

A number of other provocative tests are in use and may be helpful in expert hands.

Treatment. Unless von Gierke's disease is suspected, or the coma has been long-standing or very severe the patients may be revived with

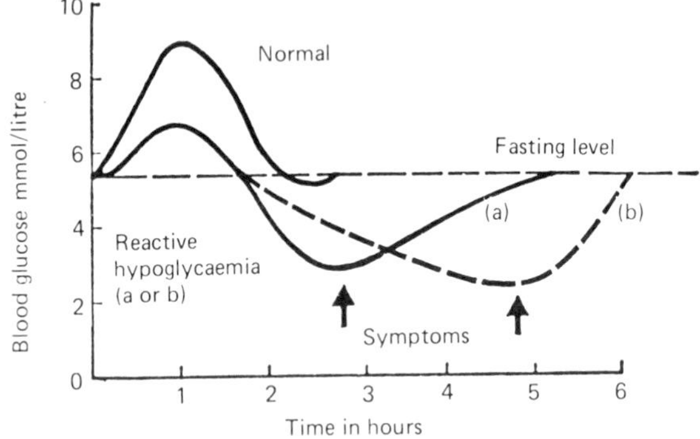

Fig. 12.4 Glucose tolerance tests in normal subject and in spontaneous hypoglycaemia.

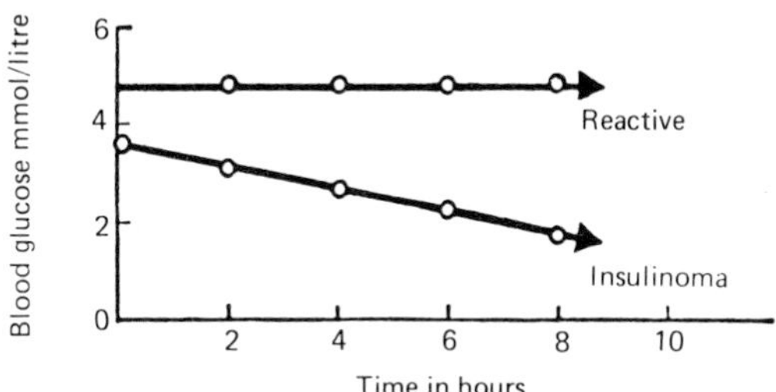

Fig. 12.5 Repeated fasting blood sugar levels in spontaneous hypoglycaemia.

glucagon. A sugar-containing drink—hot sweet tea or sugar in hot water—is prepared, and an injection of glucagon 1–2 mg IM is given. This produces a transient hyperglycaemia, with partial recovery of consciousness, during which the sweet drink can be given. Failing this, a stomach tube can be passed and the sweet drink given through this. It is better to give an IV injection of 20 ml of 50% glucose solution.

Subsequent treatment depends on the cause of the hypoglycaemia. If it is due to an insulin-secreting tumour (extremely rare) this should be removed surgically. If due to 'reactive hypoglycaemia' then best results are obtained with a high-protein diet and small frequent meals.

DISORDERS OF FAT METABOLISM

OBESITY

This is a serious disease, common in prosperous communities. It results from eating more food than is required. The common cause accounting for over 90% of cases of this hyperphagia is gluttony, but it may also occur in hypothalamic disorders or as a sequel to severe emotional stress. The rate of weight gain is proportional to the extent of dietary excess over requirement; once obesity is established, however, it may be maintained by quite small food intake. Fat can only be removed by eating less food than is required. Actuarial studies suggest that obesity is associated with a decrease in life expectancy (Table 12.7). Weight is gained in myxoedema, but is not due to fat.

Obesity may occur at any age; it is most common in the prosperous years of life, and the appearance of the plump matron or city alderman is familiar. Rarely the distribution of fat is unusual. In Cushing's syndrome (p. 571) it affects the head, neck, and shoulders chiefly, and spares the legs; the reverse is true in *lipodystrophia progressiva*. This is most common in women, who show little fat above the waist, but are

Table 12.7 Mortality rates and body weight expressed as percentage deviation from the average

	Bodyweight	Mortality		Bodyweight	Mortality
Men	−20	110	*Women*	−20	100
	−10	100		−10	95
	− 0	100		− 0	100
	+10	107		+10	108
	+20	121		+20	123
	+30	137		+30	138
	+40	162		+40	162
	+50	210		+50	200
	+60	—		+60	—

(Modified from Bray, 1979)

obese about the buttocks and legs. There is a rare association of obesity with cystic disease of the ovaries. Many fat women have menstrual irregularities which usually remit when ideal weight is achieved.

The appearance of fat is due to hypertrophy of fat-bearing cells. If obesity appears early in life, then the actual number of fat bearing cells may be greatly increased. In some cases local hyperplasia occurs, causing painful fatty lumps in the adipose tissue (*Dercum's disease*). Obesity may occur in children, most frequently the young child of elderly parents. Fat accumulates generally, but is well marked in the mons pubis; this sporran of fat overhanging normal genitalia (where there is no subcutaneous fat) often leads wrongly to a diagnosis of *Fröhlich's syndrome*, an extremely rare condition.

The effects of obesity are widespread. Extra effort is required for all activity, and extra blood and energy for the metabolism of fat. This increases the demands on the heart and lungs, and excess obesity may itself cause heart failure from restriction of respiratory excursion. The appearance of these grotesquely bloated patients in severe congestive cardiac failure, markedly cyanosed, with polycythaemia rubra, and gross oedema (*Pickwickian syndrome*) is unforgettable. Even minor degrees of obesity may induce failure in an already diseased heart.

Direct mechanical effects of obesity too must be considered. Joints and ligaments suffer from the extra weight that they are called upon to support. Osteoarthritis is common in the knees, and skeletal pains from undue tension in ligaments are the rule. The skin creases are exaggerated, and become keratinised. They are difficult to keep clean, and fungus infection and other skin sepsis is common. Because of the insulating effect of fat it is difficult for the body to lose heat. In spite of profuse sweating discomfort may be acute in hot weather. Added to these are the more mundane difficulties of obtaining appropriate clothes, rising from chairs, and entering and alighting from vehicles.

There also exists a predisposition to certain diseases. Diabetes mellitus (p. 526) is much commoner in the obese, and there is increased tendency to atheroma. Hypertensives are commonly overweight, and the risks of anaesthesia and surgery are greatly increased in the obese.

Treatment. The energy equivalent of adipose tissue is so great that exercise is of little value in treatment. It is calculated that a pound of fat would be lost for every 25 miles run! There is no benefit from hot baths, purgation, or massage. Nor is there any place for thyroid extract, which may cause irreversible exophthalmos. It may be that a few patients are helped a little by diuretics, but undoubtedly the main treatment is simply dietary restriction.

Many suitable diets for the treatment of obesity are available. Mild cases may follow a quite simple diet, merely avoiding fat and carbohydrate in normal meals. This may be reinforced by a day's starvation during the week. Drastic restriction is required in more severe degrees of obesity. The most extreme cases resemble the addiction states, and are best admitted to hospital, and supplied with only 200 calories daily; extra vitamins and iron should be given if this is undertaken. Most patients will tolerate this for 2 to 3 weeks, after which the diet may be increased to 400 calories daily. After a week or so apparent constipation occurs, from reduced faecal residue. This may be treated with methyl cellulose and liquid paraffin 15.0 ml at night. The ultimate objects are to restore the patient to his ideal weight, to enable him to conquer his hyperphagia, and to be discharged content to eat a normal diet. These may imply a profound alteration in his way of life; simple psychotherapy and supportive interviews may be necessary for some months.

ATHEROMA AND HYPERLIPIDAEMIAS

Introduction. Arterial disease as a sequel to atheroma is a major cause of ill health. Deaths attributable to it are increasing exponentially in all civilised countries. There are many features which make it probable that it is of environmental origin. For example, man is the only mammal in which atheroma is significant; it is rarely present at birth, but increases in extent and severity throughout life. It may, however, be modified by endogenous factors. It is rarely severe in healthy women until the menopause; it is more extensive and has more complications in patients with certain maladies, for example diabetes mellitus, familial xanthomatosis, myxoedema and nephrosis. It results in either abrupt or slow closure of arteries, with consequent deprivation of vital tissues of blood. It is ubiquitous and is a major cause of hospital admissions. It is the underlying cause of angina pectoris, and coronary artery disease, of cerebral vascular disease, intermittent claudication and gangrene, of retinal disease and most mesenteric thromboses.

Aetiology. The development of atheroma is a multifactorial process and there has been a great deal of investigation of the causative factors involved. The exogenous risk factors are considered on p. 204. The hyperlipidaemias are important endogenous factors. The plasma lipoproteins are large molecules formed of lipids and protein and are largely concerned with lipid transport. Lipoproteins can be classified either as a result of ultracentrifugation or plasma electrophoresis. Table 12.8 shows the main fractions together with the proportion of triglyceride and cholesterol in each fraction.

In general, high levels of HDL (α lipoprotein) exert some protective effect against atheroma whereas high levels of LDL (β lipoprotein) and VLDL (pre-β lipoprotein) are associated with an increased incidence of atheromatous vascular disease.

Type I (Exogenous Hypertriglyceridaemia)

This is a rare disease affecting chiefly children, and inherited as an autosomal recessive. In the few adult cases recorded, no relationship with atheroma has been demonstrated. It is characterised by creamy plasma from excess of chylomicrons following about 15 hours after a fatty meal.

Type II (Hyperbeta Lipoproteinaemia)

A common disease of adult life, inherited as a Mendelian dominant character. It is strongly associated with the development of atheroma. In the heterozygotes subcutaneous xanthomata of the elbows, hands, knees and heels may occur. It may occur as a secondary phenomenon to a variety of diseases, for example, myxoedema, nephrosis, myeloma, and liver disorders.

Type III ('Broad Beta Disease')

A disease, occurring chiefly in men aged 20–40 years and inherited as an autosomal recessive. It is characterised by the appearance of flat linear deposits of lipids in the subcutaneous tissues, usually of the hands (planar xanthomas), and of lumpy deposits at the elbows, knees, and buttocks (tubo-eruptive xanthomas). It too is strongly associated with the early appearance of atheroma.

Table 12.8 Lipoprotein fractions in normal subjects

	Normal % of Total Lipid	
	Triglyceride	*Cholesterol*
Pre-β Lipoprotein, Very low-density lipoprotein (VLDL)	55	15
β Lipoprotein, Low-density lipoprotein (LDL)	6	60
α Lipoprotein, High-density lipoprotein (HDL)	6	40
Chylomicrons	90	3

Type		Normal	I	II	III	IV	V
Electrophoretic lipoprotein patterns	Chylomicrons Origin Beta lipoprotein Pre-beta lipoproteins Alpha lipoprotein	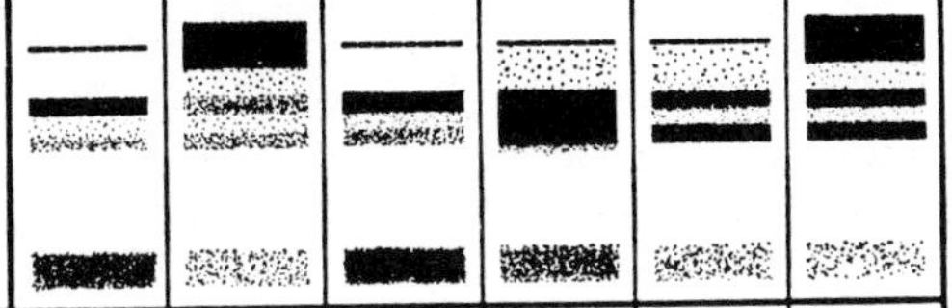					
Cholesterol mmol/litre		4.7–5.7	+	+	++	Normal or little +	+
Triglycerides mmol/litre		0.4–1.7	+++	Normal or little +	+	+	++
Glucose tolerance test		Normal	Normal	Normal	40% impaired	Impaired	Impaired
Urate mmol/litre		0.20–0.43	Normal	Normal	+	+	+

Fig. 12.6 Plasma electrophoretic patterns, cholesterol, uric acid and triglyceride levels, with glucose tolerance tests in normal and hyperlipidaemic subjects.

Type IV (Endogenous Triglyceridaemia)

This is the commonest of the five groups described. It occurs in adult life, but neither its cause nor its inheritance are currently known. It is believed to reflect an imbalance between the endogenous synthesis and removal of glycerides, and is frequently unmasked by obesity. It is often seen in association with other diseases, for example, diabetes mellitus and the nephrotic syndrome and excess ethanol consumption. There is a strong association with early atheroma. On examination, lipaemia retinalis, eruptive xanthomata, and hepatosplenomegaly may be found.

Type V (Mixed Hyperlipidaemia)

This is an uncommon lipid pattern seen usually between 10 and 30 years. It is commonly secondary to other diseases, for example, nephrosis, diabetic acidosis, and myxoedema. Clinically it resembles Type IV but recurrent bouts of abdominal pain are common. The nature of its inheritance is not yet known nor is its relationship to Type IV at all clear. No certain association with early atheroma has been found.

Treatment

(1) *Control of Plasma Lipids*

Type I — Diet with fat reduced to 50 g daily.

Type II — Diet should be low in cholesterol and high in unsaturated fatty acids. This means a diet low in dairy produce, eggs and meat together with the use of cooking oil and margarine made from unsaturated fats.

Cholestyramine in doses 12–30 g daily binds with cholesterol and decreases absorption and

	is useful when diet alone fails. Alternatively clofibrate 1.5 g daily which also lowers serum cholesterol.
Type III	Diet should aim to lose weight and alcohol must be avoided. Clofibrate as above is a useful adjunct.
Type IV	Low carbohydrate diet.
Type V	Low carbohydrate and fat so as to produce weight loss.

(2) *Local*

In some cases parts of arteries may be resected and replaced by grafts. This is almost confined to the larger vessels, for example, the carotid and lower aorta or femoral arteries.

(3) *General*

(a) Control of predisposing factors such as heavy smoking, obesity, arterial hypertension, and lethargy.

(b) When symptoms appear, e.g. in coronary heart disease (p. 203) and arterial disease (p. 228).

THE PORPHYRIAS

Haem is a constituent of haemoglobin, myoglobin and cytochromes. The important early step in its synthesis is the production of δ amino-laevulinic acid (δALA) which is catalysed by the enzyme δALA synthetase; this is the rate-limiting step in the synthesis of haem and is controlled by a negative feedback mechanism related to the concentration of haem. Following this step various porphyrins are produced and ultimately converted to haem (Fig. 12.7).

In each of the porphyrias the production of haem is reduced by a defect in enzyme action further along the pathway with a resulting fall in haem concentration and induction of δALA synthetase. There is thus an overproduction and accumulation of porphyrins. Porphyrias can be divided into:

Acute Porphyrias. The most common of these is acute intermittent porphyria.

Non-acute Porphyrias. These are predominently dermal photosensitive reactions.

Acute Intermittent Porphyria

This is an autosomal dominant disorder which usually appears in the third decade of life.

Clinical Features. It usually presents with recurrent episodes of abdominal pain which are often severe and combined with constipation and vomiting. Examination of the abdomen shows only some general-

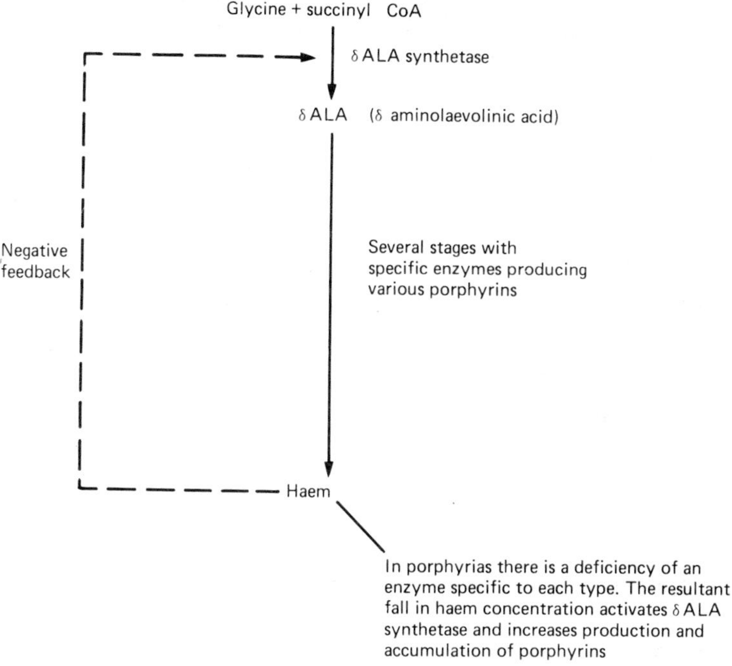

Fig. 12.7 The pathogenesis of the porphyrias.

ised tenderness. About 60 % of patients develop polyneuritis during the attack with both sensory and motor disturbance. Sometimes this may be extensive enough to cause respiratory embarrassment. Tachycardia, fever and hypertension are often features. Mental changes with hallucinations may overshadow the physical manifestation of the attack and obscure the diagnosis.

Episodes of this type are recurrent and there are often precipitating factors. These include various drugs, i.e. barbiturates, ethanol, oral contraceptives, chlorpropamide, imipramine, methyldopa and many anticonvulsants. Other factors are pregnancy and infection.

Diagnosis depends on the demonstration of excess porphyrins in the urine, blood or faeces. A simple screening test is to add Ehrlich's aldehyde reagent to a sample of urine. Excess porphobilinogen produces a pink colour which, on the addition of chloroform, remains in the aqueous layer. The urine also turns a port wine colour on standing.

Treatment

(a) Remove any precipitating factors.
(b) Relieve pain by aspirin, pethidine or morphine as appropriate.
(c) Restore water and electrolyte deficiencies.

(d) A high carbohydrate intake helps to relieve symptoms—Hycal is useful.
(e) If polyneuritis is a problem assisted respiration and physiotherapy may be required.

Attacks should be prevented by avoiding precipitating factors and by a high carbohydrate diet.

Non-acute Porphyrias

(1) **Cutaneous Hepatic Porphyria**
This eruption occurs in the areas exposed to sunlight i.e. face, neck, hands and arms. It starts as an erythema and ultimately becomes bullous, healing with scar formation. Precipitating factors are ethanol and occasionally drugs. Treatment consists of avoiding these factors, the use of barrier creams and regular venesection which produces mild iron depletion.

(2) **Erythropoietic Photoporphyria**
It appears in childhood or adolescence and its hallmark is dermal photosensitivity, presenting as solar urticaria or solar eczema. Skin reactions usually start within minutes of exposure to sunlight and subside within 24 hours without permanent damage to the skin.

(3) **Variegate Porphyria**
This is common in South Africa. It is strongly familial and its outstanding feature is skin sensitivity to both sunlight and mechanical trauma. Acute abdominal and neurological episodes may occur and the excretion of photoporphyrin and coproporphyrin in the faeces is continuously raised.

(4) **Congenital Erythropoietic Porphyria**
It appears in childhood usually in the male. Porphyrins are deposited in the bones and teeth which are stained violet and which fluoresce with UV light. Porphyrins in the skin lead to light sensitivity with blistering and subsequent scarring. The urine is port wine coloured.

Treatment. Avoidance of sunlight.

CARCINOID TUMOUR

The argentaffin cells of the appendix (and elsewhere) may give rise to tumours which appear histologically to be malignant but which clinically seem relatively benign; hence the name, carcin-oid.

The tumours secrete a substance named *serotonin* (5-hydroxytryptamine, 5HT) which stimulates smooth muscle. Normally it is detoxicated in the liver and probably the lungs, but if secondary hepatic carcinoid deposits have occurred, then high levels of 5HT appear in the blood. This causes widespread disturbance of smooth muscle. In the bowel, watery diarrhoea is provoked. There is generalised cutaneous suffusion, most marked in the face, and punctuated by attacks of vivid flushing, lasting for a minute or two and often precipitated by alcohol. Stimulation of the smooth muscle in the bronchi may cause asthmatic spasm, with persistent wheezing. A thick white layer of fibrous tissue is deposited on the endocardium of the right side of the heart, causing pulmonary and tricuspid stenosis, and eventually leading to cardiac failure.

Some of the 5HT in the body is converted into 5 hydroxy-indole acetic acid (5HIAA), which is excreted in the urine and may be detected with Ehrlich's aldehyde reagent.

Treatment is unsatisfactory. Occasionally it is justified to remove as much of the tumour as possible as this will reduce the production of 5HT. Intestinal symptoms can sometimes be controlled with methysergide which blocks the action of 5HT. The dose is 1–2 mg three times daily. Flushing may respond to a combination of an H_1 blocker (antihistamines) and an H_2 blocker (cimetidine). The course is variable, and patients may survive for ten years or more; the disease is always ultimately fatal.

AMYLOID DISEASE

Amyloid is an abnormal protein which may accumulate in the tissues. Some amyloid is composed of light chain residues from gamma globulins. It may be secondary to long-standing inflammation, for example, rheumatoid arthritis or tuberculosis, when it is perireticular in distribution. It may also complicate myelomatosis (p. 634). Amyloidosis can also occur as a primary condition, although a number of these cases show a slight increase in plasma cells in the bone marrow.

(1) In secondary amyloidosis infiltration occurs in the liver, spleen, kidneys, small intestines, arteries and skin. The heart is spared. More rarely endocrine glands, such as the adrenals are involved. The patient's already bad health grows worse, the skin takes on a waxy appearance, and diarrhoea and polyuria appear. Treatment is of the primary cause. There is some evidence that amyloidosis may be reversible in its early stages.

(2) When it complicates myelomatosis the kidney is specially involved, and a nephrotic syndrome may result.

(3) Primary amyloidosis affects men and women equally, and is occasionally familial. It occurs between 20 and 40, and may involve the heart, kidneys, muscles of swallowing and breathing, the peripheral nerves or the brain, the lymph nodes, liver and spleen, either singly or together. No treatment is very satisfactory but steroids are worthy of trial.

WILSON'S DISEASE (Hepatolenticular Degeneration)

Wilson's disease is a recessive metabolic disease which is characterised by degeneration of the basal ganglia, cirrhosis of the liver, and a brownish pigmented ring at the limbus of the cornea (Kayser–Fleischer rings). The disease is due to an increased absorption and/or a decreased excretion of dietary copper which leads to a progressive increase in the total body copper with consequent damage to the tissues of the brain, liver, and renal tubules.

Clinical Features. Wilson's disease is slightly more common in males than females and usually becomes clinically recognisable between the age of 15 and 30 years. Except in young children in whom symptoms of cirrhosis of the liver are common, neurological symptoms predominate. Tremor and rigidity of the limbs are common presenting symptoms. Dysarthria is a frequent early symptom. Rarely, symptoms of cirrhosis of the liver may predominate and the patient dies of liver failure in the absence of neurological signs. The disease is usually fatal within fifteen years of onset.

Laboratory Investigation. A decreased level of serum copper and ceruloplasmin associated with an increased urinary copper excretion is diagnostic. A normal level of ceruloplasmin does not exclude the diagnosis if Kayser–Fleischer rings are present. A low serum uric acid is common. Increased amino-aciduria is usual but not invariable.

Differential Diagnosis. The disease should be suspected in all disturbances of basal ganglion function and in all cases of juvenile cirrhosis of the liver. The presence of a Kayser–Fleischer ring is pathognomonic. Slit lamp examination is necessary in doubtful cases.

Treatment. This is directed towards removing the excess copper and decreasing dietary intake of copper. Penicillamine increases the urinary excretion of copper and is the treatment of choice (1.0–2.0 g daily). Treatment may have to be continued indefinitely. Improvement in some patients may be striking.

FURTHER READING

Krall, L. P., (ed.), *Joslin's Diabetic Manual*, 11th edition, Lea and Febiger, Philadelphia, 1978.

Oakley, W. G. and others, *Diabetes and its Management*, 3rd edition, Blackwell, Oxford, 1978.

CHAPTER 13

ENDOCRINE DISORDERS

The system of endocrine secretions, acting in one sense as another nervous system, coordinates and controls a wide variety of functions. As in the nervous system, positive and negative feedback is crucial in its operation, and this feedback is exerted either by hormones themselves or the metabolic effects of hormones. Top level control, in the hypothalamus, integrates both these forms of feedback and the signals related to the subject's environment, such as dark or light, sleep or wakening, stress and excitement. The network of endocrine control is also held together by influences between the different hormone 'channels', both at hypothalamic-pituitary level and at the periphery where hormones act. Table 13.1 outlines the principal control mechanisms of the pituitary gland.

The variety of levels at which modulation or feedback can occur deserves emphasis. Some hypothalamic factors act on tissues other than the pituitary, e.g. LHRH influences the mood (a cerebral effect) and the uterus; somatostatin occurs in high concentration in the islet cells of the pancreas and the wall of the gut. Pituitary hormones may act directly on tissue receptors (e.g. prolactin on milk-producing cells), on 'non-endocrine' tissues to release secondary 'hormones' (e.g. GH on the liver to release somatomedin), or on other endocrine glands (e.g. TSH on the thyroid). The hormones secreted by target glands in their turn activate receptors which usually elicit the cellular response through a mechanism involving a second messenger, in many cases cyclic-AMP, as shown in Fig. 13.1. The 'adrenergic' effects of thyroid hormones are a result of interaction at this sort of level, and it is likely that local factors such as prostaglandins also act here.

The nervous and endocrine systems also share evolutionary origins in primitive chemical mediators, and even in man the borderline between the two systems is often academic. The 'posterior pituitary' hormones oxytocin and vasopressin (ADH, p. 458) are synthesised in the hypothalamus and secreted down axons of the nerve fibres, to be released in the posterior lobe. Adrenaline at the nerve endings is a neurotransmitter; adrenaline released from the adrenal medulla is a hormone. Hormones of the gut and pancreas, responsive particularly to stimuli from the gut and to levels of various substrates in the blood, are strongly influenced by autonomic nervous signals and themselves influence the gastrointestinal response to the vagus nerve.

Table 13.1 Anterior pituitary and hypothalamic hormones and factors*

Anterior Pituitary Hormone		*Hypothalamic Hormone or Factor**
ACTH (adrenocorticotrophic hormone) and, as byproducts, α and β lipotrophins. (Note: MSH is *not* found in human plasma except as an artefact.)	*released by*	CRF (corticotrophin releasing factor). (The negative feedback here is through cortisol.)
FSH (follicle stimulating hormone), which in the male stimulates spermatogenesis	*released by*	LHRH (LH and FSH releasing hormone, or LRH), a decapeptide (The negative feedback here is through gonadal hormones.)
LH (luteinising hormone), which in the male stimulates interstitial cells to produce testosterone	*released by*	
GH (growth hormone, somatotrophin), which stimulates production of somatomedin (sulphation factor) by the liver	*released by*	GHRH (growth hormone releasing hormone), the dominant control
	inhibited by	GHRIH (growth hormone release inhibitory hormone, SOMATOSTATIN) which also inhibits TSH release and several pancreatic hormones
TSH (thyroid stimulating hormone, thyrotrophin)	*released by*	TRH (thyrotrophin releasing hormone), a tripeptide, the dominant control
	inhibited by	GHRIH (and by the thyroid hormones)
PROLACTIN	*inhibited by*	DOPAMINE, the dominant control, thus allowing marked increase in prolactin secretion if control is 'impaired'
	released by	TRH. A prolactin releasing factor other than TRH may exist

* The term hormone is reserved for those substances which have been well characterised and shown to have a role in human physiology.

GOITRE

A goitre is an enlarged thyroid gland. If it occurs in the absence of thyrotoxicosis it is a **non-toxic goitre**. The term **simple goitre** is used for the diffuse non-toxic goitre that is not uncommon in adolescent girls; it usually resolves spontaneously. In the context of thyroid disease the word **toxic** means thyrotoxic, in other words a thyroid condition

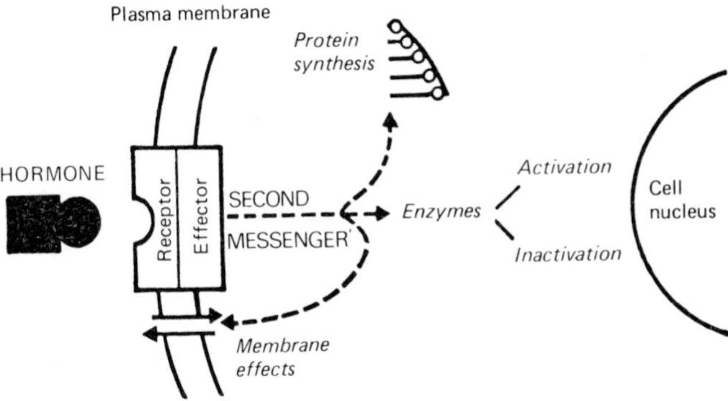

Fig. 13.1 Typical scheme of peptide hormone action. Note the many points at which the effect of the hormone could be modified.

accompanied by the disorder of function known as thyrotoxicosis. This is defined and discussed in more detail below.

Iodine deficiency is a potent cause of non-toxic goitre, and goitre is or was *endemic* in certain areas where the levels of iodine in the drinking water are low or the iodine is diverted from the thyroid gland by pollutants, fluorine or other factors. Endemic goitre has been eliminated in many areas by iodination of table salt. For reasons unknown, endemic goitre is much more frequent in women than men. The incorporation of iodine into thyroid hormone may also be blocked by antithyroid drugs, phenylbutazone, sulphonylureas or PAS (which are therefore goitrogens), or by congenital deficiencies of the enzymes involved in thyroid hormone synthesis, resulting in so-called *goitrous cretinism.*

THYROTOXICOSIS

This is the clinical state associated with raised circulating levels of free tri-iodothyronine (T3) and usually thyroxine (T4). The metabolic rate is increased, and the patient's resting state may mirror that of an athlete after a run—hot, flushed, sweaty, with a fast pulse. In adults it is due to one of two disorders: **Graves' disease**, which would classically be accompanied by a **diffuse toxic goitre**; or **toxic nodular goitre**.

Clinical Features of Thyrotoxicosis

Behaviour: nervousness and irritability; inability to relax or stay still and visible hyperkinesia; shaking and fine tremor; rarely, psychotic states.

Hypermetabolism: weight loss with increased appetite; warm moist skin (with or without fever); diminished tolerance of warm temperatures.

Muscles: general weakness and fatigue; muscle weakness and sometimes myopathy, especially of proximal muscles; some dyspnoea on exertion.

Eyes: a staring appearance as eyelid retraction widens the palpebral fissure; when the patient looks up and then down a rim of white sclera appears over the cornea (so-called *lid-lag*).

Bowels: diarrhoea (increased frequency and/or looseness) is common; nausea and vomiting, but rarely.

Cardiovascular: palpitations, tachycardia persisting during sleep or occurring in paroxysms, and atrial fibrillation; angina and high-output state with flow murmurs, bounding pulse, and sometimes heart failure.

Osteoporosis or *myasthenia gravis* may occur.

Graves' Disease

In this condition the goitre is usually diffuse and there are changes outside the thyroid gland which are *not* a direct consequence of elevated levels of T3 and T4, as if some unknown factor was acting both on the thyroid and on those other tissues. Many years ago it was shown that pituitary TSH was not the factor, and indeed the concentrations of TSH are suppressed to low or undetectable levels in all forms of thyrotoxicosis. The factor appears to be an IgG immunoglobulin, or a group of such immunoglobulins. The plasma of most patients with Graves' disease contain immunoglobulins of which some stimulate *mouse* thyroid tissue at a slow rate in the TSH bioassay system (LATS, long acting thyroid stimulator), some fail to stimulate but share binding properties with LATS (LATS-protector), some bind specifically to *human* thyroid membranes and can be displaced by TSH (TDA, thyrotrophin-displacing activity), and some activate adenylate cyclase in *human* thyroid preparations (HTS, human thyroid stimulator; TSI, thyroid-stimulating immunoglobulin). The values obtained by the various systems vary within the same plasma; this might be explained by the existence of a large variety of potentially stimulating immunoglobulins, some binding very specifically to human receptors and some non-specifically (so as to include the mouse receptor), some being biologically active in activating the receptor and some not.

Specific Features of Graves' Disease

(1) The disorder particularly affects women aged between twenty and forty, but the age range is wide and men are sometimes affected.
(2) One third of patients remit spontaneously within one or two years.
(3) The thyroid is diffusely enlarged (see Fig. 13.2), but if the condition

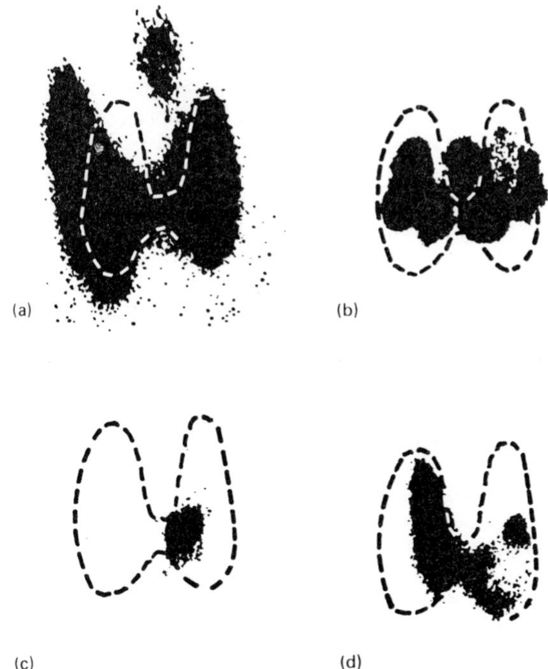

Fig. 13.2 Typical thyroid isotope scans. The dashed line indicates the outline of a 'normal' thyroid gland, which is of course variable.

(a) Graves' disease, diffuse toxic goitre with obviously active left pyramidal lobe.
(b) Multinodular toxic goitre, with several adenomata (nodules).
(c) Autonomous toxic nodule in left lobe, suppressing the remainder of the gland.
(d) 'Cold nodule'—the white area of low uptake within the left lobe. As 10 % are malignant lesions, surgery is indicated unless an ultrasonic scan suggests that it is cystic and needle aspiration of the cyst confirms its benign nature.

occurs in a previously lumpy gland (with previous non-toxic nodules) then one may find what is *clinically* a 'toxic nodular goitre'. It is important to distinguish this descriptive term, literally 'a clinically nodular goitre in a thyrotoxic patient', from the aetiologically distinct disorder described below.

(4) A systolic bruit is sometimes audible over the gland.
(5) *Exophthalmos*, protrusion of the eyeball, may aggravate the staring appearance associated with both forms of thyrotoxicosis. Infiltration of the extra-ocular muscles may occur, with consequent diplopia and/or paralysis of upward gaze. In severe cases, con-

junctival irritation, chemosis (inflammation of the eyelids) and even corneal ulceration may occur. *Malignant exophthalmos* is the progression of these changes to a condition of raised intraocular pressure, with pain, fall in visual acuity and a risk of permanent damage to the optic nerve. Guanethidine eye drops and systemic steroids at high doses may reduce the intra-ocular pressure, but if sight is seriously threatened then surgical decompression may be necessary. In *Ophthalmic Graves' Disease* the eye changes occur in the absence of thyrotoxicosis, levels of T4 and T3 being normal. About half these patients progress eventually to thyrotoxicosis.

(6) *Pretibial myxoedema*, mucopolysaccharide infiltration under the skin of the shin, and *thyroid acropachy*, a form of finger clubbing which is secondary to periosteal new bone formation and soft tissue thickening, are rare but pathognomonic signs of Graves' disease.

Toxic Nodular Goitre

A disorder which is essentially 'local' in origin, the toxic nodule is an actively secreting thyroid adenoma which has become autonomous, i.e. independent of control by the pituitary. Early in its development the levels of T4 and T3 will be normal but not influenced by changes in circulating TSH. The patient usually presents when T4 and T3 are elevated, with features of thyrotoxicosis, and by this time the TSH levels are suppressed by the high thyroid hormone concentrations, with a consequent 'suppression' of the normal thyroid tissue around the adenoma (see p. 561). On palpation, such a thyroid gland may feel lumpy, one or more nodules enlarging part or parts of the gland. The nodule may be immersed in the gland and any goitre may seem clinically 'diffuse'.

Because this form of thyrotoxicosis affects an older age group than Graves' disease, and the eye signs are less noticeable, its presentation is often more subtle. Thus many older patients present with cardiac or bowel symptoms, unexplained weight loss, or myopathy, and they may be lethargic or depressed rather than overactive and anxious (*apathetic thyrotoxicosis*).

Investigation and Diagnosis of Thyrotoxicosis

Tests of thyroid function are summarised in the Table on p. 564. The serum T3 (tri-iodothyronine, not the resin uptake) is a more reliable index than T4 in diagnosing thyrotoxicosis because the T4 is normal in some patients with thyrotoxicosis. Suppression of TSH, measured before and after injection of TRH (see graph on p. 566), is the most sensitive indicator of excessive or autonomous thyroid acitivity, but the test will only be necessary in borderline cases. Over-secretion of TSH by pituitary tumours is extremely rare.

Treatment

The fact that Graves' disease may remit spontaneously, and that in this condition surgical or radio-iodine therapy which restores normal thyroid function is accompanied by the later emergence of hypothyroidism in about 3% of patients per year of follow-up, argues for a trial of drug therapy in such patients. In contrast, the toxic 'hot nodule' will not remit spontaneously and so merits definitive treatment as soon as convenient. Having temporarily suppressed any iodine uptake by the normal thyroid tissue a hot nodule will take up virtually the whole of a dose of therapeutic radio-iodine, leaving the normal thyroid to resume normal function. But these comments and the following are in the nature of general guidance, the actual choice of treatment being tailored to the clinical state, age and circumstances of each patient.

Surgery (Thyroidectomy). This is appropriate in these situations:

(a) A significant possibility of carcinoma;
(b) Very large goitres;
(c) Pressure symptoms whatever the apparent size of the goitre e.g. deviation or compression of the trachea, or dysphagia;
(d) Alternative methods of treatment refused or impossible (e.g. allergies to antithyroid drugs, or radio-iodine contraindicated).

Patients must be rendered euthyroid by carbimazole and Lugol's iodine before operation, and the use of propanolol considered.

Radio-iodine. In most cases this is the standard method of definitive therapy, either at the time of diagnosis or after an appropriate trial of antithyroid drugs. The full effect of the radiation will not be seen for several months, during which time antithyroid drugs should be prescribed. It is contraindicated in patients who are, or may be, pregnant and those in younger age groups. Although the theoretically increased risk of subsequent thyroid cancer has not been substantiated, there are additional arguments against applying radiation to fertile subjects.

Antithyroid Drugs. The drugs in common use are carbimazole (40 mg daily, reducing to 5–15 mg daily) and propylthiouracil (100 mg q.d.s., reducing to 50 mg daily). Carbimazole is the less toxic but even so causes skin rashes in 3%, neutropenia in 1–2%, and agranulocytosis in about 0.5% of cases. Several weeks will elapse before the clinical improvement is complete. At the end of one or two years of treatment of Graves' thyrotoxicosis the drug may be discontinued and the TSH response to TRH measured (see Fig. 13.3). If this is normal then remission has probably occurred and no further treatment is necessary, but careful and prolonged follow-up is advisable.

Propranolol acts peripherally to give rapid relief of many toxic symptoms; although the levels of T3 are slightly diminished, the blocking effect is largely independent of thyroid hormone concentrations. It may be of special value in three situations:

Table 13.2 Thyroid function tests

This is a selection of the most useful tests of thyroid function. Tests now superseded by improved methods, or appropriate only in very special circumstances, are omitted from this list.

Both thyroxine (T4) and tri-iodothyronine (T3) are largely in bound form in the plasma, the main carrier protein being 'thyroid binding globulin' (TBG). The *total* concentration of T4 and T3 is therefore increased when the TBG level is increased (as during pregnancy and treatment with oestrogens), and decreased when TBG is decreased. The physiologically important levels are those of the *free* unbound hormones (FT4, FT3) but these are very much more difficult to measure directly. The T3 Resin Uptake is valuable in overcoming this difficulty because the test actually 'reads' the number of binding sites on the patient's TBG which are *not* occupied by T4 or T3; the *more* such *unoccupied* sites there are, the *lower* the 'reading' of thyroid hormone concentration. With an *increase* in the number of *unoccupied* binding sites, the T3 Resin Uptake will give a falsely *low* estimate of the effective free concentration of thyroid hormones. The Free Thyroxine Index (FTI), a product of T4 × T3 resin uptake, combines the bias in each direction to produce a reading that is less affected by the TBG concentration than either measurement alone.

Abbreviation	*What Does It Measure?*	*Normal Range*	*Comment*
FT4	Free unbound T4	8–22 pmol/l	Low in hypothyroidism. Limited availability
FT3	Free unbound T3	3–10 pmol/l	High in thyrotoxicosis. Limited availability
T4	Total T4, including bound T4	70–190 nmol/l	Increased by increased TBG (see above)
T3 (RIA)	Total tri-iodothyronine, by radio-immunoassay	1.2–3.0 nmol/l	Particularly valuable in diagnosing thyrotoxicosis (T4 may be normal)
TBG	Thyroid binding globulin	12–28 μg/ml	See discussion above
T3 resin uptake	Binding sites on TBG occupied by T3 or T4 (see above)	90–120 % of normal	Decreased by increased TBG (see above)

FTI	Free thyroxine as an index, 'T4 × T3 resin'	70–180 nmol/l	Not significantly affected by TBG, correlates with free unbound T4 (see above)
ETR	Effective (i.e. free) thyroid ratio: T4 available in the presence of the patient's plasma	90–110 % of normal	In vitro test—gives same information as FTI but in one test
TSH	Hypothalamic-pituitary function, or the degree of suppression by T4 and T3 secreted autonomously	1–6 u/l (see Fig. 13.3)	Low in pituitary failure. High in 1° hypothyroidism. Response to TRH 200 μg increased in 1° hypothyroidism, suppressed in thyrotoxicosis, diminished in hypopituitarism
Scan (^{99}Tc or ^{131}I)	Localisation of trapping of I (if ^{131}I, also rate of total uptake)	Symmetrical, each lobe approx. 2.5 cm × 4.0 cm (see Fig. 13.2)	May suggest size and location (e.g. retrosternal) of gland, or nature of disease

Note on drug interference with test results:
By displacement of T4 and T3 from TBG, salicylates and other non-steroidal anti-inflammatory drugs may lower total T4 and T3 while free levels—and the TSH—remain normal. Phenytoin may also have this effect but additionally shares with phenobarbitone a hepatic enzyme induction which increases the rate of clearance of T4; the TSH may rise slightly and those with limited thyroid reserve may be made hypothyroid.

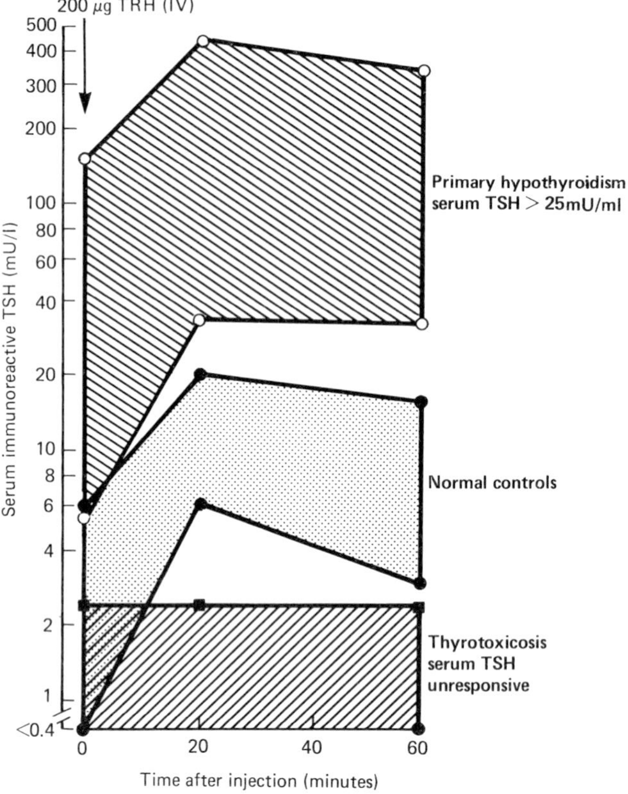

Fig. 13.3 The TRH stimulation test: range of responses.

(1) For rapid control of cardiac effects of T4 and T3.
(2) For symptomatic relief while investigations proceed.
(3) For rapid preparation of the thyrotoxic patient and the thyrotoxic gland for thyroidectomy, as a fast acting supplement to *Lugol's iodine* and/or *carbimazole*.

Thyroxine 0.1–0.2 mg daily is sometimes prescribed during or after antithyroid treatments to protect the patient from iatrogenic hypothyroidism. It will always be required if an ablative dose of radio-iodine is employed as standard therapy for Graves' disease.

Treatment of thyrotoxicosis in pregnancy is best managed with carbimazole, using the minimum dose which will keep the Free Thyroxine or Free Thyroxine Index (Table 13.2) just inside the normal range. The baby may be born with maternal thyroid stimulator in the circulation, causing *neonatal thyrotoxicosis*; this needs immediate and careful control by those with special experience, so delivery should be arranged in an appropriate centre. As carbimazole is excreted in breast milk, the baby must not be breast fed.

Thyroid Crisis

Also known as thyroid 'storm' this consists of an acute exacerbation of thyrotoxicity, with especially marked hyperpyrexia and tachycardia. It can occur after thyroid surgery (or occasionally radio-iodine therapy) but is rare since patients have been rendered scrupulously euthyroid before surgery. Treatment may include physical cooling (*not* aspirin which may unbind even more T3 and T4), Lugol's iodine, carbimazole, propranolol and hydrocortisone.

THYROIDITIS

Hashimoto's Disease (Autoimmune Thyroiditis)

A diffuse firm goitre develops, usually insidiously but sometimes in a subacute manner with pain and tenderness, characteristically in a middle-aged woman. Lymphocytic infiltration of the gland, and auto-antibodies to thyroglobulin and thyroid microsomes are to be expected. Early in the disease mild thyrotoxicosis may transiently occur, but 20 % present with, and many more progress to, overt hypothyroidism. Other auto-immune disorders may be associated with this disease and with those cases of Graves' disease and 'primary' myxoedema who exhibit thyroid auto-antibodies.

Subacute Thyroiditis (De Quervain's)

Although mild cases occur, the thyroid generally becomes acutely enlarged, firm, tender and painful, in a patient who is unwell and feverish. Transient hypothyroidism may be noted. There is often a history of recent respiratory infection, and the aetiology is thought to be viral. If the symptoms are not relieved by simple anti-inflammatory analgesics, prednisolone or low-dose radiotherapy may be necessary. Rarely thyroid abscess can mimic this disorder.

Riedel's Disease (Woody Thyroiditis)

The thyroid gland becomes hard as a result of intensive and locally invasive fibrosis (analogous to retroperitoneal fibrosis). It is rare, non-metastatic and can only be treated by resection. Thyroid function may be normal or, in the advanced case, slightly diminished.

HYPOTHYROIDISM

In the infant, thyroid deficiency produces **cretinism**, evident by slowing of growth, mental and physical retardation, a characteristic appearance and a hoarse cry. The adult form of the disease was first described by Sir William Gull in 1874; its name **myxoedema** derives from the mucoprotein thickening of subcutaneous tissue which is found in severe cases.

Clinical Features

Myxoedema: as mentioned above, a boggy non-pitting oedema which may be diffuse but is especially noticeable around the eyes and on the hands and feet.

Skin: cool, dry and coarse in texture, pale or faintly yellow in colour (aggravated by the anaemia which is often present); the hair is also dry and coarse and thin, with particular loss of the outer third of eyebrows.

Slowness: of thought, of action, of speech, of relaxation of the muscle after a reflex has been elicited (particularly at the ankle); the mental state may exhibit memory loss, dementia, depression or psychosis (so called 'myxoedema madness').

Hypometabolism: poor appetite yet mild weight gain; diminished tolerance of the cold; hypothermia may occur, even to the point of coma in a severe case.

Voice: may become hoarse as vocal cords thicken.

Cardiovascular: one third of patients show systolic hypertension until treated; some have angina and/or palpitations, which are not always relieved by treatment of the hypothyroidism; some are dyspnoeic on exertion; intermittent claudication has been reported.

Menorrhagia is a common complaint.

Investigation and Diagnosis. Tests of thyroid function are summarised in Table 13.2. Non-specific findings may include a normochromic normocytic anaemia, a raised plasma cholesterol, low voltage waves on the ECG, flattening of the glucose tolerance curve, and elevation of muscle enzymes. In doubtful cases an elevated TSH may provide valuable confirmation of the diagnosis (see Fig. 13.3).

Hypothyroidism may be the result of the following:

Primary failure of the thyroid gland. Even in those without a convincing history of Hashimoto's disease (p. 567) there is a high frequency of thyroid auto-antibodies, suggesting an autoimmune aetiology. Defects in thyroidal enzymes and thus thyroid hormone synthesis occur; they are rare and are usually discovered in early childhood in the form of **goitrous cretinism.** The latter, accompanied by congenital deafness, constitutes *Pendread's syndrome.*

External factors affecting the thyroid. Previous treatment for thyrotoxicosis is the commonest single cause of hypothyroidism. Severe iodine deficiency within the thyroid, associated with trapping or blocking of iodine, is a rare cause, usually presenting with a goitre (see p. 559).

The anti-arrhythmic drug amiodarone lowers T3 and T4 levels by interference in thyroid hormone metabolism; rebound thyrotoxicosis may occur if the drug is stopped abruptly. Lithium and phenobarbitone may also cause hypothyroidism, while other drugs alter binding to TBG (see Table 13.2).

Secondary failure, due to low TSH levels. This usually occurs as part of a panhypopituitary state, which is discussed on p. 594. TRH is a very potent stimulus to TSH secretion and a TSH response to TRH may persist even in the presence of a pituitary lesion; the hypothyroidism in such cases is presumed to reflect a low average level of pituitary drive.

Treatment. Whatever the cause of the hypothyroidism, most patients need to be treated by gradual restoration of normal thyroid hormone levels using oral *L-thyroxine*, commencing with 0.05 mg daily, increasing over three weeks to 0.02 mg daily, at which dose level most patients are euthyroid. Any more rapid rise in thyroid hormone activity may precipitate angina or left ventricular failure, especially in the old. The adequacy and effectiveness of treatment is best assessed on clinical grounds, and confirmed by finding the dose of thyroxine at which T4 and/or TSH levels in the normal range are restored. The patient must clearly understand the life-time nature of the medication.

In external and secondary types of myxoedema the primary cause must be remedied where possible.

Myxoedema Coma

Especially in the cold of winter, the hypothyroid condition of an elderly patient may progress to such a degree that bradycardia, shallow breathing, hypoxia, carbon dioxide retention, hypoglycaemia, hyponatraemia and hypothermia all contribute to a lapse into coma. The patient is cold to the touch, with depression of central and peripheral body temperatures, often *below the range of the standard clinical thermometer*, so that the severity of the problem is not recognised. Over half the patients die, so care must be intensive but not hasty—vigorous rewarming must be avoided, the gentle action of warm blankets being safer. Rapid-acting rapidly metabolised tri-iodothyronine 20 μg 8-hourly and hydrocortisone 100 mg 8-hourly should be administered IV, and the ECG and body functions closely monitored. As for any patient in coma and in shock, or on the brink of it, the airway, oxygenation and circulation must be maintained by appropriate means.

THYROID CARCINOMAS

Papillary, follicular and anaplastic tumours arise in the follicular epithelium of the thyroid, whereas the medullary carcinoma has a quite distinct origin in the parafollicular or 'C' cells.

Papillary Carcinoma

This tumour is the most common thyroid malignancy, occurring in the second and third decades and in later life. The solitary nodule in the thyroid gland may be unobtrusive and asymptomatic, and the first clinical sign may be enlargement of the local lymph nodes, by which time more extensive metastasis may have occurred. These tumours usually take up iodine but much less avidly than normal thyroid, so they appear as a 'cold' nodule on a thyroid scan (see Fig. 13.2) and solid or semi-solid on ultrasound examination. Any such nodule deserves excision: evidence of recent increase in size or of frank malignancy calls for total thyroidectomy and total excision of nodes or tissue involved. Some weeks later, if malignancy is confirmed, a large ablative dose of radioiodine is administered, and a whole body iodine scan is carried out. Tumour tissue (in the absence of the thyroid gland) now takes up the radioiodine, both displaying the extent of any local or distant metastases and receiving treatment by irradiation. Because the tumours are TSH-responsive in their rate of growth, thyroxine is administered from this point onwards so as to completely suppress TSH secretion. At intervals of 3–6 months, the ablative and diagnostic radioiodine scan is repeated, after a brief pause in the thyroxine suppression to allow TSH levels to rise and stimulate iodine uptake by any surviving thyroid tissue. Apart from these pauses, thyroxine should be continued for life.

Follicular Carcinoma

Histologically and functionally this tumour is closest to normal thyroid tissue. It tends to metastasise through the blood stream earlier than the papillary form, so it may be first identified through its distant metastases or by the finding of a stony hard nodule, which becomes subsequently locally invasive. The uptake of iodine may be similar to that of the thyroid gland, or even excessive, with the production of thyrotoxicosis. Management is along the lines of that for papillary carcinoma.

Anaplastic Carcinoma

The rapid painful enlargement of a 'cold' nodule may indicate the presence of this highly malignant form, which is fortunately less common than the related papillary and follicular carcinomas. Anaplastic tumours rarely concentrate radio-iodine, so following surgery consideration should be given to external radiotherapy. If there should be a recurrence, cytotoxic therapy may be useful.

Medullary Carcinoma

This C-cell tumour, which accounts for between 5 and 10% of all thyroid carcinomas, secretes calcitonin. Even so, it usually presents clinically as a malignant tumour of the thyroid, often with regional lymph-node involvement, sometimes with early extensive blood-borne metastases. The tumour carries a worse prognosis than papillary or follicular carcinomas, even if total thyroidectomy, neck dissection and radiotherapy are instituted promptly. It is therefore especially valuable to have high calcitonin levels, basal or stimulated by alcohol, as a 'marker' for the tumour.

Medullary carcinoma may occur sporadically but it tends to be familial, with an autosomal dominant pattern. In the familial cases there is a particular association with multiple endocrine adenomatosis (MEA) syndromes, both MEA Type II-A (with phaeochromocytoma and hyperparathyroidism) and MEA Type II-B (with phaeochromocytoma and mucosal neuromas). Relatives of an affected patient should therefore be screened for raised calcitonin levels; if such an elevation is found and confirmed, total thyroidectomy is appropriate before the cancer becomes clinically overt.

CUSHING'S SYNDROME

Excessive levels of glucocorticoids, if not the result of steroid treatment, arise from a disorder of the adrenal gland itself (about 20 %) or from an outside influence. The adrenal gland may harbour an adenoma or a carcinoma. The outside influence, which will induce adrenal hyperplasia, may take the form of an abnormally high level of ACTH from the pituitary—often driven by hypothalamic oversecretion of CRF (corticotrophin releasing factor) or an ACTH-like peptide secreted by a non-pituitary tumour (*ectopic*). The disease that Harvey Cushing described was that in which pituitary adenomas, usually small and basophilic, over-secrete ACTH.

Many of the clinical features of the syndrome reflect impaired protein synthesis or redistribution of fat.

Clinical Features

Those Related to the Effects of Cortisol

The face is typically plethoric and mooned as the skin gets thinner and adipose tissue rounds out the chin and cheeks; the supraclavicular notch may be filled, and posteriorly fat in the upper thoracic/lower cervical area produces the 'buffalo hump'. Obesity especially affects the trunk.

Muscle. As wasting occurs the thin legs and arms contribute to the 'lemon-on-sticks' shape, and the patient suffers from fatigue and weakness, sometimes severe (steroid myopathy).

Skin. This is thin and atrophic, so that purplish striae are seen.

Vessels. Purpura, or easy bruising, is common. The blood pressure may be moderately raised. Polycythaemia may be a feature.

Nervous System. Psychoses related to the condition are relieved as steroid levels return to normal.

Bones. Osteoporosis leads to compression fractures of the vertebrae and thus spinal curvature, and pathological fractures of the ribs.

Metabolic. Glucose tolerance is often impaired. The mineralocorticoid effects of cortisol and related compounds may result in a low serum potassium with alkalosis, but this is prominent only when very high levels of cortisol are circulating, and so more common in cases of ectopic ACTH production.

Androgenic Effects (especially if an adrenal tumour is present)

In men: impotence, increasing baldness, and acne.

In women: hirsutism (increased body and beard hair), recession of hair at the temples, menstrual irregularities or amenorrhoea, enlarged clitoris, and an increase in musculature.

Other Effects

Pituitary Tumours. Most often this is a rather small basophil adenoma, which will produce no local signs.

Adrenal Tumours. Signs related to the tumour itself are unusual but an adenocarcinoma may metastasise.

Ectopic Tumours. At least 12% of cases of adrenal hyperplasia are caused by secretion of an ACTH-like peptide by a tumour outside the pituitary. Typically the peptide level and therefore the adrenal output of cortisol is very high in such cases, the result being a severe Cushing's syndrome with hypokalaemic alkalosis and pigmentation. Oat-cell carcinoma of the bronchus, bronchial adenoma, carcinoid, thymic and pancreatic islet-cell tumours are especially associated with this picture. Anaemia rather than polycythaemia may then occur.

Investigation and Diagnosis. Non-specific findings may include polycythaemia, a neutrophilia between 10 000 and 20 000, depressed lymphocyte and eosinophil counts, mild glucose intolerance with or without a raised fasting blood glucose, and hypokalaemic alkalosis.

This is one of several endocrine disorders in which the diagnostic process divides into two quite separate phases: first, 'Is the hormonal function normal (physiological) or abnormal (autonomous)?' . . . a *biochemical* question; second, 'Once an abnormality of function is proven, what is the source of abnormality?' . . . a *pathological* and *anatomical* question. A basic scheme is shown in Fig. 13.4, the normal ranges are listed in Table 13.3, and specific tests are discussed below.

Plasma Cortisol. This is often the most convenient measurement, and a low or low normal level virtually excludes Cushing's syndrome. The levels may be misleadingly high in the anxious or obese subject, or in patients with high levels of the carrier protein transcortin in the blood such as those on 'the pill' or pregnant. A useful screening test for outpatients requires blood samples at 9.00 a.m. and 6.00 p.m. on the first day and 9.00 a.m. on the second day; dexamethasone 2 mg is taken by mouth at 11.00 p.m. on the first day. In Cushing's syndrome and in some stressed patients the normal diurnal variation is lost and the second

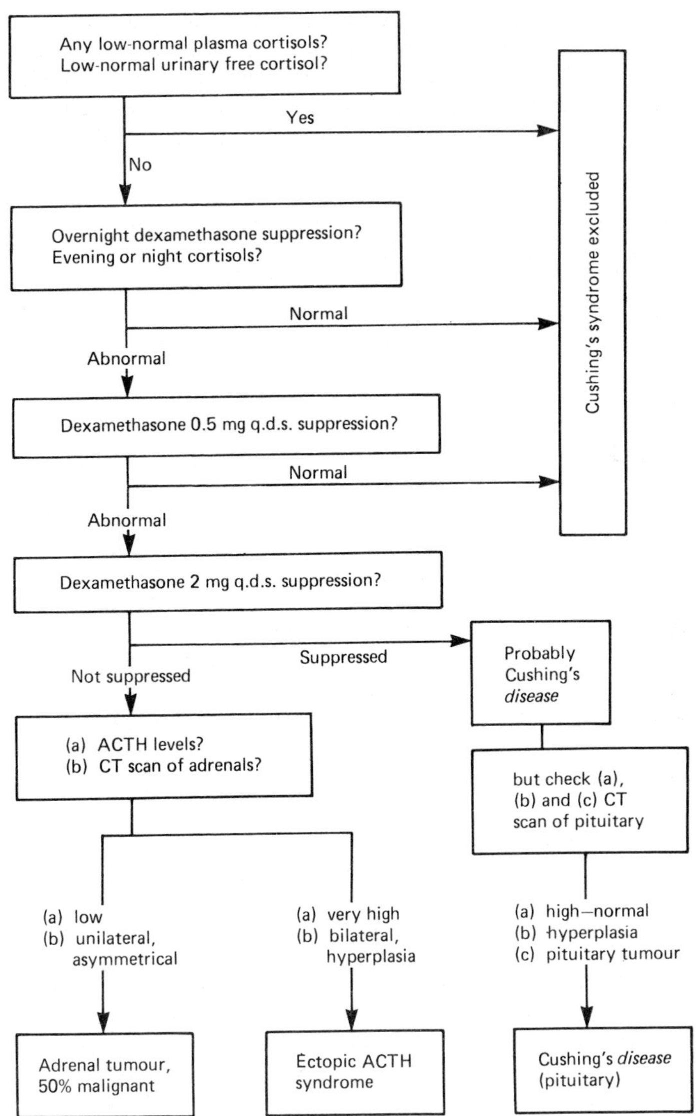

Fig. 13.4 Diagnostic flow-chart for suspected Cushing's.

9.00 a.m. cortisol is not suppressed to less than 150 nmol/litre as it should be in a normal subject. If the result of this study is not completely normal then further investigation is required.

Urinary free cortisol is unaffected by transcortin concentrations and

Table 13.3 Adrenal function tests

PLASMA CORTISOL, nmol/l

	09.00 h	*24.00 h*	*09.00 h after Dexamethasone 2 mg at 23.00 h of preceding evening*
Healthy non-stressed subjects	150–700	80–220	5–150
Cushing's syndrome	400–2400	400–2400	more than 300

Response to Synacthen (tetracosactrin) 250 μg IM	0 min	30 min	60 min
Healthy non-stressed subjects	150–700	more than 800	more than 800
Adrenal insufficiency	30–150	30–400	30–400
Disuse atrophy (chronically low ACTH)	30–150	30–400	30–400

Response to Insulin-induced hypoglycaemia: see Combined Pituitary Test (Table 13.5)

PLASMA ACTH: normal range: 10–80 ng/l at 09.00 h; less than 10 ng/l at 24.00 h

URINARY STEROIDS: OUTPUT/24 HOURS

	Male (normal)	*Female (normal)*	*Suppressed by Dexamethasone 2 mg/day for 3–5 days*
Free cortisol, nmol	130–600	130–600	less than 150
17-Hydroxycorticoids, μmol	11–45	11–30	less than 9
17-Oxogenic corticoids, μmol	15–60	11–48	less than 11
17-Oxosteroids, μmol	18–64	11–51	less than 11
Pregnanetriol μmol	1–3	1–3	less than 0.7

The normal ranges vary slightly between laboratories. The urinary output of steroids should be interpreted in the context of the patient's weight.

accurately reflects the secretion rate of cortisol. It is diagnostically more precise than measurements of 17-hydroxycorticoids, and even more useful than plasma cortisol, provided the urine collection is accurately timed. It may be mildly elevated by illness or continued stress.

17-Oxogenic corticoids include not only cortisol but several precursors and a metabolite, cortilone. While it is a more sensitive test for abnormalities of steroid synthesis such as congenital adrenal hyperplasia (adrenogenital syndrome, p. 581), it is less generally useful because high levels occur in some hirsute patients with increased androgen production but normal cortisol levels.

17-Oxosteroids mainly reflect the androgenic steroid precursors.

These are pathologically elevated in some patients with Cushing's syndrome, especially if associated with adrenal carcinoma when very high levels may occur, and in some patients with benign forms of hirsutism, including some with congenital adrenal hyperplasia (p. 581).

Dexamethasone Suppression Test. Urinary steroid excretion is suppressed in most normal or obese subjects by dexamethasone 0.5 mg q.d.s. and in most patients with adrenal hyperplasia due to pituitary ACTH by dexamethasone 2 mg q.d.s. (but not 0.5 mg q.d.s.); in most patients with adrenal tumours or an ectopic source of ACTH-like substance it cannot be suppressed even by the higher dose. However, the localisation suggested by this test can be unreliable, and it is most useful in confirming the pathological nature of borderline hypercortisolism.

Plasma ACTH levels are depressed in the presence of adrenal carcinoma or adenoma, and modestly elevated in Cushing's syndrome of pituitary or hypothalamic origin. Most ACTH assay systems give very high readings in cases of *ectopic* peptide production.

Anatomical Localisation. Computerised tomographic (CT) scan of the suprarenal area will usually define the adrenal glands and/or an adrenal tumour (Fig. 13.5), while an isotope uptake adrenal scan

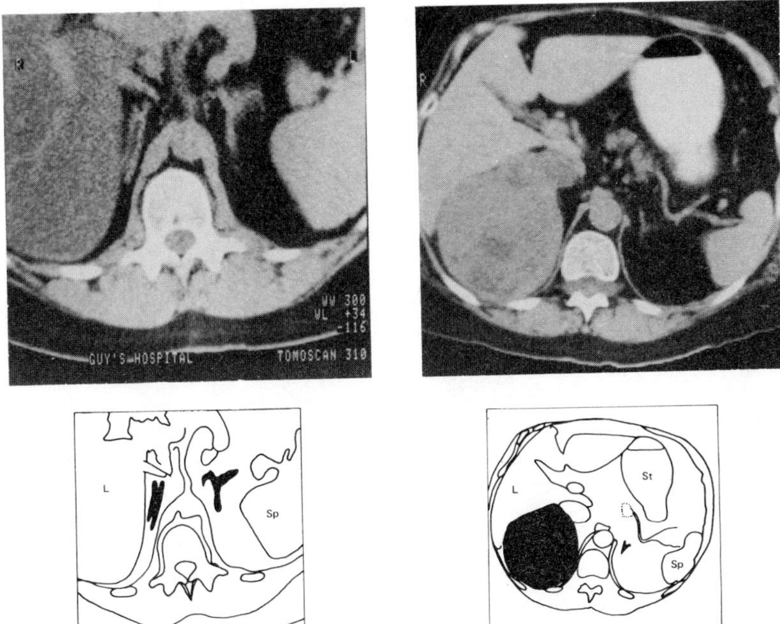

Fig. 13.5 CT scans of normal adrenal glands (on the left) and large adrenal tumour causing Cushing's syndrome (on the right). On the line diagram below each scan the adrenal tissue is shown by the solid black.

employing labelled cholesterol will show the level of activity of one or both glands and/or tumour(s). The investigation of the adrenals may then be taken further by arteriography or venography. *Bilateral* enlargement and active function favour hyperplasia secondary to an excess of ACTH, whereas *unilateral* 'suppression' as reflected by atrophy and loss of function, with marked enlargement and/or activity on the other side, suggest a primary adrenal tumour. The search for the source of excess ACTH may require X-rays and CT scans of the pituitary gland and the chest, the latter because so many of the ectopic sources are bronchial or thymic. Selective venous sampling may suggest the source of the ACTH by the finding of an especially high concentration of ACTH in a particular vein.

Treatment. An adrenal tumour must be removed with the whole of the affected gland and the other gland must be carefully inspected. In the case of inoperable adrenal carcinoma, the excessive steroid synthesis may be controlled by the drug o-p̀-DDD, which is unfortunately too toxic to use in other situations. Any non-pituitary tumour secreting an ACTH-like peptide is resected.

When adrenal hyperplasia is secondary to pituitary overproduction of ACTH the choice lies between pituitary ablation (by Yttrium implant or trans-sphenoidal hypophysectomy) and bilateral adrenalectomy, with pituitary irradiation when indicated. The advantages of the latter approach are the immediate reduction in cortisol levels, the temporary maintenance of pituitary function and in particular fertility if that is appropriate, and the positive exclusion of an adrenal tumour. The disadvantage is the risk of developing *Nelson's syndrome* (in which an ACTH-secreting tumour of the pituitary produces generalised pigmentation and local signs of expansion) during the period before the pituitary gland is irradiated. Maintenance therapy with corticosteroids and other hormones will be necessary following some of these forms of treatment.

If eradication of tumour producing ACTH is not possible, or the source of the ACTH cannot be identified, the drug *metopirone* may be valuable in diminishing cortisol synthesis. This will usually relieve symptoms but androgen levels will rise, a particular problem in female patients. The long-term objective is removal of the ACTH source.

ALDOSTERONISM (see also p. 167)

In its *primary* form this is related to an adenoma or hyperplasia of the adrenal cortical zona glomerulosa, producing a raised level of aldosterone in plasma and urine and—to a variable degree—hypertension, low serum potassium, metabolic alkalosis, and thus polyuria, periodic paralysis and paraesthesias. The frequency of the condition is controversial but between 1 and 10% of 'essential' hypertensive patients may have the condition. About 20% of hypertensive patients exhibit low plasma renin, a result of suppression by high aldosterone in some and of unknown mechanisms in others. The condition is diagnosed by the finding of persisting suppression of renin and high levels of aldosterone which cannot be suppressed by loading the patient with sodium.

Aldosterone excess *secondary* to high renin and angiotensin levels is well documented in malignant hypertension (p. 167), heart failure, cirrhosis of the liver, nephrotic syndrome, salt depletion and conditions of low blood volume.

ADRENAL INSUFFICIENCY (Addison's Disease)

Atrophy of the glands in the presence of auto-antibodies to adrenal tissue is the most common cause of deficient corticosteroid production. Tuberculous infiltration was once more common, and even now this aetiology may be betrayed by adrenal calcification and an appropriate history. Rare causes include carcinoma, various infiltrations, and haemorrhage in the gland in the course of meningococcal septicaemia (Friderichsen–Waterhouse syndrome, p. 364). The circulating levels of ACTH are high in these conditions, which constitute true 'Addison's disease', but *secondary* adrenal insufficiency may occur with low ACTH levels in hypopituitary states (p. 594). In patients with diminished adrenal reserve, *rifampicin* may cause insufficiency by induction of liver enzymes which increase the rate of metabolism of circulating cortisol and thus shorten its half-life.

Clinical Features

Chronic Insufficiency

Pigmentation is increased (an effect of ACTH), especially in skin creases, flexures, over the elbows and knuckles, in scars, on the gums and on the buccal mucosa.

Weakness, fatigue and lassitude are described and may be evident on examination.

Anorexia (apart from a specific craving for salt, which may be caused by the altered taste threshold in this disorder) is accompanied by weight loss and a decreased muscle mass. Nausea, vomiting and diarrhoea may also occur, and the patient may become clinically dehydrated.

A low blood pressure which falls further on standing may lead to dizziness and faintness.

Clinical features which, though important, occur less frequently, include the following: hypoglycaemia, hypothermia, vitiligo, hair loss, lymphadenopathy, asthma, rhinitis, mental aberrations.

Acute (*Addisonian Crisis*). This often occurs on a background of chronic deficiency, and it may therefore include any of the features described above, particularly severe hypotension, fever, profound weakness, nausea, vomiting and diarrhoea, progressing if untreated to coma. The coma may be complicated by hypoglycaemia or hypothermia. The precipitation of the crisis in a patient with chronic insufficiency may be provoked by some major stress (e.g. an infection, an accident, an operation), or by increased salt loss (e.g. in sweat).

Investigation and Diagnosis. During the acute illness the patient is in danger of fatal collapse, so treatment should not be delayed. In the stress of any severe acute illness *other* than adrenal insufficiency the plasma corticosteroids will be elevated, so plasma cortisols on samples of blood taken on admission will confirm or refute the diagnosis of Addisonian crisis. The plasma ACTH, if available, indicates directly whether the condition is that of hypothalamic-pituitary failure or that of primary adrenal failure with consequent ACTH hypersecretion. The clinical clue to the level of ACTH is the degree of pigmentation, the pallor of chronic pituitary insufficiency contrasting with the 'tan' of chronic adrenal failure. It should be born in mind, however, that increased pigmentation may also occur in chronic renal failure, hepatic cirrhosis, malabsorption, haemochromatosis, collagen disorders, folate or B_{12} deficiency, acromegaly and chronic skin infestation.

If the situation is not acute, or if a loss of adrenal reserve rather than manifest insufficiency is suspected, the diagnostic tests fall into three groups:

(1) Baseline measurements, of plasma cortisol or urinary free cortisol, which are persistently depressed in adrenal insufficiency (Table 13.3).

(2) The response to ACTH, for safety and convenience in the form of the synthetic analogue tetracosactrin (Synacthen), provides a test of adrenal function which is independent of the hypothalamic-pituitary axis. A normal response in the *Synacthen test* (Table 13.3) indicates adequate function of adrenal cortical tissue. A poor response indicates *either* adrenal gland destruction *or* a state of disuse atrophy because ACTH secretion has been chronically low (e.g. hypopituitarism, or use of oral corticosteroid drugs). If the response is poor, a three-day course of intramuscular Synacthen-depot 2 mg daily is followed by a second 60-minute Synacthen test. A marked improvement over the result of the first test suggests that disuse atrophy was the cause of the poor response; a persistently poor response points to primary adrenal disease.

(3) If the adrenal gland is not primarily at fault, the response of the entire system, hypothalamus-(CRF)-pituitary-(ACTH)-adrenal-cortisol, can then be tested by inducing hypoglycaemia with soluble insulin, 0.2 units/kg body weight intravenously. Hypoglycaemia should cause sharp rises in ACTH and plasma and urinary levels of cortisol. The 'metopirone test' may precipitate acute adrenal crisis as it lowers cortisol levels even lower than they already are, and this

method of testing the system should be avoided in cortisol-deficient patients.

Aldosterone secretion is usually reduced, as well as cortisol, and a considerable loss of sodium and water with shifts across cell membranes produces a low plasma sodium and chloride, a raised blood urea and often a high potassium, in a hypovolaemic patient. ADH secretion may be increased and aggravate the lowering of the plasma sodium. The blood sugar may be low.

Diagnostic procedures will include, where appropriate, a search for infective and neoplastic conditions which can destroy the adrenals. Only the auto-immune type of adrenal atrophy leaves adrenal medullary secretion intact, but it is not necessary to measure catecholamines in the average case.

Treatment. The acute Addisonian crisis requires immediate and generous infusion of normal saline and dextrose, to restore circulating volume and correct hypoglycaemia. Hydrocortisone sodium succinate 100 mg IV is administered stat and 6-hourly or as required. Infections must be vigorously treated. The patient's blood pressure and salt-fluid status must be carefully followed.

The long-term treatment should be based on oral hydrocortisone, between 20 and 40 mg daily, and fludrocortisone at a dose between 0.1 and 0.2 mg daily to supplement the mineralocorticoid effect. In establishing the proper maintenance dose, these factors should apply: the patient's subjective response, the supine and erect blood pressure, the absence of oedema, plasma cortisol levels and possibly the ACTH level. These patients are absolutely dependent on their steroid medication, which should be trebled in dose in the event of transient illness or stress and then gradually restored to normal levels. They must understand their condition and carry a card stating their situation, maintenance dose and procedure in the event of accident, and/or wear a Medic-Alert bracelet or necklace.

VIRILISATION

This is the clinical state associated with excessive androgenic effect in the female. While commonly of adrenal or ovarian origin, an abnormal end-organ sensitivity to androgens may also be important in many patients. Hirsutism (increased body and facial hair) is marked, pubic hair becomes masculine in distribution, and recession of the hairline at the temples occurs. The voice becomes deep, muscles increases in size and the clitoris enlarges. In post-pubertal women there is amenorrhoea, reduced fertility and shrinkage of the breasts. This picture may be associated with:

(1) Adrenal tumours, often with Cushinoid clinical features (see p. 571); indicated by high levels of 17-oxosteroids in the urine, particularly if

the tumour is an adrenal carcinoma, and high levels of free cortisol.

(2) Congenital adrenal hyperplasia (see below).

(3) Arrhenoblastoma of the ovary (high plasma testosterone with normal urinary 17-oxosteroids).

Hirsutism with no major virilisation, but often with menstrual irregularities and acne, is more common. Major causes include those of virilisation and:

(4) Polycystic ovaries.

(5) Mild androgen excess (compensated partial enzyme defects along the pathways of synthesis of cortisol or oestrogens in the adrenal gland or ovary).

(6) Simple familial hirsutism (diagnosed by family history) or 'constitutional' hirsutism with no obvious cause. Certain races, families and individuals are naturally more hirsute than others, and the problem is often as much a cultural or social problem as it is hormonal.

Investigation and Diagnosis. This is especially directed at the identification of patients with tumours. Both ACTH and the gonadotrophins stimulate the adrenal glands *and* the ovary to produce androgens, and in the absence of an obvious mass on examination (which will include a full gynaecological examination) localisation of the source of the androgen can be difficult. Free testosterone is the most relevant hormone in this condition, but other specific androgens (such as androstenediol) are said to correlate highly with hirsutism, and sex hormone binding globulins (SHBG) levels are consistently low. 17-oxosteroids tend to be especially high in adrenal disorders. Ultrasound examination of the ovaries and laparoscopy may be appropriate in doubtful cases.

Treatment. Apart from those patients in whom a tumour can be identified and removed, the long-term response to treatment is generally disappointing. Tumours should be resected, and polycystic ovaries should always be assessed by laparoscopy. Corticosteroids, for example prednisolone 5 mg at night, and cyclical oestrogen therapy—separately or together—may be effective in reducing plasma testosterone levels. Courses of at least six months should be given, and management based on the clinical response and a change in the plasma testosterone levels. Cyproterone acetate, an agent which blocks the effect of androgens on the androgen receptor, is now being used cyclically with low dose oestrogens by specialist clinics, with some excellent individual responses. This is one of the conditions in which it is particularly important to treat the patient and not just the 'disease'.

CONGENITAL ADRENAL HYPERPLASIA
(Adrenogenital Syndromes)

In these disorders there are enzyme defects along the pathway of :ortisol synthesis. In the absence of a feedback system the cortisol levels would fall markedly, but plasma cortisol is protected by a very efficient homeostatic mechanism, and indeed this hormone is the only major restraint on the secretion of CRF and hence ACTH. The result of the enzyme deficiency is therefore an increased ACTH drive, which has the effect of increasing the concentration of cortisol precursors 'proximal' to the 'block', so restoring towards normal the concentrations of substances 'distal' to the block (including cortisol itself). Some of the common levels of 'block' are illustrated in Fig. 13.6. In every case the accumulating precursor steroids have an androgenic effect overall, and in some syndromes potent mineralocorticoids are also formed in excess. While a common feature, valuable diagnostically, is the increased concentration of 17-OH-progesterone and hence urinary pregnanetriol, the presentation depends not only on the level of the 'block' but also on severity and age at presentation.

Typical clinical presentations include:

1) Perinatal and infantile: *Male*: phallic enlargement, 'infant Hercules' (musculature over-developed). *Female*: pseudohermaphroditism

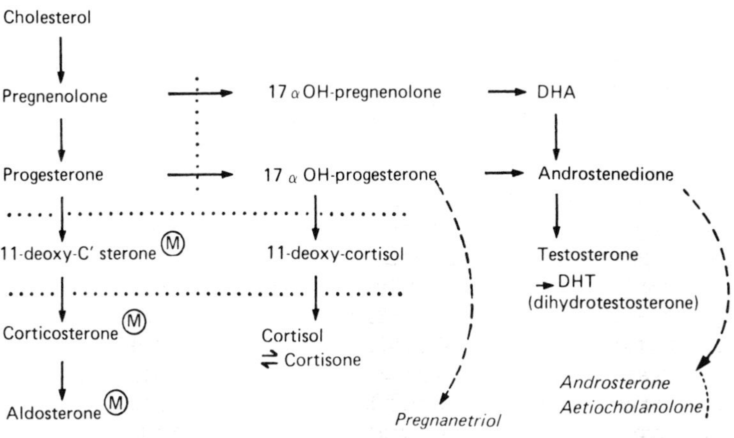

Fig. 13.6 Outline of adrenal steroid synthesis. The dotted lines indicate levels at which enzyme deficiencies may occur, acting as a block to synthesis and so causing accumulation of precursors 'above' the block. The upper horizontal line indicates C-21 hydroxylase level; the lower indicates C-11 hydroxylase level. The dashed lines indicate metabolites excreted in urine.

with genital abnormalities. *Both*: early fusion of epiphyses; adrenal insufficiency depends on severity of block.

(2) Delayed female puberty, primary amenorrhoea.

(3) C-21 hydroxylase partial block: high levels of 17-OH-progesterone etc. produce virilisation, high levels of ACTH produce pigmentation.

(4) C-11 hydroxylase partial block: as C-21 with the addition of hypertension, produced by high levels of 11-desoxycorticosterone (a potent mineralocorticoid).

(5) Compensated enzyme deficiencies responsible for some cases of 'constitutional hirsutism'?

Treatment. Corticosteroids will abolish the excessive ACTH drive in these patients and restore normal androgen levels. If adrenal insufficiency is present this is treated as would be a case of Addison's disease (p. 577).

PHAEOCHROMOCYTOMA

This very rare tumour of the adrenal medulla is important as a curable cause of hypertension, and as a 'mimic' of anxiety neurosis, thyrotoxicosis and diabetes mellitus. About 10% of the tumours are malignant and bilateral, and about the same proportion are associated with parathyroid adenomas or medullary carcinoma of the thyroid. The clinical features are related to the effects of excess adrenaline and/or noradrenaline.

Clinical Features. Most patients are hypertensive and complain of headaches. The hypertension is usually constant, but there occurs sometimes a characteristic picture of paroxysmal hypertension, with concurrent headaches, nose bleeds, or pulmonary oedema. Palpitations with or without tachycardia are common. Increased perspiration is a frequent complaint. Tremor, weakness, weight loss, feeling of warmth, even psychosis, with an increased metabolic rate, may at first suggest thyrotoxicosis. Anorexia and constipation are not uncommon. Although few patients complain of postural symptoms, the blood pressure may drop sharply on standing.

Investigation and Diagnosis. Tests currently in use include:

(1) As a screening test: vanillyl-mandelic acid (VMA) in urine: normally less than 25 μmol/24 hours (2.4 mmol/mol creatinine excreted); slightly higher in patients with hypertension, renal artery stenosis, or thyrotoxicosis, or those on tricyclic or related antidepressant drugs, usually over 50 μmol/24 hours (4.8 μmol/mol creatinine) in cases of phaeochromocytoma.

(2) As definitive tests: adrenaline and noradrenaline in plasma and/or urine.

Suppression and provocation tests, such as those employing phentolamine or glucagon, are potentially dangerous and rarely indicated. Levels of blood glucose, free fatty acids and the haematocrit may be elevated. Calcium and calcitonin levels should be checked, to exclude parathyroid adenomas and medullary carcinoma of the thyroid.

Treatment. Radiological investigations and surgery should be preceded and covered by combined adrenergic blockade, anti-α (phenoxybenzamine) and anti-β (propranolol). During surgery both adrenal glands must be inspected.

MENOPAUSE (Female Climacteric)

This can be regarded as physiological ovarian failure, leading to cessation of menstruation (menopause), sometimes preceded by menstrual irregularity. Episodes of 'hot flushes', with sweating and warmth, and symptoms of anxiety or depression may be prominent. LH and FSH levels are high. The psychological support of husband and physician is most important, with emphasis on the transient nature of the symptoms. If symptoms are severe then a combined or sequential low-dose preparation of oestrogen and a progestogen may be prescribed. Changes consequent upon the drop in oestrogen production include osteoporosis, which may become severe, a rise in the risk of cardiovascular disease, a reduction in vaginal secretions (thus a proneness to vaginitis and dyspareunia), and some involution of the uterus and breasts.

DELAYED PUBERTY IN THE FEMALE

Regular menstruation normally commences between the ages of 10 and 16, with a mean of 12.9 years, the so-called *menarche*. The other major changes of puberty include breast development and nipple pigmentation, growth of pubic hair of increasingly coarse dark curled type, axillary hair growth, thickening of the vaginal epithelium and growth of the genitalia; the pelvis gradually becomes gynaecoid in shape and the subcutaneous fat assumes the typical female distribution. Delayed puberty may be physiological and/or familial, especially in the presence of obesity. In *primary* ovarian failure the delay in fusion of the epiphyses eventually leads to overgrowth of the long bones, such that span exceeds height, and 'bone age' on X-ray may for a time be less than actual age.

Investigation and Diagnosis. Any major disease, particularly thyroid disorders, diabetes, renal failure or chronic infection, may be contributory to such a delay. As discussed on p. 581, the barrage of androgens secreted in congenital adrenal hyperplasia may impair female development. Beyond these possibilities, the main question is whether a primary ovarian defect or a failure of gonadotrophin secretion exists. If plasma and urinary FSH levels are low, the possible causes of hypopituitarism (p. 593) are pursued. Isolated gonadotrophin deficiency may be found, usually responsive to LRH, suggesting that the basic problem may be LRH failure; the line between such patients and 'late developers' is often indistinct and the initial treatment should be conservative.

High levels of FSH are consistent with:

(1) The first hint of puberty.
(2) Absence of ovaries, as in *Turner's syndrome* or *testicular feminisation.*
(3) Damage to the ovaries by cysts, tumours, trauma, surgery or irradiation.

Turner's Syndrome (Gonadal Dysgenesis)

The patients appear, act and think as women, but they are genetically male, with an XO or XO-mosaic karyotype and consequent dysgenesis of the testes. Having neither ovaries nor testes they develop into phenotypic females (as do all mammals lacking testosterone in utero, whatever their genetic sex). Secondary sexual characteristics and the normal menstrual cycle do not appear spontaneously.

They usually present as short women or girls, under 5 feet tall, who have failed to undergo sexual maturation. Numerous other clinical features occur but are variable in their expression, as might be expected from the variety of karyotypes found in the syndrome. The features may include: webbing of the neck, a short neck, increased carrying angle at the elbow (cubitus valgus), widely separated nipples, shield-like chest, coarctation of the aorta (20%), abnormalities of the urinary tract (on investigation, 60%), recurrent otitis media and sometimes deafness, lymphoedema especially of the feet, hypoplastic nails and numerous pigmented naevi. Mild mental handicap with well-preserved verbal ability is not uncommon.

Ethinyloestradiol 0.02 mg daily, given cyclically with norethisterone 5 mg daily on the last ten days of the cycle, will induce menses and sexual characteristics without over-rapid fusion of the epiphyses. Higher doses of oestrogen will improve the rate of sexual development but may reduce the patient's final height.

Androgen Resistance Syndromes (Testicular Feminisation)

Several syndromes exist but in the classical form most patients present as females, seeking medical advice because of primary amenorrhoea or infertility. They are genetic males with an XY karyotype, whose testes may be located in the abdomen, inguinal canal or 'labia'. Breasts and external genitalia are female in development with occasional slight enlargement of the clitoris, and only on investigation does it become apparent that the vagina ends blindly and there is no uterus. Testosterone production is normal in these patients, and the condition represents a diminished response to testosterone, a result of diminished conversion of testosterone to the more active dihydrotestosterone and/or a deficiency of the appropriate receptors.

AMENORRHOEA

The failure to initiate menstruation is termed by convention *primary* amenorrhoea, and it is usually accompanied by the other deficiencies in sexual development discussed above ('delayed puberty in the female'). Mechanical factors obstructing menstrual flow may also require exclusion, and a gynaecological assessment is essential.

Secondary amenorrhoea implies the *cessation* of menstruation; the condition represents the end of a spectrum that runs from regular ovulatory menstruation, through regular menses that are often anovulatory, through irregular and/or infrequent cycles (*oligomenorrhoea*) that are all anovulatory, to amenorrhoea. Conditions that give rise to amenorrhoea may cause the lesser disorders in their early stages or milder forms. These various conditions are classified in Table 13.4.

SUBFERTILITY

The availability of new modes of investigation and successful treatment, both hormonal and surgical, has transformed this subject in recent years. Nevertheless, the enthusiasm of patients and doctors should be restrained, because a large proportion of couples who have failed to achieve conception after six months 'trying' will be successful without treatment within the following year or so. It is also important to confirm that 'trying' includes normal coitus of reasonable frequency, an assumption that proves to be untrue in a surprising number of cases.

In genuinely subfertile couples a reproductive problem of some sort will be found in 65–85% of the women and about a third of the men, while in some a partial deficit is identified in both partners. The partners should be interviewed and examined independently in every instance. A cost-effective approach is then to:

(a) follow any leads given by the history or physical signs;
(b) check the sperm count on semen analysis;
(c) establish the presence or absence of ovulation.

If a normal sperm count is confirmed and regular ovulation is occurring, further investigation should take place; this might include hysterosalpingography, laparoscopy, ovarian biopsy, and studies of

Table 13.4 Scheme for main causes of secondary amenorrhoea

	Hormone lack	*Hormone block*
CENTRAL	DIMINISHED OR DISORDERED FUNCTION OF HYPOTHALAMUS AND/OR PITUITARY *Specific Conditions*: Functional (any major physical or psychological stress) Anorexia nervosa Isolated LH, FSH deficiency Panhypopituitarism, idiopathic or secondary to . . . Pituitary tumour, trauma or infarct Pituitary irradiation or surgery *Major hormonal findings* : LH, FSH (basal, and/or after LRH): LOW	HYPERPROLACTINAEMIA (see text for discussion) *Specific Conditions*: Tumours, including Prolactinomas Drugs Hypothyroidism Renal/hepatic failure, etc. *Major hormonal findings*: PROLACTIN: HIGH LH, FSH: NORMAL OR SLIGHTLY LOW
PERIPHERAL	DIMINISHED FUNCTION OF OVARIES *Specific Conditions:* Mild forms of ovarian dysgenesis or testicular feminisation (see text) Premature menopause (autoimmune?) Mumps oophoritis Ovarian irradiation or surgery *Major hormonal findings*: OESTROGENS: LOW	EXCESS OF ANDROGENS OR THYROID HORMONES (see text regarding virilisation and hirsutism) *Specific Conditions*: Adrenal tumours Congenital adrenal hyperplasia Arrhenoblastoma of ovary Polycystic ovaries Thyrotoxicosis

'mucous hostility' to the sperm (post-coital examination of the cervical mucus and *in vitro* studies).

FEMALE SUBFERTILITY

The occurrence of ovulation may be suggested by a history of transient mid-cycle ovarian pain, by a modest elevation of the basal body temperature during the luteal phase, by characteristic changes in the vaginal lining (hence 'serial smears') and the cervical mucus, or by more direct evidence of the hormonal changes illustrated in Fig. 13.7 such as a mid-luteal plasma progesterone exceeding 30 nmol/litre. The absence of ovulation, or amenorrhoea, may be secondary to any of a large number of conditions, which have been listed under the heading of secondary amenorrhoea (p. 586). Prolactin is particularly important in subfertility, because even moderate elevation of prolactin may prevent ovulation or proper luteinisation of the follicle.

Treatment. Hyperprolactinaemia is corrected by removal of the cause, or use of bromocriptine, as discussed on p. 593. Specific treatments of the other conditions listed are discussed in the relevant parts of the text. Ovulation may be provoked in some cases by the use of clomiphene, which blocks the oestrogen receptors of the hypothalamus, and induced in most by the programmed administration of human menopausal and human chorionic gonadotrophins or synthetic LHRH (LH and FSH releasing hormone).

Causes of female subfertility in the presence of ovulation include genital tract abnormalities such as blockage of the Fallopian tubes secondary to past or present infection, disease of the endometrium preventing implantation, and abnormalities of the cervical mucus or the sperm which impair penetration; some of these are now treatable by specialist techniques.

MALE SUBFERTILITY

Although sperm counts as low as 10 million/ml have been associated with fertility, the normal range for fresh semen lies between 50 and 150 million/ml, in at least 2 ml, of which at least 60 % of sperm are motile and normal in morphology. A low count (*oligospermia*) or total absence of motile sperm (*azoospermia*) may rarely be accompanied by impotence and signs of feminisation, such as gynaecomastia and small soft testes, suggesting androgen deficiency or oestrogen excess. Usually the problem is confined to the germinal cells of the testis, and levels of testosterone and the oestrogens are within normal limits: a raised level of FSH is then a useful indicator of germinal cell failure or aplasia. Sometimes the process of spermatogenesis is normal but the delivery of

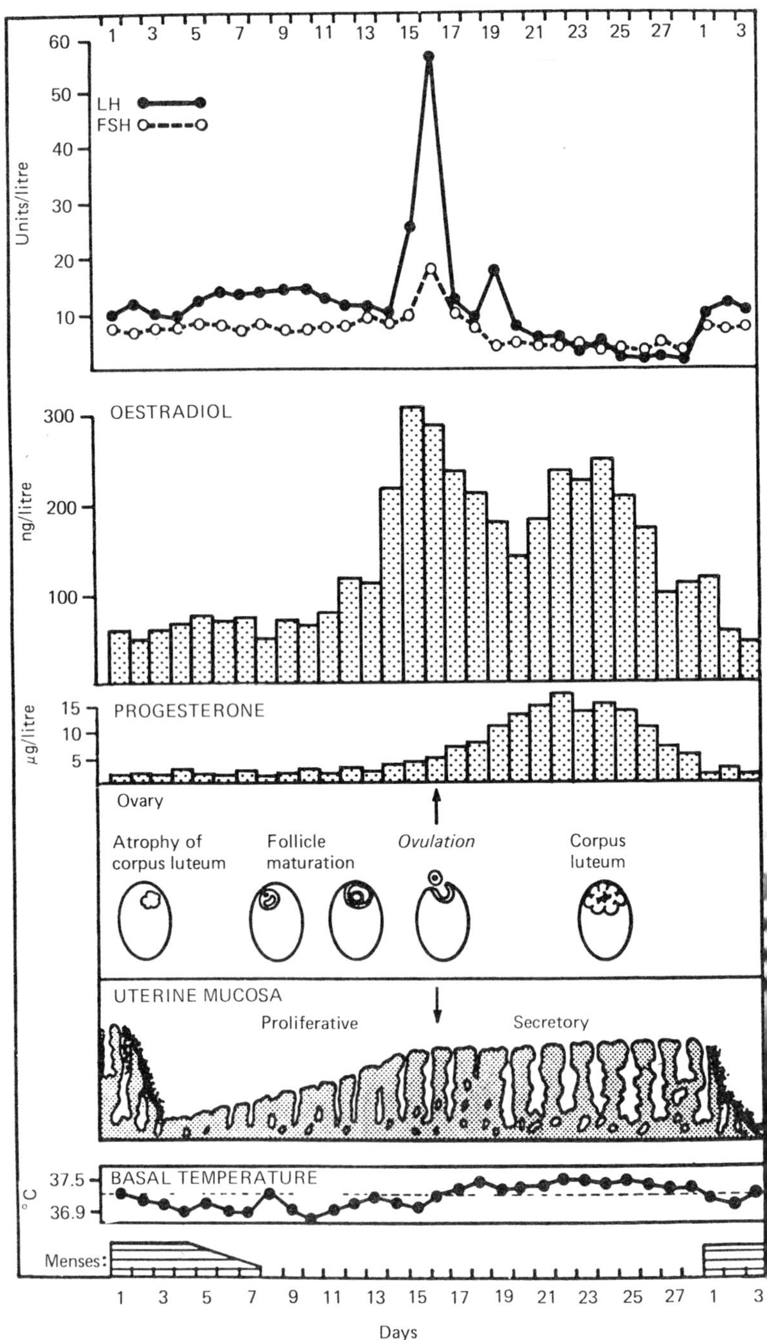

Fig 13.7 Hormonal patterns during a normal menstrual cycle.

sperm is obstructed by a lesion of the vas deferens, and this possibility needs consideration if the FSH level proves to be normal despite the occurrence of azoospermia.

The more common specific causes to be considered are these:

With gynaecomastia: Klinefelter's syndrome (described on p. 590); testes damaged by trauma, surgery or irradiation or drugs; chronic liver disease; androgen resistance syndromes (see p. 584).

Germinal cell failure or aplasia: Idiopathic ('Sertoli cell only syndrome'); cryptorchidism (undescended testes); maturation arrest; mumps orchitis; cytotoxic drugs; varicocele; any chronic endocrine or debilitating disease.

Hypothalamic/pituitary deficiency: Hypogonadotrophic hypogonadism, either selectively (such as in Kallmann's syndrome, see below) or as one feature of panhypopituitarism.

Treatment. Unless a particular hormonal deficiency can be identified and corrected, or a disorder such as obstruction of the vas or a varicocele put right surgically, treatment has little to offer. Traditional advice includes maintenance of a cool scrotal environment, hence loose underwear and cold douches, and intermittent androgen therapy (such as mesterolone). Recent work supports the use of clomiphene for patients with the less severe degrees of oligospermia. The fertile effectiveness of a semen in which the sperm count is borderline can be enhanced by the use of artificial insemination, a fresh sample of the husband's semen being applied direct to or through the os of the uterine cervix (AIH), or in vitro fertilisation of the ovum.

DELAYED PUBERTY IN THE MALE

In normal boys the earliest changes include enlargement of the testes and growth of coarse hairs in the pubic region. The scrotum develops rugal folds and darkens, the penis enlarges, axillary and then facial hair appears and the voice deepens. A mild degree of gynaecomastia is not uncommon. When the patient or his parents complain of 'delay' a family history of late puberty may be reassuring. In true gonadal failure the 'bone age' by X-ray falls behind actual age and—in the absence of epiphyseal fusion—the *eunuchoid* physique emerges, span exceeding height, ground to pubis exceeding pubis to crown.

Investigation and Diagnosis. Any endocrine disorder or debilitating illness may delay puberty. When those are excluded, the diagnosis lies between a primary gonadal disease, with high levels of FSH and LH, and a hypothalamic–pituitary disorder, with low levels of gonadotrophins and bilaterally small soft testes (see hypopituitarism, p. 593). An isolated deficiency of the hypothalamic factor LHRH may indicate **Kallmann's Syndrome**; anosmia is a useful clue to the presence of this disorder.

The only cause of primary testicular failure to commonly affect puberty is **Klinefelter's Syndrome,** in which very small firm testes are associated with variable degrees of eunuchoidism, gynaecomastia, impairment of intelligence, azoospermia, sterility and typically an XXY karyotype. Very rare versions of Turner's syndrome (p. 584) also occur in the phenotypic male.

TUMOURS OF THE TESTIS

These are rare, but occur particularly in the 20–35 age group. If the tumour is functional gonadotrophin secretion is suppressed and the other testis may be atrophied.

Type	*Five-year Mortality*	*Special Features*
Seminoma	10 %	FSH frequently raised
Teratoma	30 %	Spread by blood not lymph
Choriocarcinoma	100 %	Raised HCG; gynaecomastia
Leydig cell (IC) tumours	± benign	Oestrogens or androgens

TUMOURS OF THE OVARY

Most cysts and neoplasms of the ovary are non-secretory, but the following tumours usually secrete hormones:

Androgens secreted	*Oestrogens secreted*
Arrhenoblastoma	Granulosa cell tumour
Hilus cell tumour	Theca cell tumour
	Luteoma (and → progesterone)
	Teratoma, chorionepithelioma (and → HCG)

PITUITARY HYPERSECRETION

For discussion of hypersecretion of these hormones refer to the appropriate page: ACTH, p. 571; ADH, p. 597.

GIGANTISM AND ACROMEGALY

The syndromes of growth hormone (GH) excess are usually related to an *eosinophil adenoma* of the pituitary, characteristically slow in growth and insidious in clinical presentation. Only in retrospect may it be realised that the disease has been active for 20 or more years before the patient presents.

Gigantism results from excessive GH effect before the epiphyses are fused, producing the features of acromegaly but in addition long limbs and abnormal height. The all-time record for height was held by a Robert Wadlow of Illinois, who died in 1940 at an authenticated height of 8 feet 11 inches; the better known case of Goliath is not well documented! These patients especially suffer from muscular weakness and arthritis. The total effects of the tumour may include hypothalamic irritation and so hyperphagia, and compression of the remaining pituitary and so hypogonadism.

Acromegaly: Clinical Features

Headache; sometimes visual field defects, especially temporal.
Excessive tiredness, lips thick, nose bulbous, supra-orbital ridges enlarged.
Muscular aching, proximal muscle weakness.
Excessive sweating, skin thick, sebaceous, wrinkled.
Tingling in the fingers, carpal tunnel syndrome.
Progressive enlargement of hands and feet and head (perhaps noticed by change in size of gloves, shoes or hat), spadelike hands, soft and mushy grip, big feet.
Dentures stop fitting, bite over-rides, teeth become separated as the mandible enlarges.
Arthritis and backache, kyphosis, enlarged vertebrae.
Loss of secondary sexual characteristics. In women: menstrual irregularities, amenorrhoea. In men: loss of libido, impotence.
Hoarseness of voice, larynx enlarges, vocal cords thicken.
A few patients have galactorrhoea, or uncinate fits, or rhinorrhoea.
Soft tissue enlargement may include thyroid (goitre), liver and spleen.
Excessive pigmentation is frequently present.

Investigation and Diagnosis. X-rays of the hands show increased soft-tissue thickness, tufting of the tips of the distal phalanges, increased width of phalanges and exostoses. Skull X-rays show an enlarged mandible, prominence of all the sinuses but notably the supraorbital, and in most cases enlargement of the sella. CT scan of the pituitary usually demonstrates the tumour (Fig. 13.8). The calcaneal skin pad may exceed 30 mm in thickness. Over 10% of patients are frankly diabetic, and most have an impaired tolerance of glucose. Levels of GH in plasma are elevated even at rest and are not suppressed by oral glucose, the ultimate diagnostic test for this condition.

Treatment. Transphenoidal hypophysectomy, Yttrium implantation and proton beam irradiation are effective treatments. Bromocriptine, an ergotamine derivative with dopaminergic properties, will

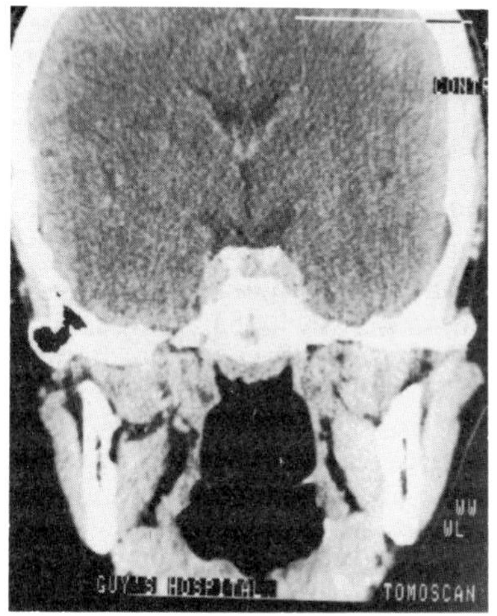

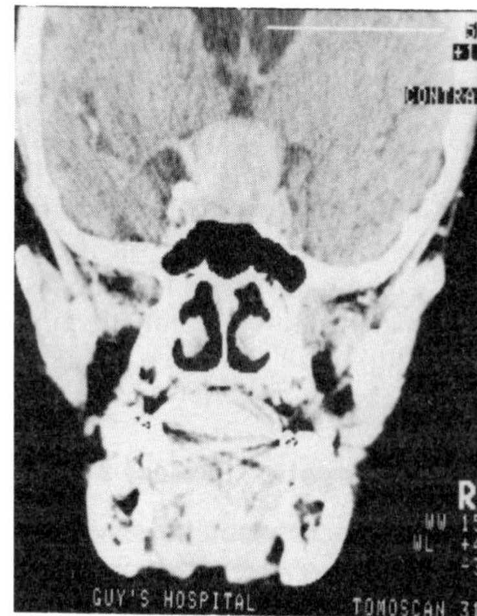

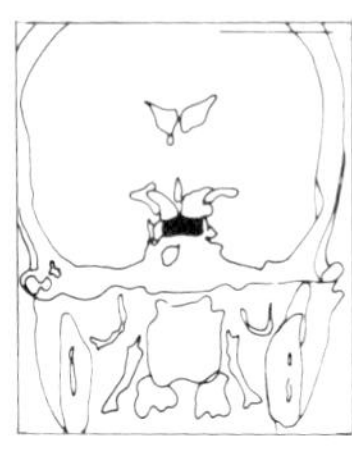

Fig. 13.8 CT scans of normal pituitary gland (on the left) and large non-functioning pituitary tumour (on the right). On the line diagram below each scan the pituitary tissue is shown by the solid black.

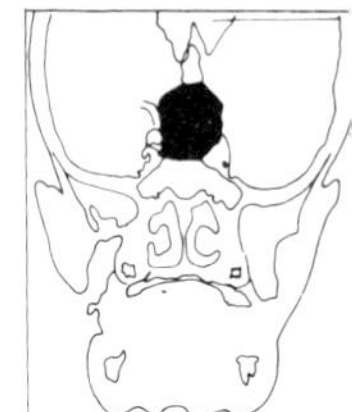

usually suppress high levels of GH, and is especially valuable for the occasional patient in whom pituitary 'ablation' fails to control the GH hypersecretion.

HYPERPROLACTINAEMIA (With or Without Galactorrhoea)

The only effects of hyperprolactinaemia recognised as clinically important are: the stimulation of lactation, the inhibition of ovulation (with or without amenorrhoea), and the inhibition of spermatogenesis (with or without impotence). An elevated prolactin level may assume greater significance as a sign of some other pathology or disorder previously unsuspected:

(1) Secretion of prolactin by a pituitary adenoma or micro-adenoma

(e.g. a 'pure' *prolactinoma*, or an eosinophilic tumour also producing GH).

(2) Interference by a tumour, trauma or inflammatory disease in the normal transmission of dopamine, the prolactin inhibitory hormone, between the hypothalamus and the pituitary, so 'releasing' the prolactin-secreting cells.

(3) Pharmacological interference in the synthesis, release or activity of dopamine, with effects analogous to (2), by phenothiazines, methyldopa, reserpine, tricyclic antidepressants, opiates, oral contraceptives, chlordiazepoxide and perhaps diazepam.

(4) Secretory response to increased levels of TRH, thyrotrophin-releasing hormone, such as occurs in the presence of hypothyroidism.

(5) Prolactin levels raised by chronic renal failure, hyperparathyroidism or hepatic cirrhosis.

If the cause of the hyperprolactinaemia cannot be removed, corrected or identified, dopaminergic agents such as bromocriptine usually suppress prolactin levels to within the normal range.

HYPOPITUITARY STATES

For purposes of discussion these can be classed as:

(1) *Isolated hormone deficiencies*, e.g. of TSH, ACTH, FSH, and GH (producing dwarfism in an otherwise normal person).

(2) *Pituitary chromophobe adenoma* producing varying degrees of hypopituitarism and hypothalamic disorder.

(3) *Panhypopituitarism*, juvenile and adult.

PITUITARY CHROMOPHOBE ADENOMA

Tumours of chromophobe histology often secrete prolactin and occasionally secrete ACTH (especially following adrenalectomy) or GH, but typically act as space-occupying lesions within the sella and then the brain.

The pressure within the sella may cause a classical 'bursting' bitemporal headache and radiologically visible expansion of the sella with erosion of the clinoid processes. The pressure on the optic chiasma causes loss of visual acuity, bitemporal hemianopia, and optic atrophy. Olfactory nerves may be involved with consequent anosmia. Signs of raised intracranial pressure may appear.

Local effects on the pituitary include progressive failure of most of the hormones of the anterior and posterior lobes, and the clinical picture may gradually move towards adult panhypopituitarism (see below).

Pressure on the hypothalamus may aggravate the pituitary failure, and also provoke characteristic hypothalamic features of weight gain, somnolence and polydipsia.

Investigation and Diagnosis. For these and other tumours in the region of the sella turcica special investigations should include:

(1) A combined pituitary test (see Table 13.5).
(2) Full visual testing including perimetry for visual fields.
(3) Skull X-rays.
(4) Computer tomography (CT scan) of the pituitary area (Fig. 13.8).
(5) Arteriography if an aneurysm must be excluded.

Treatment. Surgery and/or radiotherapy will be advised depending on the position and extent of the adenoma.

PANHYPOPITUITARISM

This condition may be congenital, then causing pituitary dwarfism with adult body proportions and combined failure of thyroid, adrenal and gonad function; this is rare and it is discussed fully in specialist and paediatric texts.

In the adult, panhypopituitarism (*Simmonds' disease*) may be caused by infiltration of the pituitary, by neoplasms or granulomas, by trauma or by infarction. The latter is the major cause, being especially associated with major haemorrhage at the time of parturition (*Sheehan's syndrome*).

Clinical Features.

History of ante- or post-partum haemorrhage.

Failure of lactation and failure to resume menstruation (FSH, LH failure), uterus and vagina shrink, vaginal secretions reduced, secondary infertility.

Loss of libido, reduced pubic and axillary hair, impotence (FSH, LH and ACTH).

Mild adrenal deficiency may occur; depigmentation and pallor (ACTH).

Secondary myxoedema (TSH).

Skin characteristically soft, fine and wrinkled.

Hypoglycaemic episodes may occur (ACTH, GH).

Mineralocorticoid function is well maintained by the reninangiotensin system.

Investigation and Diagnosis. The several gland deficiencies should be quantitated by appropriate tests. Basal levels of anterior pituitary hormones may be low, but deficiencies will be more obvious under the conditions of a combined pituitary test (Table 13.5).

Treatment. Substitution by hydrocortisone 20 to 40 mg daily, regular androgens, and cyclical oestrogens are advisable. Thyroxine may be

Table 13.5 The combined pituitary test

This is a combination of the insulin hypoglycaemia, TRH and LRH tests. In its complete form, the test measures the capacity of the anterior pituitary to secrete all the anterior pituitary hormones. In some patients a more selective test may be adequate.

THE FOLLOWING ARE INJECTED INTRAVENOUSLY AT ABOUT 09.00 h:

1. *Soluble insulin:* 0.1 units/kg body weight in suspected hypopituitarism, 0.3 units/kg in conditions of insulin resistance, 0.2 units/kg otherwise. (The blood glucose must fall to 2.5 mmol/l or below for the test to be valid. It is necessary for a doctor to be present or immediately available throughout in case severe hypoglycaemia occurs and administration of glucose becomes necessary.)
2. *TRH:* 200 μg
3. *LRH:* 100 μg

NORMAL ADULT LEVELS AND RESPONSES (typical ranges)

	GH	*Cortisol*	*TSH*	*Prolactin*	*LH (male)*	*FSH (male)*	*LH (female)*	*FSH (female)*
Sample	mu/l	nmol/l	u/l	u/l	u/l	u/l	u/l	u/l
Basal	1–10	150–700	'0'–6	'0'–0.5	3–10	1–8	3–10*	3–8*
30′			6–20	0.3–3.0	8–35	15–11	8–25	4–11
60′ 90′ 120′	peak exceeds 12	peak exceeds 800	4–18	0.2–3.0	6–35	1–11	6–20	6–12

* Figures obtained in the follicular phase of the cycle. Levels are generally lower than this during the luteal phase, having risen to a peak at mid-cycle (see Fig. 13.5).

added gradually, when the adrenal insufficiency has been abolished. As the best treatment for the pituitary remnant is another pregnancy, a trial of gonadotrophins may be in order. Patients should take the same precautions as those with Addison's disease (p. 579).

Hypopituitary Coma

This rare event, which should be prevented by good management, is dangerous in that it may involve the conjunction of hypoglycaemia, hypoadrenalism, hypothyroidism and hypothermia. The patient is treated specifically for these conditions and generally for shock.

HYPOTHALAMIC DEFICIENCIES

In generally, the characteristics are:

(1) Diabetes insipidus may occur in association with the anterior lobe hormone deficiencies (p. 544).
(2) Visual defects tend to occur early.
(3) In a small minority only, hyperphagia, weight changes, temperature disturbance and drowsiness occur.
(4) Hyperprolactinaemia, with or without galactorrhoea.

The pathological lesions include, amongst others:
Tumours
Craniopharyngioma (calcification visible on skull X-ray; common in children)
Chromophobe adenomas (early visual changes usually occur)
Granulomas
Sarcoidosis (look for disease elsewhere)
Tuberculosis (look for disease elsewhere)
Hand-Schüller-Christian disease
Trauma of various kinds.

PLURIGLANDULAR DISORDERS

Disease states in which two or more endocrine glands are involved in the same patient:

Combined Gland Failures

(1) Hypopituitary states (p. 593)
(2) Auto-immune group (associated with HLA-DW3 and DW4):
    Hashimoto's, Graves', myxoedema
    Pernicious anaemia
    Addison's disease
    Insulin-dependent diabetes mellitus.

Combined Gland Hypersecretion

Multiple endocrine adenomatosis (MEA), which may occur sporadically or as a familial disorder:

MEA Type I: especially pituitary, parathyroid and pancreatic adenomas;

MEA Type II-A: parathyroid adenomas, phaeochromocytomas and medullary carcinoma of thyroid.

MEA Type II-B: phaeochromocytomas, medullary carcinoma of the thyroid, and mucosal neuromas.

OTHER ENDOCRINE FUNCTIONS

The kidney is responsible for the secretion of three substances which are hormonal in character: (a) *erythropoietin*, controlling red cell production; (b) *renin*, controlling angiotensin production (p. 462) and (c) *1-25-OH-vitamin D3*, the active form of vitamin D3 (a pro-hormone?). The synthesis of 1-25-OH-vitamin D3 is governed by intracellular calcium and phosphate concentration in renal tubular cells, and influenced by levels of parathyroid hormone.

The gut secretes a number of identified peptides, such as pancreozymincholecystokinin, gastrin, secretin, gastric inhibitory polypeptide, vaso-active inhibitory polypeptide, enteroglucagon and glucagon of pancreatic type, and many others yet to be characterised.

Prostaglandins are modified long-chain fatty acids which are synthesised close to their site of action and are then very rapidly inactivated. They have powerful modulating influences on many processes, with effects in the inflammatory reaction, in pyrexia, in spontaneous abortion, gastric secretion, control of blood pressure, platelet aggregation and smooth muscle contractions.

ECTOPIC SECRETION OF HORMONES

Many tumours arising in apparently non-endocrine tissues are found to contain or secrete peptide hormones or biochemically similar peptides. A wide variety of tumours and peptides have been associated, but the more common and important syndromes include:

Ectopic Cushing's. Very high levels of 'ACTH' typically produce marked hypokalaemia and weakness: sources include oat-cell carcinoma of the bronchus, bronchial adenomas, thymomas, carcinoids, and carcinomas of the stomach, colon, gall-bladder and ovary.

Inappropriate ADH Secretion. Results in a dilutional hyponatremia, sometimes severe: sources include oat-cell carcinoma of the bronchus and lymphomas.

Hypercalcaemia. Non-metastatic, related to parathormone or other chemical factors: sources include squamous-cell carcinoma of the bronchus, hypernephroma, and carcinoma of the ovary.

Polycythaemia. Secondary to erythropoietin secretion: sources include hypernephroma, fibromyoma of uterus, and stomach cancer.

FURTHER READING

Felig, P., Baxter, J. D., Broadus, A. E. and Frohman, L. A., *Endocrinology and Metabolism*, McGraw-Hill, New York, 1981.

Griffin, J. E., *Manual of Clinical Endocrinology and Metabolism*, McGraw-Hill, New York, 1982.

Hall, R., Anderson, J., Smart, G. A., and Besser, M., *Fundamentals of Clinical Endocrinology*, 3rd edition, Pitman Medical, London, 1981.

Lee, J., and Laycock, J. F., *Essential Endocrinology*, 2nd edition, Oxford Medical Publications, Oxford, 1983.

CHAPTER 14

DISORDERS RESULTING FROM VITAMIN DEFICIENCIES

INTRODUCTION

Serious illnesses from vitamin deficiencies are rare in the Western world today. They are still sadly common in the underdeveloped countries. In this country their appearance is usually conditioned by some extra factor, neglect of an infant or elderly person, insanity, gastrointestinal disease causing impaired absorption, alcoholism, or drug addiction. Deficiency of the accessory food factors known to be synthesised by bacteria in the gut (folic acid, nicotinic acid, riboflavin, and Vitamin K) may be induced by antibiotic therapy. Certain groups of the population, for instance pregnant or lactating women, growing children, or children suffering from protracted febrile illnesses are specially at risk. Closed communities are at the mercy of cooks.

Although described separately they commonly occur together. Treatment must always include the resumption of a normal diet, and where doses of vitamins for treatment are quoted they are intended as supplements to such a diet.

VITAMIN A DEFICIENCY

Deficiency occurs endemically in the Middle East, rarely in this country. Symptoms are (1) *Night blindness* (Nyctalopia) from affection of visual purple; (2) *Xerophthalmia*, drying and thickening of the conjunctiva, progressing to (3) *Keratomalacia*, softening and inflammation of the cornea, leading to opacity and blindness; (4) *Follicular keratosis* (phrynoderma), the blocking of skin follicles with horny plugs leading to dryness and roughness of the skin surface. Similar changes are seen in myxoedema.

For details of treatment, etc., see Table 14.1.

VITAMIN D DEFICIENCY

Introduction

In infants deficiency causes rickets, in adults osteomalacia. It is known that cholecalciferol (Vitamin D) after absorption is hydroxylated in the liver; further hydroxylation occurs in the kidney to form 1, 25-

Table 14.1 Vitamin deficiencies and their treatment

Vitamin	*Solubility*	*Clinical Deficiency Disorder*	*Test for Deficiency*	*Prophylaxis (Daily)*	*Therapy (Daily)*	*Natural Sources*
A	Fat	Xerophthalmia, Keratomalacia, Night blindness, Follicular keratosis	Serum carotene levels	2500–5000 i.u.	10–25 000 i.u.	Eggs, milk, butter, vitamin-ised margarine, fish liver oils, coloured vegetables
D	Fat	Bone changes, Hypotonia, Tetany	Radiography of bones, serum alkaline phosphatase serum calcium serum phosphate	Calcium and Vit. D tablets (NF) 1 tablet (500 i.u.) daily	500–5000 i.u.	Eggs, milk, butter, vitamin-ised margarine, fish liver oils
K	Fat	Hypoprothrom-binaemia	Serum prothrombin time	1–2 mg	5–10 mg	Spinach, cabbage, kale, cauliflower, synthesised in gut
B	Water	Beri-beri, dry or wet,	Pyruvate tolerance test	1–1.6 mg	50–100 mg	Whole grain cereals, yeast,
Thiamine (B_1)		Wernicke's encephalopathy (p. 389)				liver

Riboflavine (B_2)	Water	Rubiolation of cornea, Kerato-malacia, Cheilosis Angular stomatitis Magenta tongue, Seborrhoeic dermatitis	Slit-lamp microscopy of cornea	1.4–2.5 mg	5–15 mg	Milk, eggs, butter, liver, yeast
Nicotinic acid (Niacin)	Water	Pellagra		10–16 mg	100–500 mg	Whole grain cereals, excluding maize
Pyridoxine (B_6)	Water	Peripheral neuritis, Anaemia in infants		1–2 mg	10–50 mg	Whole grain cereals, yeast
Cyanocobalamin (B_{12})	Water	Pernicious anaemia (p. 613)	Serum B_{12}	2–4 μg	(see p. 614)	Whole grain cereals
C	Water	Scurvy	Vit. C content of white blood cells	70–150 mg	500–1000 mg	Green vegetables, fresh fruit, oranges, tomatoes, blackcurrants

hydroxycholecalciferol which is highly active in promoting absorption of calcium from the gut.

Deficiency can therefore be caused by inadequate diet, lack of sunlight (Vitamin D being formed in the skin), failure of absorption as in the malabsorption syndrome or severe renal damage (renal osteodystrophy).

Clinical Features. Osteoid is prepared at the growing ends of bones, where it heaps up and causes tender swellings which do not become calcified. This is particularly apparent in the skull (*fronto-parietal bosses*), the ribs (*rickety rosary*), and the distal ends of the long bones, particularly at the wrist. Failure of calcification also causes softening of the bones so that they bend under stress; this shows clearly as a sulcus at the line of attachment of the diaphragm (Harrison's sulcus), and in the legs (*genu valgum*, or *varum*). *Dentition* is similarly delayed and defective. The muscles are generally hypotonic; there is delay in walking and standing, with weakness, lordosis, and abdominal protuberance. If the serum calcium is low, *tetany* may result.

For details of treatment, etc., see Table 14.1.

Overdosage

Symptoms are anorexia, nausea, thirst, vomiting, polyuria and drowsiness. Calcium and phosphorus levels in the serum and urine may be elevated, and tissue calcification may occur. Calcification of the kidneys leads to hypertension and uraemia.

VITAMIN K

Deficiency causes hypoprothrombinaemia.

VITAMIN B DEFICIENCY

(a) **Thiamine deficiency** is much more likely to occur in the presence of achlorhydria and when a high proportion of the dietary calories are provided by carbohydrate.

Clinical Manifestations

(1) *Polyneuritis* (Dry beri-beri) (p. 389), less commonly myelitis. The neuritis is always associated with extreme tenderness of muscle.

(2) *Cardiac failure* with oedema, cardiac enlargement, usually regular rhythm, and circulatory hyperkinesis (high output failure) (Wet beri-beri).

(3) *Wernicke's encephalopathy* (p. 389), in which confusion, ataxia, nystagmus, squint, and diplopia are common, often secondary to alcoholism.

(Treatment, etc., see Table 14.1.)

(b) **Riboflavine deficiency** causes widespread affection of the mucous membranes and skin, presenting as:

(1) *The tongue is sore and magenta coloured.*
(2) *Angular stomatitis*, painful red fissures at the angles of the mouth.
(3) *Cheilosis*, a stripping of the superficial epithelium at the line of closure of the lips.
(4) *Vascularisation of the cornea*, spreading in from the periphery and visible initially only on slit-lamp microscopy, later to the naked eye.
(5) Eventually *keratomalacia* with corneal opacity may develop.
(6) *Seborrhoeic dermatitis* of the naso-labial folds, ears, and chest.

(c) **Nicotinic Acid deficiency** causes the clinical syndrome of *pellagra*.

Clinical Features
(1) *Dementia.*
(2) *Diarrhoea*, which is intractable and may lead to potassium deficiency.
(3) *Dermatitis*. This consists of a scaly pigmentation of the exposed skin surfaces. The tongue is affected, and has been likened to 'raw beef'. Pellagra is a disease of maize eaters. Secondary deficiency may occur in gastro-intestinal disorders and with carcinoid tumours. (Treatment, etc., see table.)

(d) **Pyridoxine deficiency** is a rarity. Artificially fed infants given a pyridoxine deficient diet develop an anaemia with all the characteristics of iron deficiency except that it responds only to pyridoxine. They may also have convulsions. In adults, where deficiency may occur as a side-effect of *isoniazid* administration, cheilosis, glossitis, weakness, peripheral neuritis and increased susceptibility to infection may occur.

(e) **Cyanocobalamin deficiency** causes pernicious anaemia (p. 613). Peripheral neuritis, subacute combined degeneration of the cord, optic atrophy, and dementia may also occur, either in association with the anaemia or separately.

VITAMIN C DEFICIENCY

Introduction

Scurvy is seen mainly nowadays in elderly people living alone on a diet which contains no fruit or vegetables. The diet must be grossly deficient in ascorbic acid for some six months before symptoms appear.

Clinical Features. Patients feel generally ill. Signs are produced by *spontaneous haemorrhages*. These occur most frequently in the gums, which bleed at a touch, especially the interdentate papillae (*scurvy buds*). *Teeth* become loose and infected, and *foetor oris* is marked. Perifollicular haemorrhage may cause *skin purpura*, and derangement of the hairs (corkscrew hairs). Later there may be large spontaneous haemorrhages, into muscles or joints, or subcutaneous (*ecchymoses*). There is deficient haemoglobin synthesis, causing anaemia, and impaired collagen formation which gives rise to delayed wound healing.

(Treatment, etc., see Table 14.1)

CHAPTER 15

DISORDERS OF THE BLOOD

ANATOMY AND PHYSIOLOGY

Blood contains three types of cell, red blood corpuscles (erythrocytes), white blood corpuscles (leucocytes), and platelets (thrombocytes). These cells are formed mainly in the bone marrow and normally the speed of production is regulated to ensure that just sufficient numbers of each type of cell are delivered into the peripheral blood each day to replace those which have worn out and have been removed.

Red Blood Cells

The parent cell in the bone marrow is the erythroblast, a large cell which has deeply basophilic cytoplasm, contains no haemoglobin and has one or more nucleoli in its nucleus. In the presence of adequate supplies of Vitamin B_{12} and folic acid the erythroblast produces by division a smaller cell with a denser nucleus; this is the early normoblast, which still has basophilic cytoplasm. Haemoglobinisation of the cell occurs at this stage and the cytoplasm changes from the blue colour of the primitive cell through a polychromatic phase to the pink of the mature normoblast, which now has a very dense pyknotic nucleus. Disintegration of the nucleus transforms the normoblast into the young erythrocyte or reticulocyte, so-called because supra-vital staining with cresyl blue reveals a fine reticulum of polychromatic material in the cytoplasm. The fully mature erythrocyte contains no such reticulum and therefore a reticulocyte count gives a valuable indication of the rate of new red cell production. In health no nucleated red cells appear in the peripheral blood.

In the absence of adequate supplies of Vitamin B_{12} or folic acid there is failure of maturation beyond the erythroblast-early normoblast phase and these large primitive cells become prematurely haemoglobinised. Anaemia characterised by large cells and a high haemoglobin content (macrocytic and hyperchromic) is the result. Iron is an essential element in the haemoglobin molecule so that iron deficiency leads to shortage of haemoglobin, but it does not interfere with the normal maturation of the red cells. Although less haemoglobin is put into each cell, the cells are smaller and thinner than normal, and the cell haemoglobin *concentration* is unaltered. The cells appear small and pale (microcytosis and hypochromia).

Small amounts of thyroid hormone, ascorbic acid, and copper are also required for efficient red cell production.

The life of each red cell in the circulation is about 120 days. At the end of that time it is broken down by cells of the reticulo-endothelial system, mainly in the bone marrow, spleen, and liver, the haemoglobin being split into two fractions. One of these contains the iron atoms and is returned to the bone marrow for resynthesis into new red cells, forming by far the biggest source of the iron used for this purpose; the non-iron-containing fraction constitutes the bile pigment bilirubin and is transported in the blood to the liver for excretion.

White Blood Cells

(1) The Granular Series

The parent cell in the bone marrow is the myeloblast, a large cell with basophilic non-granular cytoplasm and a nucleus containing several nucleoli. From this is formed a smaller cell without nucleoli called the myelocyte, which acquires granules in its cytoplasm as it matures. The nucleus gradually condenses, becoming first kidney-shaped (at which stage the cell is known as a metamyelocyte) and then lobulated. The cell is now a mature granulocyte, and is classified as neutrophil, eosinophil, or basophil according to the staining reaction of the granules in its cytoplasm. As the cell becomes older it acquires more lobes in its nucleus.

Normal blood contains 2.0–7.5 $\times 10^9$/litre neutrophil granulocytes, 0–0.4 eosinophils and 0–0.2 basophils $\times 10^9$/litre.

(2) The Lymphocyte Series

The parent cell is the lymphoblast, found in lymphoid tissue throughout the body as well as in the bone marrow. It looks very like a myeloblast, but can usually be distinguished by the company it keeps: i.e. it breeds lymphocytes and not granulocytes. From the lymphoblast are derived the large and small lymphocytes, cells with clear blue cytoplasm and dense nuclei; the small ones are probably the more mature cells.

It is now realised that there are functionally distinct classes of lymphocyte which are discussed in Chapter 7.

The normal lymphocyte count is 1.0–3.5 $\times 10^9$/litre.

(3) The Monocyte Series

The monoblast, which also closely resembles the myeloblast, is derived from reticulum cells and gives rise to the monocyte, a cell with cloudy blue cytoplasm containing a few small red granules, and a kidney-shaped nucleus.

The normal monocyte count is 0–0.8 $\times 10^9$/litre.

The Platelets

The parent cell is the megakaryocyte found in the bone marrow, a very large cell with multilobulated nucleus and granular cytoplasm. The platelets formed from it are small (2–4 μm) bodies containing blue or purple granules but no nucleus.

The normal platelet count is 150–350 × 10^9/litre.

ANAEMIA

Definition

Anaemia is a condition of diminished oxygen-carrying capacity of the blood due to a reduction in the numbers of red cells or in their content of haemoglobin, or both.

Symptoms and Signs of Anaemia

The symptoms and signs due to the diminished oxygen-carrying capacity of the blood are common to all types of anaemia. They include general tiredness, shortness of breath on exertion, giddiness, headache, pallor (especially pallor of the mucous membranes and of the palms of the hands), palpitations, oedema of the ankles, and occasionally in older people angina pectoris.

Causes of Anaemia

The anaemias can be classified primarily into two groups:

(1) Those due to some failure in the quality or quantity of new red cells being produced in the marrow, and

(2) Those due to excessive loss of red cells from the circulation, either from acute or chronic haemorrhage or from abnormal haemolysis.

There is frequent overlap between these two groups since haemorrhage leads to iron deficiency, which is by far the commonest cause of the anaemias in group (1). The classification is useful for descriptive purposes, however, and can be amplified as follows:

(1) Deficient Red Cell Production

(a) Iron deficiency anaemia.
(b) Vitamin B_{12} or folic acid deficiency.
  (i) Pernicious anaemia (Addison's anaemia).
  (ii) Failure of absorption of Vitamin B_{12} or folic acid due to disorders of the gastrointestinal tract such as sprue, idiopathic steatorrhoea, and after gastrointestinal operations.
  (iii) Tropical nutritional macrocytic anaemia.
  (iv) Macrocytic anaemia of pregnancy.
(c) The anaemia of myxoedema from lack of thyroxine.
(d) The anaemia of scurvy from lack of Vitamin C.
(e) Impairment of erythroblastic activity in bone marrow:
  (i) Aplastic anaemia.

(ii) Invasion of bone marrow in leukaemia, metastatic malignant disease, Hodgkin's disease, myelomatosis, and myelosclerosis.
(iii) Probable toxic effect on erythroblasts in uraemia, chronic infections, malignant disease, and certain collagen diseases.

(2) Excessive Loss of Red Cells

(a) Haemorrhage.
(b) Abnormal haemolysis:
(i) Due to congenital defects in the red cells, in familial acholuric jaundice, and sickle-cell anaemia.
(ii) Due to acquired haemolysis in the blood, either of unknown cause or in incompatible blood transfusions, septicaemias, malignant disease, and erythroblastosis foetalis.

INVESTIGATION OF ANAEMIA

Haemoglobin

The average haemoglobin content of normal blood is 14.8 g per dl. (range 13.5–18.0 g in men; 11.5–16.0 g in women), which is consequently taken as the arbitrary 100 % level in most laboratories. There is still no general agreement on this point, however, and to prevent confusion the haemoglobin should always be expressed in grams per dl, the percentage figure being given in addition if desired.

Red Blood Count

The red count has a wide physiological range between about 4.0–6.0 $\times 10^{12}$/litre. Calculation of the haematological indices outlined below is based on the assumption that the normal red count is 5.0 $\times 10^{12}$/litre and that 100 % haemoglobin is 14.8 g/dl.

Haematocrit Value (or packed-cell volume)

This is the volume occupied by the red cells in 1.0 dl of centrifuged blood and is normally about 45 ml per cent.

Mean Corpuscular Haemoglobin Concentration (MCHC)

This value has been used for many years as a measure of concentration of haemoglobin within the red cells and a low value was taken as an indication of iron deficiency anaemia.

It is obtained from the formula

$$\frac{\text{Hb in grams/1 dl}}{\text{Packed cell volume/1 dl}} \times 100.$$

The low values found in iron deficiency have however been shown to be due to loose packing of the irregularly shaped erythrocytes when the packed cell volume is estimated by centrifugation. It is not really an estimate of cell haemoglobin concentration. If the packed cell volume is obtained from the red cell count and the mean corpuscular volume (as occurs with the Coulter 'S' Counter), a normal MCHC will be found in iron deficiency.

The haematological diagnosis of iron deficiency anaemia depends on the findings of a low MCV and MCH which is associated with small and irregular hypochromic erythrocytes on the stained smear (due to cells being small and thin, rather than having a low haemoglobin concentration). In addition the serum iron will be low and the bone marrow will show absence of stainable iron.

Mean Corpuscular Haemoglobin (MCH)

Is derived from the red cell count and the haemoglobin level and is normally 27–32 pg.

Mean Corpuscular Volume (MCV)

This is the average volume of a single red cell in cubic micrometers and is obtained by dividing the packed-cell volume in ml per litre of blood by the red cells in millions per mm^3. The normal range is 78–94 fl. With the Coulter 'S' counter the MCV is measured directly and is not derived from the packed cell volume obtained by centrifugation. The MCV gives an indication of the size of the red cell in three dimensions.

The **Mean Corpuscular Diameter** (MCD), on the other hand, being obtained by measurement of the diameter of the red cells in a stained film, gives an indication of the size of the cells in two dimensions only and takes no account of their thickness. The average normal MCD is 7.2 μm, with a range of 6.7–7.7 μm.

Serum Iron

Normal range men 14–31 μmol/l.
women 11–29 μmol/l.

Total Iron-binding Capacity (TIBC)

Normal range 54–80 μmol/l.

Serum B_{12}

Normal range 150–850 ng/l.

Serum Folate

Normal range 3–18 μg/l.

IRON DEFICIENCY ANAEMIA

Iron Metabolism

In normal men the amount of iron excreted daily does not exceed 1–1.5 mg. Iron is absorbed from the upper small intestine. After entering the cell it is transferred to the plasma where it is transported by a specific fraction of β globulin called *transferrin*. A considerable amount of this absorbed iron remains in the cells lining the small intestine in the form of *ferritin* and these cells are shed into the gut lumen. The body has no way of excreting iron, the uptake is controlled so that iron loss is replaced but accumulation does not occur. The mechanism controlling this delicate balance is unknown. If transferrin were fully saturated the plasma would contain 54–80 μmol/litre (total iron-binding capacity). The normal plasma iron level, however, is 12–26 μmol/litre, which represents approximately one third saturation of the iron-binding capacity of the plasma. The body's reserve stores of iron, contained mainly in the liver, are about 1.5 g; this provides enough iron for the replacement of about 1.5–2.0 litres of blood. Normally the iron used in haemoglobin synthesis for new red cells is nearly all provided by the catabolism of haemoglobin from old red cells and very little has to be drawn from the reserve stores.

The average daily loss of iron is at least doubled in women during the reproductive period of life by menstruation, pregnancy, and lactation. To remain in iron balance they must therefore absorb daily some 2–3 mg instead of 1–1.5 mg and to ensure this absorption a diet containing at least 15 mg iron is essential. A similar iron intake is advisable for growing children, but for everyone else 5–10 mg daily is probably adequate.

Aetiology

(a) The most important cause of iron deficiency is *haemorrhage*. If a pint of blood is withdrawn weekly from a healthy young man the blood count remains normal for about a month. By that time, however, the reserve stores of iron are exhausted and if bleeding continues at the same rate there is a shortage of iron and therefore of haemoglobin for the new red cells being poured out by the marrow. Signs of iron deficiency, therefore, rapidly appear in the blood. Clinical iron deficiency may be the result of acute haemorrhage of the same order, frequently from haematemesis or melaena, but much more often it is a consequence of chronic blood loss. Menorrhagia is by far the most important factor and its ill-effects are commonly enhanced by previous depletion of the reserve stores of iron by pregnancy and lactation. This is why iron deficiency anaemia is seen mainly in women.

(b) *Dietary deficiency of iron* occurs in those who, usually from either poverty, ignorance, or food-fad, do not eat enough of the main iron-containing foods, meat, eggs, and green vegetables. The deficiency is serious particularly in women who, as explained above, have high iron requirements.

(c) Impaired absorption of iron may be the result of achlorhydria, gastrectomy, and short-circuit operations involving the small intestine, or the malabsorption syndrome (coeliac disease, sprue, idiopathic steatorrhoea, and Crohn's disease).

Clinical Features. In addition to the usual symptoms and signs of anaemia, patients with iron deficiency often have brittle, spoon-shaped nails (*koilonychia*) and a very smooth tongue. The latter change is due to atrophy of the filiform papillae. Similar atrophic changes in the mucous membrane in the upper part of the oesophagus, and the development of a curious 'web' of delicate tissue which partially obstructs the lumen and causes dysphagia, occasionally develop and complete the picture of the *Plummer–Vinson syndrome*. The spleen is sometimes palpable.

Blood Count. Since lack of iron leads to shortage of haemoglobin but does not retard the production of red cell envelopes, less haemoglobin is put into each red cell. The red blood count is only slightly lowered, therefore, but the haemoglobin content of blood is reduced because the red cells are smaller and thus contain less haemoglobin (low MCH). The haemoglobin concentration of the red cell is unaltered. In a patient with unaltered iron-deficiency anaemia a reticulocyte count above 1 %, indicating increased turnover of red cells, suggests that haemorrhage has been an important aetiological factor. The untreated patient is also likely to have a fasting serum iron level below 50 μg per dl and the unsaturated iron-binding capacity of the serum will be in the range of 300–400 μg per dl.

Treatment. It is important wherever possible to deal with the various factors which have led to the iron deficiency at the same time as the latter is corrected. In practice this usually means arranging appropriate treatment for menorrhagia or gastrointestinal bleeding and giving advice about diet. For correcting the iron deficiency it is nearly always satisfactory to give *iron by mouth* and since ferrous sulphate is the cheapest effective preparation it is the one which should be chosen for routine use. There is some evidence that absorption of iron is better if it is not given on a full stomach, so that a good prescription is tab. ferrous sulphate 200 mg three times daily between meals. Ascorbic acid 50 mg twice daily, is sometimes given in the belief that it aids iron absorption. If ferrous sulphate causes gastrointestinal upset (nausea, diarrhoea, or constipation) tab. ferrous gluconate 600 mg three times daily may be given instead. Treatment must be continued for at least several months to replenish iron stores.

Parenteral iron therapy is indicated:

(1) when there is a serious impairment of absorption,

(2) when severe iron deficiency has to be corrected quickly during pregnancy, and

(3) rarely when real or imagined intolerance of oral preparations makes effective treatment by mouth impracticable.

Either iron sorbitol citric acid complex (Jectofer) or iron dextran

(Imferon) may be given intramuscularly and are usually effective and well tolerated. Each contains 50 mg iron in 1 ml. The injections cause local pain and may result in staining of the skin which is transient with Jectofer but permanent with Imferon. After a test dose of 25 mg injections of 100 mg may be given daily or at longer intervals to a total of 1–2 g. Total dosage is calculated from the fact that about 50 mg is required to raise the haemoglobin by 0.2 g dl. Toxic effects are rare if single doses do not exceed 100 mg, but Jectofer may cause fever, vomiting, disorientation, temporary loss of taste, a metallic taste in the mouth and local urticaria, and Imferon fever, allergic reactions, lymph-node enlargement and arthralgia.

SIDEROBLASTIC ANAEMIAS

These are rare disorders in which varying numbers of hypochromic microcytic red cells are found in the blood and normoblasts containing an excess of iron-containing granules appear in the marrow. There are also increased iron stores in the reticulo-endothelial system and in parenchymatous organs such as the liver, pancreas and heart; the serum iron level is raised and there is complete or almost complete saturation of the iron-binding protein. Kinetic studies may show increased iron turnover but impaired iron utilisation.

Congenital Sideroblastic Anaemia

This is usually inherited as an X-linked trait and is therefore seen mainly in male patients; it sometimes responds to large doses of pyridoxine, though there is no evidence of pyridoxine deficiency.

Acquired Sideroblastic Anaemia

This may be related to underlying disease such as carcinomas, Hodgkin's disease, leukaemia or rheumatoid arthritis, or may be a side-effect of drugs such as isoniazid and cycloserine which interfere with pyridoxine metabolism.

Treatment. Pyridoxine 50–200 mg daily should always be given for 2 months and then if there is no response steroid therapy may be tried. Since the iron overload may have serious consequences (see Haemochromatosis, p. 115) iron therapy should be avoided and blood transfusions should be given sparingly.

ANAEMIAS DUE TO VITAMIN B_{12} OR FOLIC ACID DEFICIENCY

PERNICIOUS ANAEMIA (Addison's Anaemia)

Aetiology. This is primarily a disease of the gastric mucosa, which in middle age or beyond fails to produce hydrochloric acid, pepsin and Castle's intrinsic factor. The cause of this failure is not known, but present evidence suggests that it is probably due to an inherited constitutional weakness; thus there is a significant familial incidence and the disease has been shown to be commoner in people of blood group A than blood group O. Gastric cytoplasmic antibodies can be demonstrated in over 80 per cent of patients, indicating a defect in the body's 'self-recognition system'. Vitamin B_{12} in the diet is not absorbed in the absence of gastric intrinsic factor. The disease is very rare below the age of thirty. These patients often have prematurely grey hair.

Clinical Features. The onset is very insidious and frequently the patient does not consult his doctor until the red cell count has fallen to $1–2 \times 10^{12}$/litre or even lower. This observation alone may suggest the diagnosis, since counts as low as this in the absence of severe symptoms are very rarely found in other anaemias. In addition to the symptoms common to all anaemias (p. 607), the patient may complain of recurrent soreness of the tongue and very rarely the symptoms of subacute combined degeneration of the cord (p. 390) may be the first indication of the disease. Fever is often present, but significant loss of weight is unusual. Abdominal pain and diarrhoea are common.

Examination shows pallor and in advanced cases the faint lemon-yellow colour of haemolytic jaundice due to rapid breakdown of the abnormal red cells in the circulation. About half the patients have a red raw-looking and smooth tongue. A haemic cardiac murmur, nearly always systolic in timing, can often be heard and retinal haemorrhages are sometimes present. The spleen is palpable in about 60 % of patients.

Investigations. *Gastric analysis* invariably reveals pentagastrin-fast achlorhydria, so that if any HCl is found in samples aspirated from the stomach after the subcutaneous injection of pentagastrin 6 μg/kg or histamine 40 μg/kg the diagnosis must be discarded.

Blood Picture. There is severe reduction in the red count but only moderate reduction in haemoglobin percentage, so that the MCH is high, and raised MCD and MCV values (p. 608) show that the cells are macrocytic. Examination of the stained film shows abnormal variations in size, shape, and staining reaction and immature nucleated cells, usually normoblasts but sometimes haemoglobinised megaloblasts, may be seen. There is usually a low total white count of about 3.0–4.0 $\times 10^9$/litre, the reduction affecting mainly the granulocyte cells, which also show a shift to the right (a predominance of older cells). In severe cases the platelets may also be decreased.

Bone marrow examination shows the presence of large numbers of haemoglobinised megaloblasts.

The Schilling Test. Vitamin B_{12} labelled with radioactive cobalt is given by mouth and within an hour 1 mg of ordinary B_{12} is injected intramuscularly to flood the body's stores and ensure excretion by the kidneys of any of the B_{12} absorbed. The urine is collected for 48 hr and its content of radioactive B_{12} estimated. Normal people eliminate 15–50% of the given dose in the urine, but patients with pernicious anaemia less than 10%.

The serum level of Vitamin B_{12} is reduced (normal 150–850 ng/l).

Treatment must continue for life since the gastric atrophy is permanent. This fact should be impressed on the patient as soon as the diagnosis is made, for if the blood count is allowed to fall below normal at any time there is grave danger that irreversible changes of subacute combined degeneration of the cord will develop. Vitamin B_{12} is administered intramuscularly as hydroxycobalamin. There is a good deal of individual variation in the dosage required, but average doses are 100–1000 μg of Vitamin B_{12} (hydroxycyanocobalamin) every day until the blood count is normal, followed by a similar amount once every 2–4 weeks for maintenance. The patient's progress must of course be followed by regular blood counts. At the start of treatment there is an outpouring of new young erythrocytes into the circulation, so that the reticulocyte count rises sharply to reach a peak by about the seventh day. The degree of rise in the reticulocyte count varies with the severity of the anaemia before treatment; when the initial red count has been very low it may reach 40–50%. If no reticulocyte crisis occurs in response to treatment the diagnosis should be reconsidered.

Complications. *Subacute combined degeneration of the spinal cord* is by far the most important complication and is discussed on p. 390.

Carcinoma of the stomach occurs more often in patients with pernicious anaemia than in the general population and some authorities advocate annual barium meal examination or even annual gastroscopy for its early detection in such patients. It is probably an adequate precaution, however, to perform such investigations only when there is some special indication such as an unexplained rise in the sedimentation rate.

Other Macrocytic Anaemias

Macrocytic anaemia, haematologically similar to pernicious anaemia, and resulting also from lack of adequate supplies of Vitamin B_{12} or folic acid in the bone marrow, may be seen under the following circumstances:

(a) Dietary deficiency, mainly of folic acid but affecting Vitamin B_{12} too, occurs only in association with gross general malnutrition and has been reported mainly from India as tropical (or nutritional) macrocytic anaemia (Hindus are often strict vegetarians with very low Vitamin B_{12} intake).

(b) Lesions of the gastrointestinal tract may impair the absorption of B_{12} and folic acid. Thus macrocytic anaemia is sometimes found in patients with carcinoma of the stomach, after total gastrectomy, after operations on the small gut, particularly when multiple anastomoses or blind loops have been formed, and in patients with the malabsorption syndrome (coeliac disease, sprue, and idiopathic steatorrhoea).

(c) Alcohol is a marrow toxin and chronic alcoholism causes macrocytosis and later folate deficiency and megaloblastic anaemia.

(d) Macrocytic anaemia, which usually responds to treatment with tablets of folic acid 10 mg daily, sometimes occurs for reasons unknown during the later months of pregnancy.

(e) Phenytoin and methotrexate sometimes causes macrocytic anaemia due to folate deficiency.

HAEMOLYTIC ANAEMIAS

Abnormally rapid breakdown of the red cells in the circulation leads to an increase in the level of bilirubin in the serum, causing latent or overt jaundice, and to an increased excretion of urobilinogen in the urine and faeces. The compensatory increase in the rate of erythropoiesis in the bone marrow causes an outpouring of new red cells into the circulation, so that a high reticulocyte count is another characteristic feature of haemolytic anaemia.

Causes. Excessive haemolysis may be due to:

(1) hereditary abnormalities in the erythrocytes, as in acholuric jaundice,
(2) haemolysins in the blood, or
(3) toxic or infective factors.

HEREDITARY ABNORMALITIES IN THE RED CELLS

(1) HEREDITARY SPHEROCYTOSIS (ACHOLURIC JAUNDICE)

This rare disease is usually inherited as a Mendelian dominant, being passed directly from parent to child. The sexes are affected equally. Red cells from a patient with acholuric jaundice are destroyed at a greatly increased rate when transfused into normal people, whereas normal red cells survive for the expected time when transfused into patients with acholuric jaundice. Furthermore haemolysins cannot be demonstrated in the blood. The defect therefore lies in the red cells themselves, which are smaller in diameter (about 5.6–6.2 μm) and more spherical in shape than normal erythrocytes (*microspherocytes*) and remain in the circulation on an average for only fifteen days instead of the normal 120 days. The mean corpuscular volume and mean corpuscular haemoglobin concentration are usually normal. There is always a high reticulocyte count of 10–20%, rising to 50% or more during haemolytic crises. The red cells show an increased fragility in salt solutions, haemolysis starting at a salt concentration of 0.75% and being complete at 0.4% (normal range 0.45–0.3%).

Clinical Features. Yellowness of the skin is usually noted during the first few years of life, but apart from this symptoms are few and slight except during the so-called haemolytic crises when the patient becomes pale, weak, and febrile. Slow spontaneous recovery usually occurs in about a month. It is now thought that some of these attacks are not episodes of increased haemolysis but of temporary marrow aplasia, since the reticulocyte count may fall and the jaundice become lighter.

The spleen is nearly always palpable and may extend to the umbilicus. About 60% of patients have gallstones of 'metabolic' type, which are precipitated from the excess of bilirubin excreted in the bile; they contain pigment and calcium but no cholesterol. Cholecystectomy is, however, rarely necessary. A curious but important symptom is intractable ulceration of the legs which heals only after splenectomy.

Treatment. Splenectomy is a very satisfactory treatment which nearly always leads to permanent symptomatic cure.

(2) NON-SPHEROCYTIC HAEMOLYTIC ANAEMIA

These may be due to inherited enzyme defects.

(a) Deficiency of red-cell pyruvate kinase is an autosomal recessive disorder which presents as a haemolytic anaemia with splenomegaly in childhood. Splenectomy may improve the symptoms.

(b) Deficiency of Glucose-6-Phosphate Dehydrogenase (G6PD)

This inherited disorder is due to a sex-linked gene of irregular dominance which is found among Africans and their descendants, Indians and those from Far Eastern and Mediterranean countries. There is reduced activity of the enzyme G6PD in the red cells which leads to haemolysis when the cells are exposed to oxidising agents. Agents which precipitate haemolysis include:

Broad bean (Favism)	Probenecid
Aspirin	Sulphonamides
Primaquine	Sulphones
Pamaquin	Chloramphenicol
Quinine	PAS
Quinidine	Vitamin K

Haemolysis may also occur with acute infections.

There is no specific treatment for the haemolysis but if it occurs hydrocortisone should be given intravenously and the urine made alkaline to prevent deposition of the haematin in the tubules.

(3) THE HAEMOGLOBINOPATHIES

(a) Sickle-cell Anaemia

This disease, which is practically confined to negroes, is inherited as a Mendelian dominant. The essential fault is an abnormal haemoglobin (HbS) in the red cells which causes the latter to assume a sickle shape at the lower end of the physiological range of oxygen tension. The abnormal shape of the red cells leads to increased blood viscosity and tends to promote capillary thrombosis.

The illness presents as a chronic haemolytic anaemia, sometimes with acute crises and sometimes with thrombotic episodes. Crises are usually precipitated by infection. The patient is feverish with severe pain in the back and limbs. There may also be abdominal or neurological symptoms and the anaemia becomes worse. Thromboses can cause splenic infarcts and avascular necrosis of the femoral or humeral heads. The diagnosis is confirmed by demonstrating sickling of the red cells in a sealed preparation of blood in which the oxygen tension has been reduced, and the abnormal haemoglobin can be shown by electrophoresis.

Treatment. There is no curative treatment. Transfusions may be required to control the anaemia. During the crises analgesics are necessary and oxygen can be given in an attempt to prevent further sickling.

(b) Thalassaemia

The haemoglobin molecule contains at least six different globin polypeptide chains. Normally synthesis of the alpha and non-alpha chains is balanced as in foetal Hb ($\alpha_2\gamma_2$) and adult Hb ($\alpha_2\beta_2$); thalassaemia is characterised by imbalance in globin production due to absence or reduced expression of one or more of the globin genes. The resulting syndromes are classified according to the specific globin whose synthesis is depressed; the majority are of the alpha or beta type.

β *Thalassaemia* is seen mainly in Greeks, Italians, blacks and people from India and South-East Asia.

β *Thalassaemia Major* presents as a severe anaemia in an infant both of whose parents have β thalassaemia minor. Death usually occurs in childhood from haemolytic anaemia.

β *Thalassaemia Intermedia* is clinically less severe and most patients survive into adult life. The Hb level is usually 7–10 g/dl and the red cells are microcytic (MCV < 75 fl); distinction from iron deficiency is based on normal iron studies and failure to respond to iron therapy.

β Thalassaemia Minor is usually symptomless but the blood picture reveals minimal anaemia and microcytosis.

Hb S β Thalassaemia is the combination of sickle cell disease and thalassaemia and is usually characterised by mild microcytic anaemia, periodic pain crises and splenomegaly.

α Thalassaemia presents in different degrees of severity depending on how many of the four alpha genes are missing. Clinically the most important is *Hb H disease* due to loss of three of the alpha genes; the syndrome is similar to *β* thalassaemia intermedia.

Treatment. Anaemia may have to be corrected by transfusion, but blood must be given as sparingly as possible in view of the danger of iron overload. Splenectomy may be needed if there is evidence of hypersplenism. The temptation to treat the microcytic anaemia with iron must be resisted unless there is clear evidence of iron deficiency.

HAEMOLYTIC ANAEMIA DUE TO CIRCULATING HAEMOLYSINS

Auto-Immune Haemolytic Anaemia (AIHA)

AIHA is due to an antibody directed against an antigen on the red-cell membrane. These antibodies (apart from those associated with drugs or infections) presumably arise as a result of changes in the red cell membrane or from an abnormality in the immune system which no longer recognises 'self' antigens.

AIH anaemias are classified into warm and cold according to the temperature at which the antibody is most active. *Warm antibodies* (which are usually of IgG type) react best at 37° C. No underlying cause is found at the onset in 50% of patients; the rest are associated with diseases such as lymphomas, chronic lymphatic leukaemia, collagen diseases and viral infections and on follow-up half the idiopathic group fall into one of these categories also. *Cold antibodies* (which are usually IgM) react better at temperatures below 37° C. They occur most often after infections such as mycoplasma pneumonia and infectious mononucleosis and spontaneously in chronic cold haemagglutinin disease (CHAD).

Treatment. The abnormal haemolysis can usually be controlled by giving corticosteroids, which are therefore life-saving in this disease. The drug may have to be continued indefinitely, however. Dosage is very variable; the smallest daily dose which will prevent haemolysis and therefore drop in haemoglobin should be given. Splenectomy is of benefit in some patients. The abnormal haemolysis sometimes stops if the underlying cause can be treated.

Toxic and Infective Haemolytic Anaemia

Very rarely haemolytic anaemia may occur in association with severe infections, such as streptococcal or staphylococcal septicaemia or as a result of poisoning with lead or dinitrobenzene or from idiosyncrasy to drugs such as sulphonamides, amphetamine, or potassium chlorate. The presence of large numbers of Heinz bodies in red cells strongly suggests haemolytic anaemia due to chemical poisoning.

THE HAEMORRHAGIC DISEASES

A tendency to abnormal bleeding may result from:

(1) **A coagulation defect,** or lack of one of the various substances in the blood which are necessary for the formation of a firm blood-clot when blood is shed (e.g. haemophilia).

(2) **Thrombocytopenia,** which may be either idiopathic or symptomatic of some disease of the bone marrow such as leukaemia or aplastic anaemia, or

(3) Some abnormality in the **capillaries.**

Diseases in group (1) lead to persistent bleeding after injury or trauma; groups (2) and (3) constitute the *purpuras*, which are characterised by spontaneous bleeding from mucous surfaces and into the skin, causing a purpuric eruption (petechiae or ecchymoses). Purpuric spots are easily recognised since, the blood being extravascular, they do not fade on pressure.

COAGULATION DEFECTS

Physiology of Blood Coagulation

The immediate arrest of haemorrhage after injury to small blood vessels is due to vasoconstriction and plugging of the leaks by aggregations of platelets which control the bleeding until a firm blood-clot forms. Coagulation is a complex process initiated by contact of the blood with a water-wettable surface and involves the interaction of many coagulation factors; the nomenclature of these factors has now been standardised internationally, using Roman numerals:

Factor	*Synonym*
Factor I	Fibrinogen
Factor II	Prothrombin

(Factor III was originally tissue thromboplastin; Factor IV calcium; and Factor VI the activated form of Factor V; these terms are now seldom used.)

Factor V	Labile factor
Factor VII	Stable factor
Factor VIII	Anti-haemophilic globulin
Factor IX	Christmas factor
Factor X	Stuart-Prower factor
Factor XI	
Factor XII	Hageman factor
Factor XIII	Fibrin stabilising factor

Contact with a water-wettable surface leads to a molecular rearrangement of Factor XII which thus acquires enzymatic properties and by interaction with Factors XI, IX and VIII converts Factor X to its active form. Activated Factor X with Factor V and the platelet factor form prothrombinase, which converts prothrombin to thrombin; interaction of thrombin with fibrinogen in the presence of Factor XIII leads to the formation of fibrin, which provides the framework of the blood clot. Retraction of the blood clot, which helps to draw the edges of the wound together, is due to shortening of the fibrin strands by the action of a protein liberated from the platelets.

Prostacyclin, a prostaglandin which inhibits platelet aggregation, is produced by blood vessel endothelium and it may be that the balance between it and platelet prostaglandin is a vital factor in the maintenance of normal blood flow. Local trauma alters the balance in favour of platelet adhesion and aggregation.

In haemophilia and allied states the initial arrest of haemorrhage takes place normally but failure of a firm blood clot to form results in bleeding an hour or so after the injury when the vasoconstriction passes off. This also explains why in these conditions the coagulation time is prolonged, but the bleeding time is typically normal.

INVESTIGATION OF PATIENTS WITH A HAEMORRHAGIC DISEASE

Hess's Tests. The sphygmomanometer cuff is placed round the upper arm and the pressure maintained halfway between the systolic and diastolic pressures for five minutes. A positive test, shown by the appearance of more than 5 purpuric spots on the arm below the level of the cuff, is found in patients with capillary defects and with severe thrombocytopenia.

Platelet Count. Purpura is usually present when the platelet count is below about 40×10^9/litre. Such patients also have a prolonged bleeding time and poor clot retraction.

Clot Retraction. Poor clot retraction is seen in patients with low platelet counts or more rarely when there is deficient blood fibrinogen.

Bleeding time is increased when the platelets are deficient. The lobe of the ear is pricked with a needle and the blood absorbed every 30 seconds on a piece of blotting paper which is not allowed to touch the skin. By this method the normal bleeding time is two to five minutes.

Coagulation time is increased in haemophilia and the allied coagulation-defect states. By *Lee and White's* method, using venous blood, the normal coagulation time is four to ten minutes, but a control with normal blood should always be performed as there is a wide variation in results according to the precise conditions of the test. The *partial thromboplastin time* (normal 25–55 seconds) is a more sensitive test now usually preferred to the whole blood coagulation time.

HAEMOPHILIA

Haemophilia is due to abnormality of the X chromosome and is inherited as a sex-linked character, appearing only in males and transmitted to them by clinically normal female carriers. Two types are recognised: *Haemophilia A* is due to deficiency of Factor VIII and *Haemophilia B* (Christmas disease) to deficiency of Factor IX. All the sons of haemophiliacs are free from the haemophiliac gene and all the daughters are carriers. When a female carrier marries a normal man half the sons are haemophiliacs and half the daughters are carriers. In practice only two out of three haemophiliacs know of other bleeders in their families so that a typical pedigree must not be regarded as an essential diagnostic criterion.

The common **symptoms** are persistent bleeding after cuts and abrasions and after extraction of teeth (of either first or second dentition) and bleeding into joints, particularly the knee joint. The severity of the haemophiliac state is very variable, depending on the degree of deficiency of the clotting factor concerned. The normal blood level is above 50 i.u./dl: patients with levels from 0–1 i.u./dl have severe haemophilia, with frequent spontaneous bleeding; those with levels 2–5 i.u./dl have fairly severe disease, with occasional spontaneous bleeding; those with levels 5–25 i.u./dl have mild disease, but bleed after minor surgery or accident; those with levels 25–50 i.u./dl bleed only after major surgery or accident.

Treatment. In the UK there are designated centres for the management of haemophilia where patients can obtain treatment without appointment 24 hours a day. Every haemophiliac should register at one of these centres which will supply him with a Haemophilia Card and a list of the other centres in the UK. Treatment consists of the IV administration of a concentrate of the appropriate Factor in dosage adequate to control the bleeding. Regular injections may be needed for patients with severe disease and prophylactic injections are given before surgical operations or dental extractions. Patients should be warned that intramuscular injections may cause serious haematomas and that aspirin and the non-steroidal anti-inflammatory drugs should be avoided in view of the risk of gastric haemorrhage.

The development of antibodies to the injected Factor concentrates seriously reduces the effectiveness of treatment in some patients, who may require plasma exchange or immunosuppression. All concentrates are now screened for Hepatitis B surface antigen, but non-A non-B Hepatitis is an important complication of therapy.

The address of the Haemophilia Society is P.O. Box 9, 16 Trinity Street, London, SE1 1DE (Telephone: 01 407 1010).

Von Willebrand's disease is a rare disorder inherited as an autosomal dominant trait (and occurring therefore in both sexes) in which there is deficiency of Factor VIII, but in contrast to true haemophiliacs the patients also have purpura of the skin and mucosae and a prolonged bleeding time, due to associated deficiency of the VW factor which is necessary for normal adhesion of platelets to subendothelial structures. Treatment is as for haemophilia.

Factor V deficiency is inherited in some families as a dominant trait but is extremely rare.

Factor VII deficiency is seen in patients under anticoagulant therapy and occasionally in advanced liver disease.

Prothrombin is produced in the liver from Vitamin K. Vitamin K is synthesised by certain bacteria in the intestines and is also present in a number of vegetable foods; it is not absorbed properly in the absence of bile salts. Clinical prothrombin deficiency is seen in two groups of patients: newborn babies in whose intestines the Vitamin-K-forming organisms have not yet become established (*haemorrhagic disease of the newborn*); and patients with *obstructive jaundice* whose intestine contains no bile salts. The former variety can be largely prevented by giving Vitamin K 5 mg intramuscularly daily to the expectant mother for a few days before delivery. Patients with obstructive jaundice should receive similar treatment, particularly if any surgical operation is contemplated, as otherwise serious haemorrhage may occur.

THE PURPURAS

IMMUNE THROMBOCYTOPENIC PURPURA (ITP) (Idiopathic Thrombocytopenic Purpura)

It has been established that platelet destruction in ITP is the result of an immunological process and Immune Thrombocytopenic Purpura has become the preferred name.

Acute ITP is a disease of childhood and will not be described here.

Chronic ITP is a rare disease seen mainly in adolescents and young adults, particularly girls, characterised by episodes of skin purpura and bleeding from such sites as the nose, uterus and alimentary tract. Absence of joint pains is a useful point of distinction from anaphylactoid purpura. The platelet count is low (usually below 40×10^9/litre), the bleeding time is prolonged, clot retraction is poor, but the coagulation time is normal. Hess's test is strongly positive. Gross enlargement of the spleen is uncommon, but in about one-third of the patients it becomes just palpable. As a result of haemorrhage haematological signs of iron deficiency often develop. Cerebral haemorrhage may occur.

Aetiology. Present evidence suggests that circulating antibodies interact with megakaryocytes and the resulting sensitisation of platelets leads to their premature destruction by the spleen. There may also be a defect in capillary endothelium. ITP is sometimes drug-induced, most commonly by quinine and quinidine.

Treatment. The effect of steroid therapy should first be tried, but if a complete remission does not occur or if relapse follows withdrawal of the drug splenectomy should be performed without delay. Results of operation are less satisfactory when the disease has been present for more than 12 months.

PURPURA DUE TO CAPILLARY DAMAGE

Purpura may be seen in any of the *acute specific fevers*, particularly meningococcal infections. It may also result from *drug sensitivity*; sedormid is the most notorious offender, but other well-known drugs which may cause it are quinine, quinidine, belladonna, phenobarbitone, thiouracil, chlorpromazine, isoniazid, sodium salicylate, carbromal, and the heavy metals. In certain drug purpuras a circulating antibody causing lysis of platelets has been demonstrated; such patients have a thrombocytopenia. Withdrawal of the drug is usually sufficient treatment, but if not, steroid therapy may be helpful. *Senile purpura* is common in elderly people, possibly as a result of degenerative changes in the capillary endothelium. The purpura of *scurvy* is due to nutritional changes in the capillary endothelium.

Anaphylactoid purpura (the Schönlein-Henoch syndrome) is characterised by purpura and allergic manifestations, namely urticaria, joint pains and swelling, and angio-neurotic oedema which affects not only the subcutaneous and submucous tissues but also the gut, causing intestinal colic and sometimes rectal bleeding. Classically Henoch's purpura was associated with abdominal colic and Schönlein's purpura with joint pains, but it is now recognised that the two groups often overlap.

Treatment. Subcutaneous adrenaline, 0.5 ml of 1/1000 solution, and oral antihistamines should be given. If the symptoms persist corticosteroid therapy is usually effective.

APLASTIC ANAEMIA AND AGRANULOCYTOSIS

This rare disease, which usually occurs in young adults, is the result of destruction of those cells in the bone marrow which produce the red cells, the white cells, and the platelets. A similar process affecting only the granular leucocytes is termed *agranulocytosis*. Death or destruction of the parent bone marrow cells is sometimes a toxic reaction to certain drugs, notably amidopyrine, sulphonamides, heavy metals such as gold or arsenic, thiouracil, chloramphenicol, or tridione; or to certain industrial poisons such as benzole and its derivatives. It may also result from excessive exposure to X-rays or radioactive materials. Frequently, however, the cause is unknown (idiopathic aplastic anaemia, or idiopathic agranulocytosis).

Clinical Features. Failure in production of red cells causes the gradual development of the symptoms and signs of anaemia; diminished or absent output of granulocytes impairs the body's defences against infection, leading to painful ulceration of the throat and fever; and scarcity of platelets in the blood causes purpura and bleeding from different parts of the body.

Treatment consists in removal of the cause, if possible; fresh blood transfusion repeated as often as necessary for the correction of the anaemia; and the administration of penicillin or other suitable antibiotic to combat infection. Recovery of bone marrow function may be assisted by androgen therapy: oxymetholone 3–5 mg/kg by mouth should be continued for 4–6 months before being abandoned as ineffective.

Hypersplenism is a condition in which there is progressive decline in the numbers of red cells, white cells, and platelets in the peripheral blood (or any combination of the three) associated with splenomegaly of varied aetiology. The bone marrow shows not aplasia but hyperplasia. The spleen appears to be exerting some inhibitory effect on the maturation or release of cells from the bone marrow and splenectomy is frequently followed by clinical cure.

THE LEUKAEMIAS

Leukaemia is a disease characterised by abnormal proliferation of leucopoietic tissue throughout the body. The cause is not known, but it is now generally regarded as a neoplastic process. The risk of developing it is increased by exposure to excessive radiation: there was a twenty-fold increase in its incidence among survivors of the Hiroshima and Nagasaki atomic explosions; the incidence is some six times higher in patients with ankylosing spondylitis who have been treated with radiotherapy than in the general population; and radiologists have an incidence several times higher than other doctors. The risk to doctors generally, however, appears to be about twice that to the general population and in the latter the number of cases per million has doubled in the past twenty years.

Leukaemia is classified according to the type of leucocyte affected into lymphatic, myeloid, and monocytic varieties. It is also subdivided into acute and chronic types according to the speed of the clinical course.

ACUTE MYELOID LEUKAEMIA

This type of leukaemia occurs at any age.

Clinical Features. The onset is acute or subacute with malaise and fever. Suppression of normal bone marrow function leads to anaemia, leucopenia with infection and thrombocytopenia with bleeding. Splenomegaly is quite common but lymph node enlargement is unusual. The diagnosis depends on finding myeloblasts in the peripheral blood and in the bone marrow. Some patients are aleukaemic in the early stages of the disease so that there are no blast cells in the peripheral blood and bone marrow examination is essential to establish the diagnosis.

Treatment. This is less satisfactory than for acute lymphoblastic leukaemia of childhood. Several combinations of cytotoxic drugs may be used and a remission can be induced in about 70 % of patients using a combination of:

daunorubicin;
cytarabine;
thioguanine;
prednisolone.

These drugs are given in two or three 5-day courses. Consolidation is achieved by further courses of the same drugs but when a remission has been fully established further drug therapy does not seem to prolong it. In remission the blood count and bone marrow appear normal although leukaemic cells must be present in small numbers. Remissions usually last for 10–18 months, but occasionally much longer. Relapses are treated with the same drugs but at this stage they are rarely as effective. The cytotoxic drugs used cause profound depression of the bone marrow with severe leucopenia and thrombocytopenia; supportive measures are therefore required, with platelet and whole blood transfusion and rigorous treatment of any developing infection. This can be undertaken only in units experienced in this type of treatment.

In a few specialised units bone-marrow transplantation is being used after complete ablation of the malignant cells and results are encouraging.

ACUTE LYMPHOBLASTIC LEUKAEMIA (ALL)

This is predominantly a disease of childhood. The cause is unknown but there is an increased incidence in Down's syndrome. The malignant cells may have no surface markers or may be either T or B cells.

Clinical features are due to infiltration of bone marrow and interference with normal marrow function. They consist of anaemia, bleeding due to platelet deficiency often combined with purpura and infections due to leucopenia. Lymph nodes, liver and spleen are usually enlarged. Without treatment the course is rapidly downhill to death within a few weeks or months.

Diagnosis is confirmed by finding lymphoblasts in the peripheral blood and bone marrow. Occasionally these cells are confined for a time to the marrow.

Treatment

(a) *Induction of Remission.* Prednisolone 40 mg/m^2 orally daily with vincristine 2.0 mg/m^2 weekly will induce remission in 80–90% of children, but in adults it may be necessary to add adriamycin and l-asparaginase to the regime. Unfortunately leukaemic cells may find sanctuary in the CNS and of patients surviving for more than two years 50% relapse with neurological symptoms. It is therefore necessary to eradicate the disease from this site. Most cytotoxic drugs penetrate the CSF very poorly and the usual practice is to combine irradiation of the cranium with intrathecal methotrexate. The testicles may also be a sanctuary site in a few patients.

(b) *Maintenance.* For this purpose various cytotoxic drugs are used, including 6 mercaptopurine, methotrexate, adriamycin, cyclophosphamide and cytosine arabinoside in different combinations. The most effective regime has not yet been decided and it is important that the treatment be directed by a physician with special experience in this field.

Prognosis. The treatment requires great courage on the part of the patient and perseverence by the doctor, but cure can now probably be achieved in about 40% of patients.

CHRONIC MYELOID LEUKAEMIA

Chronic myeloid leukaemia occurs mainly between early adult life and middle age and is rather more common in men than in women. Slowly progressive tiredness due to anaemia is usually the presenting symptom, or the patient may complain of a dragging sensation in the abdomen due to the enlarged spleen. The spleen attains a larger size in this disease than in any other seen in temperate climates and may extend into the right iliac fossa. The BMR is increased and this may partly explain the nervousness, night sweats, and loss of weight which are sometimes prominent symptoms. Leukaemic infiltration of the skin sometimes occurs, and pruritus may be a troublesome symptom even when no lesions can be seen or felt. In men painful priapism, due to thrombosis in the corpora cavernosa, may be an early symptom. *Blood count* typically shows a total white count between 100×10^9/litre and 500×10^9/litre of which some 50–70% are polymorphonuclears and 10–20% myelocytes, and there is always moderate to severe anaemia. The *diagnosis* is usually easy in view of the enormously enlarged spleen and typical white count, but confirmation may be obtained by marrow examination. The Philadelphia chromosome is usually present, the leucocyte alkaline phosphatase is reduced or absent and the serum B_{12} and B_{12}-binding proteins are greatly raised.

Treatment. Chronic myeloid leukaemia is ultimately a fatal disease and treatment aims at producing a remission and relieving symptoms.

The most effective drug is busulphan. The initial dose is 0.06 mg/kg daily (maximum 4.0 mg) and this is maintained until the white count drops to 20×10^9/litre or the platelets drop below 100×10^9/litre. In view of the massive cell breakdown early in treatment with the risk of precipitating gout, allopurinol 300 mg daily should be given. Treatment is then stopped. Further courses may be given at intervals or maintenance treatment given at a lower dosage. Market myelosuppression is a serious risk and the blood count must be monitored. Other side-effects include pulmonary fibrosis and pigmentation. Alternatively the spleen may be irradiated, but this is not quite as effective as chemotherapy.

Although treatment produces a remission in about 90% of patients, relapses occur and after about 2–3 years a blast-cell crisis develops with the appearance of more primitive cells in the marrow and peripheral blood and at this stage response to treatment is usually poor. Symptomatic treatment is needed in the final stages of the disease.

CHRONIC LYMPHATIC LEUKAEMIA

Chronic lymphatic leukaemia is nearly always seen in men of late middle age. The patient complains of slowly developing tiredness, due to associated anaemia, and the spleen, liver, and lymph nodes in the neck, axillae, and elsewhere are found to be enlarged. The spleen, however, does not attain the enormous size seen in chronic myeloid leukaemia. As in the latter disease the BMR is raised. Priapism does not occur, but impotence is a common symptom. Infiltration of the skin may result in eruptions of various types. The blood count usually shows a total white count of up to 200×10^9 of which 80–90% are small lymphocytes and there is always an associated anaemia.

Treatment. The median survival is about 4 years and many patients live very much longer. Treatment is not curative and is given to relieve symptoms.

Chemotherapy is indicated for relief of pressure from enlarged lymphnodes or a big spleen and to reduce bone marrow infiltration causing suppression of haematopoiesis. A lymphocyte count above 100×10^9/litre is often taken as evidence of widespread infiltration requiring treatment. Chlorambucil 8 mg/m^2 daily for 10 days every month for six months with regular monitoring of the blood count is usually satisfactory. Prednisolone 40 mg daily can be added to the chlorambucil if there is evidence of bone-marrow suppression. Prednisolone is also helpful in controlling complicating haemolytic anaemia. Radiotherapy is used to reduce the size of lymph node masses which are causing symptoms: they are usually very radiosensitive. In patients with very large spleens but very little other evidence of disease radiotherapy is useful in shrinking the spleen. Infections are common, notably by organisms such as *pneumocystis carinii* or fungi, and require appropriate antibiotic therapy.

POLYCYTHAEMIA RUBRA VERA (Erythraemia)

This is a disease of middle age and is commoner in men. It is characterised by hyperplasia of the erythroblastic, leucoblastic, and megakaryocytic tissue of the bone marrow; and although the clinical picture is dominated by the greatly increased number of red cells in the peripheral circulation, there may eventually be exhaustion of the marrow cells, leading to myelofibrosis, or the leucoblastic tissue may continue to proliferate as the erythroblasts die out, so that the final picture may be that of frank leukaemia.

It is now recognised that in a small proportion of patients with polycythaemia (about 9%) there is an underlying renal lesion, neoplasm, cyst or hydronephrosis. In such patients there is presumably increased production of erythropoietin by the kidney. Nephrectomy may cure the polycythaemia.

Clinical Features. The patient usually complains of headache, dizziness, and tiredness and has a very plethoric cyanosed appearance. The spleen is nearly always palpable. Congestion of the capillary bed leads to haemorrhage from various sites (for example, after dental extraction), while arterial thromboses in the brain, limbs, and elsewhere are also common, no doubt as a result of the increased blood viscosity. There is also an increased incidence of peptic ulcer and of gout.

The *red count* may be up to 10×10^{12}/litre or even higher with an equivalent increase in the haemoglobin level. The white count is usually raised to about 20×10^9/litre and the platelet count to 500×10^9/litre or more.

The development of myelofibrosis is suggested by a fall in the haemoglobin level and increase in the size of the spleen. Diagnosis can be confirmed by trephine biopsy of the bone marrow.

Treatment. The raised haematocrit can usually be reduced to normal

Table 15.1 Some drugs used in treating leukaemias

Drug	*Mode of action*	*Administration*	*Main uses*	*Main side-effects*
Cyclophosphamide	Alkylating agent	IV or oral	Variable	BMD, vomiting, cystitis, hair loss
Chlorambucil	Alkylating agent	Oral	CLL	BMD
Busulphan	Alkylating agent	Oral	CML	BMD, pigmentation, pulmonary fibrosis
Methotrexate	Antimetabolite	IV, oral, intrathecal*	AL	BMD, liver & renal damage, stomatitis, vomiting
6-Mercaptopurine	Antimetabolite	Oral	AL	BMD, jaundice
Cytosine arabinoside	Antimetabolite	IV	AML	BMD, vomiting, stomatitis
6-Thioguanine	Antimetabolite	Oral	AML	BMD, jaundice, vomiting
Daunorubicin	Acts on DNA and inhibits RNA synthesis	IV	AML	BMD, cardiotoxic, hair loss
Vincristine	Spindle poison	IV	ALL	BMD, neurotoxic, constipation and ileus
Prednisolone	Lymphotoxic	Oral	ALL	See steroids

Dose depends on the regime used. Doses are usually given in terms of body weight (dose/kg) or body surface area (dose/m^2).

AL = Acute Leukaemias
ALL = Acute Lymphatic Leukaemia
AML = Acute Myeloid Leukaemia
CML = Chronic Myeloid Leukaemia
CLL = Chronic Lymphatic Leukaemia
BMD = Bone Marrow Depression

*Special Preparation Required

levels by repeated venesection and sometimes this level can be maintained by removing 500 ml of blood every two to four weeks. If this method is unsatisfactory control may be achieved over long periods by giving radioactive phosphorus ^{32}P 3–5 millicuries intravenously. If a relapse occurs the dose of ^{32}P may be repeated but the total cumulation dose should not exceed 30 millicuries of ^{32}P as there is some evidence that larger amounts are associated with an increased incidence of leukaemia.

MYELOFIBROSIS

The essential features of this disease are progressive obliteration of the bone marrow by collagen and new bone formation and the development of haematopoiesis in the liver and spleen, and rarely in other organs.

Myelofibrosis may be idiopathic or may result from the infiltration of the bone marrow by carcinoma, lymphoma or tuberculosis, and occasionally it complicates primary bone disorders such as Paget's disease. Myelofibrosis may also be part of the clinical picture of myeloproliferative disorders, namely chronic myeloid leukaemia and polycythaemia rubra vera.

Patients are usually middle-aged or elderly and present with anaemia, weakness and splenomegaly. Bone marrow aspiration is often unproductive; trephine biopsy reveals increase in reticulin with collagen and new bone formation. Hyperuricaemia and clinical gout are common. The white blood count may be raised to 20–30 × 10^9/litre. The absence of the Philadelphia chromosome, normal leucocyte alkaline phosphatase and normal serum B_{12} and B_{12} binding proteins help to distinguish the disease from chronic myeloid leukaemia. There is no specific treatment. Occasionally if hypersplenism is believed to be playing a part in depressing the blood count or if the enlarged spleen is causing great discomfort, splenectomy provides relief. Increasingly frequent blood transfusions are usually needed and the disease runs a progressive course over three to five years.

THE LYMPHOMAS

HODGKIN'S DISEASE (Lymphadenoma)

The cause of Hodgkin's disease is unknown, but it is probably a malignant process. Most of the patients are young adults, though it can occur at any age, and men are affected about twice as often as women.

Four histological types are recognised and are important in that they have some bearing on the prognosis of the disease.

(a) *Lymphocyte predominant*—very slowly progressive and usually remains localised for a long while. Good prognosis.
(b) *Lymphocyte depleted*—usually rapidly progressive and may be widespread from the start. Poor prognosis.
(c) *Nodular sclerosing* } intermediate outlook.
(d) *Mixed cellularity* }

Clinical Features. The first symptom is usually the painless enlargement of a group of lymph nodes, particularly in the neck but sometimes in the axillary or inguinal regions. At first the nodes feel firm, rubbery, and discrete, but later they often become matted together. The disease may remain localised in one node or group of nodes for long periods of months or even years before further spread occurs and symptoms develop. In other patients mediastinal or abdominal lymph nodes enlarge before those in accessible peripheral situations and the patient may present with cough, dyspnoea, or pain in the chest or abdomen; such patients may have fever of the Pel–Ebstein type, which occurs in waves lasting a week or two separated by afebrile intervals of varying length, although almost any type of fever may occur. As the disease progresses general symptoms appear; these include itching, night sweats, fever, general malaise and anaemia. In general the development of symptoms implies a worse prognosis, but itching is an exception to this rule. Involvement of the spleen often occurs early and may be present even in the absence of splenic enlargement. Later the disease may spread to the liver; to bone, leading to severe pain in the spine, pelvis or ribs; to the nervous system, causing various symptoms including nerve palsies and cord compression; or to the lung.

Diagnosis can be established with certainty only by lymph node biopsy.

Staging. The extent of the disease is determined by clinical examination, radiography, lymphangiography, isotope or CAT scanning, and usually by laparotomy.

Stage 1 Disease confined to one lymph node site.
Stage 2 Disease in more than one lymph node site, all either above or below the diaphragm.
Stage 3 Involvement of nodes on both sides of the diaphragm.
Stage 4 Sites involved outside the lymphatic system:
A = symptom free.
B = with symptoms.

Treatment. *Radiotherapy* is the treatment of choice in Stage 1, 2, and 3A. Patients with 3B and Stage 4 disease are best treated with chemotherapy from the start. It is important that not only the affected nodes should be irradiated but all contiguous groups of lymph nodes as well.

With radiotherapy the enlarged lymph nodes nearly always disappear. In a few patients they recur, occasionally in the treated area but more frequently elsewhere. Recurrence can sometimes be treated with further radiotherapy but usually cytotoxic drugs are necessary. Cytotoxic drugs are given from the start if the disease is widespread (stages 3B and 4).

Cytotoxic drugs are given in repeated courses; a number of drugs may be given together and the course of treatment repeated at intervals, even if the patient appears to be in a remission. This method gives superior results and is the treatment of choice. A typical course for an adult is:

Mustine 6 mg/m^2 IV on days 1 and 8.
Vinblastine 10 mg IV on days 1 and 8.
Procarbazine 100 mg orally on days 1–14 inclusive.
Prednisolone 40 mg orally on days 1–14 inclusive.

The courses are repeated at four to six week intervals to a total of six courses. Smaller doses are required if the white count is low.

If this combination fails to control the disease or relapse occurs other drug combinations are available. These will include CCNU combined with vincristine, bleomycin and prednisolone (CVB regime) or adriamycin combined with bleomycin, vinblastine and DTIC (ABVD regime). In addition symptomatic treatment may be required, such as transfusion for anaemia and analgesics for pain.

Prognosis. The prognosis depends on the extent of the disease at diagnosis, on the presence or absence of symptoms, and on the histology.

Of patients whose disease is localised and who are therefore treated with radiotherapy about 80% survive 5 years and about 50% 10 years or longer. Of those who require treatment with cytotoxic drugs about 50% survive 5 years.

NON-HODGKIN'S LYMPHOMAS

They can be divided on the basis of the cell type and of the cell architecture. The lymphoid cells may be either well or poorly differentiated and the architecture may show a nodular (follicular) or a diffuse pattern. The Rappaport classification is:

Cell Type	*Architecture*
Lymphocytic—well differentiated	nodular^x or diffuse^x
Lymphocytic—poorly differentiated	nodular^x or diffuse^o
Mixed lymphocytic and histiocytic	nodular^x or diffuse^o
Histiocytic	nodular^o or diffuse^o

x = favourable prognosis
o = unfavourable prognosis

This classification is helpful in determining the natural history of the disease. In patients with a favourable histology the disease often progresses slowly and may not cause symptoms for years. After a long period of indolent spread it usually becomes more aggressive and unless eradicated will ultimately be fatal. In patients with an unfavourable histology the disease is often widespread from the start, symptoms appear early and few patients survive more than two years, although vigorous treatment with cytotoxic drugs improves this outlook and long remissions and even cures are now possible.

Clinical Features. These are very like those of Hodgkin's disease and range from an isolated enlarged lymph node to generalised lymphadenopathy in a very ill patient. Involvement outside the lymphatic system may occur early, particularly in the liver and bone marrow but often affecting other organs. Sometimes malignant lymphocytes appear in the peripheral blood in quite large numbers and this may make the distinction from chronic lymphatic leukaemia difficult.

Treatment depends on the histology and the extent of the disease.

Localised disease in the favourable histology group usually responds well to radiotherapy and this may be all that is needed. If the disease is localised but histologically unfavourable, radiotherapy should be followed by chemotherapy.

Generalised disease should be treated with chemotherapy. Those with favourable histology can be treated with:

(a) Chlorambucil 10 mg daily for 2 weeks in every month, or
(b) The COP regime:
Cyclophosphamide 600 mg/m² IV on days 1 and 8,
Vincristine (Oncovin) 1.5 mg IV on days 1 and 8,
Prednisolone 40 mg orally daily on days 1–8.

After 2 weeks without drugs the course is repeated. Both regimes are usually given over a period of one year.

Most patients respond well to one or other of these regimes but relapses occur in about 15% of patients per year. Further treatment may be successful but ultimately the disease becomes unresponsive. In elderly or frail patients drug treatment or radiotherapy may not be necessary if the disease is not causing any symptoms.

In patients with generalised disease caused by less favourable pathologies vigorous chemotherapy is required. The CHOP regime is widely used:

Cyclophosphamide 400 mg/m² IV on days 1 and 8,
Adriamycin 50 mg/m² IV on day 1 *only* (Maximum total accumulative dose 500 mg/m²),
Vincristine 1. 5 mg IV on days 1 and 8,
Prednisolone 40 mg/m² orally daily for 5 days.

The cycles are given every 3 or 4 weeks and are continued for a minimum of six cycles.

Although the prognosis for this group of non-Hodgkin's lymphomas is very poor if they are not treated, it is possible with chemotherapy to obtain a remission in about 60% of patients, the histiocytic group responding particularly well, and in some of these a cure is possible.

PLASMA CELL MALIGNANCIES AND RELATED CONDITIONS

Neoplasm arising from plasma cells may be of several types with differing natural histories. They usually produce an abnormal gamma globulin. The following will be considered:

multiple myeloma;
localised plasmacytoma;
Waldenström's macroglobulinaemia;
benign monoclonal gammopathy.

Multiple Myeloma (Myelomatosis)

The malignant cell in myeloma is probably derived from a B lymphocyte. These cells originate from a stem cell in the bone marrow and enter the lymphocyte pool as a clone of small lymphocytes. They re-enter the bone marrow again where they differentiate into plasma cells causing osteolytic change and producing a monoclonal immunoglobulin.

Clinical Features. The commonest initial symptom is bone pain, often of a rib or vertebra, but sometimes the first indication is an unexplained anaemia or fever. More rarely the disease presents with symptoms of spinal-cord compression causing bladder and bowel disturbances and lower limb weakness.

Impaired renal function and proteinuria are quite common and may be due to several causes:

(a) damage to the tubular epithelium by light chain fragments;
(b) amyloidosis;
(c) hypercalcaemia which occurs in 10–20% of patients and may produce polyuria, thirst, anorexia, constipation and sometimes a confusional state.

As a result of bone marrow involvement, anaemia is usual and may be either normocytic or occasionally macrocytic. Leucopenia and thrombocytopenia are rare in the early stages of the disease but may develop late in the disease or as a result of treatment. Occasionally plasma cells appear in the peripheral blood. Enlargement of the spleen or lymph nodes is very rare.

The plasma proteins show a distinct and discrete band on electrophoresis which may be associated with any of the major immunoglobulin groups and is due to an abnormal protein produced by the myeloma cells. Light chain fragments are also produced by the malignant cells and appear in the urine as Bence–Jones protein which is present in about 90% of patients. Although there is excess production of abnormal protein, the synthesis of normal immunoglobulins is depressed and this results in an increased tendency to intercurrent infections.

As a result of changes in the plasma proteins, the ESR is often very high.

The diagnosis depends upon:

(a) demonstration of excess plasma cells in the bone marrow;
(b) an abnormal immunoglobulin found on plasma electrophoresis together with low levels of normal immunoglobulins;
(c) the presence of Bence–Jones protein in the urine;
(d) osteolytic bone lesions which can be demonstrated on X-ray but only rarely by bone scanning.

Staging and Prognosis. Attempts have been made to stage the disease using such criteria as haemoglobin levels, amount of abnormal protein in the blood and the extent of the bone lesions. In general the immediate response to treatment is not related to the stage of the disease but the more widespread the disease at the time of diagnosis, the shorter the life expectancy. The outlook is also related to the type of immunoglobulin produced by the malignant cells, being best in patients with an excess of IgM. Survival is variable and is usually between 4 months and 4 years.

Treatment. *Chemotherapy*. There is as yet no agreement as to the most effective regime.

Melphalan 10 mg/m^2 with prednisolone 40 mg, both orally daily for 4 days, given at monthly intervals, produces a remission in about 60% of patients.

Multiple drug regimes are also used:

Cyclophosphamide 250 mg/m^2 daily for 3 days orally;
Melphalan 6 mg/m^2 daily for 3 days;
Prednisolone 40 mg daily for 3 days;
CCNU 50 mg/m^2 on day 4 *only*.

The course is repeated every four weeks.

Whether results are better with more complicated regimes has yet to be determined.

Symptomatic treatment is usually required. Blood transfusion may be necessary to treat anaemia and analgesics to relieve bone pain. Hypercalcaemia is quite a common and dangerous complication and its management is considered on p. 446.

Localised Plasmacytoma

A small number of patients have an isolated plasma-cell tumour with minimal changes in immunoglobulins. They are best treated by local radiotherapy. The prognosis is variable. A number of these patients rapidly develop evidence of widespread myelomatosis with the usual changes in plasma protein and in fact probably had myelomatosis from the start.

In a few, however, long survival and even apparent cures have been recorded, so presumably in these cases the myeloma was indeed solitary.

Waldenström's Macroglobulinaemia

In this rare disease there is infiltration of the lymphatic system and bone marrow by lymphoid cells which produce IgM.

Clinical Features. These may be general symptoms of tiredness and weight loss and this may be associated with a normocytic anaemia. A further group of symptoms can be related to the hyperviscosity of the blood and consists of spontaneous bleeding, various visual abnormalities due to the disturbances of retinal circulation and nervous system disorders including focal symptoms and signs and a peripheral neuropathy. Examination may show widespread lymphadenopathy and hepatosplenomegaly.

Treatment. Hyperviscosity can be relieved initially by plasmapheresis. The disease process can be controlled in some 40 % of patients by chlorambucil 8.0 mg/m^2 daily for 2 weeks with prednisolone 40 mg daily for 1 week, and the course repeated at 8-week intervals. Survival varies considerably but the average is about 3 years.

Benign Monoclonal Gammopathy

Plasma electrophoresis may occasionally show a monoclonal protein band in patients who have no other evidence of multiple myeloma. The abnormal protein is usually of the IgA type and serum concentration is less than 3.0 g/100 ml. There is no decrease in the concentration of the normal plasma proteins.

The prognosis in such patients, who are usually elderly, is good and they rarely develop myelomatosis. No treatment is required.

FURTHER READING

Wintrobe, M. M., *Clinical Haematology*, 8th edition, Lea and Febiger, Philadelphia, 1982.

CHAPTER 16

INFECTIOUS DISEASES

DEFINITION

Although the term 'infectious disease' might logically be applied to any illness which results from invasion of the body by a micro-organism, its use is customarily restricted to those diseases which spread by direct contact from patient to patient. This chapter therefore deals mainly with those diseases for which isolation or 'barrier nursing' is required to prevent spread of infection.

INFECTION AND IMMUNITY

The result of any infection depends partly on the virulence and numbers of the invading organisms and partly on the state of the patient's defences against them. The state of his defences depends partly on his *natural immunity*, which may be good or bad according to his race and heredity and may have been reduced by such factors as malnutrition, worry, and overwork, and partly on *acquired immunity* resulting from previous infection or prophylactic inoculation with this particular organism. Such inoculations given to stimulate the formation of antibodies constitute *active immunisation*, and are widely used in the prevention of such diseases as smallpox, diphtheria, tetanus, enteric fever, and poliomyelitis. *Passive immunisation* means conferring temporary protection against a disease by injecting serum containing the specific antibodies; such serum is obtained from humans who have recovered from the disease or from horses actively immunised for this purpose.

Carriers. Some people after recovering from an infectious disease continue to harbour the specific organisms and may transmit them from time to time to susceptible persons, either by direct contact or by infecting food or water. This carrier state is particularly important in the spread of enteric fever.

Routes of Infection. The invading organism usually gains access to the patient either in inspired air ('droplet infection') or in contaminated food or drink.

Incubation Period. This is the time which elapses between the access of organisms to the tissues of a susceptible individual and the onset of the first clinical symptoms. Its duration varies widely in the different infectious diseases, but remains fairly constant in each of them. The approximate length of the incubation period of the common specific fevers is:

Less than 7 days	Cerebrospinal meningitis
	Diphtheria
	Scarlet fever
10 to 14 days	Measles
	Whooping cough
	Small pox
	Enteric fever
14 to 21 days	Chicken-pox
(usually nearer *21*)	German measles
	Mumps

The incubation period is occasionally helpful in diagnosis if the date of exposure to a particular infection is known. The period of *quarantine* or isolation of contacts, used in serious diseases such as smallpox and where there is some special risk, is obtained by adding a few days (to be on the safe side) to the known incubation period.

Stage of Invasion. At the end of the incubation period the infecting organism or its toxic products become distributed throughout the body and give rise to the symptoms and signs of the disease. Common to all infectious diseases are fever, headache, general malaise, loss of appetite, dry furred tongue, hot dry skin, and scanty highly coloured urine; but in addition each has special features, which in many include a typical rash, which enable diagnosis to be made.

Barrier Nursing

To prevent direct transmission of organisms from patients with proven or suspected disease to other patients the technique known as 'barrier nursing' is employed. Preferably the patient is isolated in a separate room; if he must remain in a general ward the space between the adjoining beds is increased and a screen placed at the foot of the bed serves as a reminder that barrier precautions are being observed. Gowns are provided for all medical and nursing staff attending the patient; these may be hung within the 'barrier' with the 'dirty' side outermost or outside the barrier with the 'dirty' side turned inwards. The hands must be washed before removing the gown and again after leaving the barrier. For diseases spread by droplet infection masks should also be worn. To prevent indirect transmission of infection the patient's cutlery, crockery, and linen are kept separate, everything that has been near him being considered a possible source of infection.

Precautions

Routine vaccination of children against smallpox is no longer recommended in the UK since the risk of contracting the disease is now less than the risk of developing a serious complication of vaccination. *Encephalopathy* is a rare complication of whooping-cough vaccination

Table 16.1 Scheme of prophylactic inoculations for children

Age	*Vaccine*	*Interval*	*Notes*
During first year of life	Diph/Tet/Pert and first dose of oral Polio vaccine		The first dose should not be given before 3 months; a better immunological response is obtained if it is not given until 6 months of age.
	Diph/Tet/Pert and second dose of oral Polio vaccine	Preferably after an interval of 6–8 weeks.	
	Diph/Tet/Pert and third dose of oral Polio vaccine	Preferably after an interval of 6 months	
During second year of life	Measles vaccine	After an interval of not less than 3–4 weeks.	
At 5 years old or school entry	Diph/Tet and oral Polio vaccine		These may be given at 3 years to children at nursery school, day nurseries or homes.
Between 10–13 years of age	BCG vaccine		For tuberculin negative children.
At 15–19 years or on leaving school	Polio vaccine Tetanus toxoid		

Antigens for primary immunisation are now given later, at an age when antibody responses are no longer depressed by the presence of maternal antibody and the child is able to make antibody more efficiently.

and it is more likely to occur in infants with a history of convulsions; such children should be given combined diphtheria and tetanus vaccine instead of triple vaccine. Children with a history of asthma, hay fever, or eczema have a high incidence of *allergic reactions* after injections; they must be kept under observation for an hour after inoculation, therefore, and adrenaline must be immediately available for injection if needed. When a severe local reaction occurs after the first injection of triple vaccine it is probably the whooping-cough component which is responsible and for the subsequent injections it may be advisable to use only the combined diphtheria and tetanus vaccine.

When Does the Rash Come Out?

It is important to remember the day of the disease on which the specific eruption usually appears in the exanthemata. The following is a useful mnemonic:

	Disease	*Rash appears on*
Really	**Rubella**	1st day
Sick	**Scarlet Fever**	2nd day
People	**Small Pox**	3rd day
Must	**Measles**	4th day
Take	**Typhus**	5th day
No	**Nil**	—
Exercise	**Enteric**	7th day

BACTERIAL INFECTIONS

DIPHTHERIA

Diphtheria is an infection of the throat, nose or larynx (or occasionally the skin) and although the organism, *C. diphtheriae*, remains localised to this site, it produces a powerful exotoxin which becomes widely distributed and may cause serious or fatal effects on other parts of the body. The amount of exotoxin produced by different strains of the organism varies a good deal and that is one reason why some patients are much more serverely ill than others. Another reason for the variation in clinical severity is the state of the patient's immunity at the time of infection.

Immunity. Immunity to diphtheria may be acquired in three ways:

(1) After recovery from an attack of the disease.
(2) After repeated subclinical infection, that is, as a result of coming into contact from time to time with organisms insufficient in either numbers or virulence to cause a full-scale attack of diphtheria.
(3) As a result of active immunisation by inoculation. It is because of the widespread inoculation of children that this killing disease is much less common than it used to be; if immunisation were universally practised, as it should be, there would be no cases.

The Schick Test is used to detect whether an individual has immunity against diphtheria. Diphtheria toxin 0.2 ml is injected into the skin of the left forearm and 0.2 ml of the same toxin which has been heated to 70° C. to destroy its potency is injected into the skin of the right forearm as a control. The result is read in 5 to 7 days, as follows:

Positive. An area of redness and swelling at the site of injection on the left arm, with no reaction on the right (control) arm. This indicates that the person tested has no antitoxin with which to neutralise the toxin injected; in other words, he is *susceptible* to diphtheria.

Negative. No reaction in either arm. The injected toxin has been neutralised by antitoxin and the subject is therefore *immune* to diphtheria.

Positive plus 'Pseudo Reaction'. There is redness and swelling on both arms, but more on the left (test) arm than on the right (control) arm. The reaction on the right arm and part of the reaction on the left are due to some factor in the injection other than the actual toxin; the extra reaction on the left must be due to unneutralised toxin and the subject is therefore *susceptible* to diphtheria.

Negative plus 'Pseudo Reaction'. There is equal redness and swelling on both arms; the subject is *immune* to diphtheria.

Active Immunisation

All children should be immunised against diphtheria. The Schick test is used on adults who are exposed to special risk of infection, for example nurses and medical students, and those shown to be susceptible are immunised.

Immunisation of children may be effected by three injections of alum-precipitated toxoid (APT), but it is better to give a combined triple vaccine against diphtheria, whooping cough, and tetanus. The first dose of 0.3–0.5 ml of APT is given between three and nine months, the second of 0.5 ml is given four weeks later and the final boosting dose of 0.2 ml at the age of four. Adults are immunised in the same way, but if the preliminary Schick tests show a 'positive plus pseudo' result unpleasant reactions may follow the use of APT and it is better to use toxoid-antitoxin floccules (TAF). This is given in three doses of 1 ml each at intervals of two weeks and rarely causes any side effects.

Clinical Features of Diphtheria. Diphtheria is classified clinically according to the exact site of infection. The commonest variety is *faucial* diphtheria, in which the characteristic membrane of the disease forms in the throat. There is a short incubation period of only three or four days from exposure to infection. Points which help to distinguish diphtheria from streptococcal tonsillitis are:

(1) The throat is not so sore and the temperature usually not so high, but the general exhaustion and toxaemia are much greater.
(2) The lymph-nodes in the neck are usually enlarged to a greater extent, in severe cases causing a collar of swelling sometimes referred to as the 'bull-neck'.
(3) The exudate in the throat is not confined to yellowish spots on the tonsils, but forms a continuous greyish sheet of membrane which often extends forwards over the soft palate and backwards on to the pharyngeal wall and is so firmly adherent that any attempt to wipe it off leaves a bleeding surface.

Less common and more difficult to diagnose is *nasal diphtheria*, in which the membrane is confined to the nose, where it may lead to a bloodstained nasal discharge; and *laryngeal diphtheria*, a very dangerous form in which the membrane on the larynx may obstruct breathing and necessitate emergency tracheotomy. *Cutaneous diphtheria* is very rare in this country, but in troops serving in the East during the war it was a common cause of so-called 'jungle-sores' or 'desert-sores', the true nature of which was often not appreciated until the development of post-diphtheritic paralysis.

Complications. The complications of diphtheria are due to the effects on the heart and nervous system of the exotoxin absorbed from the lesions in the upper respiratory tract or skin.

Carditis may occur during the second week and is characterised by vomiting, a greyish pallor, a weak rapid pulse, low blood pressure, diminished urinary output, usually with some albuminuria, and sometimes pain over the heart. Conduction defects such as heart block may be found. Sudden death is not uncommon in these cases, but no permanent cardiac lesion results in patients who recover.

Paralysis. Paralysis of the palate is the commonest type and causes a nasal voice and regurgitation of food through the nose. It usually appears in the second or third weeks and may extend to the pharyngeal muscles, causing difficulty in swallowing, or rarely to the intercostal muscles or diaphragm, causing weakness in breathing and necessitating treatment with a mechanical respirator. There is sometimes paralysis of the ciliary muscle, causing difficulty in reading, and lateral rectus (sixth nerve) palsy is not uncommon. Towards the fifth or sixth weeks peripheral neuritis may occur, causing weakness in the limbs of varying degree. Complete recovery from all types of diphtheritic weakness occurs, but may take as long as six months.

Treatment

Antitoxin and Antibiotics

Although a throat or nasal swab should always be taken whenever diphtheria is suspected, the disease is so dangerous that treatment must invariably be started at once without waiting for the result of the culture. The most important measure is the immediate administration of antitoxin. The dose varies from about 8 000–100 000 units, according to the severity of the infection and it is usual to give half the total dose intramusculary and then if there has been no serum reaction within 15–30 minutes to give the remainder, warmed to body temperature, by slow intravenous injection. The latter route should be avoided, however, in patients giving a history of allergic phenomena, owing to the serious risk of fatal anaphylaxis; and any patient who develops vomiting, wheezing, urticaria, or collapse must be given 0.5 ml of 1 : 1000 adrenaline subcutaneously without delay and an antihistamine, for example promethazine 25 mg, by slow intramuscular injection. It is usual also to give intramuscular benzylpenicillin, 100 000 to 500 000 units every 4 hours with erythromycin 250 mg 4-hourly, but it should be stressed that these are less important than the antitoxin.

Nursing

The patient is nursed flat in bed with only one pillow and as complete rest is essential everything, including feeding, must be done for him. In patients with acute carditis these conditions may have to be maintained for some two or three months. Local treatment of the throat probably does more harm than good, but ordinary cleanliness of the mouth is important. If palatal and pharyngeal paresis occur tube-feeding may become necessary.

Control of Outbreaks

When a case of diphtheria occurs in a closed community such as a school or a hospital ward the parents and District Community Physician are notified and the patient is transferred to an infectious diseases unit. The parents of contacts are also notified and combined active and passive immunisation of the latter is carried out. Antitoxin 1000 units is given into the deltoid of one arm and the first 0.5 ml of APT into the other. Four weeks later the second injection of 0.5 ml of APT completes the procedure.

Sometimes an outbreak of diphtheria can be traced to a healthy *carrier* and it is important that his infection be eradicated to prevent further spread of the disease. This can sometimes be achieved by giving large doses of penicillin, 2–4 million units daily, combined with sulphadimidine 4–6 g daily for up to a week. If the infection persists tonsillectomy may be indicated.

WHOOPING COUGH (Pertussis)

Whooping cough is an infection of the respiratory tract by either *Bordetella pertussis* or a virus. In this country at present it is the most serious of the acute specific fevers of childhood, not only causing many deaths in young children, particularly under the age of twelve months, but also occasionally leading to serious damage to the bronchi and lungs (see bronchiectasis, p. 264). Asthma in childhood also sometimes dates from an attack of whooping cough. Infants receive no passive immunity from the mother and are therefore susceptible to the infection from birth.

Clinical Features. After an incubation period of about 7–14 days the child develops what is thought at first to be an ordinary cold on the chest, but within a week of onset the paroxysms of coughing have usually become so severe and typical that the diagnosis is obvious. A characteristic paroxysm consists of a deep inspiration followed by a rapid series of explosive coughs during expiration. The tongue protrudes, the face and lips become deeply cyanosed and the attack may end with the inspiration of air through a partially closed glottis, producing the classical whoop. Paroxysm may follow paroxysm until a little sticky mucus is expectorated or until the child vomits and sinks back exhausted. During the spasms of coughing the tongue may be abraded against the lower incisors, causing a traumatic ulcer on the fraenum; rectal prolapse, hernia, and haemorrhage, particularly under the conjunctiva, may also be induced.

In young infants, however, cough is often not such a prominent symptom. Instead, procedures such as feeding or changing may induce cyanotic attacks, in which the child becomes flaccid, blue, and alarmingly lifeless. There may also be frequent vomiting. Furthermore, immunised subjects may have a mild form of the disease without the typical paroxysmal cough or whoop. The diagnosis may remain very obscure until the appearance of a few feeble whoops at the end of attacks. The preliminary catarrhal stage is short in duration but highly infectious; the paroxysmal stage and whooping may continue for many weeks but the infectivity is now very slight.

Diagnosis. The paroxysmal coughing is virtually diagnostic, but bacteriological confirmation may be obtained by isolation of *B. pertussis* on 'cough plates' (a Petri dish held in front of the patient's mouth) or better, by taking a post-nasal swab. *B. pertussis* does not grow readily, however, and special culture media are essential. It is now thought that patients with negative cultures have virus infection. The blood count shows a lymphocytosis, but young children have a high lymphocyte count in health so that no significance should be attached to a count of less than 70% of 20 000.

Complications. *Acute bronchitis* and *bronchopneumonia* are the most serious complications and account for most of the deaths which occur in infancy and in old age. *Collapse* of bronchopulmonary segments, or less often of lobes of the lung, from plugging of bronchioles or bronchi by sticky mucus may lead to bronchiectasis if allowed to persist. A radiograph should be taken, therefore, and appropriate physiotherapy instituted if necessary. *Otitis media* is the other common infective complication. *Convulsions* occur more often in whooping cough than in any of the other specific fevers. *Spontaneous pneumothorax* may occur.

Treatment. Erythromycin 12.5 mg/kg body weight orally four times daily in the first week of infection may attenuate the symptoms and should be given to infants under one year old. Feeding is often a problem; the diet is most likely to be retained if given after an episode of vomiting. Cyanotic attacks in infants should be treated by freeing the airway and re-establishing breathing by gentle pressure on the chest. It may also be advisable to nurse such a child in an oxygen tent. Chlorpromazine or promethazine in small doses may help to reduce the frequency of paroxysms.

Prophylactic Inoculation. Suspended whooping cough vaccine may be given subcutaneously or intramuscularly. It is best given as a combined triple vaccine against diphtheria, whooping cough, and tetanus (p. 639).

SCARLET FEVER

When seen in historical perspective many infective diseases go through periods of increased or decreased severity, and scarlet fever at the present time is a much less serious illness than it was in the first two decades of this century. It is a haemolytic streptococcal infection which is distinguished from other diseases due to the same organism by its typical rash; this rash indicates that the streptococcus concerned is of a strain which produces a special erythrogenic toxin and that the patient is susceptible to its action.

The **Dick test** is performed by injecting 0.2 ml of erythrogenic toxin into the skin of the forearm, no control injection in the other arm being necessary. A red swollen area at the site of injection in 24 hours shows that the person tested is *susceptible* to the toxin (Dick positive); no reaction shows that he is *immune* (Dick negative). The test is little used at the present time.

Clinical Features. After a short incubation period of less than a week the illness starts abruptly with sore throat, fever, shivering, and often vomiting. Small children may not complain of sore throat, but examination shows that the tonsils and fauces are very red and swollen and the tonsils may be covered with patches of soft, yellowish exudate. At first the tongue is covered with a white fur, which peels off from the edges during the next two or three days, leaving a clean surface with enlarged red papillae—the 'strawberry' or 'raspberry' tongue.

The *rash* appears on the second day and is described as a punctate erythema; the skin is a bright scarlet colour and on close inspection is seen to be covered with minute red spots. It appears first behind the ears and on the side of the neck and spreads rapidly over the whole body, but avoiding the area round the mouth (giving the so-called 'circum-oral pallor') and tending to be particularly heavy in flexures such as the axillae, cubital fossae, and groins. After about a week 'pin-hole desquamation' of the skin starts: little round pieces of dead skin flake off, temporarily leaving small holes in the superficial layers of the epidermis.

Septic Scarlet Fever, in which there is suppuration of cervical lymph nodes as well as extensive septic infection in the throat, and **Toxic Scarlet Fever,** in which there is overwhelming toxaemia characterised by circulatory failure, delirium and stupor with minimal faucial reaction and rash, are severe and often fatal forms of the disease fortunately rare at the present time.

Complications. Local spread of infection may cause peritonsillar abscess (quinsy), retropharyngeal abscess, sinusitis, and cervical adenitis while aspiration may cause bronchitis and pneumonia, but none of these is common nowadays.

Late complication, occurring some three weeks after the original illness, are those which may follow any streptococcal tonsillitis, namely acute nephritis, rheumatic fever and anaphylactoid purpura.

Treatment. For the mildest form of the disease oral penicillin (phenoxymethyl penicillin) 250 mg four times daily or phenethicillin 125 mg four times daily is satisfactory. For more severe infections benzyl penicillin 250 000–1 000 000 units should be given 6-hourly IM for the first two days, followed by oral penicillin. To ensure eradication of haemolytic streptococci and minimise the risk of acute nephritis and rheumatic fever it is wise to continue penicillin therapy for ten days. Patients allergic to penicillin may be given erythromycin 250–500 mg orally every 6 hours for 10 days.

ENTERIC FEVER

Enteric is the name applied to a group of diseases which consists of *typhoid fever* and *paratyphoid A, B, and C*. They are due to closely related salmonella organisms, short thick motile Gram-negative bacilli which can be distinguished from most of the non-pathogenic organisms of the colityphoid group by their inability to ferment lactose. Typhoid and paratyphoid B occur all over the world, the latter being the most common of the enteric fevers in this country; paratyphoid A is found mainly in the East; paratyphoid C is rare.

Method of Spread. Enteric fever is spread by contamination of food or water by excreta from carriers or from patients with the disease. It is therefore prevalent in countries whose standards of sanitation are low and armies on active service in the tropics are at special risk. The sharp reduction in the incidence of the disease which occurred in this country at the end of the nineteenth century was due to the introduction of methods of sewage disposal which prevent access to the water supplies. In countries with good sanitation outbreaks can usually be traced to unsuspecting carriers of the disease who are engaged in the handling of foodstuffs.

Clinical Features. After an incubation period of about a fortnight there is usually a gradual onset of *headache, aching* in the limbs, *tiredness, cough,* and *fever*, which typically rises in 'step-ladder' fashion by about half a degree (C) daily to reach a height of perhaps 39–40° C towards the end of the first week. For the next week, or sometimes much longer, the temperature continues at this high level, showing very little variation throughout the twenty-four hours. The pulse usually does not show the increase in rate which accompanies most febrile illnesses, a *relative bradycardia* of less than 100 per minute being frequently maintained through the whole course of the illness. *Cough* and signs of bronchitis or even bronchopneumonia are common in the first few days and may dominate the clinical picture at this stage.

In suspected cases watch must be kept about the end of the first week for the appearance of the characteristic *rash*. In typhoid this consists of a few 'rose-spots', which can easily be overlooked but which nevertheless are very typical of the disease. They occur particularly on the abdomen or chest and appear for a few days in a succession of crops of tiny pink spots, each not more than 1–2 mm in diameter and each one lasting for only 24 hours or so. It is useful, therefore, to make a ring with a skin pencil round each spot seen so that the next day if any new ones have appeared it is clear at a glance that they are a new crop. In paratyphoid the rash is often much more profuse and may be composed of much larger less clearly defined elements which tend to coalesce with each other, producing an eruption rather like that of measles. The spleen often becomes palpable at about the same time as the rash appears.

Most patients are constipated during the first few days, but towards the end of the second week the abdomen becomes distended and *diarrhoea* sets in. By this time if the attack is a severe one the patient is very gravely ill and may pass into the 'typhoid state', in which he remains throughout the 24 hours in what has been called a 'coma-vigil', drowsy and confused but continually muttering to himself, plucking at the bedclothes, and groping for non-existent objects. The faeces are now fluid and light yellow in colour ('pea-soup stools') and up to twenty may be passed in 24 hours.

Gradual improvement usually occurs during the third and fourth weeks; the temperature settles by lysis, the diarrhoea stops, the mind becomes clearer and the other symptoms also slowly disappear. Very occasionally relapse occurs in convalescence: the writer has seen one patient before the antibiotic era who went through the whole course of typhoid fever three times within six months before making a complete recovery.

Diagnosis

Blood culture is by far the best way of establishing the diagnosis, and as the organisms circulate in the blood only during the first week it is extremely important that blood should be taken for culture as early as possible, preferably during the first three days.

Blood count typically shows a leucopenia, but this is not a constant finding, particularly in paratyphoid, and in the presence of bronchitis or other complication there may even be a slight leucocytosis.

Agglutinations (Widal test). As a rise in the agglutinin titre during the illness is the most important evidence of active infection, blood should be taken for this estimation at the same time as the initial blood culture during the first few days, and again during the second week. Quite high titres of 'H' (flagellar) agglutinin may be found in the blood of healthy people who have been inoculated with TAB, but a rising titre of 'O' (somatic) agglutinins is usually indicative of enteric infection. A high titre of 'Vi' (virulence) agglutinin is also usually significant.

Complications. The two most serious complications of typhoid are liable to occur during the third week of illness, when sloughs separate from the Peyer's patches in the ileum leaving deep ulcers which may *perforate* or cause serious *haemorrhage*. Such *perforations* are easily overlooked clinically. By the time they occur the patient is in such a weak state that very little peritoneal reaction takes place and nothing approaching the dramatic pain and tenderness of the patient with a perforated peptic ulcer is to be expected; the only clue may be a sudden worsening of the general clinical condition, with a fall in the temperature and a rise in the pulse and respiration rates and the appearance of minimal abdominal tenderness. Before the days of antibiotics surgical closure of the perforation gave the only hope of recovery, but patients receiving chloramphenicol can usually be treated conservatively. *Haemorrhage* is more common than perforation; it is suggested by sudden faintness, pallor, and sweating, and diagnosed by the appearance of bright-red blood in the next stool passed. Transfusion is occasionally necessary but surgery never.

Venous thrombosis, particularly in the femoral vein, is common.

Parotitis is a dangerous complication which should be prevented by careful attention to the hygiene of the mouth.

Cholecystitis, with the subsequent formation of gall-stones containing *Salmonella typhi*, and *acute arthritis*, are rare complications.

Typhoid abscesses in bone and periostitis causing the stiff and painful *typhoid spine* are very rare sequelae which may appear years after the original infection.

Treatment. The prognosis of typhoid has been greatly improved since the introduction of chloramphenicol, which is usually very effective. A satisfactory scheme of dosage for an adult is 1.5 g twice daily for the first five days, then 0.75 g twice daily for a week, and finally 1 g daily for a few more days. Agglutination titres are lower and relapses more common than in untreated patients but the relapses usually respond satisfactorily to further courses of chloramphenicol. Subsequent development of the carrier state is no commoner in treated than in untreated patients, but chloramphenicol usually fails to eradicate the organisms from carriers and for this purpose cholecystectomy remains the most useful measure.

Ampicillin, in doses of 8 g daily, is also effective but rather slower in producing a response than chloramphenicol.

Patients with typhoid must of course be nursed with strict barrier precautions. They should be given a high-calorie low-roughage diet.

Prophylactic immunisation against the enteric fevers is achieved by giving TABC vaccine intramuscularly, 0.5 ml, followed a week later by a second inoculation of 1 ml. Those living in endemic areas should receive 'booster' doses of 0.5 ml annually.

STAPHYLOCOCCAL FEVER

Staphylococci may invade the bloodstream from abscesses in any part of the body, the most common primary lesions being skin boils and carbuncles, lung abscess, osteomyelitis, and renal carbuncle. Factors tending to promote bloodstream invasion are the early incision of abscesses and attempts to evacuate pus by squeezing, and general debility due to chronic fatigue, malnutrition, or serious underlying disease such as diabetes or leukaemia.

Outbreaks of antibiotic-resistant staphylococcal infection have become a serious menace in hospital wards in recent years, the organism being disseminated by contact with such articles as blankets and bed-curtains, and by healthy carriers.

Clinical Features. The initial staphylococcal lesion may be an apparently trivial one, unsuspected by the patient as the source of his subsequent severe illness. The onset of septicaemia is heralded by *rigors* and *fever* which is usually high and remittent or intermittent in type. Profuse *sweats* are common and sometimes there is a relative bradycardia. Metastatic *abscesses* develop in various sites, notably the lungs, joints, muscles, and skin, and purpura is also common. Bacterial endocarditis should be suspected when there are changing cardiac murmurs and when septicaemia persists in the absence of obvious staphylococcal lesions elsewhere. Some anaemia and leucocytosis are usual and the diagnosis is clinched by a positive *blood culture*.

Treatment. In spite of modern antibiotic therapy the mortality rate is still high. When staphylococcal septicaemia is suspected clinically, blood should be taken for culture and treatment started with benzylpenicillin 10 mega units daily together with flucloxacillin 2.0 g daily. Treatment should be continued for at least two weeks (six weeks if endocarditis is suspected). If a satisfactory response is not obtained, sodium fusidate 500 mg thrice daily can be added to the treatment. If blood culture reveals other organisms antibiotic treatment should be adjusted accordingly.

CEREBROSPINAL FEVER (Meningococcal Meningitis)

This disease is endemic throughout the world and in this country it is seen mainly during the winter months. From time to time epidemics occur, usually localised ones in residential institutions such as military barracks. Sporadic cases are commonest in infancy, while outbreaks affect adolescents and young adults.

Transmission is by droplet infection from patients and carriers and in susceptible contacts the meningococcus enters the bloodstream from the nasopharynx, causing a septicaemia. Usually, but not always, the infection then becomes localised to the meninges.

Clinical Features

(1) **Usual Meningitic Form.** After an incubation period of two or three days the illness starts rather suddenly, often with a shivering attack or rigor, followed by fever, severe headache, and vomiting. Convulsions

are common in children. Within a few days signs of acute meningeal irritation develop: these are *neck rigidity* and a positive *Kernig's sign.* About 30% of patients have a macular rash which rapidly becomes purpuric and is of great help in clinical diagnosis. Although the eruption may be profuse, there are frequently only a few lesions which are easily overlooked unless a careful search is made for them.

Diagnosis is established by lumbar puncture, which reveals turbid fluid under increased pressure. The fluid contains large numbers of polymorphs, and meningococci can be demonstrated either by microscopy of a stained film or on culture.

(2) **Fulminating Meningococcal Meningitis.** This rapidly fatal but fortunately rare form starts very abruptly with high fever and within a few hours the patient is in coma with signs of acute meningitis and a profuse petechial rash. In spite of treatment death usually occurs within 24–48 hours.

(3) **Friderichsen–Waterhouse Syndrome.** Also fortunately rare, this syndrome is the result of bilateral adrenal haemorrhages accompanying the purpura of acute meningococcal (and other) septicaemias and is usually seen in children. Acute adrenal insufficiency leads to vomiting, collapse, and low blood pressure. Cortisone 200–300 mg daily must be given in addition to antibiotic therapy but rarely averts the fatal outcome.

(4) **Chronic Meningococcal Septicaemia.** This curious, recurrent, and often puzzling disease, which has become much rarer since the introduction of the sulphonamides and antibiotics, causes little constitutional upset but presents with bouts of low fever, accompanied by headache, joint pains, and a maculopapular rash on the trunk and limbs. On the legs the eruption may mimic erythema nodosum and sometimes, though not always, it contains purpuric elements. Such attacks may recur at varying intervals over a period of many months. The diagnosis is confirmed by isolation of the meningococcus on blood culture.

Treatment. Sulphonamides should no longer be used alone as many strains of meningococci are now resistant to them and benzylpenicillin is the drug of choice. Penicillin crosses the blood–brain barrier better when the meninges are inflamed and adequate concentration can be achieved in the CSF when large doses are given intravenously. Adults should be given 20–30 mega units daily in divided doses 6-hourly by rapid IV infusion over 20–30 minutes. Treatment should continue for 5–7 days. Sulphadiazine may be given in addition by mouth, 1.5 g 4-hourly for 2 days, then 1.0 g 4-hourly for 2 days and finally 1.0 g 6-hourly for 3–4 days.

VIRUS INFECTIONS

SMALLPOX (Variola)

It may well be possible to omit this section from future editions since it is believed that smallpox has now been eradicated from the world. The accidental transmission of the virus to laboratory workers in Birmingham in 1978, however, suggests that it may be wise not to discard it too quickly.

There are three varieties of the smallpox virus. The first causes true Asiatic smallpox (*variola major*), which has a high mortality rate; the second causes a much milder disease (*alastrim* or *variola minor*); and the third is the one used for vaccination, which, though it retains the power to stimulate immunity against smallpox, can no longer itself cause a serious disease.

Routine vaccination against smallpox is no longer practised.

Clinical Features. After an incubation period of about a fortnight (exactly 12 days in most patients) there is sudden onset of headache, fever, shivering, severe pain in the back, and generalised aching in the limbs. In the most severe cases a prodromal purpuric rash may be seen almost from the start, but the true eruption of smallpox does not appear until the third day. Mucosal lesions are often the first to appear and may be very extensive in the mouth and throat. When the disease is very severe the skin of the whole body may be covered by the rash (confluent smallpox), but usually it can be seen that the peripheral parts of the limbs are more thickly covered with spots than the proximal limb segments and the trunk. Each spot starts as a red discoloration (a *macule*), but within about 24 hours it becomes thick and raised so that it can be felt with the finger (a *papule*). About three days later the centre of the papule becomes soft and filled with clear serous fluid, so that it is now a *vesicle*; and secondary infection of the fluid with pyogenic bacteria changes it in a few days into pus, so that the lesion now becomes a *pustule*. All the spots go through this series of changes at approximately the same time. A day or two after the appearance of the rash the patient's temperature may come down and his general condition improve, but a few days later, when the lesions have become pustular, the fever returns and he again becomes gravely ill. Most of the deaths (up to 25% of the patients in some epidemics of variola major; 16 out of 64 patients in one outbreak dealt with by the writer) occur during the pustular stage, though in the most severe but fortunately rare form of the disease (*haemorrhagic smallpox*) death occurs within 48 hours of the onset with signs of bleeding into internal organs and from various mucosal surfaces. In patients who recover, the temperature slowly settles over a period of a week or so as the pustules gradually dry off into crusts and scabs. Since the crusts contain living virus, the patient has to be kept in isolation until they have all come away: this may take several weeks, the last to separate being the deep-seated scabs in the palms of the hands and soles of the feet.

Modified Variola Major and Variola Minor. Variola major modified by partial immunity from past vaccination and variola minor are relatively trivial illnesses with only slight constitutional upset and a rash which may be very difficult to distinguish from that of chickenpox.

Diagnosis. In distinguishing mild smallpox from chickenpox the following points are helpful:

(1) The lesions of chickenpox are set more superficially in the skin and tend to be smaller.
(2) In chickenpox the lesions are more profuse on the trunk than on the extremities; the reverse is true of smallpox,
(3) In chickenpox the eruption appears in a series of crops, so that at any one time lesions at different stages of maturity can be found; in smallpox the lesions are all at the same stage.
(4) Recent successful vaccination excludes smallpox.
(5) The diagnosis of smallpox can be confirmed within a few hours by electronmicroscopy of scrapings from the base of a lesion.
(6) Virus culture on the chorio-allantoic membrane of a chick embryo is the only positive proof of smallpox, but takes 72 hours.

Complications include bronchopneumonia, otitis media, conjunctivitis, corneal ulceration and resultant opacity, cardiac failure, and encephalitis.

Treatment. There is no specific therapy against the virus of smallpox, but the stage of secondary pyogenic infection can be cut short by the administration of a suitable antibiotic. Penicillin by injection or one of the tetracyclines by mouth may be given for this purpose and if necessary changed later when the *in vitro* sensitivities of the organism isolated from the lesions have been established. Skilled nursing is of great importance, particular attention being paid to the care of the mouth, eyes, and skin.

Action to be Taken when Smallpox is Suspected

(1) The District Community Physician must be notified immediately.

(2) If the diagnosis is confirmed the patient is transferred at once to a special smallpox hospital.

(3) All members of the hospital staff and all who have been in contact with the patient must be vaccinated or revaccinated. N-methylisatinthiosemicarbazone (Marboran) given by mouth to contacts within the incubation period has been reported as giving remarkable protection and may replace vaccination for this purpose. The dose is 1.5–3 g twice daily for four days.

In addition the District Community Physician will take further action to trace the source of infection and to prevent further spread; this will include disinfection of the patient's house and keeping his family and other contacts under supervision for at least 16 days.

Prevention by Vaccination

Edward Jenner introduced vaccination at the end of the eighteenth century after noting that milkers who had had cowpox (vaccinia) appeared to be immune to smallpox. This is because the virus of smallpox is attenuated by passage through the cow, though it retains its antigenic properties.

Technique of Vaccination. Fresh glycerinated calf lymph is obtained from the public health laboratory service and stored in a refrigerator. Secondary infection is least common when the vaccination is performed over the deltoid area. The skin at the chosen site is cleaned with soap and water and dried with a sterile towel; alternatively ether or acetone may be used, but spirit and iodine should be avoided as they may kill the virus and so prevent the vaccination taking. Using a rubber bulb a drop of lymph is ejected from the capillary tube on to the prepared area of skin and a sterile Hagedorn needle, held parallel to the skin, is moved rapidly up and down through the lymph, just sufficient pressure being applied to penetrate the epidermis at the point of the needle. This is the *multiple pressure technique*, which is superior to the old scratch method as it limits the depth of penetration of the virus into the skin and reduces the incidence of complications. About 10 pressures are recommended for primary vaccination and 30 pressures for revaccination. After a few minutes (during which time the area should not be exposed to direct sunlight) excess lymph is dabbed off and a dry sterile dressing is applied.

Results of Vaccination. Successful vaccination may be indicated by three types of reaction:

(1) The *primary reaction* (obtained in people who have not been vaccinated before) is the appearance by the third or fourth day of a papule which develops through a vesicular stage to become a pustule by the seventh day (when the result is read). During this week there may be fever, malaise, and axillary adenitis. A scab forms in the second week and separates in the third week, leaving a permanent pitted scar.

(2) The *accelerated reaction* is seen in people with partial immunity. The lesion goes through its stages more quickly and may never become pustular.

(3) The *immune reaction*, seen in people with a higher degree of immunity, consists simply of a small itchy papule on the second or third day which disappears without becoming vesicular.

Contraindications to Vaccination. Vaccination should be avoided in infants with eczema since it may cause a generalised pustular rash which may be fatal (eczema vaccinatum); it should be postponed if possible in patients with septic skin lesions; and it should be avoided if possible in people with conditions predisposing to generalised vaccinia (hypogammaglobulinaemia, long-term steroid therapy and blood dyscrasias such as leukaemia).

Complications of vaccination are very rare and particularly so in infancy.

Encephalitis (see p. 366) is much the most serious and has a mortality of about 50%. Its incidence is about 1 in 100 000 vaccinations.

Generalised vaccinia, in which lesions occur on the skin all over the body from widespread dissemination of the virus, is also very rare except in people with eczema, who should not be vaccinated unless exposed to special risk.

Secondary infection of the vaccination site and *accidental inoculation* of other areas of skin by scratching are commoner and less serious complications.

Foetal mortality is high in women vaccinated during the first three months of pregnancy and this time should consequently be avoided for vaccination whenever possible.

CHICKENPOX (Varicella)

The virus of chickenpox is identical or closely allied to the virus of herpes zoster (shingles); susceptible children who come into contact with shingles frequently develop chickenpox, while less often adult contacts of the latter disease may develop shingles.

Clinical Features. After an incubation period of up to three weeks the illness may start with a day of vague malaise, headache, fever, and a transient prodromal rash, before the specific eruption appears, but more often the rash is the first sign of the disease. Vesicles appear first in the mouth and throat and soon rupture, leaving ulcers which may cause a good deal of pain and difficulty in swallowing. The skin rash, unlike that of smallpox, is most profuse on the trunk and sparsest at the periphery of the limbs; and instead of all the lesions going through their various stages together, the spots appear in a succession of crops over several days, so that at any one time papules, vesicles, pustules and crusts can be seen together. The papules develop within a few hours into small round vesicles containing clear fluid set in the superficial layers of the skin. Within two or three days they become pustules and then dry up into crusts.

Constitutional upset is usually slight, though the enanthem (mucosal lesions) may cause much discomfort and the exanthem (skin rash) much itching. The disease is more severe in adults, who may develop patchy consolidation in the lungs and may subsequently be found to have scattered calcified opacities on chest X-ray.

Complications are unusual. Secondary infection may lead to boils, impetigo, cellulitis, or conjunctivitis. More serious but very rare are polyneuritis, transverse myelitis, and encephalitis.

Diagnosis from smallpox; see p. 651.

Treatment is purely symptomatic. Irritation of the skin can be relieved by the application of calamine lotion containing 1–2% phenol, or by warm boracic baths, and antihistamine tablets may be helpful.

MEASLES (Morbilli)

Next to whooping cough this is the most serious of the infectious fevers of childhood at the present time. Passive immunity from the mother prevents infection in the first three months of life, but thereafter the child becomes highly susceptible.

Clinical Features. About 10–14 days after exposure to infection there develops what appears to be a common cold, with fever, running nose and eyes, sneezing, and cough. Examination of the mouth, however, reveals an eruption of tiny white spots like grains of salt set on a slightly reddened base, usually best seen on the mucous membrane inside the cheeks opposite the molar teeth. These are *Koplik's spots* and they are diagnostic of measles. If they are overlooked the erroneous impression that the child simply has a cold may appear to be confirmed on the third day, when the temperature may come down to normal, but this opinion is finally refuted on the fourth day, when the rash appears on the skin.

Transient prodromal rashes are sometimes seen during the first three days, but the true *morbilliform eruption* appears on the fourth day as pink macules, about 3–5 mm in diameter, which first appear behind the ears and quickly spread over the face, trunk, and limbs. Within a day or two the lesions enlarge and become papular, many of them coalesce into large, irregular, blotchy areas, and their colour gradually changes to a darker red. The temperature rises again with the appearance of the rash and continues for several days before finally subsiding as the lesions fade.

Complications are mainly due to secondary bacterial infection of the respiratory tract. *Bronchopneumonia* is the most serious of them, particularly in very young children, and should always be suspected in a severely ill child with a persistent cough. *Otitis media* is fairly common. *Corneal ulceration* and potential blindness should be prevented by careful treatment of any conjunctival inflammation which occurs.

Treatment. The virus of measles is not susceptible to any form of specific treatment, but antibiotics are of value for the prevention and cure of secondary bacterial complications. Save in the mildest cases it is probably wise to give a course of penicillin, starting with the appearance of the rash and continuing for up to a week. Procaine penicillin 300 000 units twice daily may be given intramuscularly, but phenoxymethyl penicillin 250 mg 6-hourly, is almost as satisfactory and avoids the necessity of injections.

Prevention. Effective measles vaccines are now available and the best course for inducing *active immunity* is probably to give 0.5 ml killed vaccine intramuscularly followed by 0.5 ml of live vaccine one month later. A rise in temperature may occur after live vaccine and it should not be given to children under 9 months, to pregnant women or to patients with infective or neoplastic disease. Rapid *passive immunisation* lasting two or three weeks can be achieved by the intramuscular injection of gamma globulin, from 150–900 mg during the first five days after exposure to infection. Large doses prevent the attack of measles; smaller doses have the advantage that, although an attack of measles may occur, it will be a mild one and recovery from it will leave lifelong immunity.

Subacute Sclerosing Panencephalitis (SSPE) (see p. 368)

GERMAN MEASLES (Rubella)

This is a less infectious disease than true measles and even in towns many people reach adult life without acquiring it. It causes little constitutional upset and is never fatal, but when acquired by women in the first four months of pregnancy it may lead to development defects in the foetus. Cataract, glaucoma, disorders of retinal pigmentation, deaf mutism, and congenital heart disease are the lesions commonly caused. There is also an increased incidence of abortion, miscarriage, and stillbirth, but fetal injury is not inevitable and a proportion of women who have had rubella early in pregnancy do produce healthy live babies. It is now recommended that girls who have not had rubella should be given a single dose of live attenuated rubella virus, Cendehill strain, between the ages 11–14. No other vaccine should be given within 3–4 weeks. This vaccine must not be given to pregnant women because of the risk of foetal damage, or to patients with Hodgkin's disease or leukaemia or to those on immunosuppressive therapy..

Clinical Features. After an incubation period of two to three weeks the rash is usually the first indication of the disease, and takes the form of small pink macules and papules which remain distinct units and do not run together as in true measles. There are no Koplik's spots in the mouth. The only other notable feature is generalised lymph node enlargement, affecting particularly the nodes at the back of the neck. There are rarely any general symptoms of illness and the rash usually fades in two or three days. In adults a transient mild arthritis is common.

No **treatment** is needed. The disease may be prevented in women in early pregnancy who have been exposed to infection by giving high-titre immunoglobulin if available; protection lasts for three weeks. Ordinary gammaglobulin is of little value.

MUMPS (Epidemic Parotitis)

Mumps is a relatively trivial illness in young children, but if contracted after puberty it may have serious complications. There are undoubted advantages, therefore, in 'getting it over with' early in life, and only if a child is in a weak state of health from some other illness should any steps be taken to isolate him from this infection.

Clinical Features. After an incubation period of three weeks or a little longer the patient develops fever, malaise, and stiffness in the jaw, and examination reveals swelling of one or more of the salivary glands. Usually the parotid glands are affected and fill out the hollow between the angle of the jaw and the mastoid process. Sometimes the submandibular glands are affected too, or occasionally they are involved alone. There is no rash and usually the fever and glandular swellings subside within a few days.

The *diagnosis* is usually easy, but if there is doubt it can be confirmed by isolation of the virus from saliva, or by demonstrating a rising antibody titre in two specimens of serum taken at the onset of illness and a fortnight later.

Complications are almost confined to adolescent and adult patients and usually arise a few days after the swelling of the salivary glands.

Orchitis is the commonest complication, being seen in about 25% of patients. It is usually unilateral and causes severe pain and swelling of the testicle. Very rarely it may be bilateral and result in sterility.

Oophoritis is less common and causes severe lower abdominal pain and vomiting.

Prostatitis should be suspected in patients with unexplained fever and perhaps some frequency of micturition.

Mastitis, causing pain and swelling of the breast, may be seen in either sex.

Pancreatitis is characterised by severe upper abdominal pain, fever and vomiting.

Meningitis. Routine lumbar puncture in patients with mumps usually reveals a pleocytosis in the CSF, so that invasion of the nervous system by the virus is common, but in only about 10% of cases is there clinical evidence of meningitis (headache, fever, vomiting, and neck rigidity). These symptoms usually subside within two or three days and the prognosis is excellent.

Encephalitis, characterised by severe headache, fever, vomiting, perhaps cranial nerve palsies, drowsiness, and coma, is much more serious and carries a mortality of about 50%.

Treatment. There is no specific treatment and no method of inducing either active or passive immunity has yet been shown to be effective. However, patients with orchitis gain relief from systemic steroids.

ORNITHOSIS (Psittacosis)

This virus is acquired by contact with infected birds, who do not themselves necessarily appear ill. Originally described in parrots, it can, however, be transmitted by other birds, including canaries and budgerigars.

Clinical Features. After an incubation period of 1–2 weeks there is gradual onset with cough, fever, headache, backache, and general malaise. The pulse usually remains low in relation to the temperature, but in fulminating cases with high fever and delirium rising pulse and respiratory rates indicate a poor prognosis. Though clinical signs of pulmonary consolidation are often absent, radiographs usually show evidence of pneumonia spreading out from the hilum of the lung. The white blood count is low or normal.

The disease acquired from parrots is often more severe than that spread by other birds. Convalescence is usually slow and prolonged.

Diagnosis may be confirmed by a complement fixation test using psittacosis antigen.

Treatment. Tetracycline is the drug of choice and should be given in doses of 0.5 g 4-hourly for a week. In view of the possibility of case to case transmission by droplet infection the patient should be nursed on barrier precautions.

ACUTE INFECTIOUS MONONUCLEOSIS (Glandular Fever)

An infective agent which fulfils Koch's postulates has not yet been found, but there is strong evidence linking the disease with the Epstein–Barr (EB) virus, which is also associated with Burkitt's lymphoma and acute leukaemia. Rarely, an attack of infectious mononucleosis is followed by Hodgkin's disease.

It is a common disease, seen mainly in young adults, but its infectivity is low, though small outbreaks occur quite often in hostels and similar institutions. There is evidence that the virus is transmitted in saliva, either by kissing, or sharing of drinking vessels.

Clinical Features. The main symptoms are fever, which is usually low and long-continued, lassitude, general malaise, and sometimes sore throat, but the severity and course of the disease are very variable. Some patients simply feel a little tired for a week or two, while others are gravely ill with high fever, headache, and severe sore throat; and although this acute stage does not usually last for more than a week or so, general debility and depression may persist for up to six months. The prognosis, however, is excellent; the disease is never fatal and all patients make a complete recovery. Examination usually reveals enlarged lymph nodes in the neck and elsewhere and the spleen can often be felt. Many patients have a transient macular rash and palatal petechiae are common.

Subclinical hepatitis is very common but actual jaundice infrequent. ECG evidence of myocarditis has been reported in 16% of patients.

Acute abdominal pain simulating appendicitis, benign lymphocytic meningitis, transient thrombocytopenic purpura and rupture of the spleen are rare manifestations.

Diagnosis depends on:

(1) The *white blood count* which after an initial leucopenia is usually raised with an excess of monocytes and lymphocytes, many of which are seen in the stained film to have a characteristic abnormal appearance ('glandular fever cells').
(2) The *Paul–Bunnell* test is positive in about 90% of cases. It depends on the fact that in glandular fever the serum contains an unknown factor which agglutinates sheep's red cells. Occasional false positive results occur, but a titre of 1:64 or higher, and particularly a rising titre during the illness, may be taken as significant. If the Paul–Bunnell test is negative, the possibility of toxoplasmosis or cytomegalovirus infection should be considered.
(3) Antibodies against the EB virus found in the IgM fraction of the plasma proteins are evidence of recent infection by the virus and are found in a high proportion of cases.

Treatment. The duration of fever and debility may be reduced by a week's course of prednisolone, starting with 40 mg daily, but this should be reserved for severely ill patients. There is no specific treatment, and prolonged convalescence is often necessary.

CYTOMEGALOVIRUS INFECTION

Intra-uterine infection with this virus causes severe generalised disease at birth or severe brain damage some months later; infection later in childhood or in adult life is common but usually remains subclinical. Sometimes, however, it causes fever and lymphocytosis with many atypical lymphocytes, but the Paul–Bunnell test and tests for Epstein–Barr virus antibody (both positive in infectious mononucleosis) are negative. The diagnosis may be confirmed by isolation of the virus, usually from the urine, or by demonstrating antibody to cytomegalovirus by complement fixation and indirect haemagglutination tests.

INFLUENZA

Of the three strains of influenza virus, A is more common than B and C is rare. There is no correlation between the clinical severity of the illness and the strain of virus and no cross-immunity between the strains. Variation in the antigenic structure of the virus occurs from time to time and limits the effectiveness of vaccines. Epidemics of influenza A tend to occur every two to three years and influenza B every four to five years.

Factors leading to occasional pandemics, as in 1918 and 1957 (the 'Asian flu') are unknown. Between epidemics the virus is probably kept going in a chain of sporadic infections in man; some of these may be subclinical. Transmission is by droplet infection.

Clinical Features. After an incubation period of one to two days there is sudden onset with fever, shivering, headache, profound malaise, and severe aching in the back and limbs. Cough, sneezing, and upper respiratory catarrh are usually relatively slight. Remittent fever and general prostration continue for up to a week and the temperature settles by lysis. In some patients convalescence is very slow and post-influenzal debility and depression may persist for months.

Influenzal pneumonia. Particularly in the 1918 pandemic pneumonia was a common complication and a common cause of death, but in recent years it has been comparatively rare. It is due to secondary bacterial infection with *H. influenzae*, staphylococci, streptococci or pneumococci.

Treatment. There is no specific treatment, though the appropriate chemotherapy should of course be given for any bacterial complication. Aspirin 0.6 g 4-hourly helps to relieve symptoms during the febrile stage.

Prophylaxis. Vaccines containing inactivated strains of A and B virus give partial immunity for about six months and are of limited value if given just before an epidemic.

EPIDEMIC VOMITING

This very common virus infection typically causes small outbreaks of several cases in a family.

Clinical Features. Onset is abrupt with nausea and vomiting and sometimes there is mild fever and diarrhoea as well. Constitutional upset is very mild and complete recovery usually occurs within two days.

Diagnosis is usually obvious from the occurrence of multiple cases and the short duration of symptoms and no *treatment* is necessary.

OTHER VIRUS CONDITIONS

In addition to the well-recognised virus diseases, it is now realised that there are several groups of viruses which may cause a variety of clinical syndromes. Among the most common are:

COXSACKIE AND ECHO VIRUS GROUP

These viruses may cause:

(a) **Meningitis** (Benign lymphocytic)

This presents with fever, headache, nausea and a stiff neck. The cerebrospinal fluid contains a hundred or so cells per mm^3 which are predominantly lymphocytes.

(b) **Epidemic Myalgia** (Bornholm disease) (p. 310).

ADENOVIRUS GROUP

An acute upper respiratory tract infection which is sometimes no more than a common cold, but it may be a more severe influenza-like illness with fever, sore throat, cough, and sometimes painful enlargement of the lymphatic glands. Areas of pneumonic consolidation and concomitant conjunctivitis have been reported.

HAND, FOOT AND MOUTH DISEASE

This infection with Coxsackie A viruses is distinct from foot and mouth disease of animals, which is caused by another picornavirus. It is seen mainly in young children, but adults in the family are often affected too. It occurs mainly in summer and autumn.

Clinical Features. After an incubation period of 3–6 days there is a mild febrile illness lasting only a few days. On the second or third day a maculopapular rash, later becoming vesicular, appears on the fingers, toes and lateral borders of the feet and painful ulcers develop in the mouth. These lesions heal within about a week.

Diagnosis. The clinical picture is quite characteristic but if necessary the diagnosis can be confirmed by virus studies. The virus may be present in the faeces for several weeks after infection.

POST-INFECTIOUS ENCEPHALITIS AND ENCEPHALOMYELITIS

This condition is a very rare sequel to acute specific fevers such as whooping cough, measles, and mumps and less often to others such as chickenpox, German measles, scarlet fever, and glandular fever; it is no commoner after severe than mild attacks. It also sometimes follows vaccination and other immunising procedures. It has been suggested that the underlying cause may be an antigen-antibody reaction and sometimes improvement does seem to follow treatment with ACTH or cortisone.

Clinical Features. Symptoms appear within a week or two of the onset of the original infection or vaccination. Headache, malaise, vomiting, irritability, drowsiness, or coma are common; other patients present with fits or sudden paresis mimicking a cerebral vascular accident; while in others the clinical picture is dominated by signs of meningitis, cranial nerve palsies, and transient lower motor neurone weakness in the limbs. Mortality is highest, above 50 %, in encephalitis following smallpox or vaccination, but even in the other groups it does not fall below 10 % and is often higher. Moreover, many of those who recover are left with a disability such as hemiplegia, cranial nerve palsies, mental defect, or a Parkinsonian syndrome.

OTHER INFECTIONS

WEIL'S DISEASE (Epidemic Spirochaetal Jaundice)

The causal organism, *Leptospira icterohaemorrhagica*, is excreted in the urine of infected rats. Man acquires the infection either by ingesting food or drink contaminated by rat urine or by immersion in contaminated water, since the spirochaete is able to gain entry through the nasal mucosa or through minor skin abrasions. In this country leptospirosis is therefore mainly seen as an occupational disease of people working in damp rat-infested places, notably sewer workers, miners, canal and dock-workers, farm-hands and fish-cleaners.

Clinical Features. After an incubation period of between one and two weeks there is rapid onset of fever, headache, pains in the back and limbs. Injection of the conjunctivae is often a very striking feature. The name 'icterohaemorrhagiae' implies jaundice and purpura, but clinical jaundice is seen in only about 75 % of patients; it appears during the first week. Features which help in distinguishing the disease from infective hepatitis are the profound prostration, heavy albuminuria, purpuric rash, and sometimes haemoptysis, haematemesis, melaena, or bleeding from the gums. There is usually a leucocytosis. Some patients develop signs of meningeal irritation and some proceed from oliguria to anuria and uraemia; the mortality rate is about 15 %.

Diagnosis is established by identifying the spirochaete by dark-ground illumination of specimens of blood taken during the first few days or urine during the third week. The organism can also be isolated by intraperitoneal inoculation of guinea-pigs with blood or urine. A rising titre of serum agglutinins also occurs but does not give diagnostic information until the clinical illness is more or less over.

Treatment. To be effective penicillin must be given early in the illness, in large doses such as 3 million units 6-hourly. If there is no improvement after three days oxytetracycline 1.5 g 6-hourly may be given a trial.

CANICOLA FEVER

This is due to infection with *Leptospira canicola* and is acquired by contamination of skin lesions by urine from infected dogs. The clinical illness is similar to Weil's disease but less severe, though headache and weakness may persist for 2–3 months.

BRUCELLOSIS (Undulant Fever; Malta Fever)

The causative organism is a Gram-negative coccobacillus which is transmitted to man in infected milk. In this country the usual infecting organism is *Brucella abortus*, which is prevalent throughout the world and is transmitted in cow's milk. *Brucella melitensis* is transmitted in goat's milk and is found particularly in the Mediterranean area, where it causes Malta fever. *Brucella suis* infects pigs and is rarely transmitted to man.

The disease is an occupational hazard of farm workers and slaughtermen since infection can be acquired through the skin and mucosae, but others may be infected by drinking unpasteurised milk. There is reason to think it may be more common in this country than is generally realised.

Clinical Features. Typical undulant fever has an incubation period of between one and three weeks, followed by headache, malaise, anorexia, constipation, and a bout of fever which usually settles by lysis after about ten days. Cough and profuse sweating are common and the spleen is usually palpable. After the temperature has been normal for a few days another bout of fever begins and these febrile episodes may continue recurring at short intervals for many months. During the course of the illness arthritis is common. One joint is usually affected at a time, the pain and swelling subsiding after a few days and then appearing elsewhere. The joints most often affected are the hip, knee, shoulder, ankle, and wrist, but occasionally the small joints of the fingers and toes or of the spine may be involved. Peripheral neuritis, orchitis, and albuminuria are less common complications.

Abortus fever as seen in this country is on the whole clinically milder and sometimes takes such a prolonged and insidious course that the more appropriate label *chronic brucellosis* is often used. Recurrent bouts of drenching night sweats without serious general ill-health should always suggest this diagnosis and the other clinical features mentioned above may also be seen.

Diagnosis. *Blood culture* is the most satisfactory way of establishing the diagnosis, but the organism is difficult to isolate (even under increased CO_2 tension) so that sterile cultures do not rule out this disease. *Urine culture* is occasionally positive. A rising *agglutinin titre* during the illness is helpful; dilutions up to 1:5000 should be tested, since agglutination may be found in the higher dilutions but absent in the lower ones. The brucellin skin test is of doubtful value. The *blood count* usually shows a leucopenia and perhaps mild anaemia.

Treatment. Tetracycline 0.75 g 6-hourly and intramuscular streptomycin 0.75 g twice daily, with a Vitamin B preparation such as Becosym Forte two tablets three times daily, should be given for two weeks. A second course of treatment may be necessary for patients with chronic brucellosis.

Prevention of infection may be achieved by attention to personal hygiene by those handling cattle, pigs, and goats; pasteurisation of milk; a clean water supply; and disinfection of excreta, particularly urine, from patients with the disease.

TETANUS

It is estimated that in Britain each year this preventible disease is contracted by 200–300 people and kills half of them. *Clostridium tetani* is a normal inhabitant of the alimentary tract of horses and sheep, so that its spores are particularly prevalent on cultivated land, and as it is a strict anaerobe it thrives especially in deep penetrating wounds contaminated with soil or road dust. The wound, however, may be a trivial one which heals before the tetanic symptoms appear. These are due to a powerful exotoxin which is absorbed by muscle end-plates at the site of infection and travels along motor nerves to the central nervous system.

Clinical Features. The incubation period is very variable and is important in prognosis: tetanus appearing within a few days of a wound is usually fatal, while if symptoms are delayed for two or more weeks the disease is likely to be mild. Local muscular weakness near the site of infection, attributable to the action of the toxin on the motor end-plates, may precede the generalised spasms. These are usually heralded by trismus (hence the term lockjaw), which may be accompanied by spasm of the facial musculature causing the classical *risus sardonicus*. Tonic spasm spreads to the trunk, causing opisthotonus and board-like rigidity of the abdomen. Fever is commonly present.

The *paroxysmal stage* starts in severe cases within two days of the appearance of trismus; the longer it is delayed the better the prognosis. Paroxysms are precipitated by stimuli such as feeding and other nursing attentions, clinical examination or even simply external noises. The whole body is thrown into painful spasm, with arching of the back, extension of the limbs and clenching of the teeth; this may subside after a few seconds or persist for several minutes. In severe cases the paroxysms recur with increasing frequency until death occurs from exhaustion.

Treatment. Specially staffed and equipped tetanus units have been established in Britain and strenuous efforts should be made to have the patient transferred without delay to the nearest of these. The patient should be nursed in a quiet room with shaded light.

(a) Human antitetanus immunoglobulin (Humotet, Wellcome) is the antitoxin of choice since it avoids the serious allergic reactions which may follow horse serum antitoxin; the dose is 30–300 units/kg body weight given intramuscularly. Even though the neurotoxin is fixed to the nervous tissue by the time clinical signs of tetanus appear, it is important to give antitoxin to deal with toxin still circulating in the blood or being produced at the wound site.

(b) *Wound Toilet.* An hour after the antitoxin has been given, surgical debridement of the wound should be carried out under light general anaesthesia.

(c) *Antibiotic therapy.* As a prophylaxis against bronchopneumonia procaine penicillin 450 000 units and benzylpenicillin 500 000 units should be given twice daily.

(d) *Control of Muscular Spasms.* For successful management of severe cases continuous skilled medical supervision throughout the 24 hours is necessary. Intravenous succinylcholine 0.2% at a rate of 1–1.5 ml (2–3 mg) per minute controls most of the spasms, but occasionally much faster administration is needed for a few seconds and at these times respiration ceases and the lungs must be inflated with oxygen delivered through an anaesthetic machine. For the latter purpose tracheal intubation should be carried out as soon as satisfactory relaxation has been obtained and later a tracheotomy may be done. The foot of the bed should be blocked to prevent accumulation of secretions in the air passages, which are cleared every hour by a sucker attached to a catheter which is passed through the tracheotomy tube. From time to time the patient is allowed to come round so that an attempt may be made to feed him, but in the early stages this must be done through an intragastric tube. Intravenous therapy to maintain fluid and electrolyte balance is also essential.

Prophylaxis. *Active immunisation* if generally adopted could wipe out this disease. Tetanus toxoid should be given to all children in the combined triple vaccine with diphtheria and pertussis (see p. 639). Alternatively tetanus toxoid alone may be given in three doses of 1 ml, the second 6–12 weeks after the first and the third six to twelve months after the second. If an individual actively immunised in this way receives a wound he should be given a further dose of toxoid instead of antitetanic serum.

Passive immunisation. All non-immunised patients with tetanus-prone wounds should be given antitoxin. Human antitetanus immunoglobulin (Humotet, Wellcome) should be used, since it provides better protection and has none of the disadvantages of horse serum antitoxin; the dose is 250–500 i.u. intramuscularly. At the same time the first immunising dose of absorbed toxoid should be given.

TOXOPLASMOSIS

Infection with the protozoon *toxoplasma gondii* is common, but only rarely causes clinical disease; it is mainly acquired by eating undercooked meat from infected animals.

Congenital toxoplasmosis may lead to choroido-retinitis, or less often to lesions in the brain which may calcify and may cause hydrocephalus.

Acquired toxoplasmosis causes lymphadenopathy and may mimic infectious mononucleosis, or Hodgkin's disease. The *diagnosis* may be suspected from the histology of a node removed by biopsy and the toxoplasma may be isolated by mouse inoculation. Antibody tests, particularly the dye test, and a skin test may also help; intradermal inoculation of toxoplasma antigen causes a reaction which is maximal in 24–48 hours.

Treatment. Spiramycin (50–75 mg/kg daily) may give good results in children with ocular infections, but has little effect on lymphadenopathic toxoplasmosis.

CAT-SCRATCH FEVER

This disease, whose causative organism has not yet been isolated, is transmitted by the scratch of apparently healthy cats.

Clinical Features. A few days after the scratch a small indolent ulcer or sore may appear at the site of inoculation and a week or two later the regional lymph nodes become very enlarged. There may be some fever at this stage but constitutional upset is slight. The affected lymph nodes sometimes suppurate, but recovery without serious complications or sequelae is the rule though adenitis may persist for some months. The white blood count is normal and aspirated pus is sterile.

Treatment. A course of tetracycline, 250 mg 6-hourly for five days, may prevent suppuration.

ACTINOMYCOSIS

The organism *Actinomyces bovis* occurs in pus as 'sulphur granules' of up to 1 mm in diameter and is anaerobic. The disease is much more common in men than in women.

Clinical Features. There are three clinical varieties:

(1) *Actinomycosis of the jaw* is the commonest type. Infection through the mucous membrane of the gum leads gradually to woody induration of all the tissues of the jaw and overlying skin, through which multiple sinuses eventually discharge. There is little pain or constitutional upset and the regional lymph nodes are not usually involved.

(2) *Ileocaecal actinomycosis* causes a hard irregular mass in the right iliac fossa and in time fixation to the overlying skin and sinus formation occurs. The disease may spread to the liver, spleen, and other organs and is frequently fatal.

(3) *Actinomycosis of the lung* is the least common type. Cough, dyspnoea, fever, and pain in the chest occur and in the later stages induration and sinuses appear in the chest wall.

Diagnosis depends on identification of the 'sulphur granules' in the pus.

Treatment consists of the administration of penicillin in high dosage for a prolonged period and surgical eradication of the disease wherever possible.

FURTHER READING

Christie, A. B., *Infectious Diseases*, 3rd edition, Churchill Livingstone, Edinburgh and London, 1980.

Mims, C. A., *Pathogenesis of Infectious Disease*, 2nd edition, Academic Press, London, 1982.

CHAPTER 17

TROPICAL DISEASES AND HELMINTHIC INFECTIONS

PROTOZOAL INFECTIONS OF THE TROPICS

MALARIA

Malaria is probably the most important infective disease found in man and even today is responsible for more deaths than any other infection. In parts of Africa mortality from it in early childhood is as much as 10% per annum and at all ages significant morbidity and mortality are caused by it. In the Far East and in India seasonal epidemics of malaria are responsible for most of the very great mortality which it causes there. In Britain up to 2000 cases have been imported in some recent years and there have been up to 10 deaths caused by it annually. It should always be considered as a possible cause of fever when the patient has lived in tropical or sub-tropical countries. In those who have recently arrived in temperate regions from Africa, malaria should be regarded as an acute emergency for such patients are liable to go rapidly downhill and die.

Aetiology. Malaria in man is acquired either from the bites of mosquitoes of the genus *Anopheles* or by transfusion or inoculation of blood containing the parasite. On biting man, mosquitoes inject sporozoites which circulate in the blood for approximately one hour by which time they have entered parenchymal hepatic cells. There they develop in six to ten days and on re-entering the blood stream multiply in erythrocytes and cause the malarial attack. Four malarial parasites affect man: *Plasmodium (P.) falciparum, P. vivax, P. ovale* and *P. malariae*. No symptoms are produced by the presence of the developing parasites in the liver. The parasitic forms which emerge from the liver cells and invade the blood cells are known as merozoites and measure approximately 2 μm in diameter. Merozoites of *P. vivax* and *P. ovale* emerging from liver cells may, it is thought, enter not only erythrocytes but also other liver cells in which they may mature after a period varying from weeks to several years. Maturation of these forms, known as exo-erythrocytic forms, is responsible for long-term relapses of malaria. Only *P. falciparum* and probably *P. malariae* have no exo-erythrocytic cycle; all the pre-erythrocytic forms of these parasites developing in liver cells mature after 6–10 days, enter the blood and persist there until eradicated by treatment or by the patient's acquired immunity or until they cause the death of the patient. The pre-erythrocytic forms of the other species mature after approximately 8 days but some of the merozoites so produced are presumed to enter into other liver cells.

Clinical Features. The early clinical features of all forms of malaria consist of fever with malaise, chilly sensations and headaches. In all malaria other than that caused by *P. falciparum* the fever may initially occur daily; however regular periodicity soon becomes established. *P. falciparum* malaria often continues to produce irregular fever throughout its course but a 48-hour periodicity commonly develops. *P. malariae* causes fever at 72-hour intervals and *P. vivax* and *P. ovale* at 48-hour intervals.

Attacks of fever occur at the time of maturation of parasites within erythrocytes which consequently rupture. The parasites which are then liberated enter further red blood cells within which they first appear as rings about 2 μm in diameter; these grow into amoeboid forms within which, when mature, the protoplasm divides into segments each of which contains a red-staining chromatin particle. The protoplasm and chromatin is known as a merozoite. After several cycles of this type, some parasites differentiate into sexual forms known as gametocytes. These produce no symptoms and do not develop further in man but if taken up by a mosquito will develop into sporozoites within the mosquito's body. They will be injected into the next person whom the mosquito bites and in this way the infection is normally transmitted.

In persons with low immunity to malaria *P. falciparum* infections which have persisted for approximately one week may suddenly cause delirium and a profound shock-like state in which there is oliguria or anuria associated with coma, uraemia and death. Such a reaction occurs particularly in those who are relatively new arrivals into a malarial area or in young children born in such an area. Even adults who have lived their lives in hyperendemic malarial zones may become affected in this way if their immunity drops as a result of pregnancy, intercurrent infection or immuno-suppressive therapy. Infections with *P. vivax*, *P. ovale* or *P. malariae* are seldom associated with such severe shock-like states unless there is other coincident disease. *P. malariae* infections however tend to be very persistent and the immunoglobins produced may be deposited in the renal glomeruli with the production of a nephrotic syndrome. Such infections may also be associated with gross splenomegaly, the 'big spleen disease' encountered in some parts of the world. All forms of malaria may produce anaemia, partly as the result of the growth within, and consequent destruction of erythrocytes, and partly as the result of a haemolytic mechanism of immunological origin.

Relapses. *P. falciparum* infections, if properly treated, do not relapse, for exo-erythrocytic forms do not persist in the liver. For the infection to continue, survival of parasites in the blood is necessary and this will not occur if proper treatment is administered. In the absence of such treatment however, relatively short-term relapses may develop and if the patient has acquired some degree of immunity to malaria, reproduction of parasites in the blood may be inhibited by the immunoglobulins so that the development of the relapse is delayed for weeks or even in some cases for months. The latter type of case is usually in a person who has lived many years in a highly endemic region and has acquired a considerable degree of immunity. The relapse in these cases may sometimes follow reduction in the immunity from intercurrent infection or, in the case of women, from pregnancy.

P. vivax. This infection may relapse for approximately 3 years.after the last infective mosquito bite and results from maturation of exo-. erythrocytic forms which have been persisting in the liver. These relapses are usually slightly less severe than the initial attack from which they are otherwise indistinguishable.

P. ovale. This may relapse for up to 18 months or so after acquiring the infection. Relapses are usually, though not always, relatively mild.

P. malariae. Relapses of this infection have been known up to 20 years. It is, however, now generally believed that they, like those of *P. falciparum*, result from persistent blood-borne forms of the parasite and not from exo-erythrocytic forms continuing in the liver.

Diagnosis. Malaria should be considered in all febrile persons who have been to the tropics or sub-tropics. Such consideration will be almost automatic if in taking the history the question is first asked 'have you travelled recently, and if so where?' Once the disease is thought of diagnosis is rarely difficult. It is when it is overlooked that tragedies occur. In all suspected of malaria a blood film should be taken and stained by one of the Romanowsky methods. The malarial fluorescent antibody test if positive indicates past infection; as the test only becomes positive a week or two after infection, serious errors can result from assuming that a patient's fever, in the presence of a positive fluorescent test, results from malaria.

Differential Diagnosis. Lassa fever must be considered in those who have been to West Africa within the preceding three weeks. It is more probable in those who have been in rural areas of West Africa and is still more probable in those who have worked in hospitals or been in contact in West Africa with patients who had fever. This diagnosis is unlikely among those who have only visited large towns. In dealing with patients who could have Lassa fever it is important to wear protective clothing, to wear gloves when taking the blood film and to stain the film in a safety cabinet. Where these precautions are impossible care should be taken to avoid contamination of the fingers with the patient's blood and to avoid droplet infection from the patient.

Influenza, dengue, sandfly fever, enteric and typhus fevers may have to be considered, and when there is jaundice, infective hepatitis or yellow fever. In patients with coma, cerebral haemorrhage, meningitis, diabetes, alcoholic intoxication and drug ingestion may be suspected. Malaria giving rise to severe symptoms will almost invariably also give rise to the presence of parasites in the peripheral blood and this examination together with a consideration of the clinical features and geographic origin of the patient enables the diagnosis to be made.

Treatment. For acute attacks chloroquine is the most generally useful drug and to patients who are not vomiting and who are able to swallow it should be given initially in doses of 600 mg (base) followed by 300 mg (base) 3–6 hours later and 300 mg on each of two successive days. Amodiaquine is an alternative that may be given in doses of 600 mg (base) initially and 400 mg (base) on each of 2 successive days. In areas of the Far East and South America, resistance has emerged; it has also been reported in a few cases in Africa. Quinine is valuable in such cases and may be given in doses of 600 mg thrice daily for 3 days or until the fever subsides followed by 600 mg daily for 6–8 days. Sulfadoxine (1 g) with pyrimethamine (50 mg) (Fansidar) is also useful for the treatment of chloroquine-resistant strains of *P. falciparum* and may be given as a single dose combined with one of the other standard regimes.

Cerebral and Severe Forms of Malaria. To patients from Africa or regions where chloroquine resistance has not emerged, chloroquine may be given intravenously in doses of 200 mg (base) repeated in 2–3 hours if necessary. This dose is best given in a drip infusion of physiological saline administered over 30–60 minutes. Patients with severe malaria are almost invariably dehydrated. Alternatively the 200 mg dose may be diluted to 20 ml and injected very slowly. Children may be given 5 mg (base) chloroquine per kg body weight. Quinine is an alternative to chloroquine and is given in doses of 600 mg of dihydrochloride in a drip infusion, or if this is not available, dissolved in 20 ml distilled water and injected slowly.

In patients with cerebral features 10 mg dexamethasone may be given intravenously or 100 mg hydrocortisone intramuscularly and often rapidly improves consciousness by, it is believed, reducing cerebral oedema.

Long-term Relapses. For preventing long-term relapses a drug that acts on the exoerythrocytic forms of *P. vivax, P. ovale*, and possibly *P. malariae* is needed. Primaquine in doses of 15 mg (base) daily for 14 days is the most widely used and satisfactory of such drugs.

Prophylaxis. Proguanil is the least toxic of all antimalarials and may be given in doses of 100 mg daily throughout the period of residence in the malarial area and for two weeks after leaving the area. Alternatively chloroquine may be given in doses of 300 mg (base) weekly or pyrimethamine in doses of 25 mg weekly. In areas where chloroquine resistance occurs Maloprim (Wellcome) a combination of dapsone with pyrimethamine may be given in doses of one tablet weekly.

BLACKWATER FEVER

This is an acute and often profound haemolytic anaemia probably due to a dual sensitivity to *P. falciparum* and quinine. It is usually encountered in those who, having been sensitised to quinine are later treated for an acute or chronic *P. falciparum* infection with quinine, often in small and inadequate dosage. In many instances the quinine is taken for suppression. Sometimes the quinine is taken in very small amounts perhaps even inadvertently in tonic water, bitter lemon drink or in tinned grapefruit, in all of which quinine is commonly used for flavouring. The severe intravascular haemolysis leads to excretion of haemoglobin in the urine which becomes dark brown or black from the presence of methaemoglobin. Clinically the condition is ushered in by a rigor, sweating, collapse, vomiting and later oliguria or anuria. Administration of steroids such as dexamethasone in doses of 10 mg intravenously may be lifesaving. Renal failure may require haemodialysis to maintain life until the kidneys recover. Tubular necrosis is the usual histological change found in the kidneys.

LEISHMANIASIS

Leishmania are flagellate protozoa, transmitted by sandflies and causing either systemic illness with visceral involvement or infection localised to the skin and mucocutaneous tissues.

VISCERAL LEISHMANIASIS (Kala-Azar)

Aetiology and Epidemiology. The causative agent *Leishmania donovani* is an intracellular parasite measuring 2.5–3.5 μm. It invades reticulo-endothelial cells especially those of the spleen, liver, lymph nodes and bone marrow. It may occasionally be found within leucocytes in the blood.

Visceral leishmaniasis is widely distributed in the Old and New World. Many of the epidemiological features are explained by the knowledge that around the Mediterranean, in the Middle East, Central Asia and China canines are the reservoir of infection. In Eastern Africa and the Sudan the reservoir is in rodents and in Burma and North-Eastern India it is in man.

Clinical Features. The onset is usually with fever which may be of insidious or abrupt onset and usually occurs between one and four months after infection although incubation periods of up to ten years are known. The fever is usually irregular and commonly there are two pyrexial peaks in each twenty four hours. Sweating is profuse after each bout of fever. The general condition of the patient is often better than might be expected in view of the degree of fever sustained. After two or three weeks of irregular fever an apyrexial period usually follows and later there will be relapses of fever lasting days or weeks.

The skin becomes duskily pigmented and from this feature the name kala-azar, meaning black fever, is derived. The spleen becomes greatly enlarged and the liver too enlarges. Splenic enlargement partly results from parasitisation of the spleen's reticulo-endothelial cells and partly from phagocytosis of erythrocytes which are damaged as a result of the immunological process which leads to anaemia, in which a large haemolytic component has recently been demonstrated. The hypergammaglobulinaemia which develops is largely the result of an enormous increase in immunoglobin G in the serum. Leucopenia becomes associated with the anaemia in well developed cases.

Diagnosis. Until the parasite is demonstrated the diagnosis remains in doubt. Parasites may occasionally be identified in stained blood films but they are much more numerous in marrow aspirates. Splenic aspiration is sometimes performed but is dangerous and should only be carried out by those who have experience of the procedure and where there is full surgical backing. Arrangements for blood transfusion should always be made before splenic aspiration is attempted. Ideally parasites should be demonstrated in culture on rapid-blood agar (NNN medium). Valuable supporting evidence of the diagnosis may be obtained from identification of leishmanial antibodies in the serum using the fluorescent antibody test. In former years the aldehyde test was much used and in this a positive result depends on a great increase in the gammaglobulins within the patient's serum. The test is carried out by adding one drop of formalin to 1 ml of serum, shaking and allowing to stand when the serum becomes gelatinous and opaque.

Other fevers, particularly those associated with splenomegaly must be considered within the differential diagnosis; it is important to consider malaria, tuberculosis, brucellosis, bacterial endocarditis, leukaemia, and schistosomiasis.

Treatment. Pentavalent antimonials are effective and several preparations are available e.g. Pentostam, Solustibosan and Stilbatin. These contain sodium stibogluconate and are given in initial doses of 5.0 mg/kg body weight followed by daily doses of 10–15 mg/kg which are repeated on nine to thirteen occasions so that a course consists of ten to fourteen injections. An interval of 7 days may usefully intervene between the 7th and 8th injections if 14 are given. The intravenous route is to be preferred for intramuscular injection is liable to cause necrosis with painful and sometimes chronic abscess formation. The Indian and Asian forms of leishmania are most sensitive to antimony and Sudanese, Mediterranean and Brazilian forms may be relatively resistant and require more than one course of treatment. Recently courses of up to 6 weeks duration have been used for resistant cases in East Africa.

VARIETIES AND SEQUELAE OF VISCERAL LEISHMANIASIS

Infantile Kala-Azar

Particularly in the Mediterranean, visceral leishmaniasis is most common in children aged two to five years. The causal organism is designated *L. infantum* but it is morphologically indistinguishable from *L. donovani*, from which however, it may be differentiated by its iso-enzymatic properties and by its different epidemiology.

Post-Kala-Azar Dermal Leishmaniasis

This develops one or two years after visceral leishmaniasis has seemed to be cured. Macules containing leishmania form in the skin and later become nodular. The condition is associated with failure in the acquisition of delayed hypersensitivity. This is not normally present during an attack of visceral leishmaniasis but develops as the patient is cured.

CUTANEOUS LEISHMANIASIS

Varieties of this occur in the Old and New Worlds, their epidemiology and clinical features depending on the parasite strain and its reservoir. The classical Old World variety will first be described (synonym, oriental sore, Baghdad boil, etc.)

Aetiology and Epidemiology. The causative organism, *L. tropica* is morphologically indistinguishable from that of visceral leishmaniasis (*L. donovani*) but may be distinguished by iso-enzyme studies and by the epidemiology of the condition. In this connection the areas in which cutaneous leishmaniasis occurs rarely overlap with those in which there is visceral leishmaniasis. Iraq forms an exception to this general statement for the childhood form of visceral leishmaniasis occurs there along with cutaneous leishmaniasis. Cutaneous leishmaniasis is most common in the Middle East and Northern India and Pakistan. Parasites are introduced into the skin by the bites of infected sandflies and remain locally at the site of the bite, in this respect contrasting with the situation in visceral leishmaniasis.

Pathology. The leishmaniae grow in local macrophage cells and cell-mediated immunity to them occurs.

Clinical Features. The lesions occur particularly on the parts exposed at night to the bites of sandflies; thus the face and hands are most commonly affected. On the bitten area an irritable papule develops, breaks down and on it a crust forms. Without treatment, the ulcer may take a year or more to heal and leaves a scar which is often extensive.

Diagnosis. Definitive diagnosis is by demonstration of the organism in aspirates or scrapings from nodules at the edge of the ulcer. The nodule must first be squeezed to exclude blood. Scrapings or swabs taken from the surface of the ulcer are useless.

Treatment. Best results are obtained by soaking off the crusts and applying a bland dressing such as tulle-gras; this local treatment is combined with systemic antimony as for visceral leishmaniasis. In some parts of the world only local treatment is employed, consisting in the application of CO_2 snow or local injections of berberine; such treatments however, always result in marked scarring and are also painful. The use of specially constructed electric pads to raise the temperature of the affected area to 40–43°C for several hours a day is effective.

Mucocutaneous Leishmaniasis (Espundia)

In South America, leishmanial lesions particularly affect the mucocutaneous junctions around the nose and mouth. The causative organism is designated *L. brasiliensis* and is distinguished clinically, epidemiologically and by iso-enzyme studies. It causes very extensive tissue destruction and is often resistant to treatment. Treatment with pentavalent antimony should be given for 21 days and if it fails amphotericin B is the drug of choice. It is given by slow intravenous infusion in daily doses of 250 μg to 1 mg/kg body weight for 20–60 days.

Lupoid Leishmaniasis

This is encountered in the Middle East and causes chronic circinate sores with central healing. It responds to systemic pentavalent antimonials.

Leishmaniasis Recivida

This is a chronic relapsing form of the skin infection and is associated with delayed hypersensitivity. It usually responds to systemic pentavalent antimonials.

Diffuse-cutaneous Leishmaniasis

This rare form of the disease occurs both in South Central America and East Africa. The patient lacks both cellular immunity and humoral antibody. The primary lesion fails to heal and metastatic nodules form on exposed areas, particularly the face and arms, where they have distinct edges and are shiny. In the nodules may be found macrophages whose cytoplasm is filled with amastigotes of *L. aethiopica* or *L. mexicana*. The mucous membranes are not involved and the general health remains good. The condition simulates the skin lesions of lepromatous leprosy but there is no nerve thickening; however, enlarged and palpable lymphatics may sometimes be mistaken for thickened nerves. The disease is resistant to treatment but prolonged courses of pentamidine, given once weekly, or of amphotericin B may help.

Chiclero's Ulcer (Baysore)

This is found particularly in parts of Mexico and Belize and especially affects those who collect chicle or latex from trees in the forests in which sandflies are present. The ulcer is usually very chronic and has a tendency to affect the pinna of the ear. It may respond to pentavalent antimony as given for visceral leishmaniasis (p. 673).

Peruvian-Cutaneous Leishmaniasis (Uta)

This gives rise to simple ulcers or papules which do not invade the mucocutaneous junctions. The management is as for oriental sore.

TRYPANOSOMIASIS

AFRICAN TRYPANOSOMIASIS (Sleeping Sickness)

This disease is rarely encountered outside the endemic areas in Africa but is of great importance in that its diagnosis is then usually overlooked with tragic results.

Aetiology. The causative organism is either *T. gambiense* or *T. rhodesiense* both transmitted by Glossina (Tsetse) flies.

Pathology. The organisms, introduced by the bites of the infected flies, multiply locally for some days and then are taken into the blood stream from which they are disseminated particularly to lymph nodes. After a variable period they pass the blood brain barrier and cause cerebral damage. The lymph nodes become enlarged particularly in *T. gambiense* infections and in late cases there is a characteristic meningo-encephalomyelitis. Anaemia develops and as in the case of visceral leishmaniasis a marked haemolytic component has recently been demonstrated as a factor in its causation. The plasma globulins, particularly IgG are greatly increased.

Clinical Features. At the site of the infected bite an area of induration with bruise-like discoloration develops within days or a week or two of being bitten. This resolves after two to three weeks during which time the patient has developed irregular pyrexia; transient pink circinate erythematous regions may develop on the trunk. The pulse is rapid, and the spleen becomes enlarged and there may be a curious deep hyperaesthesia known as *Kérandel's sign.*

After a period of months the cerebral manifestations develop insidiously with behaviour abnormalities and later somnolence. Finally if untreated the patient sinks into coma and dies. The symptoms develop more acutely and the cerebral manifestations develop earlier in

T. rhodesiense infections than in those with *T. gambiense*.

Diagnosis. *T. gambiense* is usually most readily found by aspirating lymph nodes. *T. rhodesiense* are more numerous in the blood. Using immunofluorescent techniques antibodies can be detected in the patients' serum three to four weeks after infection.

Prognosis. In the absence of treatment the disease is almost invariably fatal but occasionally recovery has been reported in *T. gambiense* infections.

Treatment. During the early stage of all infections the most effective drug is suramin (Antrypol, Bayer 205). It is given intravenously, initially in doses of 0.2 g and if this is well tolerated 1.0 g repeated at intervals of 4–7 days on four or five occasions. An alternative for *T. gambiense* infection is pentamidine isethionate a course of which consists of five to ten intravenous injections of 2–10 mg/kg body weight. The drug may also be given intramuscularly. Melarsoprol (Mel B) is the most effective drug for advanced *T. gambiense* and *T. rhodesiense* infections. It is given intravenously in doses of 3.0–4.0 mg/kg body weight on three occasions separated by 24–48 hour intervals. The drug is dissolved in propylene glycol to make a 5% solution. It should be noted that the therapeutic dose is not uncommonly associated with cerebral or dermatological signs of arsenical toxicity but as the condition is fatal unless treated, this risk of toxicity must be accepted.

SOUTH AMERICAN TRYPANOSOMIASIS (Chagas' Disease)

Patients with this infection are seldom encountered outside of South America where it is transmitted by flying bugs of the genus *Triatoma*. These live in cracks in mud and among straw. The persons usually infected live in mud walled huts with thatched roofs in which straw mattresses are used.

The bitten area becomes inflamed and swollen; adenitis and irregular fever then develop. The spleen and liver enlarge and there may be meningeal symptoms. The febrile phase lasts a few weeks and is followed by a chronic phase in which symptoms eventually result from damage to cardiac and smooth muscle of the digestive tract and later to peripheral autonomic nerve ganglia caused by the trypanosomes. There may be intermittent pyrexial episodes and the neuronal damage later causes cardiomegaly, dilatation of the oesophagus and other hollow viscera. Trypanosomes may occasionally be demonstrated in the blood; other diagnostic methods include a fluorescent antibody test, complement fixation test and xenodiagnosis.

Treatment is unsatisfactory. Nifurtimox administered orally in doses of 8–10 mg/kg body weight for 60–120 days reduces circulating trypanosomes to undetectable levels but has no effect on chronic infections in which the trypanosomes are within cells especially cells of the heart and in smooth muscle. Benznidazole has also recently been used orally in doses of 5 mg/kg body weight. Among its possible side-effects are peripheral neuritis and dermatitis.

HELMINTHIC INFECTIONS

DISEASES CAUSED BY CESTODES

Cestodes are flat tapeworms of which the principal varieties in man are *Taenia saginata*, the beef tapeworm, *Taenia solium*, the pork tapeworm, and *Diphyllobothrium latum* (synonym *Dibothriocephalus latus*) the fish tapeworm. In addition man is a host of the larval form of the dog tapeworm *Taenia echinococcus* (synonym *Echinococcus granulosus*) and in man this larval infection is known as hydatid disease.

TAENIA SAGINATA INFECTION

Man is infected by eating undercooked infected beef in which the larval cysts of the parasite *Cysticercus bovis* occur. The beef has become infected by cattle consuming *Taenia saginata* eggs from pastures in regions where hygiene is poor and ova from infected humans reach the soil.

Clinical Features. Symptoms are usually few and in most instances the infection declares itself by the passage of segments in the faeces.

Diagnosis. The segments (synonym proglottids) are distinctive and may be identified by placing some between two microscope slides and examining them with a hand lens. Each segment contains several thousand ova but these are not liberated into their surroundings unless they rupture or disintegrate; hence the faeces of infected persons do not usually contain free ova.

Treatment. Therapeutically nothing is more effective than aspidium oleoresin (extract of male fern). This is given after the patient has fasted for 24–36 hours, and, for adults 2 ml of the extract (BP) are given on three occasions separated by 30-minute intervals. Children of two years may take up to 2 ml extract in divided doses. The extract is best made into a draught flavoured with syrup. After administration, stools are saved until the head of the worm is recovered or until 24 hours have elapsed, whichever is the shorter period. A mild saline purgative may usefully be given half an hour after the last dose of anthelmintic. Faeces should be searched for the head of the worm, for unless this is dislodged and passed, a new tapeworm will grow from it in approximately three months.

Niclosamide (Yomesan) is an alternative drug and after similar preparation of the patient may be given to persons over the age of eight years in a dose of 1.0 g (two tablets) followed in half an hour by a further gram. Half this amount may be given to those aged 2–8 years. The drug causes considerable disintegration of the worm so that identification of the head is seldom possible.

TAENIA SOLIUM INFECTION

Infection with the adult *Taenia solium* is acquired by eating undercooked pork or pork products, and the clinical manifestations are similar to those of infection with *Taenia saginata*. An important difference between this infection and that with *Taenia saginata* is, however, that the ova of *Taenia solium* are infectious to man in whose tissues, after ingestion, they produce cysticercosis. It is important therefore that the patient with *Taenia solium* should be barrier nursed or nursed in isolation and that the patient's faeces should be burnt or autoclaved before disposal. It is also important that the anthelmintic used should not cause disintegration of the adult worm with consequent liberation of its contained *Taenia solium* ova; these render the faeces more dangerous than they otherwise would be, and if the patient should develop retrograde peristalsis and the ova be carried into the upper part of the intestine the patient could then develop a heavy cysticercoid infection. For these reasons treatment with extract of male fern (**BP**) as described under *Taenia saginata*, is recommended.

Cysticercosis

Aetiology. This occurs when *Taenia solium* ova contaminating food, fingers or water are swallowed, or when such ova are liberated from *Taenia solium* segments within the intestine and are taken by reverse peristalsis into the upper intestine. There they are acted upon by digestive juices; their shell then weakens and their contained larvae thus escape. The released larva burrows into the intestinal wall, circulates in the blood and is ultimately held up in capillary plexuses within any of a wide variety of organs or tissues. It there develops into a cyst measuring up to approximately one centimetre in diameter, the *Cysticercus cellulosae*.

Pathology. Remarkably little inflammatory reaction occurs around the cysticerci until they die and this may not take place for several years. A zone of polymorphonuclear infiltration then develops and eosinophil cells are numerous. It is at this time that irritative phenomena are likely to occur, especially around cysticerci in the brain. Ultimately the cysticercus collapses and after several years is marked only by cells lining the remains of its wall. The cysticerci may enter the ventricular system of the brain and by obstructing the flow of cerebrospinal fluid cause internal hydrocephalus.

Clinical Features. The presence of cysticerci may cause swelling of any tissue or organ and in the subcutaneous tissue cystic localised swellings. The symptoms depend upon the organ or organs invaded but symptoms resulting from cysticerci in the brain usually overshadow those produced by the cysts elsewhere. One of the commonest results of cerebral involvement is epilepsy which may be of any degree of severity from mild petit mal to severe grand mal. The symptoms of internal hydrocephalus may also occasionally be encountered. Cysts are known occasionally to involve the eye and to damage sight or cause blindness of the infected eye.

Diagnosis. If possible a cyst should be excised and identified histologically. Biopsy procedures are of course most readily carried out when cysts are superficial as in the subcutaneous tissues. A complement fixation test for cysticercosis is available. When the cysts are dying, the patient may exhibit an eosinophilia. In those with cerebral cysticercosis the spinal fluid may contain an increased amount of protein and some eosinophil cells.

Treatment. The treatment is symptomatic for it is not possible to locate all the cysts present and to remove them. In most cases this amounts to control of epilepsy. Standard drugs are employed as described in the section on epilepsy (p. 372).

DIBOTHRIOCEPHALUS LATUS (Diphyllobothrium latum)

The infection is conveyed to man by consumption of undercooked fresh water fish in which the infective larval forms of the parasite are present. It is, therefore, in regions well supplied with fresh water lakes and rivers that the infection occurs most commonly and such regions include Finland and the Baltic countries, parts of central Asia and the Far East. The worm may grow to a length of 8–9 m and if its head is anchored high up in the small intestine it may successfully compete with its human host for Vitamin B_{12} and in this way be responsible for development of a megaloblastic anaemia. The segments are broader than long, measuring 10 × 12 mm, and in their centre there is a rosette shaped uterus. The treatment is as for *Taenia saginata*.

HYDATID DISEASE

Aetiology. This disease results from the development in man of the larval or intermediate stage of *Taenia echinococcus* (synonym *Echinococcus granulosus*). It is thus the counterpart in this infection of the development of the larval forms of *Taenia saginata* in cattle, i.e.

Cysticercus bovis and of the larval forms of *Taenia solium* (*Cysticercus cellulosae*) in man and pigs. The adult worm measures only 5–8 mm in length and lives in the intestines of dogs. Ova leave the dog in faeces and contamination of uncooked vegetables or other food with ova is the usual means of infection although water-borne spread is also possible. Lettuce and other salad vegetables are those most usually responsible for transmission.

Pathology. The ova, on being swallowed, are acted upon by digestive juices, their shell is weakened and the contained embryos escape and burrow into the wall of the host's intestines. They are carried first to the liver and most are there retained in the sinusoids thus resulting in the liver being the most commonly affected organ. Others pass to the lungs which are the second most common organs to be involved. A smaller proportion pass the lungs and reach the systemic circulation whence they may travel to any organ in the body. Cysts may grow to a diameter of up to 25 cm and contain many daughter cysts, much fluid and thousands of heads of immature *Taenia echinococcus*. These immature heads settle in the dependent part of the cyst and become known as hydatid sand. After growing for several years the cyst dies, its fluid content is absorbed and the wall becomes calcified.

Clinical Features. Symptoms depend on the situation of the cyst and whether it becomes infected. If infected the signs and symptoms are those of an abscess of the organ involved. Pressure symptoms depend on the location of the cyst.

Allergic manifestations result from absorption of the fluid contents when the cyst dies and they also develop in an acute and sometimes fatal form if the cyst ruptures as the result of trauma and the fluid is rapidly absorbed parenterally.

Diagnosis. Cysts in the lung are readily outlined radiographically; those in the liver, however, are rarely visible in this way until they have calcified. For those in the liver therefore, scintillography using radioactive material or examination by ultrasound are very valuable. In the blood there may be eosinophilia and the serum often gives a positive complement fixation test for hydatid disease.

Differential Diagnosis. Carcinoma of the liver, amoebic abscess of the liver, pleural effusion, bronchial neoplasm, hydronephrosis, distension of the gall bladder, pancreatic and other cysts all have to be considered in the differential diagnosis. Hydatid cysts of the brain simulate a cerebral tumour and those in bone cause pathological fractures which must be differentiated from other causes of fracture. Hydatid cysts in the vertebral bodies lead to a collapse of the infected bone, and usually to paraplegia from other causes of which the condition must be differentiated.

Treatment. Systemic treatment may be required for allergic reactions and following rupture of a cyst the injection of dexamethasone intravenously in doses of 10 mg may be lifesaving. From the lungs and from bones, cysts may be removed surgically. Removal from the liver is usually more hazardous and should only be carried out in centres where there is experience of this procedure. The aspiration of cysts, except under direct vision at a surgical operation, is dangerous, leading to leakage of fluid and contamination of the surrounding tissues with daughter cysts. The daughter cysts may later develop into full-sized cysts. Shrinkage, and even death of cysts has been claimed following long-term oral mebendazole treatment. There is however considerable doubt regarding these claims.

DISEASES CAUSED BY NEMATODES

ASCARIS LUMBRICOIDES (Round Worm Infection)

Aetiology. This worm measures up to 25 cm in length and lives in the intestine of man. Its ova meausre 0.08 by 0.06 mm and have an irregularly bossed cortex. They are directly infectious to man after maturing outside the body, usually in soil. Upon being ingested, the embryos penetrate the mucous membrane of the intestine, enter the bloodstream and are taken to the liver and later reach the lungs. They pass up the bronchial tree till they reach the pharynx, are swallowed with food or saliva and enter the intestine again. The usual mode of infection is by eating uncooked vegetables contaminated with ova.

Clinical Features. Urticaria may develop during the migration of the larvae, probably because many of them die during this process and on being absorbed provide the equivalent of a parenteral injection of helminthic protein. If many larvae pass through the lungs at one time pneumonitis with cough, and sputum, fever and eosinophilia may result.

Symptoms resulting from the presence of adult worms in the intestine vary with their number; if there are only two or three present, occasional attacks of mild colic may be all that is experienced. In heavy infections, particularly in children, intestinal obstruction may result. Heavy infections may also cause or aggravate malnutrition.

The worms may migrate and very occasionally have caused appendicitis by entering the appendix or obstructive jaundice by entering the common bile duct.

Diagnosis. The distinctive ova may be recognised by microscopic examination of the faeces.

Treatment. Piperazine compounds are commonly employed and for persons of all ages 4 g of the hydrate may be given and repeated after 24 hours. A saline purge administered 2 hours after taking the piperazine is useful in expelling worms. Tetrachlorethylene has long been used and is highly effective and cheap. It is the commonest drug used for ascariasis in many tropical countries. To adults it is given in doses of 4 ml, to children aged 7–14 in doses of 2 ml and to those aged 1–7 in doses of 1 ml. Other drugs which may be used include bephenium hydroxynaphthoate, thiabendazole, pyrantel embonate (Combantrin), see pp. 684 & 685. Levamisole in a single dose of 2.5 mg/kg body weight is also favoured by many.

TOXOCARIASIS

This disease is caused by infection in man with the larval stage of worms of the dog and cat ascarids, *Toxocara canis* and *Toxocara cati*. The adult worms, which resemble *Ascaris*, live in the intestines of these animals and it is their ova which are infective to man. These ova are usually transmitted to the mouth on soil-contaminated fingers or food. In the intestines they hatch and larvae which are liberated burrow into the intestinal mucosa. Being smaller than larvae of *Ascaris lumbricoides*, they may be transported to any organ in the body. Most damage is caused if larvae enter the eye where they cause choroidoretinitis and commonly damage sight. They may also enter the brain and produce encephalitis or epilepsy. In the lungs they may give rise to pneumonitis or asthma. Children are commonly infected, probably because they often put soil-contaminated fingers into their mouths.

Diagnosis. Immunofluorescent techniques are used to detect toxocaral antibodies in the serum. There is often an associated eosinophilia. Toxocaral lesions in the eye must be distinguished from retinoblastoma and toxoplasmal choroidoretinitis; these however, are not to be expected to be associated with eosinophilia or with the presence of toxocaral antibodies in the serum.

Treatment. Diethylcarbamazine in doses of 3 mg/kg body weight administered 3 times daily for 21 days will kill the larvae but cannot be expected to undo damage to vital structures which the larvae may have caused.

ANCYLOSTOMIASIS (Hookworm Infection)

Aetiology. This worm lives in the upper small intestine of man; the male is approximately 10 mm long and the female between 10 and 18 mm. Ova are passed in the faeces of the infected person and require moist earth for the development of the contained larvae. The infection then occurs by penetration of the skin by the larvae. This often occurs when walking barefoot on contaminated earth but any form of exposure of the skin to such earth can result in infection. Larvae can also penetrate the buccal mucosa to which they may be carried on contaminated salad or other vegetables. Two species of the parasite occur, *Ancylostoma duodenale* and *Necator americanus*. The latter is not confined to the New World as its name suggests. After penetrating the skin or mucosa, the larvae are conveyed in blood to the lungs and there enter alveoli, migrate up the pulmonary tree and reaching the pharynx are swallowed in food or saliva. They are carried to the upper intestine where their mouthparts become attached to the mucosa and they live for several years drawing blood from the host.

Clinical Features. Larvae penetrating the skin cause irritation and if numerous, may give rise to an eruption known as 'ground itch'. In this, small tracks of the larvae may be outlined by the inflammatory reaction which they stimulate. The eruption lasts for a few days and settles down as the larvae leave the area. Unless several or many larvae enter the skin at one time a discernible eruption may not develop.

In the lungs larvae produce small areas of pneumonitis and if several are present at the same time, clinically detectable pneumonitis may result. This phase of the infection is usually associated with a pronounced eosinophilia.

In the established infection the small daily blood loss caused by each parasite may lead to hypochromic anaemia. The development of the anaemia is dependent upon several variables, including the number of worms present, the type of worm, the duration of infection, the amount of iron in the diet and the absorbability of that iron from the intestine. It is estimated that each *Necator americanus* causes a daily loss of approximately 0.02 ml and that each *A. duodenale* causes a loss of approximately 0.1 ml daily. Iron in animal products is much more readily absorbed from the intestine than is that contained in vegetables. In infected persons living on a poor, mainly vegetarian diet iron deficiency is therefore particularly likely to develop. In them too the protein also lost in the blood drawn by worms may aggravate hypoproteinaemia or malnutrition.

Diagnosis. This is usually straightforward, the ova measuring 60–75 μm by 35 μm being readily detectable in the patient's stool.

Treatment. Bephenium hydroxynaphthoate (Alcopar), is probably the drug most widely used for hookworm infection. It is given in doses of 5.0 g washed down by a glass of water; for those aged less than twelve years 3.0 g may be given. The treatment should be repeated after 24–48 hours. Pyrantel embonate given in doses of 10–20 mg/kg body weight is also highly effective. One of the most widely used drugs is however tetrachlorethylene. It is given by mouth in doses of 0.2 ml for each year of age up to 15; for adults 5 ml is administered and a mild saline purge should be given 3–4 hours after the anthelminthic. The dose is repeated after 1–3 days.

It is important not only to eradicate the worms from the intestines but also to treat any anaemia or nutritional defect which coincidentally may be present.

STRONGYLOIDIASIS

Aetiology. The causative agent *Strongyloides stercoralis* is common in the tropics generally and in the Far East in particular.

Adult females measure 2 mm × 50 μm and live in the mucosa and submucosa of the duodenum and small intestine. Their eggs contain short rhabditiform larvae which emerge in the intestine and are passed in faeces. In soil these may develop into elongated filariform larvae which are free living and produce further progeny which become filariform and are capable of penetrating human skin and mucous membranes thus causing infection. They are then carried in blood and lymph to the lungs where they may mature into adults or may migrate up the broncho-tracheal tract, be swallowed in food or saliva and, on reaching the intestine, burrow into mucosa. Rhabditiform larvae in the intestine may also occasionally metamorphose into the filariform variety and penetrate the bowel wall or peri-anal skin. Rhabditiform larvae cannot penetrate tissues. Auto-infection with filariform larvae enables the parasites to remain many years in the human host.

Pathology. In the intestinal mucosa larval tracks and granulomatous reaction associated with many eosinophils develop and may be the basis of malabsorption which occurs in this infection. In the lungs the worms and larvae produce pneumonitis.

Symptoms. Few symptoms occur in the majority of cases though there may be intestinal colic and intermittent bowel looseness. In heavier infections the malabsorption syndrome (q.v.) is now well recognised.

Adults and larvae encysted in the lungs and producing pneumonitis are responsible for cough and sputum. In the latter larvae may occasionally be demonstrated.

Filariform larvae, by penetrating peri-anal skin, cause a form of cutaneous larval migrans which gradually extends from the buttocks to the trunk and unless treated may be of great chronicity.

Diagnosis. Larvae may be demonstrated in the stool and occasionally in sputum. An eosinophilia usually accompanies the infection. Antibodies, some of which may cross-react with filarial antibodies may be demonstrated in serum.

Treatment. Thiabendazole is administered orally in doses of 25 mg/kg body weight for 3–5 days.

THREADWORMS (*Enterobius vermicularis* or *Oxyuris vermicularis*)

Aetiology. The worms live in the lower bowel and the female migrates through the anus at night to lay ova on the peri-anal skin. These ova are directly infectious to man and auto-infection occurs when they are carried to the mouth on fingers, contaminated food or dust which is swallowed.

Clinical Features. These are principally produced by the worm and its eggs on the peri-anal skin; pruritus ani results and this plays a part in the life cycle of the parasite by stimulating scratching whereby ova are collected on the fingers and particularly behind the finger nails. Sleep may be disturbed by the pruritus ani. Occasionally worms enter the appendix and encyst in the submucosa producing acute or subacute appendicitis.

Diagnosis. Ova are not usually present in the stool for they are laid on the peri-anal skin; diagnosis is, therefore, usually most successfully made by swabbing or scraping this skin and examining for ova, the material so obtained. Another useful method is to apply strips of adhesive transparent tape to the peri-anal skin and after a few seconds remove them and use the adhesive side to stick them to microscope slides. Ova adhere to the adhesive material and may be recognised microscopically.

Treatment. Anthelmintics are relatively ineffective against threadworm infection and failure or relapse is common following their use. Successful elimination of the worms is best obtained by preventing auto-infection which, if successfully carried out, will lead to elimination of the infection in three to six weeks. With this objective, patients should be instructed to wash their hands and scrub the finger nails before each meal and after each visit to the toilet. A bath taken immediately on rising in the morning will rid the skin of any ova laid there during the night and further prevent contamination of fingers and clothing. These measures alone are successful in the majority of cases.

Of the drugs, piperazine compounds are those most commonly used and are usually dispensed as the hydrate containing 750 mg/5 ml of elixir or in tablets containing the equivalent of 500 mg piperazine hydrate. For adults 15 ml elixir or 4 tablets are given daily for 7 days. The equivalent doses for children between 5 and 12 years are 10 ml elixir or 3 tablets and for those 2–4 years 5 ml of $1\frac{1}{2}$ tablets daily. Vipyrnium embonate (BP) is also used. It is prepared in a suspension containing 10 mg/ml and in tablets containing 50 mg. For adults a single dose of 8 tablets or 40 ml suspension is given and for children one tablet or 5 ml suspension per 10 kg body weight, until the adult dose is reached.

TRICHINELLA SPIRALIS INFECTION

This worm was first named *Trichina spiralis* and the disease it causes was referred to as trichinosis. The parasite was later named *Trichinella spiralis* and the disease it causes trichiniasis; occasionally and most correctly it is named trichinelliasis.

Aetiology. The adult male measures approximately 1.5 mm and the female 3–4 mm. They develop and live in the upper intestine and produce embryos which penetrate the intestinal mucosa and are carried to many tissues throughout the body of the animal harbouring the adult worms. This animal may be man but is more usually a pig or rat. Transmission of infection occurs when larvae encysted in the muscles or other tissues are eaten in an undercooked state by a potential host such as man. The larvae are then freed from the muscle during the process of digestion, develop rapidly in the intestine and attach themselves to the intestinal wall. The parasite is found widely dispersed in nature and is particularly common in East Europe including Poland. It is also found in Africa, Canada and in the Americas. Not uncommonly outbreaks have followed hunting for wild pig or bear the flesh of which on being barbecued in camp is eaten inadequately cooked.

Pathology and Pathogenesis. The freed ingested larvae become mature worms in three days. By the sixth or seventh day females are producing embryos and continue to do so for five or six weeks. These embryos enter lymphatics or veins and are dispersed widely in the body of the host where they encapsulate.

The presence of adults in the intestine may give rise to gastrointestinal irritation with abdominal pain, vomiting and often diarrhoea, but except in known outbreaks or epidemics this stage is often overlooked.

A stage of myositis and allergic reaction occurs from the seventh day of infection onwards and corresponds to the arrival in muscles and other tissues of embryos. The muscle becomes swollen and tender and movements are painful. The diaphragm and the muscles of respiration and of mastication in particular cause symptoms. Oedema of the face and eyelids may be apparent and almost invariably there is leucocytosis with eosinophilia. In heavily infected patients there may be drowsiness and meningeal irritation. Occasionally there is oedema glottidis and this if not treated with great urgency may be fatal.

Diagnosis. The diagnosis is suggested by the history of myositis with oedema and is supported by the presence of eosinophilia. Special investigations include haemagglutination and complement-fixation tests which are available in special laboratories and biopsy of affected muscle, usually the biceps, which is then examined histologically for the presence of encysted embryos.

The differential diagnosis has to be made from rheumatic fever, pleurisy, dermatomyositis and typhoid fever. In differentiating the condition from rheumatic fever an important point is that trichiniasis causes myositis not arthritis. Although pleurisy may be simulated, the pain results from the involvement of intercostal muscles not the underlying pleura; a pleural rub does not develop. The absence of rose spots, marked headaches and splenic enlargement help to distinguish trichiniasis from typhoid fever. Dermatomyositis may clinically resemble trichiniasis but the specific tests for trichiniasis help to differentiate.

Treatment. If trichiniasis is suspected early enough, removal of worms from the intestines should be attempted in order to reduce the number of embryos which will find their way to the tissues. Thiabendazole may be used for this purpose in doses of 25 mg/kg body weight twice daily for five days. The judicious use of corticosteroids will alleviate allergic manifestations and for oedema glottidis their use parenterally may be life saving. Analgesics such as paracetamol or codeine compound tablets are helpful in controlling muscle pain.

FILARIASIS

This group of diseases is due to infection with a number of closely related nematode worms of the family Filarioidea. Seven types are known according to the subspecies of filaria.

Species	*Disease*
Wuchereria bancrofti	Bancroftian filariasis
Brugia malayi	Brugia filariasis
Loa loa	Loiasis
Onchocerca volvulus	Onchocerciasis
Dipetalonema perstans	*Dipetalonema perstans* infection
Mansonella ozzardi	Mansonelliasis
Dipetalonema streptocerca	Streptocerciasis

Bancroftian Filariasis

This disease is widespread in the tropics and is caused by *Wuchereria bancrofti*. In the human host adult worms produce microfilariae which are taken up by feeding culicine mosquitoes in which they develop into infective larvae. When the mosquito next bites, the larvae are transmitted to the new host. The microfilariae reside in the lungs during the day but at night they circulate in the peripheral blood. The disease is caused by the adult worms which invade the lymphatics, producing recurrent episodes of inflammation until finally the affected lymphatics become obliterated by fibrosis.

Clinical Features. The incubation period is about three months. In the early stages there are episodes of lymphangitis and lymphadenitis with fever. The blood shows an eosinophilia. After some years lymphoedema progressing to elephantiasis may become a feature and this may be accompanied by hydrocele and serous effusions.

Diagnosis. In the acute stage of the disease microfilariae can be found in the blood, but the blood sample should be taken between 10.00 p.m. and 2.00 a.m. A complement-fixation test is available. It covers all pathogenic filariae but is only positive in about 50 % of infected patients.

Treatment. Diethylcarbamazine is the most effective drug and is given in doses of 3 mg/kg three times daily for 3 weeks. Acute allergic reaction may occur during treatment but this can be controlled by steroids and antihistamines. This treatment will not improve elephantiasis.

Prevention. Anti-mosquito measures offer the best hope of success.

Brugia malayi

This parasite is found in Asia and it produces a clinical picture similar to bancroftian filariasis. It may also be responsible for tropical pulmonary eosinophilia (see p. 305).

Loa Loa

This parasite is found in Central and West Africa. After an incubation period of three months to one year clinical manifestations develop. These are caused by the worm migrating to various parts of the body particularly to the subcutaneous tissue around medium sized joints and the eye. When this occurs it produces a local erythematous swelling (Calabar swelling) together with fever and eosinophilia.

Treatment. Diethylcarbamazine as for bancroftian filariasis is effective.

Onchocerciasis

This infection is caused by *Onchocerca volvulus* transmitted by flies of the genus *Simulium* which breed in well oxygenated streams and rivers. The disease is endemic in the greater part of tropical Africa and Guatemala and in localised areas in South Arabia, Mexico, Venezuela, Colombia and Brazil.

Clinical Features. After an incubation of two to three months the disease presents with pruritus and later there may be painless subcutaneous nodules. Late in the untreated disease there is necrosis of elastic fibres of the skin which may hang loosely (hanging groin). Microfilariae in the eye are the cause of 'African river blindness'.

Diagnosis. (1) By microscopic examination of snips of skin for microfilariae. (2) Identification of microfilariae in the eye may be possible. (3) The filarial complement-fixation test is positive in 50% of cases. (4) An eosinophilia is often present.

Treatment. Diethylcarbamazine, in doses as for bancroftian filariasis, although effective, is liable to cause reactions. Suramin may be given by intravenous injection in doses of 1.0 g weekly for 4–6 weeks. Careful observation of the urine is necessary, as the drug is nephrotoxic.

Dipetalonema streptocerca

In Ghana and Central Africa this causes a dermatosis similar to that of onchocerciasis. It responds to diethylcarbamazine.

Dipetalonema perstans and Mansonella ozzardi

Dipetalonema perstans and Mansonella ozzardi are usually non-pathogenic. Occasionally, in a heavy infection, they may cause eosinophilia. They both respond to diethylcarbamazine.

DISEASES CAUSED BY TREMATODES

SCHISTOSOMIASIS

Four species of schistosomes (blood-flukes) produce human disease: *Schistosoma haematobium, S. mansoni, S. japonicum* and *S. intercalatum*. The first of these produces disease of the urinary tract and the others of the intestine, portal system and liver. Although other species occasionally affect man they are of much less importance. The various species can be recognised by their characteristic ova. This group of diseases affects approximately 200 million people in the tropics—especially in Africa. The world incidence is at present increasing, because the habitat of the intermediate host—various species of fresh water snail—is increasing as new irrigation schemes are constructed.

Man acquires infection when cercariae in fresh water come into contact with his skin which they penetrate. They are transported by blood or in the lymphatics till they reach blood vessels in their preferred site for development into adult worms. This site is either around the large bowel or around the urinary tract. Eggs are deposited into the bladder or intestine (depending on the species) and are excreted in urine or faeces. If the ova reach fresh water a larva (miracidium) emerges and swims around until a suitable species of snail is found. Within the snail the life cycle is completed with the production and liberation of many new cercariae.

Whenever man is exposed by wading, swimming, fishing, sailing, etc., even though briefly, to contaminated water he is in danger of infection. The duration and frequency of exposure are important in determining the severity of disease in man. Ova in tissues produce granulomata, and subsequently fibrosis and calcification cause long-term sequelae.

Urinary Schistosomiasis (*S. haematobium*)

Africa, the Middle East and Mediterranean littoral are the main endemic areas. Lesions develop in the urinary bladder and later in the ureters, seminal vesicles, prostate, uterus, vagina and kidneys. The bladder is affected first and the initial granulomatous reaction is followed by ulceration, fibrosis, loss of elasticity and incomplete emptying of the bladder, urinary infection, and in some cases calcification of the bladder wall. Carcinoma is a late sequel. Hydronephrosis and pyonephrosis may follow obstruction to the ureters, particularly as they pass through the bladder wall.

Clinical Features. Cercariae, on penetrating the skin, cause transient localised erythema but unless many penetrate at the same time this reaction may be overlooked. Between 4 and 6 weeks after heavy exposure eosinophilia with malaise, aching limbs and urticarial weals may develop and be present for several weeks. Light infections often are asymptomatic but some 6–8 weeks after heavy infection terminal haematuria may develop and ova may be detectable in the urine. In those chronically and heavily exposed, frequency and incontinence with blood clots and pus, due to secondary infection, may ensue. Progressive deterioration in health may occur if the complications, such as hydronephrosis, pyonephrosis, bladder carcinoma and lung involvement with cor pulmonale, develop.

Diagnosis depends on finding ova (terminal-spine) in the urine; the sediment of a day-time specimen is most likely to yield a positive result. Straight abdominal radiographs may show calcification in part or all of the bladder wall. Cystoscopy reveals characteristic appearances: shallow ulcers, sandy-patches, constricted (golf-hole) ureteric orifices, and later polyps and carcinoma. Bladder-biopsy reveals ova and occasionally adult worms. In advanced cases, intravenous pyelography may reveal hydronephrosis.

Intestinal Schistosomiasis (*S. mansoni*)

Parts of Africa, the Middle East, South America and the Caribbean are endemic areas. Infection with *S. intercalatum* occurs in Zaire and although the ova resemble those of *S. haematobium* the disease takes a course similar to that of *S. mansoni*. Lesions develop in the walls of the large intestine. Granulomatous reactions give rise to ulceration, bleeding papillomata and fibrosis; carcinomatous change is rare. Embolisation of ova to the liver gives rise to the main complication; granulomata precede periportal fibrosis upon which portal hypertension becomes superimposed. Splenomegaly, ascites and bleeding oesophageal varices result. Ova sometimes embolise to the lungs giving rise ultimately to pulmonary hypertension; similarly they may reach the spinal cord and occasionally the brain, causing encephalo-myelitis.

Clinical Features. Prodromal symptoms including lassitude are often more severe than in *S. haematobium* infection. After months or years, intestinal symptoms – diarrhoea with blood and mucus and tenesmus, may appear. Exacerbations may resemble amoebic colitis. The colon sometimes becomes thickened, fibrosed and tender. Colonic ulcerations may become secondarily infected, and polyps and abdominal lymphadenopathy may develop. As hepatic involvement progresses hepatosplenomegaly and evidence of portal hypertension appear. Ascites and bleeding from oesophageal varices are late manifestations of the disease. Pulmonary involvement is heralded by haemoptyses, and signs of cor pulmonale.

Diagnosis depends on finding the ova (lateral-spine) in the stool; numerous stools may have to be examined before a positive diagnosis can be made. Sigmoidoscopy may reveal ulceration or polyps. Rectal biopsy and aspiration liver biopsy are of great value in diagnosis. As liver involvement occurs, liver function tests, portal venography, and liver scans will give additional information. If pulmonary involvement is present, a chest X-ray may demonstrate right ventricular hypertrophy, an increased pulmonary artery component to the cardiac outline, and mottling of the lung parenchyma.

Far-Eastern Schistosomiasis (*S. japonicum*)

South-eastern China and the Philippines are the main endemic areas. Like *S. mansoni* infection, the disease is primarily intestinal. The superior as well as inferior mesenteric vein, and thus the small intestine and mesentery and proximal colon are involved. Liver pathology and portal hypertension are similar to those in *S. mansoni* infection. Pulmonary involvement is less common, and central nervous system involvement much more common than in *S. mansoni* infection.

Clinical Features. The allergic phase (*Katayama syndrome*) occurring 2–3 weeks after infection is severe and is followed more rapidly by symptoms of intestinal involvement than in *S. mansoni* infection. The clinical manifestations are more severe than in the other schistosomal infections.

Diagnosis is by methods similar to those for *S. mansoni* infection. The ova have a lateral knob instead of a spine.

In all forms of schistosomiasis, sero-diagnosis is of value approximately 4 weeks after infection, but is no substitute for finding the ova. Complement fixation, fluorescent antibody and precipitation techniques may be used. None of the reactions is species specific.

Treatment. The most widely used treatment is niridazole (Ambilhar) in a dose of 25 mg/kg daily for 7 days. The most successful results are in *S. haematobium* and the least successful in *S. japonicum* infections. Most complications occur in the presence of portal–systemic anastomoses when the unmetabolised compound has a direct effect on cerebral metabolism: mental confusion, hallucinations and convulsions ensue. It is therefore contraindicated in the presence of severe hepatocellular disease and known portal–systemic shunting, and also in psychotic patients. Hycanthone (Etrenol) given as a single intramuscular dose of 3 mg/kg body weight has given results, especially with *S. haematobium*, that are satisfactory for mass treatment but the cure rate is too low for reliable treatment of individuals; however, hepatocellular toxicity can be severe. Oxamniquine given orally in doses of 20 mg/kg body weight daily for 3–5 days is particularly effective against *S. mansoni*. In single doses of 40 mg/kg body weight, praziquantel has given good results in all forms of the disease. Like hycanthone it appears more suitable for mass than for individual therapy. Metrifonate is effective against *S. haematobium* in orally administered doses of 7.5 mg/kg body weight every 2–4 weeks for 2–3 doses. Assessment of cure in schistosomiasis is difficult; survival of a few adult worms can give rise to recurrent output of ova. Continued absence of viable ova 3 months after treatment suggests cure. Dead ova in urine, stool or biopsies after treatment are not indications for further treatment.

Treatment of liver disease and portal hypertension may require portacaval anastomosis and other measures for arresting bleeding from oesophageal varices. Urinary and renal infection and carcinoma of the urinary bladder are treated on their merits. Brain and spinal cord involvement may require surgery, and respiratory and cardiac complications appropriate therapeutic regimes.

BACTERIAL AND VIRAL INFECTIONS

LEPROSY (Hansen's Disease)

This is a disease of low infectivity which is endemic in many parts of the tropics. Infection with the acid-fast causative organism, *Mycobacterium leprae*, is usually acquired by close contact over a prolonged period and the incubation period is therefore difficult to determine, though it may be several years. There is no known animal reservoir or vector.

Immune Pathology. The pathology and clinical course of leprosy depend on the pattern of immune response to the *M. leprae*. If the cellular immune response predominates, tuberculoid leprosy results. The pathological lesion is a granuloma containing very few bacilli. The disease tends to be localised, and the lepromin skin test is positive. Acute inflammatory reactions (*type I* lepra reaction) may occur. When the cellular immune response is poor the disease is widespread and the lesions contain many bacilli. Acute vasculitis due to circulatory immune complexes (*type 2* lepra reaction) can occur in many organs. Most patients however, lie somewhere between these two extremes.

Clinical Features. (1) **Tuberculoid Leprosy.** This is the benign variety of the disease. The main reaction occurs in peripheral nerves and skin supplied by them: the patient complains of numbness, tingling and loss of pain and temperature sense in the affected parts, and the local nerve or nerves can be felt as hard thick cords. The great auricular nerve is very commonly affected. Circinate areas of erythema with clear cut raised edges appear in the skin, and as they extend, their centre heals and is depigmented. The disease usually runs a self-limiting course and the patient is not usually infectious. Often the lesions are rather more numerous and cellular immunity is less, and the condition is then known as borderline tuberculoid or dimorphous leprosy.

(2) **Lepromatous Leprosy.** This is the malignant form of the disease. The earliest lesion is a macular rash over the face, head, chest and extensor surfaces of the arms. The patient's resistance is low and granulomatous lesions teeming with *M. leprae* appear in the skin, particularly of the face and ears. As in the tuberculoid variety the earliest lesions are probably in the nerve fibrils, from which extension occurs to

the skin and up the nerve trunks, but as there is very little inflammatory response, nerve function is not disturbed until much later in the course of the disease. Granulomatous lesions may also appear in the lymph nodes, testes, bone marrow and upper respiratory mucosa. The general health is not usually affected, and leprosy *per se* rarely causes death.

Leprosy may be confused with pityriasis versicolor, vitiligo, post-kala-azar dermal leishmaniasis, onchocerciasis, lupus vulgaris, psoriasis and Kaposi sarcoma.

Diagnosis is established by identifying the characteristic acid-fast bacilli in scrapings from skin lesions of lepromatous leprosy, or by the characteristic histology of skin or nerve fibrils in tuberculoid and dimorphous forms of the disease.

Treatment. Patients with *tuberculoid leprosy* and those with few or no organisms demonstrable in the lesions are treated with dapsone 25–50 mg daily for months or a year or two.

It has been suggested by a WHO committee that patients with *lepromatous leprosy* may be treated with:

(1) Rifampicin 600 mg once a month.
(2) Clofazimine 50 mg daily plus a 300 mg dose once a month.
(3) Dapsone 100 mg daily.

The rifampicin and clofazimine to be given for 4 months and the dapsone until the patient's skin smears become negative or, if negative when the patient is first seen, for a minimum of 2 years.

Acute immune reactions (type 1 and 2 lepra reactions) are treated with prednisolone 40–60 mg daily.

Patients who develop severe toxic reactions to dapsone, such as hepatitis or haemolytic anaemia, or in whom the organisms become dapsone-resistant, may be treated effectively with clofazimine 100–200 mg three times weekly. It is worth remembering that treatment with dapsone is very cheap whereas the other drugs are expensive, an important factor in poorer countries.

Symptomatic treatment, attention to nutrition, orthopaedic deformities and rehabilitation will also be required.

Patients with tuberculoid leprosy are not usually infectious; those with lepromatous leprosy should be isolated for 2–3 weeks if receiving rifampicin and for 4–5 weeks if receiving dapsone only.

Notification. Leprosy is a notifiable disease in Great Britain and the help of one of the National Health Service consultants in leprosy should be obtained in managing patients.

PLAGUE

Plague is endemic in the Far East, India, Central Africa, and parts of South America. The causative Gram-negative bacillus, *Yersinia pestis*, is transmitted by fleas from rats and other rodents to man.

Clinical Features. (1) **Bubonic plague** is the most common type. After an incubation period of two to four days there is sudden fever and constitutional upset, sometimes with delirium. Enlarged and tender lymph nodes (buboes) appear after two or three days, usually in the groins but not uncommonly in the neck or axillae. Of recent years most cases have been of the pestis minor variety and constitutional upset has been relatively mild; ambulant cases are not unusual.

(2) **Septicaemic** and (3) **Pneumonic** plague are both rare; they are characterised by fever and profound toxaemia, with cough and signs of bronchopneumonia in the latter variety, but buboes do not form. The mortality rate varies in different epidemics and may be as high as 80%.

Diagnosis is established by isolating the organism from the blood or from material aspirated from a bubo.

Treatment. Combined therapy with the following drugs gives good results and in treated cases the mortality rate is low.

(1) Streptomycin 0.5 g IM 4-hourly until the temperature is normal, and then 1 g daily until a total of 15 g has been given, and
(2) Chloramphenicol *or* tetracycline 0.5 g 6-hourly for a week or 10 days.

Controls of Outbreaks. Patients must be strictly isolated and their clothes autoclaved or treated with malathion or DDT. Attendants should wear protective clothing and their clothes be treated with malathion. Contacts should take 1 g sulphadiazine thrice daily together with adequate fluid while exposed and for 6 days thereafter. If this and surveillance are not possible, vaccination is an alternative but causes severe reactions. Equally important is the energetic prosecution of campaigns against the rat and flea population of the district.

TROPICAL ULCER

Tropical ulcer is common in tropical countries. It usually follows minor trauma and is due to infection with *Fusibacillus fusiformis* or with *Borrelia vincenti*. Occasionally both organisms may be isolated from the ulcer.

Clinical Features. The ulcer usually occurs on the lower limbs. It starts acutely and after a few weeks may become chronic, covered with a slough and invade underlying tissues. It is usually solitary and has raised edges which may be thick and oedematous. Sequelae include scarring, deformity and development of epitheliomata.

Treatment. The causative organisms are sensitive to penicillin and procaine penicillin 600 mg (600 000 units) twice daily is satisfactory for treatment. Tetracycline 500 mg four times daily for seven days is an important alternative. The ulcer may be kept clean with hypertonic magnesium sulphate.

RELAPSING FEVER

The causative organisms, spirochaetes of the genus *Borrelia*, are transmitted by lice and ticks. The disease is found in southern Europe, South America, the Middle East, Africa, and India.

Clinical Features. The incubation period is usually about a week, but varies from a day or so to a fortnight. The onset is remarkably sudden, with giddiness, headache, fever and rigor, pains in the back and limbs and sometimes vomiting. There is continuous high fever for several days and the patient soon becomes gravely ill, restless, and often delirious, with enlargement of the liver and spleen, sometimes purpura, and occasionally in severe cases, jaundice. On the fifth or sixth day the temperature drops to normal and there is a sudden dramatic clinical improvement, but after a week or so the first of a series of relapses occurs, each febrile bout tending fortunately to be less severe than the last. The mortality rate is variable, but may be as high as 30%.

In tick-borne relapsing fever the febrile periods are of 2–3 days and are more numerous than in the louse-borne variety. Neurological complications may also occur.

Diagnosis is established by identifying the spirochaete in the blood during the bouts of fever.

Treatment. Tetracycline is given orally in doses of 0.5 g 6-hourly for 5 days.

YAWS

This disease, due to *Treponema pertenue*, is non-venereal but is spread by direct contact from patient to patient. The highest incidence is among children over the age of eighteen months.

Clinical Features. The first sign is a papular skin rash, which eventually ulcerates. Hyperkeratosis of the soles of the feet is common and there may be lymphadenopathy and lesions in the bones and periosteum. The disease usually runs a very chronic course over many years.

Diagnosis is established by identifying the *Treponema pertenue*. The Wassermann reaction is also positive.

Treatment. Penicillin aluminium monostearate (PAM) a slow release penicillin is very satisfactory. The dose is 1.2 mega units daily by injection for 3 days. A second course should be given if treponemal antibodies remain detectable after 3–6 months.

TYPHUS FEVER

There are several varieties of typhus caused by closely related rickettsiae. The most important is epidemic or louse-born typhus, due to

R. prowazeki. Other varieties are murine typhus, which is transmitted chiefly by fleas; Rocky Mountain fever, 'fièvre boutonneuse' (prevalent along the Mediterranean coast), and Queensland or 'Q' fever, transmitted chiefly by ticks; tsutsugamushi fever and scrub typhus, transmitted chiefly by mites.

Epidemic Louse-borne Typhus

This has been one of the scourges of armies since prehistoric times and is an aftermath of civil disasters which lead to overcrowding and destitution. Lice become infected by drawing blood from an infected person and transmit the rickettsiae in their faeces, which may be rubbed into scratches and other lesions in the skin.

Clinical Features. The incubation period is usually 12 days, with a range from 5–14 days. The onset is gradual with headache, shivering, backache, general malaise and tenderness of the eyeballs, but by about the third day the patient is more seriously ill and has a flushed face, injection of the conjunctivae and tachycardia out of proportion to the fever. Epistaxis is common. About this time the temperature rises gradually towards its maximum (which is usually between 38.5–40°C) and remains at this level with only slight morning remissions throughout the rest of the illness. The rash appears on the abdomen on the fifth day and spreads to the chest and shoulders; the limbs but not the face may also be involved. The rash takes many forms but there are usually macules of varying sizes, a subcuticular mottling and sometimes petechial elements. As the rash develops the patient becomes stuporose or delirious and is difficult to rouse. By the second week the spleen is often palpable, the urine is scanty and contains protein and casts. In patients who recover, the temperature settles by lysis during the third week. The clinical severity and mortality rate of typhus varies widely in different epidemics, but most patients recover.

Murine Typhus

This is due to infection by *R. typhi* and is widespread in tropical and subtropical areas. It is endemic in rodents and is transmitted by the rat flea. Clinically it is similar to, but milder than, louse-borne typhus.

Mite-borne Typhus (Scrub Typhus)

An infection with *R. tsutsugamushi*, syn. *R. orientalis*, transmitted by mites from rodents which are the animal reservoir. It is found in Bangladesh, South East Asia and the Far East.

Clinical Features. A papule which ulcerates with the formation of a black crust—the eschar—develops in four days at the site of the infective bite, and is associated with local enlargement of the lymph nodes.

General symptoms develop at this time with fever, headache and limb pains. There may be conjunctival injection and periorbital oedema. About the fifth day a reddish-brown macular rash develops. Death can occur as a result of encephalitis, myocardial or renal failure.

Rocky Mountain Spotted Fever

One of the varieties transmitted by ticks; the causal agent is *R. rickettsii*. It is widespread on the American continent. The animal reservoirs are wild rodents, domestic dogs and cats.

Clinical Features. The onset is sudden with fever, headache and myalgia. Conjunctival injection is usual, the rash appears about the fourth day and consists of reddish macules. In the second week CNS signs may develop in severe disease, with confusion, meningitis and occasionally focal signs. The mortality is about 20% in untreated patients and may result from cardiac or renal failure.

Diagnosis *Weil-Felix Reaction.* Serum from patients with these rickettsial infections agglutinate OX strains of *Proteus vulgaris*.

		Proteus	
	OX 19	OX 2	OX K
Louse-borne typhus	+ + +	+	
Flea-borne typhus	+ + +	+	
Tick-borne typhus	+ + +	+	+
Mite-borne typhus			+ +

False positives can occur with proteus infection, relapsing fever, leptospirosis and brucellosis.

Treatment. Tetracycline in doses of 0.75 g should be given 6-hourly for 48 hours and then 0.5 g 6-hourly until the temperature has been normal for two days. Intravenous glucose–saline may be required to combat dehydration; intramuscular chlorpromazine 50–100 mg or morphine 15 mg may be needed to control the delirium.

Control of Outbreaks

Delousing measures should be directed both to patients and to the population at risk. Clothes should be autoclaved or dusted with a DDT-containing powder. Specially exposed attendants may be vaccinated with the Cox type vaccine.

RABIES

This disease is caused by a rhabdovirus which gains access to the central nervous system and produces an encephalomyelitis. It is widespread throughout the world, but is not endemic in the United Kingdom, Scandinavia, Japan and Australasia. In Europe it is spreading westward and now occurs in animals within a short distance of the

Channel ports. Its continued existence depends on an animal reservoir of the virus. This varies in different parts of the world; in Europe the fox predominates; in Central and South America, the vampire bat; in the USA, the skunk and racoon; and in Asia and Africa, the dog. Infection is usually due to the bite of a domestic animal, commonly the dog. The virus passes in the saliva of the infected animal through the broken skin, though it can also pass through intact mucous membranes. After a variable period the virus, by travelling up the axons of peripheral nerves, ultimately reaches the central nervous system.

Clinical Features. The incubation period is from two weeks to two years. The initial symptoms are non-specific—fever, sore throat, myalgia and headache. Two clinical types of the disease are recognised:

(1) **Furious Rabies.** This is the more common variety. The striking feature is the development of painful spasms of the pharynx and larynx on attempting to drink. As the disease progresses the mere sound or mention of water can cause spasms which produce widespread opisthotonos and respiratory arrest. The spasms are associated with acute fear, and the patient may also experience hallucinations and confusion. He lapses into a terminal coma and death results from cardiac or respiratory arrest.

(2) **Paralytic Rabies.** This is a progressive flaccid paralysis starting at the site of infection and finally affecting all voluntary muscle. Death occurs in two to three weeks.

Diagnosis. *Animal Involved.* Diagnosis is confirmed by finding Negri bodies or evidence by immunofluorescent techniques of rabies antigen in the brain of the animal.

Human Involved. Specific antibodies are detectable in serum on about the 7th day of the illness and the virus has been cultured from the saliva of a patient. Fluorescent techniques may enable rabies antigen to be demonstrated in skin biopsies from the bitten area.

Treatment. *Prevention.* In areas where the disease occurs control of domestic animals is important. This consists of vaccination, muzzling of dogs and the elimination of stray animals. It is difficult to eliminate the main reservoirs as they are usually wild animals.

Vaccination. If infection is suspected the patient should be vaccinated as soon as possible. The best vaccine is the HDCS vaccine which consists of killed virus grown on human embryonic lung fibroblasts. The dose is 1.0 ml given intramuscularly on days 0, 3, 7, 14, 30 and 90. It is relatively free from side-effects. Human rabies immune globulin (HRIG) can also be used to produce passive immunity before the vaccine becomes effective. The usual dose is 20 units/kg; half into the bite and half intramuscularly.

Developed Disease. There is no cure for rabies once symptoms have developed. Treatment is symptomatic with heavy sedation and intensive care. The usual sedatives are diazepam 20–40 mg twice daily and chlorpromazine 100–200 mg three times daily. It is nearly always fatal.

YELLOW FEVER

Yellow fever is a viral infection which is found in Central and South America and Africa, but it has now become uncommon. The virus is transmitted by the mosquitoes of the genera *Aedes*. It may be transmitted from man to man but the main animal reservoir is in the monkey.

Clinical Features. After a short incubation period (usually 3–6 days) the onset of the disease is rapid with fever, headache and backache. A feature at this stage is the relatively slow pulse rate. In severe cases the disease progresses to jaundice with a tendency to bleed, leading to haematemesis (black vomit), malaena and epistaxis. Proteinuria is common and there is usually a leucopenia. The temperature may drop a few days after symptoms develop but will rise again as the disease progresses. Death occurs in about 10% of patients but the mortality is higher in epidemics. It may be due to myocardial and/or renal failure or to an encephalitis.

Diagnosis. The virus can be isolated from the blood in the first few days of the disease.

Antibodies appear in the blood in the second week.

Treatment. There is no specific remedy and treatment is symptomatic. Active immunisation with an attenuated virus is however very effective and affords protection for at least ten years.

LASSA FEVER

This disease, which is caused by an arenavirus, is found on the west coast of Africa. The incubation period is probably 3–17 days. The only natural reservoir yet discovered is the rodent *Mastomys natalensis*. Transmission from animal to man is through food and dust contaminated by infected rat excreta. Person to person infection occurs, particularly in hospitals through contact with infected blood, vomit, excretions and tissues.

Clinical Features. The disease starts with fever, headache and generalised aching. During the first week prostration is marked, with a relatively slow pulse rate and low blood pressure. A tonsillar exudate and a membrane on the pharynx are usual. In severe infection the disease progresses to coma; facial oedema and serous effusions may develop.

Diagnosis

(1) Isolation of the virus from the blood, throat or urine.
(2) Serum antibodies become detectable in a week.

See section on differential diagnosis of malaria, p. 670.

Treatment. This is mainly symptomatic but the infusion of plasma containing Lassa fever antibodies which is obtained from recovered patients appears to be useful.

MARBURG/EBOLA FEVER

This is a viral disease which first occurred in Marburg, West Germany where a small outbreak followed contact with African green monkeys. In 1976 there was a large outbreak in Southern Sudan and Zaire of a similar disease caused by a morphologically identical but immunologically separate virus now known as Ebola virus.

Clinical Features. The early symptoms are fever and headache, and this may be followed by abdominal pain, vomiting and diarrhoea. The rash which appears about the sixth day is macropapular against an erythematous background. With more severe infection lymphadenopathy, epistaxis and gastrointestinal bleeding may occur. There is leucopenia and sometimes a thrombocytopenia, and liver function tests reveal elevation of enzyme levels.

Treatment. This is symptomatic. Infusion of immune plasma may be beneficial in mild cases or in the early stages of the disease.

SANDFLY FEVER

This arboviral infection is transmitted by *Phlebotomus papatasi*, a small hairy midge about the size of a pin-head, and is prevalent in summer in Mediterranean countries, India and China. The incubation period is two to seven days. People new to an endemic area are particularly susceptible and immunity after a single attack is short-lived.

Clinical Features. Onset is sudden with high fever, headache, aching in the back and limbs and prostration. There is no rash though the sandfly bites may be vesicular and resemble chickenpox. The fever settles in three days.

Diagnosis is usually made on clinical grounds but blood films must be examined to exclude malaria. The virus can be isolated from the blood and a rising antibody titre can be demonstrated if specimens of blood are collected during and after the illness.

Treatment. There is no specific treatment.

Prevention. The phlebotomus is small enough to pass through an ordinary mosquito net, but impregnation with an insecticide helps to keep it out. Attention should also be paid to its breeding sites in cracks and crevices in walls, masonry and banks.

DENGUE

This is a group B arboviral infection transmitted by the mosquito *Aedes aegypti* and is widespread in tropical and subtropical coastal areas. The incubation period is five to nine days. Single attacks give immunity for a few months; after several attacks there is usually lasting immunity.

Clinical Features. The illness closely mimics sandfly fever but typically the fever lasts longer (a week or more instead of 3–4 days) and there is often a short second bout of fever after an afebrile period of a day or two ('saddle-back fever'). A morbilliform rash may be seen during this second phase. Leucopenia is usual and there may be enlarged cervical lymph nodes.

Diagnosis is usually easy in endemic areas. Malaria is ruled out by blood examination and anicteric yellow fever by the absence of proteinuria. Confirmation may be obtained by isolation of the virus or demonstration of a rising antibody titre.

Treatment. There is no specific treatment.

Prevention is by the use of mosquito nets and the eradication of breeding sites for the Aedes mosquito.

DIARRHOEAL DISEASES OF THE TROPICS

TRAVELLERS' DIARRHOEA

Clinical Features and Epidemiology. The commonest disorder affecting travellers to tropical regions is Travellers' Diarrhoea, the diarrhoea being a short-lived variety of this condition. It is known by many colourful local terms. Typically it affects persons who have arrived, usually from a temperate though sometimes from other tropical or subtropical regions, within the preceding three weeks. The diarrhoea commences suddenly and is often accompanied by nausea, vomiting and abdominal colic. Symptoms last a few days and usually clear up spontaneously. It often affects several persons travelling in a group, e.g. in a package tour or military operation.

Aetiology. In British Army/MRC investigations the organisms most frequently isolated were pathogenic strains of *Escherichia coli*, particularly strain 0 148. In many other cases mild *Shigella* infections were responsible. However no infective cause could be found in a considerable proportion of patients and it is probable that killed bacteria in reheated food, especially staphylococci, were responsible in the majority of these; in others intestinal viral infections may have been present.

Treatment. Only if symptoms are unusually severe and persistent is treatment required and in such cases a *Shigella* infection (q.v.) is probably responsible. Relief may be obtained from compound codeine tablets (BP) in doses of 2, taken 3 or 4 times daily. Two tablets of diphenoxylate hydrochloride 2.5 mg and atropine sulphate 0.025 mg (Lomotil) given 6-hourly is an alternative. More severely affected patients may be given Streptotriad (streptomycin 65 mg, sulphadimidine 100 mg, sulphadiazine 100 mg and sulphathiazole 100 mg) in doses of two tablets twice or thrice daily for 3 days.

Prevention. Avoidance of uncooked foods, especially salads, cream, cake fillings and meats, which, since cooking, have been handled or exposed to flies. Meat sandwiches and shellfish are obvious sources of infection. A single tablet of Streptotriad taken twice or thrice daily appears to be the most successful form of drug prophylaxis.

BACILLARY DYSENTERY (Shigellosis)

The characteristics of bacillary dysentery are the frequent passage of fluid stools often containing blood and mucus. There is associated tenesmus and colicky abdominal pain.

Clinical Features. The incubation period is short, a few hours to 3 days, rarely up to 8 days and is followed by the abrupt onset of diarrhoea which in severe cases may become almost continuous. Colicky abdominal pain occurs particularly during and just after the passage of stools. Early in the attack there is often nausea and vomiting and at that time the stools are faeculent but in severe cases later contain little other than mucus and blood. The temperature is variable and erratic. In the severer forms dehydration supervenes and the skin becomes inelastic and cold; the abdomen becomes retracted but rigidity is unusual though an acute abdomen may be mimicked. Occasionally dehydration and toxaemia precipitate renal and circulatory failure. Non-specific urethritis, arthritis with synovial effusions and conjunctivitis (Reiter's syndrome) may follow attacks of any degree of severity. Chronic bacillary dysentery is rare though symptom-free carriers occur. Complications include not only arthritis but peripheral neuritis, iritis, iridocyclitis, haemorrhoids and occasionally peritonitis with or without perforations of the gut.

Aetiology. There are three main groups of dysenteric bacilli designated by the genus name *Shigella*. *S. dysenteriae* is a specific organism without strains and is primarily separated from the others by producing neither acid nor gas in mannitol as well as being a non-lactose fermenter. It produces a powerful exotoxin. The *S. flexneri/boydii* group produce acid without gas in mannitol and does not ferment lactose. Serologically *S. flexneri* contain one or more group antigens which *S. boydii* lack but contain distinctive type antigens. Phage typing also enables separation of strains. The group produces endotoxins. *S. sonnei* is distinct from the others in being a late lactose not a non-lactose fermenter. It is also antigenically distinct and homogeneous.

Mode of infection. The disease is transmitted as a result of faecal contamination of food, water and drink by flies and carriers. Poor hygiene favours transmission.

Pathology. The organisms occur only in the intestinal tract and do not invade the mucosa or bloodstream. Pathological changes are brought about by the bacterial toxins and consist principally of hyperaemia, ulceration and thickening of the mucosa of the colon. The ileum may also be hyperaemic, the lymphoid follicles are first affected and ulcers form especially on transverse folds of the mucous membrane. Peritoneal adhesions may develop. Dehydration, shock and renal lesions follow in the severely affected.

Diagnosis is by culture of stools or preferably rectal swabs. Agglutination reactions are of limited value. The infection may be differentiated clinically from amoebic dysentery by its more acute onset, greater toxaemia, more numerous and more fluid stools with a greater content of mucus and pus cells and more diffuse mucosal inflammation when viewed sigmoidoscopically. Sigmoidoscopy should however not be performed on patients with acute, severe diarrhoea. Giardiasis (q.v.) may simulate bacillary dysentery.

Treatment. Replacement of fluid and electrolytes is of great importance and in less severe cases can be done orally. Quarter strength normal saline can be given and flavoured with fruit juice, and with potassium chloride added so that approximately 2 g are taken 8-hourly. The patient should take as much of this as possible for by the oral route it is virtually impossible to overload the circulation. Enough should be drunk to ensure that at least 1.5 litres of urine are passed daily. If there is much fluid loss intravenous therapy is required and 20 ml of isotonic saline per kg body weight are given plus any needed to replace abnormal losses. Potassium should be given orally if possible otherwise not more than 13 mEq (0.5 g) can be given intravenously per hour and not more than half that amount per hour over 24 hours. For infants and young children half-strength physiological saline brought up to isotonicity with glucose should be used (NaCl 0.9%, glucose 2.5%).

Resistance of shigellae to sulphonamides and antibiotics is now common and widespread so that whenever possible treatment should be with fluids only. Indeed *S. sonnei* infections rarely require specific drug therapy. Ideally sulphonamide or antibiotic therapy should only be started after stool cultures have been shown to be positive and have demonstrated the sensitivities of the organisms isolated. In severely ill patients however specific therapy may have to begin before cultural results are known.

AMOEBIASIS

This is common in tropical and subtropical countries. It also occurs occasionally in developed countries. Many people harbour the causative organism asymptomatically for years.

Infection takes place when the cystic form of *E. histolytica* is ingested in contaminated food (especially vegetables) or drink. Infection follows the faecal-oral route and food handlers have an important role in this. Cysts are killed at 55°C and boiled water is therefore safe. In the terminal ileum or proximal colon the cysts develop into active trophozoites—amoebae with four nuclei, which divide to form single nucleated organisms. In the presence of diarrhoea, amoebae are excreted and can be identified in the stool. If transit through the colon is slower, encystment occurs, cysts are passed in the stool, and the life cycle of the organism is complete. Differences in the pathogenicity of different strains of amoebae have been demonstrated and tropical strains are usually more pathogenic than those in temperate regions. Intercurrent bacterial enteritis may facilitate entry of amoebae into mucosa and precipitate amoebic dysentery in some who had hitherto been asymptomatic carriers.

Pathology. Multiplication of amoebae occurs in the subepithelial tissues and is dependent on symbiotic growth of bacterial flora from the colon. Shallow colonic ulcers result. After a variable period, submucosal invasion takes place, and amoebae are found mainly in the margins of the ulcers. When blood vessels are involved extra-intestinal metastatic spread occurs, most commonly to the right lobe of the liver which is involved via the portal system. Whether a transient amoebic hepatitis occurs before the development of an amoebic abscess is controversial. Although *clinical* hepatitis is not infrequent, proof that that is amoebic rather than non-specific toxic hepatitis is lacking. Local and metastatic spread to other organs occurs.

The clinical features can be divided into those associated with the colitis—with or without dysentery—and the complications either local or metastatic.

Amoebic Dysentery

Onset of diarrhoea is usually gradual and may occur within a week or so of infection or after several months. Stools (6–8 daily) are loose with blood and mucus. Fever is unusual and recovery takes place after a few days or weeks. The colon (especially the descending or sigmoid) is sometimes palpable. Following a period of constipation, a further bout of dysentery occurs. Attacks seem to be more severe in malnourished and debilitated patients. They can be acute with severe dehydration, haemorrhage or perforation, but such sequelae are unusual. Colitis without dysentery is characterised by irregular bouts of mild diarrhoea sometimes with blood and mucus. This is important in differential diagnosis, where non-specific ulcerative colitis and colonic carcinoma may be closely mimicked; all patients with intermittent diarrhoea, whether blood and mucus is present or not, who have been in a tropical country should be assumed to have this disease until it is disproved. If a diagnosis of non-specific ulcerative colitis is made and corticosteroids are administered and/or colectomy is performed the result may prove fatal. Granulomatous masses (amoebomata) occasionally form in the intestinal wall or peri-anal region. They may be palpable either per abdomen or on rectal examination and carcinoma may be closely mimicked. Complications of colitis also include haemorrhage, and perforation leading to amoebic peritonitis.

Amoebic Liver Abscess

This is not excluded by the lack of a history of diarrhoea or dysentery. Only rarely does it develop *during* an attack of dysentery. Usually one, but sometimes multiple abscesses are present, three quarters are in the right lobe of the liver. Clinically, the liver is enlarged and tender, and a high swinging fever and sweating ensue. Bulging in the right hypochondrium or over the right lower ribs may be present. Jaundice is unusual. Breathing is often painful with signs of consolidation and/or effusion in the right lower chest. If the abscess erodes the diaphragm it may reach the bronchi and classical 'anchovy sauce' (necrotic liver tissue containing amoebae) is coughed up. Local spread to the pericardium with production of amoebic pericarditis is a grave development. Spread to contiguous organs or distant metastatic spread to organs such as the brain are rare.

Investigations. Demonstration of *E. histolytica* trophozoites is needed for definitive diagnosis. In faeces, it is best that fresh warm stools are examined; motile trophozoites live for only a few hours in cold faeces. Engulfed red blood cells are present in some *E. histolytica* trophozoites. In cold specimens of faeces, mature cysts may be demonstrated, consisting of 4-nucleated structures. Sigmoidoscopy is of value in visualising amoebic colitis—shallow ulcers with undermined edges. A biopsy frequently proves of value. Barium enema gives variable results and is rarely diagnostic. In the presence of liver abscess, liver function tests are usually normal apart from a raised alkaline phosphatase concentration; there is a polymorphonuclear leucocytosis. A chest radiograph often shows a raised right diaphragm with consolidation and/or effusion at the right base. Liver 'scan' and/or ultrasound will demonstrate the site of the abscess. Trophozoites may be found in aspirate from the liver abscess or 'anchovy sauce' sputum in a proportion of cases, if examined immediately. Immuno-diagnostic methods are of value in the invasive disease only. The fluorescent-antibody-titre is raised to high concentrations in the presence of metastatic disease; antibodies persist however for some weeks after treatment of an infection and the test must therefore be viewed with caution in assessing cure. Complement fixation, gel-diffusion and haemagglutination techniques are also used.

Treatment. For amoebic dysentery or colitis 800 mg metronidazole thrice daily for 5 days, and for extra-intestinal forms of the disease the same dosage for 10 days should be given. It is important that alcohol is avoided during treatment or a severe confusional state may be troublesome. Recent reports suggest that a minority of strains of *E. histolytica* especially from India may be partially resistant to metronidazole. Liver abscesses resolve more rapidly if aspirated. That is especially so with a large abscess in a patient who shows signs of severe toxicity and pyrexia. Resolution of the 'filling defect' in the liver 'scan' and ultrasound often takes many months after successful treatment of a liver abscess. Amoebic empyema and pericarditis should be treated with aspiration or surgical drainage. In acute amoebic dysentery with dehydration, fluid replacement is indicated. For those passing only cysts diloxanide furoate (500 mg thrice daily for 10 days) is the treatment of choice. To establish cure, fresh stool specimens should be examined one month after treatment; immuno-diagnostic tests often remain positive for months, and are of no immediate value in assessing cure.

GIARDIASIS

Aetiology. *Giardia lamblia* (syn. *G. intestinalis*) is a flagellate protozoan which inhabits the duodenum and jejunum. It is pear-shaped in outline, has 4 pairs of flagella and a saucer-shaped depression on one side. The organism encysts and is usually passed in the stool in that form. The mode of infection is similar to that of amoebiasis and is by faecal-oral route. Considerable outbreaks of the infection have in recent years been associated with groups of persons on package tours, particularly to USSR, but also in USA.

Clinico-pathological Features. Many infections are asymptomatic but in many others there is diarrhoea and colic of varying severity. In recent years however the infection has gained in importance by becoming recognised as a common cause of the malabsorption syndrome (q.v.). The stools may be typical of that condition, being bulky, pale and associated with much flatus. There is often an abrupt onset and many persons in a group may be similarly affected. The mechanism whereby *Giardia* infections cause malabsorption is suspected to be by facilitating bacterial invasion of the jejunal mucosa and jejunal contents.

Diagnosis. The flagellate forms may be found in the stools, particularly if there is diarrhoea; if the stools are solid or semi-solid cystic forms usually occur. A string test is a valuable diagnostic procedure. In this a brushed nylon string, to which a gelatine capsule is attached, is swallowed and allowed to be carried into the upper intestine. After an hour or two it is withdrawn and the fluid it has trapped is squeezed onto microscope slides and examined. Mucus obtained in this way or found in stools is often a good source of *Giardia*. A fluorescent antibody test has also been divised for *Giardia* infection.

Malabsorption is recognised by the standard biochemical tests for this condition (q.v.).

Treatment. Specific treatment is with metronidazole given orally in doses of 200 mg twice daily for 10 days or 2 g daily for 3 days. Mepacrine may be given in doses of 100 mg thrice daily for 8 days.

CHOLERA

This disease, associated with poverty, overcrowding and low socio-economic status is characterised by severe watery diarrhoea, dehydration and vascular collapse. The causative organism is the *Vibrio cholerae*; most recent outbreaks have been caused by its *El Tor* variant. Infection is confined to the small intestine where functional changes in electrolyte and fluid transfer lead to net movement of fluid towards the lumen; the organism is not found in blood or urine. Cholera occurs endemically in India, Pakistan, Afghanistan and China and many other parts of the Far East; although epidemics periodically occur in the Middle East and tropical Africa they have in general been seasonal and self-limiting. The disease can today be transferred by air whereas in the past it followed the slower population movements of caravan routes, pilgrimages and sea travel.

Pathophysiology. The vibrios rapidly multiply within the intestinal lumen and cause loss of vast quantities of water and electrolytes. The morphological appearances of the small-intestinal mucosa are normal and the action of the cholera endotoxin is at a subcellular level. The equilibrium between absorption and secretion of electrolytes and fluid is grossly deranged leading to a massive net secretion into the lumen. The mucosa is able to absorb electrolytes and water normally from solutions containing glucose and glycine, and this suggests that abnormal secretion into the lumen dominates the situation. Severe dehydration with haemoconcentration and circulatory collapse result. Renal tubular necrosis with anuria and uraemia may occur.

Clinical Features. Infection is by the faecal-oral route; although rapidly killed at 55°C the organism can survive for several days on moist clothing and several weeks in contaminated water. In classical cholera the vibrios can be found in the faeces during the incubation period and for about 5 days during the attack; with the *El Tor* variety, however, the organism can persist for weeks or months. Gastric acidity has been suggested to be important in prevention of the disease and a claim has been made that blood group O is associated with a higher infection rate than group A. Protection after the disease is incomplete, and lasts only for a short period.

The incubation period is from a few hours to 5 (mean 3) days and there are no prodromal symptoms. A broad spectrum of clinical severity exists, from subclinical illness to rapid death in untreated cases. Diarrhoea is at first mild but soon increases with the painless passage of large volumes of opalescent liquid, the classical 'rice-water' stools. The stools contain very high concentrations of vibrios. Blood may be present later in the disease. Vomiting usually starts after the diarrhoea and consists of material similar to the stool, and also teeming with vibrios. This continues for 3–4 days during which dehydration may become extremely severe, with dry mouth and tongue, loss of skin elasticity, sunken eyes and hollow cheeks. Progressive dehydration leads to fall in blood pressure and circulatory failure. Body temperature is often elevated, initially mildly and more so later. Muscle cramps, tetanic spasms, confusion and disorientation may occur. Oliguria procedes to anuria and acute renal failure. The rapidity of death depends on the severity of dehydration. Mortality rate in a cholera epidemic is often 50% and even higher in children and old patients. If effective treatment is instituted early, recovery is dramatic.

Diagnosis is usually straightforward, especially in epidemics; other causes of acute diarrhoea and vomiting, and algid malaria (*Plasmodium falciparum*) should be considered. Vibrios are easily identified in stool or vomit.

Treatment. Prophylactically, vaccination with killed vibrios renders some protection; two injections 0.5 and 1.0 ml, separated by 1 week, should be given. Partial protection lasts for approximately 3 months. Treatment of the disease is aimed at repleting the water and electrolyte balance and correction of acidosis, if present.

Fluid replacement therapy has been revolutionised by the demonstration that water and electrolytes can be absorbed well from the small intestine in cholera if given as a glucose solution of the correct molar concentration (glucose-stimulated membrane-transport).

Thus an oral solution containing:

Sodium chloride	3.5 g
Sodium bicarbonate	2.5 g
Potassium chloride	1.5 g
Glucose	20.0 g

and made up to one litre, will in all but the most severe case and in the absence of vomiting produce rapid rehydration. The volume of fluid given is based on fluid loss in stools—which should be measured every 2 hours—20 litres or more may be lost in 24 hours.

For initial rehydration, intravenous fluids are necessary in a severe case. State of hydration is assessed clinically, on the basis of general appearance, skin turgor, etc. In an average case, one tenth of the body weight (kg) of fluid in litres should be given initially, i.e. for a 50 kg patient 5 litres are necessary. The first litre should be given in 10 minutes. Solutions vary in their composition; one example (used in Dacca, Bangladesh) contains:

Sodium chloride	5.0 g
Sodium bicarbonate	4.0 g
Potassium chloride	1.0 g

made up to one litre.

Other measures are directed to management of anuria and shock. Analgesics may be necessary for severe muscle cramps, and intravenous calcium gluconate for tetany. Tetracycline is of proved efficacy in shortening duration of diarrhoea and clearing the stools of vibrios in the *El Tor* variety; it is usual to start treatment 3 hours after replacement therapy has commenced, i.e. when vomiting has stopped. The diarrhoea is usually controlled within 48 hours. Careful nursing is necessary; contacts should be vaccinated and great care taken over disposal of faeces and bed linen, and the sterility of water supplies.

MALABSORPTION SYNDROMES OF THE TROPICS

Chronic diarrhoea with frothy fatty stools has for centuries been recognised as common in the tropics and the term 'sprue' was applied to this syndrome by Sir Patrick Manson. A similar condition can result from several different causes some of which have only been recognised in recent years. The conditions causing malabsorption in temperate regions can, of course, also be found in the tropics and must be considered in the differential diagnosis of patients.

Tropical Sprue (Tropical Malabsorption Syndrome, p. 95)

This is characterised by steatorrhoea with the passage of bulky pallid stools particularly in the early morning and often also glossitis, abdominal distension, loss of weight and in severe cases anaemia.

Aetiology. During the Second World War sprue was shown to be likely to follow dysentery and infective diarrhoea. A number of infective causes of diarrhoea are now well recognised as causes of malabsorption similar to the classical sprue syndrome. These include particularly strongyloidiasis and giardiasis (q.v.). Indeed the latter may cause a syndrome indistinguishable from classical sprue. Classical sprue however continues to be a clinical entity well recognised in the tropics. It may well represent the final common pathway of a number of conditions yet to be fully delineated and the use of the term sprue or tropical malabsorption syndrome does not imply that a single cause of the condition exists. Nevertheless the majority of cases follow within weeks or months of a recognised bout of diarrhoea probably of infective origin. In many patients with tropical sprue, *Enterobacteria* and *Klebsiella* have in recent years been demonstrated in the normally sterile contents of the small intestine and there is evidence that cellular absorption is impaired by these bacterial toxins. Infections in some people may lead to subsequent impairment of intestinal mobility that leads to persisting bacterial overgrowth. Much, however, remains to be elucidated before it can be fully understood why some people develop sprue particularly after intestinal infections, including travellers' diarrhoea, and some do not.

The disease is particularly common in India, the Far East and in the Caribbean, and is rare in Africa. The reason for its rarity in Africa has not been satisfactorily explained.

Pathology. Some stunting of the intestinal villi and cellular infiltration of the lamina propria occurs but severe flattening of the villi as in adult coeliac disease is unusual. Megaloblastic bone marrow change may result, usually from impaired folate absorption. Malabsorption of fat, Vitamin B_{12}, and xylose occurs. Lactase deficiency may result from severe mucosal damage and secondary hypolactasia then develops. The plasma protein and serum calcium values are reduced in longstanding cases.

Clinical Features. Diarrhoea with large, pale, fatty, frothy stools passed particularly in the early morning are typical of the disease. Because of their high fat and gaseous content the stools usually float in water. Flatulence and flatus are troublesome, there is abdominal distension and lethargy becomes marked. In untreated cases glossitis and anaemia later develop and there may be hypoalbuminaemia and oedema.

Diagnosis. A 24-hour collection of faeces from the patient will contain more than the normal 5 g fat. The blood sugar curve following administration of 50 g glucose is flat, i.e. rises by less than 30 mg %. Absorption and excretion of xylose are delayed after administration of 25 g in 500 ml water. There is impaired absorption of Vitamin B_{12} which can be revealed by the Schilling test. Jejunal biopsy will reveal changes already described (vide supra). A barium meal will reveal a loss of the jejunal mucosal pattern and loops of small bowel become dilated and the barium within them pooled into relatively large masses.

Differential diagnosis. The clinical and pathological features of steatorrhoea in other conditions have to be considered and usually enable differentiation to be made without much difficulty. These conditions include gluten enteropathy, regional enteritis, strictures of the small intestine, pancreatitis, giardiasis (q.v.), strongyloidiasis (q.v.), intestinal atrophy following severe malnutrition, radiation and prolonged use of neomycin and steatorrhoea that sometimes follows partial gastrectomy. Occasionally infection with *Capillaria phillipinensis* and *coccidiosis* (*Isospora hominis* and *I. belli*) appear to cause malabsorption.

Prognosis. This following modern treatment is good but formerly it was poor and death often resulted.

Treatment. A high protein diet should be supplemented for 3 weeks with folic acid in doses of 5 mg thrice daily. Tetracycline should be given in doses of 250 mg thrice daily for 2 weeks. If anaemia is severe a transfusion of packed red cells may be helpful and if improvement does not follow then folic acid and Vitamin B_{12} may be given, Vitamin B_{12} being injected in doses of 200 μg weekly for 2 weeks. Attention must be given to fluid balance and to plasma electrolytes.

Ileal Tuberculosis

Tuberculosis of the ileocaecal region is an important and under-diagnosed cause of malabsorption in the tropics.

Clinical Features. There is malabsorption with diarrhoea and weight loss. A low grade pyrexia is common. Lymphadenopathy is sometimes present. A mass is occasionally felt in the right iliac fossa. Barium meal and follow-through will often show multiple ileal strictures. Acid-fast bacilli are rarely identified in the stool. The diagnosis is difficult and diagnostic laparotomy is frequently necessary. It is important not to overlook this condition when considering the differential diagnosis of diarrhoea and malabsorption in indigenous inhabitants of tropical countries even when it is many years after they have left their native land.

Treatment is with antituberculous agents; resection of ileal strictures is frequently necessary.

Chronic Calcific Pancreatitis

This is common in indigenous people of tropical countries. Its aetiology is uncertain but malnutrition in infancy and alcohol have been incriminated. Clinical presentation is with symptoms suggesting malabsorption, and weight loss which is often severe, associated with diabetes mellitus and frequently severe abdominal pain penetrating to the back. Diagnosis is by demonstration on a straight abdominal radiograph of the extensively calcified pancreas.

Treatment consists of treating the diabetes mellitus and the pain (which is often very severe). Pancreatic extract may be given with meals to attempt to counteract the exocrine deficit.

Lactase deficiency

Diarrhoea, which is sometimes fatty, may be caused by lactase deficiency of constitutional origin. The prevalence of the deficiency varies in different racial groups. In some negro races and in Northern Cypriots it may reach 90 %, whereas in Northern Europe about 10 % are affected.

The **diagnosis** is suggested by abdominal symptoms related to ingestion of milk though in mild cases this may be difficult to elicit. There is a flat lactose tolerance test, normal glucose and galactose tolerance tests and normal jejunal mucosa as revealed by biopsy.

The **treatment** is to avoid milk and milk-containing foods.

Deficiency of other disaccharidases, especially sucrase and iso-maltase, occasionally causes diarrhoea in adults but is more likely to affect infants. The deficiencies are partly outgrown in later life.

PROTEIN-ENERGY MALNUTRITION

Malnutrition is common in Africa, India, the Far East and Central and South America, especially in children under five. It is responsible for many deaths in infancy and early childhood in these parts of the world. Protein-energy malnutrition covers a spectrum of deficiencies but the main groups are marasmus, which is due to lack of both protein and energy producing foods, and kwashiorkor which is due mainly to protein deficiency in the presence of a relative sufficiency of carbohydrate. Elements of both types may exist in the same patient and the clinical picture may be further modified by mineral and vitamin deficiencies and by infection.

Marasmus

This frequently occurs during the first year of life and a precipitating factor is diarrhoea or other illness which depresses the child's appetite and vigour. Social factors and parental ignorance and mismanagement are important. Early weaning is occasionally partly responsible but continuation of breast feeding in the absence of adequate milk flow is probably more important. Marasmus is caused by lack of both protein and energy-producing foods.

Clinical Features. The child appears wizened with shrunken facies and the appearance of dehydration. He is grossly underweight and growth is slowed. The child is usually apathetic, weak and languid. Hunger is not usually marked. The abdomen may be distended and diarrhoea with bulky stools is common.

Kwashiorkor

The essential cause of kwashiorkor is a diet which is predominantly deficient in protein and relatively adequate in carbohydrate. This may arise from a number of causes:

(1) *Early Weaning.* This happens in developing countries where, because of social changes, mothers are taking to Western ideas with insufficient background knowledge. After early weaning the infants are not given the correct foods, and in particular foods containing little protein.

(2) *Heavy Parasitic Infection.* Hookworm and ascariasis are known precipitating factors.

(3) *Infection.* Intercurrent infections, by impairing appetite, can decrease protein absorption in borderline cases and thus act as a precipitating factor.

(4) Three other factors may modify nutrition:

(a) Wars.

(b) Poor harvests.

(c) Customs and taboos which may forbid certain foods which are rich in protein.

Clinical Features

(1) Children are usually lethargic and have an appearance of misery. This is attributed to hyponatraemia and hypokalaemia.

(2) Loss of weight is a major feature of kwashiorkor and may be diagnostic in the early stages.

(3) Low muscle bulk especially the biceps with increased subcutaneous tissue is due mainly to deficient formation of muscle because of insufficient protein.

(4) Flaky-paint dermatitis occurs late in the disease and is due principally to stretching by oedema of superficial layers of skin. Deficiency of Vitamin A may also be partly responsible. Stomatitis and inflammation of other mucocutaneous junctions may occur as a result of multiple vitamin deficiencies.

(5) Recurrent infection is mainly due to lowered immunity. Because of protein deficiency, not enough immunoglobulin is synthesised and therefore immune mechanisms are impaired.

(6) Anaemia is usually marked and is largely due to the protein deficiency. In some cases it is aggravated by hookworm infection.

(7) Lack of protein also leads to deficiency of enzymes especially mucosal disaccharidases which are responsible for splitting sugars. This causes a malabsorption state with diarrhoea. Hypoglycaemia is also a feature of the disease and may be due to deficient glucose absorption.

(8) Oedema is a main feature of the disease. It may be attributed to two causes, hypoproteinaemia, and low grade congestive cardiac failure due to anaemia. Hookworm infection may aggravate the hypoproteinaemia.

Treatment. The essential treatment is to give adequate protein and calories in the diet. This can be achieved in various ways. Dried skimmed milk has been widely used. It can either be made up with water (60 g in 600 ml of water provides 21 g of protein and 240 calories) or sprinkled on the child's food. The aim should be to give 2–3 g/kg of protein daily. Unskimmed milk may be too rich in fat but if it can be taken 100 ml/kg/day is adequate. Milk or skimmed milk alone is not an adequate diet so it must be added to the local staple diet and recipes are available. Dietary supplements may also be required and these include potassium (8.0 mmol/kg/day), magnesium (2.0 mmol/kg/day) and iron. Multiple vitamin preparations are also important in the early stages of treatment.

Infection is frequently a complicating factor and some authorities give penicillin and/or a course of sulphonamides as a routine. The most important and most common precipitating infection however is malaria and this should be vigorously sought for and treated.

Helminthic infections are common precipitating factors and bephenium hydroxynaphthoate is a useful vermifuge with a wide range of activity. In severe cases with marked anaemia, transfusion may be required and this is best if given as packed cells for there is a risk of overloading the circulation. Although mild cases are readily treatable severe kwashiorkor carries a high mortality.

Prevention. The prevention of malnutrition is complex and involves economic, social and educational factors. In spite of the efforts of government, international agencies and other bodies, malnutrition remains a major cause of ill health in the Third World.

FURTHER READING

Cook, G. C., *Tropical Gastroenterology*, Oxford University Press, Oxford, New York and Delhi, 1980.

Woodruff, A. W., *Medicine in the Tropics*, 2nd edition, Churchill Livingstone, Edinburgh and London, 1984.

Woodruff, A. W. and Bell, S., *Synopsis of Infectious and Tropical Diseases*, 2nd edition, John Wright, Bristol, 1978.

Lucas, A. O. and Gilles, H. M., *A Short Textbook of Preventive Medicine for the Tropics*, 2nd edition, Hodder and Stoughton, Sevenoaks, 1984.

CHAPTER 18

DISEASES OF THE SKIN

If all diseases are considered together, then it will be found that the external diseases, or skin diseases, constitute a very significant proportion of the total. Many skin diseases are of minor importance, but some can give rise to significant illness or even death if untreated. One advantage that skin diseases have over other disorders is that the morphology can be examined completely in any one individual and the lesions are readily available for histological examination if this is appropriate. Wrong diagnosis is generally made because the patient is not examined carefully and completely. Well over 80% of skin disease should be easily diagnosed and treated by a general practitioner. Hospital referral is seldom necessary, but it is a fact that 1% of a population in most areas of the British Isles are seen by a Hospital Consultant per annum as new referrals. This figure could be significantly reduced, in many instances, by a simple diagnosis and application of sensible treatment by the primary health care doctor.

Most dermatologists would agree that it is better to keep treatment safe and simple. New remedies are not necessarily the most successful, and occasionally result in a dermatitis medicamentosa, that is a contact dermatitis to the topical application. Moist, exudative lesions need a lotion to dry them up, chronic, scaly lesions are best treated with an ointment or cream, and some diseases have appropriate systemic therapy.

RED SCALY ERUPTIONS

A very large proportion of skin disease comes under the heading of an erythemato-squamous dermatopathy, that is red, scaly lesions. There are seven important conditions in this group, namely all the *eczemas, superficial fungus diseases, psoriasis, pityriasis rosea, secondary syphilis, discoid lupus erythematosus* and *lichen planus*. The eczema group has six main constituents, that is *atopic eczema, contact eczema, seborrhoeic eczema, discoid* or *nummular eczema, stasis eczema* and *chronic hand and foot eczema*. These will now be considered.

ECZEMA AND DERMATITIS

The words 'eczema' and 'dermatitis' have been a source of confusion for many years. It is now generally accepted that they are synonymous and clinically and histologically refer to the same condition. However, because of long usage the two words are sometimes retained and eczema is used if the cause is endogenous, as in atopic eczema, and dermatitis is used if the cause is exogenous, such as in a contact dermatitis due to nickel.

Some substances provoke a dermatitic reaction when applied to the skin of normal people, others only when applied to the skin of a sensitised individual. The former is often referred to as a primary irritant dermatitis and the latter as a contact dermatitis followed by the name of the causative agent. A very common cause of a primary irritant dermatitis is detergents; these are often too strong to be applied undiluted to the skin.

Atopic eczema generally begins after the age of three months and before the age of two years. It is frequently associated with asthma and hay fever. The eczematous lesions may develop first on the face in very young children but subsequently the antecubital and popliteal fossae are the sites most commonly affected.

Contact eczema or dermatitis is extremely common and the substances which may provoke this reaction can be classified into the following groups:

(1) *Chemicals.* Almost any therapeutic agent applied to the skin may induce a dermatitic response, particularly if it is applied repeatedly over a period of time. Drugs such as neomycin, penicillin and streptomycin are common causes and doctors, nurses and students should be very careful when giving injections with the last two substances not to allow any of the solution to come into contact with their hands. Nickel (on rings, necklaces and brassiere clips), lipstick, nail varnish and hair dyes are common causes of a contact dermatitis and so are furs and some articles of clothing. Soaps, bleaching agents and detergents usually cause a primary irritant dermatitis rather than a true contact dermatitis.

(2) *Substances of Plant Origin.* In this country the plants which most commonly give rise to a contact dermatitis are primulas and chrysanthemums.

(3) *Micro-organisms.* Skin infections such as impetigo and ringworm (tinea) may be accompanied by an eczematous reaction. The diagnosis of contact dermatitis is usually suggested by taking a careful history and by the site and distribution of the lesions. It may be confirmed by a patch test when appropriate dilutions of the suspected substance are applied to an area of normal skin, usually on the back, covered with a micropore dressing and left for 48 hours, when it is removed. The tested area should be reviewed another 48 hours later. A positive result is seen with the development of a dermatitic response in the area of skin covered by the testing substance.

Treatment. The most important point is the removal of the cause if this is known. Contact with the offending agent must be prevented. If there are several possible causes, for example if the patient is a hairdresser or dentist, patch tests must be done to determine the exact cause. For local therapy treatment with a 1% hydrocortisone ointment is the safest remedy. However, betamethasone valerate or triamcinolone acetonide are often more effective and may be needed, but these agents can induce striae formation, atrophy of the skin and telangiectasia if they are used for too long and particularly if they are applied under polythene occlusion. The stronger steroid ointments should rarely be used in children. If the dermatitic lesions are secondarily infected, then the steroid may be combined with an antibiotic such as tetracyline. Neomycin should not be used on the skin because of the danger of sensitisation. Other antibiotics should be avoided as topical applications, because they may need to be used systemically.

Seborrhoeic Eczema or Dermatitis. It is difficult to give an exact cause of this condition and it is often considered constitutional in origin, because some individuals seem to be more prone to it than others. However, a reasonable definition might be a low-grade infected eczema, with three main clinical components: First, bad pityriasis capitis. Scaling of the scalp (dandruff) is extremely common and in most cases probably due to inadequate hygiene, that is the individual does not shampoo often enough. However an extremely crusted and infected scalp is undoubtedly pathological and called pityriasis capitis. Second, flexural infected eczema. The lesions are situated behind the ears, on the cheeks next to the nose, in the axillae and groins. Third, a presternal petaloid dermatitis. Red, scaly lesions on the front of the chest are particularly common in older men.

Discoid or Nummular Eczema. In older individuals disc-like lesions are seen predominantly on the legs, and occasionally the arms and trunk. They are notoriously unresponsive to treatment and cause a great deal of distress because of the pruritus. They are not associated with systemic disease.

The stronger fluorinated steroids, if necessary under polythene occlusion at night, are usually helpful, for instance betamethasone valerate and triamcinolone acetonide.

Stasis Eczema. Most patients with chronic varicose veins develop stasis eczema, classically just above the ankles, which, if untreated, may progress to a varicose ulcer. Similarly most chronic leg ulcers are surrounded by an area of eczema which may need different treatment to the ulcer itself. Ultimately resolution of the eczema depends on appropriate treatment for the veins which are responsible for its development.

Chronic Hand and Foot Eczema. Many patients present with this type of lesion, which is characterised by its non-responsiveness to ordinary therapy. Occasionally these individuals, in fact, have psoriasis, but often the cause is unknown because patch tests are negative and scrapings for a fungus infection are negative.

Fungus Infections. See below.

Syphilis and the Skin. The skin can be affected in all three stages of syphilis. The primary chancre is the first stage occurring at the point of infection and is a small button-like ulcer. Scrapings confirm the diagnosis by observing the spirochaete with dark ground illumination under the microscope. The secondary stage may present with an extensive eruption over the trunk which is red and scaly and may have a slightly coppery tint to the eruption. There may also be ulcers in the mouth, a lymphadenopathy, general malaise and pyrexia. Loss of scalp hair may be a feature. The third stage is characterised by gummatous lesions over the trunk, limbs or face.

PSORIASIS

The cause of this common chronic skin disorder is unknown, although heredity (polygenic inheritance) undoubtedly plays some part in its aetiology. In some patients the onset appears to be precipitated by an acute infection, by pregnancy, or by minor trauma.

Clinical Features. The typical lesion is a red spot or patch of varying size covered with a thick layer of scales, which can be scraped off with the finger nail or curette, and which exhibits a characteristic silvery sheen. Further gentle scraping of the exposed red shiny surface causes bleeding, but there is no exudation of serum. The lesions are most often seen on the knees and elbows, but practically the whole surface of the body may be involved. The scalp is a common site and there may be hyperkeratotic patches on the palms and soles. Affection of the nails causes them to be thickened, pitted and striated and onycholysis may occur. The condition may persist for life, with occasional remissions and acute exacerbations.

Arthropathic Psoriasis

Arthropathic psoriasis is often seen in middle-aged or elderly patients. There is a characteristic destructive sero-negative polyarthritis of the hands and feet, associated with the skin lesions as described above, similar to that seen in rheumatoid arthritis (p. 419).

Treatment. The appearance of the lesions on exposed parts and the profuse scaling may cause great social embarrassment and it is important to stress to the patient and his relatives that the disorder is neither contagious nor infectious. He should also be encouraged to live an active, normal life with as much sunshine as possible, though a period of bed rest may be very beneficial during acute exacerbations. At such times a 1% hydrocortisone, Ung. emulsifications (BP) baths or even yellow vaseline (Paraff. molle flav.) should be used, but in the chronic stage preparations such as 0.1% dithranol in Lassar's paste should be applied daily after a tar bath. If this causes inflammation of the skin, 3% crude coal tar in a zinc or starch paste may be more suitable. Application of the absorbable fluorinated corticosteroids under polythene occlusion at night may clear the lesions but should be used with caution because of the danger of secondary infection. It is wise to treat only one area at a time, to use the ointment sparingly and to watch for the development of striae or atrophy of the skin. Topical steroids are helpful in the treatment of psoriasis, but the lesions are more liable to relapse than if they are treated with dithranol. Newer oral therapy for psoriasis includes methotrexate, razoxane and etretinate, but all these drugs should be used with caution, only in patients who are severely affected.

PITYRIASIS ROSEA

This is probably due to a virus infection and occasionally groups of three or four cases are seen in hostels and similar institutions. It produces one of the most characteristic rashes in dermatology. The first lesion (or *herald patch*) is an oval erythematous area about an inch across with a collarette of inward facing scale. It is often situated on the front of the chest. A few days later other similar but smaller oval patches appear, mainly on the trunk with long axes in line with the ribs, though there may be a few on the upper arms and thighs. There may be slight itching but this is not a striking feature and the general health is unimpaired and complete spontaneous recovery is the rule within about 6–8 weeks. No treatment is necessary, but if irritation is troublesome 1% hydrocortisone ointment may be used.

EXFOLIATIVE DERMATITIS

Exfoliative dermatitis is a syndrome in which there is a progressive desquamation involving the whole skin. It is characterised by the shedding of large amounts of the superficial layers of the skin, and is complicated by excessive heat loss and almost always by secondary infection. There may be generalised lymphadenopathy. If of long standing the constant skin loss causes negative nitrogen balance and hypoproteinaemia, which may result in oedema. Special skin structures (sweat and sebaceous glands and hair follicles) may be destroyed, sometimes permanently. If healing occurs these structures may not regenerate, so that the patient is left hairless and unable to sweat.

Many causes of exfoliative dermatitis are recognised, and the commoner are numerated below:

(1) Medicamentosa. Arsenic, gold, streptomycin, penicillin.
(2) External applications. Penicillin, sulphonamides, dithranol, streptomycin.
(3) Generalised atopic eczema.
(4) Generalised psoriasis. Often after therapy which is too strong has been applied.

(5) Generalised erythroderma may complicate Hodgkin's disease, leukaemias and lymphosarcomas.
(6) Two rare conditions, mycosis fungoides and pityriasis rubra pilaris.
(7) Idiopathic group, which is by far the largest group.

Treatment. Secondary infection should be treated appropriately, and the patient's body kept clean and warm. All other drugs should be withdrawn. If heavy metal poisoning is suspected a course of dimercaprol (BAL) should be given (p. 753). Some cases respond well to local and systemic steroids, but with the exception of the iatrogenic group treatment often has to be continued for months or even years.

DRUG ERUPTIONS

In theory nearly every drug can produce any type of skin reaction, but in practice a particular drug often produces a particular response, such as purpura. Problems must arise when a patient is on several drugs and it is often not possible to say which is the cause of his reaction. All drug therapy may have to be stopped and re-introduced one by one, when the eruption has faded. Drug eruptions are very common and may mimic the rashes of many other disease, such as measles and scarlet fever. The *barbiturates*, *sulphonamides*, *streptomycin*, *gold*, and *aspirin* commonly do so and *para-aminosalicylic acid* (*PAS*), *isoniazid* and *phenylbutazone* may also cause skin rashes.

Iodides are usually taken in the form of potassium iodide in a cough mixture and if taken for a long time can cause remarkable, large fungating lesions. The heavy metals such as *gold* and *arsenic* may cause a severe generalised exfoliative dermatitis which can be fatal if untreated. Twenty-five per cent of the patients on gold therapy will develop a skin eruption in time. In a sensitised individual an injection of *penicillin* may cause an urticarial rash, angioneurotic oedema or even death within a few minutes from anaphylactic shock. The last complication may occur in people who are atopic, that is they have asthma, eczema and hay fever. If a patient says he has had a rash from penicillin on no account should any more be given.

Treatment. In mild cases withdrawal of the drug is all that is needed. For relief of irritation an antihistamine tablet should be given, such as promethazine hydrochloride 25 mg or mepyramine maleate 100 mg two or three times a day. Nearly all antihistamines cause drowsiness and motor-car drivers and others should be warned of this side-effect. Chlorpheniramine maleate 4 mg three times daily is an alternative which is said to cause less drowsiness. Promethazine 50 mg or chlorpheniramine 10 mg may be given intramuscularly if the need is urgent. Very severe cases should be treated with systemic prednisolone.

For anaphylactic shock following injection of a drug give an immediate injection of adrenaline 1:1000, 0.5 ml intramuscularly, after which it may be necessary to give an intravenous infusion of saline, an antihistamine or hydrocortisone may also be required. It is a very good rule never to give any drug by injection without having a solution of adrenaline ready for use if needed.

URTICARIA

In susceptible subjects local urticaria may follow trauma, stings, or insect bites. Generalised urticaria may be due to sensitivity to certain foods, particularly shellfish and strawberries, or to drugs, notably penicillin, or to parenteral serum or blood. In other patients the condition is associated with worm infestation; but in more than half of the cases seen with chronic urticaria the cause is never found.

Clinical Features: The typical lesion is an extremely itchy wheal surrounded by a zone of erythema. The wheals, which may be of any size and shape, may cover the greater part of the body. There may be associated swelling (*angioneurotic oedema*) in the subcutaneous tissue and mucous membranes, particularly in the mouth and throat. Papular urticaria without much wheal formation is common in children.

Treatment. Quick relief can usually be obtained by giving 0.5 ml 1:1000 adrenaline hydrochloride subcutaneously. An intramuscular antihistamine, such as promethazine hydrochloride 50 mg may also be given. If there is laryngeal obstruction which is not quickly relieved by these measures emergency tracheotomy must be performed. Antihistamines are given by mouth for more sustained effect; promethazine hydrochloride 25 mg or mepyramine maleate 100 mg are the most powerful of these but often cause troublesome drowsiness. Chlorpheniramine maleate 4 mg has a slightly weaker antihistamine effect but causes less sedation. The tablets are given two or three times daily. Cortisone suppresses the lesions, but its administration is rarely justified in this condition. The best local application is calamine lotion or 1% hydrocortisone ointment.

ERYTHEMA MULTIFORME

This eruption consists of raised erythematous areas of irregular outline and varying size and shape; sometimes in addition there are vesicular, bullous, or nodular lesions. There may be associated ulcerative lesions on the buccal mucosa. Sometimes it appears as a cutaneous reaction to a focus of infection in the skin or elsewhere; sometimes it is a manifestation of acute rheumatism; sometimes it is a drug reaction; but usually the cause is never discovered. It may be preceded by herpes simplex, which is often the precipitating factor.

Apart from slight fever there is little constitutional upset and spontaneous healing occurs within a couple of weeks, though recurrent attacks are common.

STEVENS–JOHNSON SYNDROME

This is the severest variety of erythema multiforme presenting acutely with fever, followed by the appearance of ulcers in the mouth and sometimes on the conjunctivae. Within a few days an erythematous and bullous eruption spreads over the body, occurring particularly on the genitalia. The patient may be gravely ill for a week or two, but rapidly recovers when the temperature settles. Ophthalmic scarring however, may lead to blindness. Prednisolone should be given, particularly if there is a rising pulse rate or falling blood pressure.

ERYTHEMA NODOSUM

Clinical Features. In this condition there are painful red, tender nodules usually affecting the front of the lower legs, and occasionally the thighs and forearms. These subside spontaneously in 3–6 weeks, with some scaling of the skin and colour changes like a bruise. The nodules do not leave permanent skin changes. Occasionally the patient is pyrexial. Women are affected more commonly than men, with a peak incidence in the third decade of life.

The commonest cause is a streptococcal infection of the throat, but it is also often due to sarcoidosis or a drug such as a *sulphanamide*. *Pulmonary tuberculosis* is no longer a common cause, but it must be excluded. Less common causes are *ulcerative colitis*, *Crohn's disease*, *deep fungus infections* such as *coccidioidomycosis and Hodgkin's disease*. In Africa and Asia *leprosy* is a common cause.

Erythema nodosum is an important condition to recognise, because most patients need further investigations. The treatment is for the underlying condition.

INFECTIONS OF THE SKIN

Infection with coagulase positive staphylococci is responsible for *furunculosis* (*boils*), *sycosis barbae* (*folliculitis of the beard area*) *carbuncles*, *axillary hidradenitis*, and *impetigo contagiosa* (which may also be due to streptococcal infection). Only the last of these will be described here.

Impetigo Contagiosa

This is a very common condition and is due to a bacterial infection of the superficial layers of the skin. If the condition does not respond to treatment, an underlying cause such as scabies or pediculosis should be suspected. As the name implies it is spread by direct contact or by the use of contaminated towels or clothes.

Clinical Features. The first lesion is a pink macule up to half an inch in diameter, but within a few hours this becomes converted into a superficial vesicle, then a pustule which soon ruptures with the formation of a typical bright yellow crust. Bullous lesions may occur in children. The face is a common site. There is rarely any fever or constitutional disturbance.

Treatment. Patients with severe infection should be given flucloxacillin 250 mg 6-hourly by mouth. The essential local treatment is to remove the crusts with 1 % centrimide (Savlon). Topical antibiotic preparations should be avoided because of the risk of sensitisation. In many cases it is essential to give a systemic antibiotic. It is important to search for and treat any associated lesion, such as scabies or pediculosis capitis. The latter is particularly likely to be found in girls with long hair. The patient must of course be kept away from other children and must have his own towel and pillow-case, which should subsequently be sterilised by boiling.

Viral Diseases of the Skin

The commonest viral disease of the skin is the common wart or verruca vulgaris. Warts can occur on any part of the skin, but are particularly common on the hands and soles of the feet (*plantar warts*). Untreated, most warts will spontaneously remit in about 18 months, because the body develops immunity to the wart virus. Warts on the genitalia are often known as venereal warts and are often due to an antigenically distinct virus. Peri-anal warts can be very difficult to treat.

Little is known for certain about the transmission of the wart virus. However, there is strong circumstantial evidence that plantar warts may be acquired at swimming pools and in changing rooms. Contact may be a factor, but their contagiousness is low.

Treatment of warts can be legion, which suggests that there is no really effective remedy. Magic-type treatments probably owe a great deal to the fact that they are given when the wart is spontaneously remitting. Surgical removal is often apparently beneficial at first, but then many warts may develop around the site of the original lesion. Carbon dioxide snow and liquid nitrogen are probably as quick and effective as any other remedy. 40 % salicylic acid plasters applied every night can be useful for their keratolytic action. Podophyllin application can be very helpful for penile, vulval and peri-anal warts, but the patient must be warned to wash off the application a few hours later or ulceration may result. If the patient can be persuaded, no treatment is often the best treatment.

Herpes Simplex (The cold sore). This very common, localised vesicular lesion must be known to everyone. The lesions are generally on the face about the lips and the virus may be activated by an upper respiratory tract infection or sunlight. However lesions can occur anywhere, for example on the ear, the point of the shoulder or the penis. The last site may be particularly difficult to treat because they often occur after sexual intercourse. 5% idoxuridine in DMSO may have some effect in cutting short an attack if applied immediately it is apparent the lesions are developing. For the developed lesion, some patients prefer a spirit lotion and others an antibiotic (chlortetracycline) cream.

Herpes Zoster. Caused by the same virus as that responsible for chicken pox and therefore commonly, but not exclusively, occurring in adults. The characteristic lesion of herpes zoster is preceded by pain, which may result in mis-diagnosis of other disorders such as acute appendicitis. However, once the vesicles have erupted in the distribution of a cutaneous dermatome the diagnosis is readily made. Treatment with intravenous acyclovir may shorten an attack, and reduce the incidence of post-herpetic neuralgia. Acyclovir tablets (200 mg four or five times a day) are also available.

RINGWORM

This is a group of common fungus infections of the skin which affect mainly the scalp, the groin and the feet.

Tinea Capitis (Ringworm of the Scalp)

The infection is seen mainly in children under ten, particularly boys, and never persists beyond adolescence. The scalp shows a number of rounded or oval patches which are covered with fine greyish-white scales and from which most of the hairs have fallen out. Infected hairs may fluoresce a bright green colour under Wood's light, and this examination is therefore helpful in diagnosis. The fungus can also be identified microscopically in stumps of hair removed from one of the patches.

Treatment. Griseofulvin 250 mg two times daily for a month or 6 weeks is now the treatment of choice. Very occasionally, it may cause headache and urticaria, and it increases the effects of alcohol. Ketoconazole (200 mg daily with food) is also an effective remedy for superficial fungal infections and has the advantage of being anti-candidal as well.

Tinea Cruris (Ringworm of the Groins)

This infection occurs mainly in young adults, particularly men, and may be acquired by direct contact, from infected clothing or spread from between the toes. It causes a red, slightly raised patch extending from the crutch for two or three inches down the inner aspect of each thigh. There is sometimes itching in the affected area. The infection is seen mainly in hot weather and is more common therefore in the tropics.

Treatment. Half-strength Whitfield's ointment is usually very effective, but relapses in subsequent spells of hot weather are common. Imidazole creams may be used. Griseofulvin may also prove effective.

Tinea Pedis (Athlete's Foot)

This infection occurs with two characteristic distribution patterns, but both may occur together, the first showing vesicles and subsequent desquamation on the sole of the foot, and the second causing fissuring and maceration of the skin in the clefts between the toes. Like tinea cruris, with which it may be associated, this infection is often seen in young adults and is acquired from the floors of swimming baths and changing rooms.

Treatment. Half-strength Whitfield's ointment, an imidazole cream, and undecenoic acid ointment are three among a number of effective remedies. Relapse is common, however, and to try to prevent it careful attention to the hygiene of the feet is important. They should be washed daily, carefully dried and powdered and the socks should be changed every day.

PARASITIC DISEASES

Scabies

The animal causing scabies is a mite (*Sarcoptes scabiei hominis*). It has four pairs of legs and the female, which causes the trouble, is about 0.3 mm long, being therefore just visible to the naked eye. The male is smaller. The female makes a burrow up to a centimetre in length in the epidermis and lays about 30–40 eggs in it. Each egg hatches out in 4–8 days into a larval form which leaves the burrow and eventually matures into the adult form.

Infection is usually acquired by contact, for example by sleeping with an infected person. It may therefore be a venereal infection, or children may acquire it from their parents or from each other. Less often, infected blankets, bedding, or clothes may transmit the infection.

Clinical Features. The burrow is the characteristic lesion of scabies and appears as a fine, often zig-zag, hair-like line in the epidermis, greyish or whitish in colour and 0.5–1 cm in length. At the far end a tiny pinhead vesicle may be seen. These burrows occur mainly in the webs and sides of the fingers, the ulnar sides of the hands, the anterior axillary folds, the lower abdomen and penis and the lower part of the buttocks. They cause intense itching, particularly when the patient is warm in bed.

As a result of scratching secondary infection is common and there may be an extensive papular and pustular eruption.

Diagnosis is usually easy from the history of intense itching and the discovery of typical burrows and may be confirmed by identifying the female acarus or its eggs in a microscopical preparation of scrapings from a burrow.

Treatment. This starts with a hot bath, the patient being instructed to scrub with a nail brush and soap all areas where there are burrows. After drying himself the patient is painted from head to foot with a 25% emulsion of benzyl benzoate sparing only the head and neck, which are never affected by scabies in adults. Next morning the lotion is applied again and allowed to dry before the patient dresses. This regime is repeated for two more days. On the third night another hot bath is taken to wash off the remains of the benzyl benzoate and a complete change of clothing and bed linen is made. Gloves and other articles which are difficult to disinfect should be laid aside for three weeks, at the end of which time all acari they contain will have died. Residual itching after benzyl benzoate treatment is quite common. It is important to treat this with calamine lotion or crotamiton lotion because further applications of benzyl benzoate will make it worse by causing a dermatitis. It need hardly be said that all contacts with the patient, particularly those within his family circle, should be treated at the same time to avoid re-infection.

PEDICULOSIS

Lice are blood sucking parasites which mainly infest hairy parts of the body. The female produces several hundred eggs, each of which is attached to a hair and is commonly known as a nit. A larva is hatched out from the egg in 6–9 days and develops into a mature louse in one to two weeks.

Pediculosis Capitis (Infestation with Head Lice)

The louse concerned is the *Pediculus humanus capitis* which is about 3 mm long and 1 mm broad. It infests the scalp, the nits being attached mainly to hairs at the back and sides of the head. Since the louse deposits the eggs on hairs close to the scalp and since they have hatched out by the time the hair has grown an inch or so, the search for nits should be concentrated on hair close to the head. The diagnosis depends usually on the discovery of nits, since the lice themselves are few in number and difficult to find. Nits are greyish-white, shiny, oval, opalescent structures firmly attached to the hairs.

Infection may be acquired by direct transmission from person to person or by wearing infected headgear; it is now often seen in young men as well as in women living under poor hygienic conditions.

However, school children are particularly liable to be infested. Patients recently infected usually complain of irritation of the scalp, but those who have had head lice for a long time often seem to suffer no inconvenience at all. When there has been much scratching septic lesions of the scalp are a common complication.

Treatment. Gamma benzene hexachloride application is effective but may have to be repeated after a week. The hair should be shampooed 12 hours after the application and combed while wet with a fine-toothed comb. It is much easier to treat short hair.

Pediculosis Corporis (Infestation with Body Lice)

Pediculus humanus corporis is similar to the head louse but slightly bigger. It normally lives in the clothes and deposits its eggs in the seams and folds of woollen undergarments.

Clinical Features. Infestation causes a variable amount of itching; scratch marks are seen mainly around the shoulders, buttocks, and the fronts of the thighs and there may be a widespread eruption from secondary bacterial infection in these situations. Tramps and vagrants after life-long infestation may develop a generalised pigmentation of the skin like that seen in Addison's disease (vagabond's pigmentation). The diagnosis is established by finding the louse or its ova in the seams of the patient's underclothes.

Treatment. Gamma benzene hexachloride should be applied as a 0.6 % dusting powder and scrubbed on to infected hairy areas as a 2 % lotion in a detergent base. Underclothes must be washed and ironed and bedding and other clothing autoclaved. It is sufficient for the patient to take a hot bath before putting on clean clothes.

In some countries, in addition to their direct effects, infestation with head and body lice is important in the spread of typhus (p. 696) and relapsing fever (p. 696).

'Pediculosis' Pubis (Infestation with 'Crab' Lice)

This louse is not in fact of the species pediculus, its scientific name being *Phthirus pubis*. Its life history is similar to that of the pediculi, but it is smaller (about 2 mm by 1.5 mm) and does not spread typhus or any other disease.

Clinical Features. It infests the pubic region, but in very hairy men the whole of the trunk, the thighs, and the upper arms may be involved. On close inspection the adult lice can be seen, lying flat on the skin and holding on to a hair at each side; the nits are very similar to those of pediculus humanus and are closely attached to the body hairs. Infection is acquired mainly by sexual intercourse and occurs usually therefore in young adults.

Treatment is as for pediculosis corporis. Crotamiton lotion or even benzyl benzoate are alternative applications.

ACNE VULGARIS

Acne is often associated with seborrhoea (that is excessive sebaceous secretion). The essential lesion is the comedo, which is a sebaceous follicle, the opening of which has been blocked with sebum mixed with epithelial debris, and these comedones frequently become pustular from infection of the retained sebaceous material. They are found on the face, chest, shoulders, and back. Their formation appears to be favoured by androgens and they appear therefore in the years following puberty and more often in boys than in girls. Adolescent acne tends to disappear spontaneously in early adult life, though when it is very severe it may persist and healing of the lesions may leave permanent scarring.

Treatment. The treatment of acne falls under two headings: those applications which de-grease the skin and those which treat the secondary infection. Natural sunlight (or ultraviolet light therapy) combines the two actions and is the best single treatment for acne. A hair style which keeps the hair from falling over the face is important. Daily washing with soap and water is a help in mild cases, and the patient should shampoo his scalp at least three times a week. Oral tetracycline 250 mg twice daily for two months or longer may be of great benefit for patients with grossly infected lesions. All patients, particularly women, must be discouraged from picking and squeezing the lesions, and they should realise there is no magic cure, but patient, persistent therapy can achieve remarkable results.

ROSACEA

This is a chronic hyperaemia of the face, particularly the cheeks and central part of the forehead, leading to permanent dilatation of capillaries and the formation of telangiectases. The patients are often middle-aged women, many of whom also have vague digestive symptoms for which no definitive cause can be found. The cosmetic disability is aggravated by the flushing associated with the menopause and with the taking of alcohol or hot spicy food, i.e. anything which tends to make the face flush. There may be associated papules and pustules and sometimes hyperplasia of the sebaceous glands. Oral tetracycline 250 mg twice daily for 2 months and application of 2% sulphur in aqueous cream may be of benefit. Increasing strengths of sulphur may be combined with 1% hydrocortisone.

LUPUS ERYTHEMATOSUS (See p. 420)

LICHEN PLANUS

The cause of lichen planus is unknown. Although it usually clears up spontaneously in 6–18 months, relapses are common, and in some patients the lesions may persist for years. A lichenoid eruption, indistinguishable from lichen planus, may be caused by some drugs.

Clinical Features. The typical lesion is a small flat-topped violaceous papule, often little bigger than a pin's head. The papules may be limited to certain situations, such as the anterior aspect of the wrists and forearms, the genitalia, or the legs, or they may be very profuse and widespread over most of the body, though the face and other exposed parts are rarely affected. Linear disposition of the lesions along scratch marks (Koebner phenomenon) is common. In some of the patients bluish-white reticulate streaks or patches may be seen on the buccal mucosa. There is usually some irritation of the skin and sometimes this is severe.

Treatment. Confinement to bed and sedation may be necessary in very severe acute cases, but usually all that is necessary is an application such as calamine lotion in order to allay irritation. An antihistamine tablet such as promethazine hydrochloride 25 mg may help in this respect. If itching continues, 1 % hydrocortisone ointment may be tried. If the mouth, scalp, or genitalia are affected about a month's course of oral steroids may be given, but is seldom necessary.

PEMPHIGUS VULGARIS

This is a very serious auto-immune disease of the skin. Fortunately rare, it occurs equally in men and women and seldom appears before late middle age. Before cortisone therapy it was nearly always fatal within 2 years.

Clinical Features. The essential lesion is a superficial bulla which appears on normal skin with no surrounding erythema. Crops of these bullae appear on the skin and mucous membranes and soon rupture and become infected. Constitutional disturbance is severe.

Treatment. Cortisone or an equivalent must be given in high dosage—for example, prednisolone 60 mg daily. The dose is slowly reduced when fresh blisters cease to appear, but at least 15 mg daily should be continued until the patient has been free of symptoms for three months, when the drug may be further reduced in dosage. With this treatment a fatal outcome is not so common.

DERMATITIS HERPETIFORMIS

This disease has a clinical similarity to pemphigus, since the lesions are predominantly vesicular or bullous, and it tends to run a chronic or relapsing course. There are however, important differences; first, the vesicles and bullae are set on erythematous base and are often accompanied by urticarial and erythematous lesions. Second, the blisters tend to appear in clusters, particularly on the elbows, buttocks and posterior aspect of the thorax. Third, there are seldom lesions in the mouth. Fourth, constitutional upset is slight and, fifth, irritation of the skin is usually severe.

About 80% of patients with this condition have a coeliac syndrome with villous atrophy which responds to a gluten-free diet.

Treatment. Dapsone is the drug of choice and so often successful that it is sometimes used as a diagnostic test in this condition. The dose is 100–200 mg a day by mouth. Prednisolone and sulphapyridine are now less often used.

FURTHER READING

Sneddon, I. B. and Church, R. E., *Practical Dermatology*, 4th edition, Edward Arnold, London, 1983.

Hall-Smith, P., Cairns, R. J. and Beare, R. L. B., *Dermatology. Current Concept and Practice*, 3rd edition, Butterworth, London, 1981.

Borrie, P. (revised), *Roxburgh's Common Skin Diseases*, 14th edition, H. K. Lewis, London, 1975.

Levene, G. M. and Calnan, C. D., *Colour Atlas of Dermatology*, Wolfe Medical Books, London, 1974.

Marks, R. and Samman, P. D., (eds.), *Dermatology. Tutorials in Postgraduate Medicine*, Vol. 6. Heinemann Medical Books, London, 1977.

CHAPTER 19

SEXUALLY TRANSMITTED (VENEREAL) DISEASES

The word venereal is derived from Venus, the goddess of love, and is applied to those diseases which are communicated by sexual intercourse. The important members of this group are syphilis, gonorrhoea and other causes of urethritis and vaginitis; rarer disorders include chancroid and lymphogranuloma venereum.

GONORRHOEA

The *Neisseria gonorrhoeae* is a delicate organism which does not survive for long outside the body, and gonorrhoea is almost invariably acquired by coitus with an infected person. Recovery confers no immunity and it is therefore possible for the same individual to have repeated attacks of the disease. Young girls may acquire the disease from infected bed-linen and towels, and outbreaks of vulvo-vaginitis in children are in fact more often due to other organisms.

The *Neisseria gonorrhoeae* is identified in smears of purulent exudates as a Gram-negative kidney-shaped diplococcus which must be seen within the cytoplasm of polymorph leucocytes before the diagnosis can be made. It is rather difficult to grow in culture unless special media and increased carbon dioxide tension are employed.

Clinical Features

(1) **In Men.** Within about three to ten days of exposure to infection the first symptom is usually slight *scalding* on micturition, soon followed by a *purulent urethral discharge* and there may be tender swollen lymph nodes in the groin. If treatment is not given the infection tends to spread to the posterior urethra, as indicated by cloudiness in the second glass of voided urine. Infection of the *prostate* may follow and may cause acute retention of urine, while involvement of the *seminal vesicles* causes several local pain and fever. Stricture in the posterior urethra is a late sequela. *Acute epididymitis*, indicated by severe pain, swelling, and tenderness which often spread to involve the testicle on the same side is a serious complication since it may be followed by sterility. With modern treatment spread beyond the anterior urethra is very rare.

(2) **In Women.** After a similiar incubation period the disease usually presents with *painful, frequent micturition*, and *vaginal discharge*, though there may be no symptoms if the infection is confined to the cervix. Two-thirds of women infected do not seek medical advice, either through fear

or lack of presenting symptoms. Involvement of *Skene's* or *Bartholin's glands* may lead to large painful abscesses, though in fact Bartholin's abscess is much more often of streptococcal origin. If untreated the infection may spread to the uterus and Fallopian tubes, leading to the formation of a *pyosalpinx*; this presents with severe lower abdominal pain and fever and a tender adnexal mass can be felt on one or both sides on pelvic examination. It may be possible to demonstrate gonococci in cervical smears. Involvement of the tubes usually leads to permanent sterility.

Complications. Metastatic lesions due to transient bacteraemia are now very rare, but a purulent arthritis is occasionally seen. Gonorrhoeal rheumatism, however, is usually not due to bacteria in situ and may be in fact an associated Reiter's syndrome (p. 419). It may take the form of a fitting polyarthritis coming on a month or so after infection, or a single joint may be involved, particularly the knee, wrist or ankle. Associated tenosynovitis is common and iritis may occur.

Treatment. A single injection of procaine penicillin of 4.8 million units is usually adequate treatment of uncomplicated gonorrhoea. This may be combined with 1.0 g of probenecid given one hour before the injection to slow the excretion of the penicillin. Women may require a higher dose as they tend to respond less well. There are now strains of gonococci relatively resistant to penicillin; but most of the patients whose symptoms persist or relapse within a few days respond to procaine penicillin, fortified, BP, 5 ml (containing procaine penicillin 1.5 g and benzylpenicillin 0.5 g). A single injection of spectinomycin 2.0 g for a man or 4.0 g for a woman given intramuscularly is useful in patients who are sensitive to penicillin. Good results have also been obtained with co-trimoxazole 4 tablets twice daily for four days. This drug will not mask the appearance of syphilis. It is important to remember that the treatment of gonorrhoea with penicillin and some other antibiotics may suppress the appearance of a syphilitic lesion acquired at the same time and serological tests for the latter disease must always be made three and six months after the gonorrhoea has been treated.

SYPHILIS

As a result of improved treatment and the consequent reduced infectivity of patients with the disease, syphilis is much less common. It remains very important, however, because of the serious lesions which may appear in almost any organ of the body many years after the primary infection.

The causative organism, *Treponema pallidum*, is a thin, actively motile spirochaete from 6–14 μm in length, which can be recognised by its characteristic movements in preparations of the serous discharge from the early infectious lesions examined by the microscopic technique known as dark-ground illumination (DGI). It cannot withstand drying and is transmitted only by direct contact.

Congenital syphilis is contracted by the foetus through the placenta in the later months of pregnancy; acquired syphilis is nearly always the result of sexual intercourse with an infected person, though occasionally extragenital infection may be acquired, for example by doctors or nurses, by handling syphilitic lesions. Congenital syphilis is fortunately extremely rare nowadays. It is a preventable disease, since if a woman with syphilis is given adequate treatment sufficiently early in pregnancy the child escapes infection. Routine serum tests should therefore be made on all women on their first attendance at ante-natal clinics.

Clinical Features. Congenital syphilis may cause intra-uterine death and result in *miscarriage* or *stillbirth*, or the child may be born apparently healthy only to develop various stigmata of the disease during childhood. Early manifestations are failure to gain weight in the first month or two of life and an infection in the nose (*snuffles*) which interferes with the development of the nasal bones and leads eventually to the depressed bridge of the nose which is one of the most characteristic signs of the disease. A scaly yellow or copper-coloured *rash* is also common. Among the many lesions which may appear later in childhood are notches in the incisor teeth of the second dentition, which also tend to be widely spaced and to taper from the gum margin to the cutting edge (*Hutchinson's teeth*); scars known as *rhagades* radiating from the margins of the lips; and opacity of the cornea due to *interstitial keratitis* (IK). Aortic lesions are very rare in congenital syphilis, but juvenile forms of *tabes* and *general paresis* are occasionally seen.

Acquired syphilis passes through three stages, known as *primary* syphilis, *secondary* syphilis, and *tertiary* syphilis. The secondary stage occurs within a few months of primary infection, but many years may elapse before a tertiary lesion appears.

Primary syphilis is characterised by the appearance of a hard chancre (pronounced 'shanker') about a month after exposure to infection. In men the chancre usually occurs on the penis; in women it appears most often on the labia or cervix and in the latter situation readily escapes notice. Much more rarely the primary sore may be on the lip, tongue, tonsil, or nipple. The chancre is a hard, painless ulcer about 1 cm in diameter, has a thin, serous discharge and is accompanied by painless enlargement of the regional lymph nodes. *Diagnosis* depends on identifying the *Treponema pallidum* in the exudate with the use of the dark-ground microscope.

Secondary syphilis may cause some constitutional disturbance with *sore throat*, low *fever* and generalised *lymph node enlargement*, but usually its manifestations are confined to the skin and the mucous membrane of the mouth. Various types of skin *rash* are seen, all having in common a symmetrical distribution over the body, absence of irritation, and a colour usually likened to raw ham. In the mouth painless, slimy, greyish patches known as '*snail-track ulcers*' are the typical lesions. Warty lesions known as *condylomata* may appear in the peri-anal and vulval regions. The cutaneous and mucosal lesions of the secondary stage are highly infective and the serum tests for antibody are invariably positive.

Tertiary Stage. A localised swelling known as a gumma may appear anywhere in the body many years after the primary infection; these lesions differ from those of primary and secondary syphilis in containing no spirochaetes and being therefore non-infective. In certain situations such as the liver, the lung, or the stomach, a gumma may be mistaken for a carcinoma; the distinction can be made by giving potassium iodide 1–2 g which causes rapid disappearance of a gumma but has no effect on a carcinoma. The centre of a gumma often breaks down and leads to the formation of an ulcer with sharply punched-out margins.

Syphilitic *aortitis* is discussed on p. 191, and *neurosyphilis* on p. 369.

Serological Tests for Syphilis. Tests for syphilis can be divided into those which test for reagin, a non-specific plasma protein fraction which is elevated in syphilis together with a number of other diseases, and other more specific tests. It is usual to perform one non-specific and one more specific test to confirm syphilis.

Non-specific Tests

(i) *Venereal Disease Research Laboratory Test (VDRL)* is a flocculation test for reagin and it can be quantified.
(ii) *The Rapid Plasma Reagin Test (RPR)* is similar.

These tests are sensitive, cheap and easy to perform and are very useful for screening large numbers of specimens. Their disadvantage is that false positive reactions may be found in patients with immune disorders such as lupus erythematosus, in conditions in which there is increased destruction of cell nuclei and occasionally in healthy people. It is usual therefore to perform also one of the specific tests employing *T. pallidum* as the antigen:

(1) *The Fluorescent Antibody (Absorbed) Test* is the first serological test to become positive in primary syphilis. It is expensive and tedious to perform and is not used for routine screening, but is very useful if dark-ground microscopy cannot be performed. False positive reactions are rare.
(2) *The Treponema pallidum Haemagglutination Assay Test (TPHA)* can be quantified, is highly specific and can be automated and used for large-scale screening.

In most patients the reagin tests become negative one year after treatment for primary syphilis and two years after treatment for secondary syphilis, but the specific tests may remain positive for many years. The reagin tests are therefore more useful than the specific ones for evaluating the result of treatment.

In general the serological tests for syphilis are also positive in patients with other treponemal infections such as yaws. When such a patient develops syphilis a rise in the reagin titre may give a clue to the diagnosis.

Treatment of Syphilis

(a) *Early Syphilis.* Procaine penicillin injection BP, 600 mg (600 000 units), should be given daily for 10 days. Alternatively itinerant or uncooperative patients may be given a single intramuscular injection of benzathine penicillin 2.4 g (2.4 mega units) as this will maintain the necessary blood level (at least 0.03 units per ml) for about 2 weeks. Patients who are sensitive to penicillin should be given tetracyline 500 mg 6-hourly for 15 days and the course repeated after 3 months. Those with early infectious syphilis should be kept under observation for 2 years by which time serological tests should have returned to normal. Sexual intercourse should not be resumed until the course of treatment is finished and lesions have healed. Cure is achieved in 90 % of patients.

(b) *Late Syphilis.* Procaine penicillin 600 000 units daily for 21 days is satisfactory. Prednisolone 30 mg daily should be given to cover the first few days of treatment to prevent a Herxheimer reaction.

(c) *Congenital Syphilis* responds to procaine penicillin 100 000 units daily for 10 days.

Acute symptoms consisting of fever, shivering, headache and malaise, and lasting for a few hours, may occur within a day or two of starting treatment. This is known as a *Herxheimer reaction* is not harmful at this stage. The Herxheimer reaction may have more serious effects in patients with syphilitic aortitis or gummata in special situations such as the larynx; penicillin therapy should be started under steroid cover in such patients.

NON-SPECIFIC URETHRITIS (NSU)

About 50 % of patients presenting with NSU (i.e. with a bacterial urethral pus) have urethritis due to *Chlamydia trachomatis*, which is now by far the most common sexually transmitted disease in the Western World. The D–K serotypes of *C. trachomatis* primarily infect the genital tract; the A, B, Ba and C serotypes cause trachoma in developing countries. There is a huge reservoir of D–K serotypes in the genital tract of both men and women. Women often have few or no symptoms so that the infection may be discovered only when some complication appears or an infant develops ophthalmia neonatorum, which is now 7 times more often due to chlamydial than to gonococcal infection.

Complications of chlamydial infection include acute epididymitis and prostatitis in men; Bartholinitis, cervicitis and salpingitis in women;

and in both sexes proctitis, conjunctivitis (due to contamination of the eye with genital secretion), perihepatitis and Reiter's syndrome (p. 419).

Treatment. Oral oxytetracycline 4 times daily for 14 days (21 days for complications) is effective. It should be taken after meals, which should not include milk or milk products. Alternatively doxycycline 100 mg 4 times daily for 14–21 days may be given. These capsules must be washed down with plenty of fluid as they may cause oesophagitis.

GENITAL HERPES

The four species of herpes virus which infect man are varicella-zoster, cytomegalovirus, the Epstein-Barr virus and herpes simplex virus (HSV); all are DNA viruses characterised by the ability to remain latent in their hosts. Genital herpes is due to infection with HSV1, or more often HSV2, acquired by sexual intercourse; its recent increase in incidence may be related to the more widespread practice of orogenital contact.

Primary Infection may be heralded by malaise, fever, headache and pain in the back and buttocks followed in the male by itching and pain usually in the glans penis and frenal area and in women by severe dysuria. Proctitis may follow anal intercourse in either sex. *Examination* reveals groups of papules which become vesicular in a day or two and then rupture forming painful ulcers. Meningeal involvement is not uncommon, causing headache, neck stiffness and photophobia for 2–3 days and spread of infection from the posterior ganglia to the sacral nerve roots may cause transient impotence and impairment of micturition.

Recurrent infection occurs in about half the patients. The relapses, which are shorter and less severe than the first attack, may be precipitated by fever, exposure to UVL, trauma, menstruation or stress.

Carcinoma of the Cervix. It has been suggested but not proved that HSV infection is a factor in the development of cervical cancer and women with genital herpes are advised to have annual cervical smears examined.

Treatment. Particularly in women with difficulty in micturition due to pain, an analgesic jelly (Lidothesin gel) may be very helpful. Specific treatment with acyclovir, either by IV infusion over 45–60 minutes every 8 hours for 5 days in a dose of 5 mg/kg or 200 mg by mouth 5 times daily for 5 days, relieves symptoms and promotes healing but does not prevent relapses.

SOFT SORE (Chancroid)

Chancroid is very rare in Britain, though it is occasionally seen in seaports. The causative organism is *Haemophilus ducreyi* (Ducrey's bacillus), a Gram-negative bacillus about 1–2 μm in length.

Clinical Features. After an incubation period of 2–14 days one or more small red papules appear on the genitalia or surrounding skin and within a few days develop into necrotic ulcers with undermined edges surrounded by an area of erythema and oedema. The inguinal lymph nodes enlarge and sometimes suppurate. The important distinction from syphilis is made by the shorter incubation period, the absence of induration in the lesions, the failure to demonstrate spirochaetes on dark-ground illumination and identification of Ducrey's bacillus in stained smears and on culture.

Treatment. Sulphadimidine 1.0 g 4-hourly (missing out the night dose) given for 2 weeks is usually successful.

LYMPHOGRANULOMA INGUINALE

This is also very rare in Britain. It is a virus infection with an incubation period of up to three weeks.

Clinical Features. The initial lesion may be a small vesicle or ulcer on the genitalia, but more often the first evidence of the disease is enlargement of the inguinal lymph nodes. The swelling may become quite massive and eventually suppuration may occur with the discharge of yellow pus through multiple sinuses in the skin. There is often severe constitutional reaction with high fever. In women proctitis and subsequent rectal stricture may occur; sequelae in men include scarring and elephantiasis of the genitalia.

Diagnosis. A positive intradermal *Frei test* indicates that the patient now has or has had the disease.

Treatment. Some success may be achieved with either the sulphonamides or the tetracyclines, or the two drugs may be combined. Sulphonamides such as sulphadimidine should be given in doses of 3–4 g daily for three to six weeks; tetracycline dosage is 500 mg 6-hourly for five days followed by 250 mg 6-hourly for 3–6 weeks or longer. Fluctuant buboes should be aspirated rather than incised.

FURTHER READING

Catterall, R. D., *Venereology and Genito-Urinary Medicine*, 2nd edition, Hodder and Stoughton, Sevenoaks, 1979.

King, A. J. and Nicol, C., *Venereal Diseases*, 4th edition, Ballière Tindall, London, 1980.

CHAPTER 20

ADVERSE REACTIONS TO DRUGS

INTRODUCTION

Drug reactions are becoming increasingly important as the range of substances used for diagnostic and therapeutic purposes multiplies. The classification of these reactions is difficult, for their underlying mechanism is often not fully understood.

A useful classification originally proposed by Rawlins and Thompson is:

Type A reactions which can be predicted from the known pharmacological action of the drug.

Type B reactions which are unpredictable and include allergies, idiosyncratic reactions and those due to some genetically determined abnormal response to the drug.

TYPE A REACTIONS

In this type of reaction the pharmacological effects of the drug are excessive. This can be due to *overdose* or to *undue sensitivity* of the patient to the drug's action—an example being the undue respiratory depression produced by morphine in a patient with long-standing respiratory disease. Pharmacokinetic factors may be important, usually because the patient is unable to eliminate the drug as a result of disease. A good example is the patient with renal failure who fails to excrete digoxin with subsequent toxicity.

Sometimes adverse effects are inherent in the action of the drug even when given in normal doses and without undue sensitivity on the part of the patient. Most people taking tricyclic antidepressants will complain of dry mouth and other anticholinergic effects and about half the patients taking the vasodilator nifedipine will develop some ankle swelling. Generally this type of side-effect can be predicted and often avoided if the possibility is considered before prescribing.

TYPE B REACTIONS

This is a more heterogenous group where the reaction is unrelated to the drug's pharmacological action and is usually unpredictable. They can be divided:

(a) Drug allergies
(b) Idiosyncratic
(c) Genetically determined

DRUG ALLERGIES

Some reactions to drugs are known to be mediated by immune mechanisms. This means that the patient has been previously exposed to the drug or to some closely related substance. Most drugs are of a low molecular weight and are therefore not antigenic. They can however combine covalently with a large molecular substance, usually a protein and the combination which is known as a *hapten* acts as an antigen.

Four types of allergic reaction are now recognised and it is possible for a single drug to cause more than one type of allergy.

Type I (Immediate Anaphylactic) Reaction

This is due to the antigen/antibody reaction occurring on the surface of the mast cells and releasing pharmacologically active substances including histamine, bradykinin and 5-hydroxytryptamine. The antibody belongs to the IgE fraction of the immunoglobulins. This type of reaction is seen typically with pencillin, streptomycin and some other drugs.

Clinical Features. The reaction occurs within a few minutes of administration of the drug. The main features are chest pain, dyspnoea, cyanosis and a rapid fall in blood pressure with collapse. The attack may be fatal.

Treatment. *Prophylaxis.* It is important to ask the patient whether he is sensitive to the drug about to be given. It is also useful to know whether he suffers from hay fever, asthma, infantile eczema or urticaria as this type of reaction is more frequent in atopic subjects.

When the serum is being given the following rules should be observed:

(1) The patient should be asked whether he has had serum before or whether he suffers from allergic diseases such as asthma, hay fever, eczema, or urticaria.

(2) If the answer to these questions is negative, 0.1 ml of serum is injected subcutaneously. If there is no local or general reaction within half an hour, the full dose of serum is given intramuscularly.

(3) If the patient has a history of allergic disease or has had serum before, 0.1 ml of serum diluted 1:10 is given subcutaneously; if there is no reaction within half an hour 0.1 ml of serum is given subcutaneously; if after a further half an hour there is still no reaction, the full dose of serum is given intramuscularly.

(4) If the patient has a history of serum reactions or has a reaction to

the test dose, he should be admitted to hospital. He is then given an antihistamine followed by the serum in gradually increasing doses. It is usual to start with 0.1 ml of a 1:100 dilution of serum and if this causes no reaction in half an hour the dose is doubled and so on until enough serum has been given. It is a very tedious process.

(5) Whenever serum is given it is essential that a syringe of fresh 1:1000 adrenaline solution be at hand and also an antihistamine suitable for IV injection (chlorpheniramine maleate 10 mg). Whenever patients are given serum they must be observed for half an hour after the injection and must be warned of the possibility of a delayed serum reaction.

(6) Intravenous injections of serum should be avoided if possible. Where they are necessary, the same precautions should be adopted. Intravenous serum should not be given to those who have previously had serum or who have allergic disorders and in addition a test dose of 0.1 ml of serum should also be given intramuscularly. As a general rule intravenous serum should be given only to patients in hospital.

(7) Following the administration of serum the patient should be actively immunised against the appropriate diseases. This should be delayed until at least one month after he has received the serum, as the circulating antibody from the serum may prevent the antigen from provoking active immunity.

Management of Reaction. Adrenaline 0.5 ml of a 1:1000 solution should be given intramuscularly together with an antihistamine (chlorpheniramine maleate 10 mg IV). Often hydrocortisone hemisuccinate 100 mg IV is required.

Type II reactions

These are due to antibodies of class IgG and IgM combining with antigens on the surface of cells and fixing complement. Reaction to quinidine and some reactions to penicillin are probably of this type.

Type III reactions

These are responsible for several clinical syndromes which are believed to be due to circulating immune complexes consisting of antigen/antibody/complement. Among them are:

Serum Sickness. This is due to a circulating antigen/antibody/complement complex which causes transient damage to certain tissues.

Clinical Features. About a week to ten days after the patient has received serum he develops a rash, usually urticarial, pain and stiffness with some swelling in the joints, and usually a fever. Sometimes there is enlargement of the lymph nodes and a transient albuminuria. Rarely, a shock-like state develops with low blood pressure. This condition usually clears up in a few days.

Treatment. Local application of calamine lotion helps to relieve the itching. An antihistamine such as chlorpheniramine maleate 4 mg t.d.s. shortens the duration of the illness. In severe or resistant cases, prednisolone 30 mg for a day or two and then tailed off will usually relieve the symptoms.

Other syndromes include:

Immune Complex Glomerulonephritis (see p. 475).

Systemic Lupus Erythematosus. A syndrome resembling this disease is caused by several drugs including procainamide, hydralazine, anticonvulsants and isoniazid. It recovers on stopping the drug.

Type IV (Delayed Hypersensitivity) Reactions

The typical example of this type of reaction is a contact dermatitis. When the drug is applied to the skin it forms an antigenic conjugate with the dermal proteins which stimulates the formation of sensitised T-lymphocytes. If the drug is applied again a rash develops.

IDIOSYNCRATIC REACTIONS

Although it has been possible to demonstrate an allergic basis for a number of drug reactions, in many cases there is no evidence suggesting allergy and other mechanisms may be involved. It is therefore better to consider these reactions on a system basis.

Blood Dyscrasias

Blood dyscrasias are among the most important drug reactions. It would seem that many of them are hypersensitivity reactions and are due to a combination of antigen, antibody and complement on the cell. Others are due to a direct effect on the blood cells or their precursors.

Agranulocytosis. This may occur with a number of drugs including amidopyrine, the sulphonamides, thiouracil, carbimazole, tridione, isoniazid, phenylbutazone, chloramphenicol, gold, and arsenic. In addition large doses of most cytotoxic drugs will produce agranulocytosis as part of their pharmacological action. With most drugs the agranulocytosis is reversible, provided the drug is not continued for too long, but with chloramphenicol recovery may not occur.

Clinical Features. There may be no symptoms and the depression in the granulocytes may be found by a routine blood count. Such patients are susceptible to infection and may present with general malaise, fever, and some infective process, usually a severe throat infection.

Treatment

(1) *Prophylaxis.* The patient should always be asked if he is susceptible to the drug before it is given. Certain drugs such as amidopyrine and chloramphenicol should be avoided if possible. It is doubtful if routine blood counts on patients taking drugs which may cause agranulocytosis are much help as the fall in granulocytes may be sudden. The patient must, however, be told to report to the doctor if he becomes ill and in particular if he develops a sore throat; a blood count must then be performed.

(2) *Curative.* The drug must be stopped immediately. If the white count does not improve within a few days, prednisolone 30 mg daily should be given. Infections should be treated as they arise with the appropriate antibiotic. The majority of patients will recover on this treatment. When granulopenia is due to heavy metals it should be treated with dimercaprol (p. 753).

Thrombocytopenia. This may occur as a result of drug administration. It has been described with sedormid, tridione, chloramphenicol, thiazide, gold, sulphonamides, and quinine. It may occur with excessive dosage of cytoxic drugs. Clinical features include purpura and bleeding from various sites.

Treatment. The drug should be stopped immediately. Prednisolone 30 mg daily sometimes helps. Platelet transfusions will raise the plasma platelet count for a few days.

Aplastic Anaemia. This is not common following the taking of drugs. It may occur with benzol and its derivatives, with chloramphenicol and with a number of other drugs including gold and the sulphonamides. It may be associated with depression of other elements of the blood.

Treatment. The drug should be stopped. Repeated transfusion may be required. Prednisolone is not usually very helpful, but it is worth a trial in patients who are not recovering. If poisoning is due to heavy metals, dimercaprol should be used. Provided the drug is stopped quickly, recovery usually occurs. The exception is chloramphenicol, which rarely causes bone-marrow dyscrasias and usually only after repeated courses; if they occur, however, they are usually irreversible and ultimately prove fatal.

Haemolytic Anaemia. Drugs can occasionally cause haemolysis. It seems that a number of mechanisms may be responsible. Quinine has long been known to precipitate the acute haemolysis occurring in association with malaria and called *blackwater fever*.

Potassium chlorate in large doses will produce haemolysis by a direct action on the cell; occasionally this occurs with quite a small dose of the drug and it can then be classed as an example of intolerance.

In about 10% of American negroes, a high proportion of Africans and some races in the Mediterranean littoral there is a *deficiency in glucose-6-phosphate dehydrogenase* which is normally responsible for the integrity of the red cells. This results in acute haemolysis when such subjects take primaquine, sulphonamides, nitrofurantoins and other drugs and is an example of a genetically determined reaction to a drug.

Methaemoglobinaemia and Sulphaemoglobinaemia. These changes in the haemoglobin may occur with certain drugs, including phenacetin, potassium chlorate, and the sulphonamides. The patient appears cyanosed, but is not distressed or dyspnoeic. The diagnosis is confirmed by finding the absorption spectra of methaemoglobin or sulphaemoglobin in the blood. The only treatment usually required is to stop the offending drug. Methaemoglobinaemia can be temporarily reversed by giving methylene blue as a 1% solution intravenously, the dose for an adult being 5 ml.

Megaloblastic Anaemia. Certain drugs including pyrimethamine and the anticonvulsants primidone and phenytoin may produce a megaloblastic anaemia which can be reversed by folic acid 10 mg daily.

Liver Damage (see p. 116)

Drug Reactions and Collagen Diseases

Although some authors include a wide variety of syndromes under the term collagen diseases, this term should be confined to rheumatic fever, rheumatoid arthritis, disseminated lupus erythematosus, polyarteritis nodosa, dermatomyositis, and giant-cell arteritis. There has been considerable discussion whether drug reactions can cause these conditions. There is no doubt that a clinical picture similar to that of disseminated lupus erythematosus can be produced by *hydralazine* and by *procainamide*, but it differs from the true disease in that recovery occurs when the drug is stopped. In addition, transient arteritis can occur in association with hypersensitivity reaction to a number of drugs, including *penicillin* and the *sulphonamides*. Whether such reactions play any part in the pathogenesis of true polyarteritis nodosa is more doubtful and it is unlikely that drug reactions are causal to any of the other collagen diseases.

Other types of connective tissue disease can be drug induced. *Methysergide* causes a retroperitoneal fibrosis which may affect the mediastinum. It is a rare cause of ureteric obstruction. *Practolol* produces various disorders including skin rashes, sclerosis of the cornea and peritoneal fibrosis. The cause of these changes is not known.

Other Drug Reactions

Fever is quite common and should always be remembered in patients with PUO.

Lymphadenopathy can be caused by drugs, particularly phenytoin, and the histological picture resembles a lymphoma.

Rashes are often caused by drugs and are considered on p. 721.

GENETICALLY DETERMINED DRUG REACTIONS

Hereditary differences in response to drugs may be due to:

(a) *Polygenic influences* when there is a continuous variation.
(b) *Polymorphism* when there are two distinct populations in terms of drug response.

Genetic polymorphism usually results in one group being deficient in specific enzymes. For example:

(i) *Acetylation.* A number of drugs are inactivated by acetylation including isoniazid, hydralazine, sulphonamides and procainamide. Peripheral neuritis is more liable to develop in slow acetylators taking isoniazid and a lupus-like syndrome appears more frequently in those taking hydralazine or procainamide.
(ii) *Cholinesterases.* The muscle relaxant suxamethonium is broken down by cholinesterases. These may be deficient due to an inherited deficiency and the paralysing effect of suxamethonium is greatly prolonged.
(iii) Some individuals are deficient in *hydroxylating enzymes* and this leads to failure to eliminate the hypotensive drug debrisoquine.
(iv) *Glucose-6-phosphate dehydrogenase* deficiency leading to haemolysis with certain drugs is considered on p. 616.

DRUG INTERACTIONS

The increasing use of drugs, particularly the prescribing of more than one drug at a time, has made drug interaction an important problem. Interaction may occur at several stages in the passage of drugs through the body:

(1) **In the gastrointestinal tract** drugs may combine or their physical state may be altered so that absorption is modified. For example, iron combines with tetracycline decreasing its absorption and leading to lower blood levels of the antibiotic.

(2) **Competition for Transport Sites on the Plasma Proteins.** Many drugs are transported to their sites of action partially or almost totally bound to plasma proteins. When bound in this way they cannot produce their pharmacological effects and are not available to be metabolised or

excreted. The activity of the drug depends on the unbound fraction.

When two drugs compete for a limited number of protein-binding sites there is a decrease in the bound fraction of each and an increase in the amount of free drug, with a corresponding enhancement of the pharmacological effect. Examples of this type of interaction are the displacement of bilirubin by sulphonamides in the new born causing kernicterus, the displacement of tolbutamide by salicylates leading to hypoglycaemia and the displacement of warfarin by salicylates causing haemorrhage.

(3) **Modification at Sites of Action.** The pharmacological action of a drug can be modified in several ways by the concurrent administration of another drug. For example:

(a) Hypokalaemia produced by *diuretics* enhances the action of *digitalis* on the heart.

(b) *Tricyclic antidepressants* reverse the effect of *adrenergic blocking hypotensive* agents, possibly by increasing the amount of noradrenaline at the adrenergic nerve endings. They also enhance the effect of *sympathomimetic amines*, which for example may be added to a local anaesthetic.

(c) The action of central nervous depressants such as barbiturates and alcohol is additive.

(d) *Monoamine oxidase inhibitors* (*MAOI*). These interact in two ways:
(i) Certain drugs, particularly sympathomimetic drugs such as phenylpropanolamine or tyramine, release the excess noradrenaline which accumulates in nerve endings of the subject taking MAO inhibitors, resulting in a hypertensive crisis. Tyramine is found in certain foods.
(ii) The effect of some central depressants, particularly pethidine, is enhanced.

(4) **Enzyme Induction.** Many drugs are metabolised by enzymes, usually in the liver. Certain drugs increase the activity of these enzymes so that drug breakdown is enhanced. For example, if a patient on an oral anticoagulant is given phenobarbitone the barbiturate increases the enzyme activity and the anticoagulant is metabolised more rapidly. An increased dose is therefore necessary to produce a satisfactory anticoagulant effect. Conversely, if the phenobarbitone is stopped enzyme activity decreases and signs of anticoagulant overdosage may appear.

(5) **Enzyme Inhibition.** Sulphonamides decrease the rate of breakdown of tolbutamide. Allopurinol decreases the rate of breakdown of 6-mercaptopurine.

(6) **Renal Excretion.** Competition for pathways in the kidney by two drugs given together may reduce the rate of excretion of both. Use is made of this phenomenon when probenecid is given with penicillin to reduce its excretion and so achieve a higher level of penicillin in the blood.

FURTHER READING

Davies, D. M., (ed), *Textbook of Adverse Drug Reactions*, 2nd edition, Oxford University Press, Oxford, 1981.

Stockley, I. H., *Drug Interactions*, Blackwell Scientific Publications, Oxford, 1981.

CHAPTER 21

POISONING

Poisoning is responsible for about 10% of all acute admissions to hospital in the UK. It may be due to:

(a) *Self-poisoning*. This may be a serious suicide attempt, or more often an attempt to draw the attention of relatives, friends or doctors to some intolerable situation in the patient's life.
(b) *Accidental.*
(c) *Rarely homicidal.*

Preliminary Assessment. When a diagnosis of poisoning is made it is important to determine:

(a) The nature of the poison or poisons. More than one poison has often been taken.
(b) Any other complicating factors such as injuries, etc.
(c) The severity of the poisoning.

The assessment of the severity of the poisoning will be based on three criteria.

(1) *Level of Consciousness.* This is usually divided into:

Grade I	Drowsy but responds to mild stimulation.
Grade II	Unconscious but responds to mild stimulation.
Grade III	Unconscious but responds to severe stimulation.
Grade IV	Unconscious and unresponsive.

(2) *Circulation.* Many drugs cause acute circulatory failure (p. 740). This can be assessed by the blood pressure and by the peripheral blood flow (temperature of extremities, etc.). An apparently normal blood pressure may however be associated with inadequate peripheral perfusion.

(3) *Respiration.* Central depression of respiration is caused by many drugs. A crude assessment may be obtained from the respiration rate and presence or absence of cyanosis. Blood gases should be measured if there is any doubt.

Treatment. *Non-specific Measures.* Certain measures are common in the management of most types of poisoning. They consist of:

(a) *Maintenance of Adequate Ventilation.* This includes keeping a clear airway in the unconscious patient and the use of a ventilator in severe poisoning.

(b) *Emptying the Stomach.* In all patients who are conscious except those who have taken corrosive poisons, vomiting should be precipitated by making the patient drink a pint of warm water and then stimulating the pharynx with fingers. This must be followed, except with corrosive poisons, by gastric lavage. A 30 English gauge Jacques tube is passed and 250 ml of warm water is run into the stomach and then syphoned out. This should be repeated at least six times. If the nature of the poison is known, a suitable antidote may be left in the stomach (see below).

It is very important to avoid inhalation of gastric contents by the patient and during gastric lavage he should lie in the prone position with the head and shoulders lower than the rest of the body.

In the unconscious patient the risk of inhalation is increased. In these patients the help of an anaesthetist is advisable for gastric lavage which should be preceded by the passing of a cuffed endotracheal tube.

After four hours most poisons have left the stomach and so very little will be recovered by gastric lavage. Salicylates however cause pyloric spasm and gastric lavage is useful for up to 24 hours.

Finally, all vomit and the first return from gastric lavage should be kept and carefully labelled for further analysis.

(c) *Forced Alkaline Diuresis.* Excretion of certain poisons (particularly phenobarbitone and salicylates) can be accelerated by producing an alkaline diuresis. A central venous pressure line is useful to guard against overloading the circulation and the bases of the lungs should be examined regularly for signs of pulmonary oedema. In the first hour 500 ml of 1.4% sodium bicarbonate (or $\frac{1}{6}$ M sodium lactate) + 20 mg of frusemide, followed by 1.0 litre of 5% dextrose + 20 mg of frusemide are given intravenously. At the end of the hour the urinary flow should be greater than 3.0 ml/min. Subsequent rate of infusion will depend on central venous pressure and urinary volume. Every third bottle (500 ml) of infusion fluid should contain 150 mmol of sodium and every bottle of infusion fluid 10.0 mmol of potassium. Diuresis can be maintained either by adding mannitol (not more than 10 g/hour) to the infusion fluid or by further injections of frusemide intravenously. The urinary pH must be kept above 7.5.

If a diuresis is not produced by the end of the first hour there is probably impairment of renal function and dialysis will be required.

(d) *Adsorbents.* Medicinal charcoal can adsorb some drugs when given orally and thus prevent absorption. They must be given within an hour of taking the drug and are therefore of limited use.

(e) *Further general measures* include maintenance of fluid electrolyte balance, adequate nutrition and treatment of infection if it arises.

Barbiturate Poisoning

Barbiturate poisoning is the commonest type of poisoning in Great Britain and stands second to carbon monoxide as a cause of death. Chronic addiction to barbiturates also occurs.

Acute Barbiturate Poisoning

Barbiturates are usually taken in a deliberate suicidal attempt; occasionally by accident. Barbiturate and alcohol poisoning may be combined; these two drugs certainly have an additive effect, and it is believed by some that their actions are synergistic.

The speed of action and duration of effect depend on the type of barbiturate used.

Clinical Features. The symptoms of mild barbiturate overdosage are mental confusion with slurred speech, nystagmus, and unsteady gait. These are followed by deep sleep from which the patient can be roused though perhaps with difficulty. The corneal and pharyngeal reflexes remain and respiration is not markedly depressed. A bullous rash occurs in about 10% of patients with barbiturate overdosage.

In severe barbiturate overdosage there is deep coma, the patient cannot be roused and the reflexes have disappeared. Finally death occurs from respiratory depression complicated by circulatory failure. The diagnosis can be confirmed by finding the drug in the urine, blood, or gastric contents.

The blood level of barbiturate is a poor guide as to prognosis as patients vary in their sensitivity to the drug.

Treatment. If the patient is conscious, no treatment will usually be required unless a large dose has just been taken, when it should be removed by gastric lavage.

In the unconscious patient management is:

(1) Ensure a clear airway, if the cough reflex is absent, an endotracheal tube should be introduced.
(2) Ensure adequate ventilation; in a cyanosed patient with respiratory depression some form of mechanical ventilation will be required.
(3) Gastric contents should be aspirated and the stomach washed out only if the drug has been taken within the previous four hours.
(4) Maintain hydration by giving 2.0 litres of intravenous fluid in 24 hours (.18% dextrose saline).
(5) Treat intercurrent chest infections as they arise.

In severe intoxication however (absent reflexes, depressed respiration), an attempt should be made to increase the rate of barbiturate elimination. Renal excretion of phenobarbitone can be increased by producing a high flow rate of alkaline urine. This is not however effective with the short acting barbiturates which are largely broken down in the liver. For method see p. 749.

The death rate from hospital admission with barbiturate poisoning is about 2–5%.

Chronic Barbiturate Addiction

Chronic barbiturate addiction is by no means uncommon. Patients may indulge in bursts of intoxication or may take the drug regularly. Most addicts suffer from some form of psychological abnormality. If the drug is suddenly stopped a well-marked withdrawal syndrome occurs with weakness, nausea and vomiting, anxiety, and often convulsions.

Ethyl Alcohol

Most subjects with acute alcoholic intoxication will sleep it off. In severe cases the stomach should be washed out if the alcohol has been taken recently, and treatment continued as in barbiturate poisoning. Forced alkaline diuresis is not used. Various substances, including Vitamins B and C and fructose, have been claimed to sober up a patient, but there is little evidence that they are of practical use in the treatment of acute alcoholic poisoning.

The combination of alcohol and barbiturates is additive and can be very dangerous.

Methanol

Methanol poisoning is serious with an overall mortality of 20 %. The lowest fatal dose is about 25 ml. It is metabolised to the toxic metabolites formaldehyde and formate and is thus associated with a metabolic acidosis.

Clinical Features. The patient is confused with abdominal pain and vomiting. Visual disturbances are common and examination of the retina may show pallor and oedema of the discs.

Treatment

(a) Treatment of acidosis, if severe, with infusion of bicarbonate.
(b) Removal of methanol and metabolites and correction of acidosis by haemodialysis. This will be required if there are visual symptoms or signs, severe acidosis or a blood methanol level of >0.5 g/litre.
(c) It is common practice to give ethanol to reduce methanol metabolism. Whether this is effective is not established.

Morphine

Acute morphine poisoning may result from overdosage during the therapeutic use of the drug or from a suicidal attempt. The lethal dose is variable, but has been given as between 60–240 mg, but it must be realised that repeated dosage quickly produces tolerance of the drug.

Clinical Features. The patient is comatose and cannot be wakened. The respiration rate is very slow. The skin is cyanosed and is cold and clammy. The pupils are pin-point in size. With severe poisoning the blood pressure may fall. Death results from respiratory depression.

Treatment

(1) If the drug has recently been taken by mouth, wash out the stomach with 1:2000 potassium permanganate solution.

(2) Naloxone is the antidote of choice. The usual adult dose is 0.4 mg IV or IM. If this does not improve respiration it may be repeated after 3 minutes. Failure to respond suggests reconsideration of diagnosis. The aim of treatment is to establish adequate respiration not to wake the patient. Naloxone is effective against a wide range of narcotics.
(3) If there is severe respiratory depression with cyanosis, oxygen should be given and artificial respiration may be required.
(4) Occasionally respiratory stimulants such as nikethamide 4 ml of a 25% solution intravenously, or aminophylline 0.5 g intravenously are useful in patients only partially relieved by naloxone.

Glutethimide

Glutethimide is occasionally used as a suicide agent. It produces deep unconsciousness with dilated pupils, in severe poisoning periods of apnoea may occur and these are associated with the development of papilloedema. The fatal dose is in the region of 10 g.

Treatment. Dialysis is not useful and treatment is largely supportive. If papilloedema develops 500 ml of 20% mannitol should be given intravenously over 20 minutes followed by 500 ml of 5% dextrose over the ensuing 4 hours.

Phenothiazines

The dose response curve of the phenothiazines is fairly flat so there is a wide safety margin. Overdosage produces unconsciousness associated with extrapyramidal signs and with torticollis. Cardiac arrhythmias, hypotension and hypothermia occur.

Treatment. If the extrapyramidal signs are severe they respond to benztropine 2.0 mg IV otherwise treatment is supportive.

Benzodiazepines

This group of drugs has a very wide safety margin so that they rarely produce anything more than unconsciousness and no specific treatment is required.

Methaqualone

This drug is a relatively mild hypnotic but is combined with diphenhydramine in the preparation *Mandrax* which is both powerful and quick acting. Overdosage produces a rather characteristic clinical state with coma combined with increased muscle tone and reflexes.

Tricyclic Antidepressants

This group includes imipramine, nortriptyline and amitriptyline. These drugs have become common agents in attempted suicide. The

clinical picture is the result of cholinergic blockade, increased adrenergic activity and direct cardiac and CNS depression. It is essentially one of excitement followed by coma. The pupils are dilated, the reflexes increased and the plantars extensor. In severe overdosage special features are hypotension, tachycardia and the occurrence of cardiac arrhythmias. Cardiac arrest may be delayed for several days after severe overdose. Frequently these drugs may be combined with a phenothiazine or with a benzodiazepine compound such as chlordiazepoxide which produces a complicated clinical picture.

Treatment. There is no specific antidote and symptoms must be treated as they arise. Fits can be controlled by diazepam. The cardiac arrhythmias should be treated along the usual lines (see p. 148). Hypotension is difficult to treat and both vasoconstriction and cautious infusion with plasma volume expanders such as dextran have been used. Forced diuresis and dialysis are *not* effective.

β Blocker Poisoning

Bradycardia and a low cardiac output are the important signs.

Treatment. Bradycardia can be reversed by atropine 2.0 mg IV or if this fails by a pacemaker.

In an attempt to raise the blood pressure hydrocortisone 500 mg is given IV and various positive ionotropic agents can be used (i.e. isoprenaline or dopamine). If bronchospasm is a problem salbutamol should be given by nebuliser.

Arsenic Poisoning

Inorganic arsenic, usually in the form of the oxide, acquired notoriety as a homicidal poison and is still sometimes taken with suicidal intent. Poisoning may also occur as a result of exposure to arsenical dusts which are produced in various industrial processes. It produces its toxic action by inhibiting the intracellular sulphydryl enzymes which are essential to metabolism.

Acute Arsenic Poisoning

Clinical Features. The main symptoms of acute poisoning by arsenic are burning in the throat, vomiting, abdominal pain, and diarrhoea. In severe cases circulatory collapse and death may follow.

Treatment

(1) The stomach should be emptied and then washed out with freshly prepared ferric hydroxide, which is made by adding 45 g of ferric chloride to 15 g of sodium carbonate (washing soda) in half a tumbler of water.

(2) *Dimercaprol* (BAL) 300 mg in oily solution is given IM 6-hourly for two days and then decreased over the next few days. The action of

dimercaprol is to offer SH groups with which the arsenic combines; it is thus unable to combine with the SH groups in intracellular enzymes.

Chronic Arsenic Poisoning

The symptoms and signs of chronic arsenical poisoning are variable, but include:

(1) Pigmentation of the skin which has a typical mottled ('raindrop') appearance.
(2) Polyneuritis.
(3) Hyperkeratosis of the palms of hands and soles of the feet.
(4) Chronic pharyngitis and perforation of the nasal septum.
(5) Chronic diarrhoea.

Treatment. The patient should be removed from exposure to arsenic and given dimercaprol as for acute poisoning.

Ferrous Compounds

This form of poisoning has become common; it is usually due to children eating sugar-coated ferrous sulphate tablets in mistake for sweets.

Clinical features. Initially there is vomiting and diarrhoea often associated with haematemesis and melaena. After a few hours the patient becomes confused and this may be followed by coma, convulsion and shock. Acute liver necrosis can occur.

Treatment

(1) Vomiting should be induced.
(2) The stomach should then be washed out with a solution containing 2.0 g of desferrioxamine per litre and 5.0 g in 50 ml should be left in the stomach in adults. Desferrioxamine is an iron chelating agent.
(3) 2.0 g of desferrioxamine are given intramuscularly twice daily. In severe cases desferrioxamine can be given intravenously in 5% glucose solution at a rate of 15 mg/kg/hour to a maximum of 80 mg/kg/24 hours.
(4) The patient must be kept in bed and under observation for at least 48 hours after apparent recovery.

Anticholinesterase

A number of these substances are used in medicine and also as insecticides. They also have a potential use in war, and are known as 'nerve gases'. They inhibit the enzyme cholinesterase either temporarily or for long periods, so that there is widespread overactivity of the parasympathetic nervous system and also neuromuscular block in voluntary muscle. Symptoms may include colicky abdominal pain, excess salivation, respiratory paralysis and the pupils are constricted.

Treatment. Atropine should be given in doses of 2.0 mg IV or IM, and repeated as required. This will not however relieve neuromuscular block. Cholinesterase can be reactivated by pralidoxime 1.0 g in 5 ml of water IV or IM, and repeated at 4-hourly intervals as required. In severe cases some form of assisted ventilation may be necessary.

Paraquat

Paraquat is normally used as a weed killer and is very toxic. More than 30 ml of the concentrated drug is dangerous. With massive overdosage, death may occur from acute renal failure, with smaller doses it is usually due to lung damage and may be delayed for one to two weeks. There is no known antidote.

Salicylate

Poisoning by salicylates is common; it may be suicidal, or in children it may be accidental. The fatal dose in adults is in the region of 25 g. Doses of 2–4 g have proved toxic in children. In addition, some subjects, particularly asthmatics, may develop an asthmatic attack with salicylates and death has occurred after as little of 0.3 g of aspirin.

Clinical Features. In mild cases the main symptoms are nausea, vomiting, tinnitus and increased respirations. After larger doses there is mental confusion, the patient is flushed and sweating with a full pulse and overbreathing is very striking. In the early stages hyperventilation lowers the $P\text{CO}_2$ of the plasma and leads to a respiratory alkalosis; with increasing absorption of salicylate there is a metabolic acidosis with a fall in plasma bicarbonate. In children acidosis is common, whereas in adults a raised blood pH is more usual. In addition vomiting and sweating lead to dehydration and oliguria.

The urine gives a positive reaction to ferric chloride and may contain protein.

Treatment

(1) In salicylate poisoning it is always worthwhile to wash out the stomach with water. If the patient is in coma a cuffed endotracheal tube should be passed beforehand to avoid possible aspiration of vomited material into the lungs.

(2) In mild cases 5% sodium bicarbonate solution should be given orally in doses of 2 g 4-hourly for 24 hours. Sodium bicarbonate, by making the urine alkaline, increases the rate of excretion of salicylate by the kidneys.

(3) In severe cases (plasma salicylate level of more than 30 mg/100 ml in children and 50 mg/100 ml in adults) treatment is aimed at correct-

ing dehydration and producing a diuresis of alkaline urine and thus rapidly clearing salicylate from the body. Owing to the complex acid/base disorder which occurs in salicylate poisoning, it is important to estimate plasma pH, bicarbonate and $P\text{CO}_2$. For method of forced diuresis see p. 749.

(4) 25 mg of phytomenadione should be injected intravenously to prevent bleeding.

By this method a majority of adult patients with salicylate poisoning can be resuscitated. In a few patients with high plasma salicylate levels (over 100 mg/100 ml) and with renal or circulatory failure, haemodialysis will be required. Children are more sensitive to the toxic effects of salicylate.

Paracetamol

Overdosage by paracetamol is dangerous and a single dose of over 15 g can produce serious liver damage and 25 g is usually fatal. With the normal therapeutic dose of paracetamol a toxic metabolite is produced which however is mopped up by glutathione in the liver. With overdose the glutathione mechanism is saturated and the metabolite combines with the liver cell macromolecules causing cell death. Liver damage is probable if the blood level of paracetamol exceeds 300 μg/ml at 4 hours or 50 μg/ml at 12 hours after ingestion.

Clinical Features. Nausea and vomiting may occur after ingestion of the drug but symptoms and signs of liver failure may be delayed for some days.

Treatment. The stomach should be washed out. There is good evidence that methionine orally or cysteamine intravenously will decrease the liver damage if given within ten hours of taking the drug. These drugs alter the metabolism of paracetamol and reduce the production of toxic metabolites.

Carbon Monoxide

Excluding road accidents, carbon monoxide is the commonest cause of accidental death in Great Britain; it is also used by the suicide. Poisoning may result from the escape of carbon monoxide from gas lights or gas fires, from car exhausts, from combustion stoves in a poorly ventilated room or from coal-mine explosions.

Carbon monoxide is odourless and lighter than air. It has a far greater affinity for haemoglobin than oxygen and forms a compound, carboxyhaemoglobin, which is bright-red colour. It cannot carry oxygen and tissue anoxia results.

Clinical Features. Symptoms are minimal if less than 30% of haemoglobin is combined with carbon monoxide and consist of nausea, lassitude and headache. With higher concentrations the onset of symptoms is rapid. There is a transient increase in pulse rate and respiration followed by weakness, dimness of vision and finally coma, respiratory depression, and death.

The patient with carbon monoxide poisoning is often pale and cyanosed. The typical cherry red colour due to carboxyhaemoglobin is usually only seen at post-mortem. The presence of this compound in the blood may be confirmed by its characteristic absorption spectrum.

Treatment. The patient must be removed from the poisoned atmosphere. Artificial respiration should be started immediately. If possible, pure oxygen should be given by the best available method. Cerebral oedema may develop in severe cases. The diagnosis is suggested by papilloedema and it should be treated by 50 ml of 20 % mannitol by infusion. Several days in bed are required after apparent recovery. Occasionally patients show evidence of permanent brain or cardiac damage after recovery.

Cyanide

Hydrocyanic acid and potassium or sodium cyanide are very powerful poisons. They act by inhibiting a number of enzymes, the most important of which is cytochrome oxidase. They are used as pesticides and in metallurgy.

Clinical Features. The inhalation of hydrocyanic acid (which is a gas) results in death within a few minutes. After ingestion of cyanide salts, death may occur in anything from a few minutes up to several hours, depending on the dose. Generally speaking the absorption of about 1 mg of cyanide is fatal.

Treatment. The aim of treatment in cyanide poisoning is to give substances which will combine with cyanide and prevent interference with enzyme systems. The following steps should be taken as rapidly as possible.

(1) Crush ampoules of amyl nitrite and allow the patient to inhale the vapour; this will form some methaemoglobin which combines with cyanide. This should be followed by sodium nitrite 0.3 g in 10 ml of water given IV over 3 minutes, to form more methaemoglobin.
(2) Sodium thiosulphate 50 ml of 50 % solution should be given IV over 10 minutes; this also combines with cyanide.
(3) The stomach should be washed out with 5 % sodium thiosulphate.
(4) Oxygen and artificial respiration may be required.

If available 20 ml of a 1.5 % solution of cobalt edetate given IV over one minute is a specific remedy. It can be repeated if the response is adequate.

Bee and Wasp Stings

Bee and wasp stings contain a number of pharmacologically active substances. Some of these only produce local reactions with pain and swelling, but there are also allergens which can cause serious reactions with urticaria, bronchospasm, hypotension, visual disturbances, diarrhoea, vomiting and collapse. Most subjects only develop local swelling and pain, but sometimes repeated stings cause increasingly severe reactions until a severe generalised response occurs which may be fatal.

Treatment. Bee stings can be removed and local swelling and pain can be treated with aspirin and local antihistamines.

If anaphylaxis develops adrenaline 0.5 ml of 1:1000 solution should be given intramuscularly together with 10 mg of chlorpheniramine intravenously. Subjects who have severe reactions should be given immunotherapy which consists of increasing doses of venom given at intervals.

Adder Bites

The adder is the only poisonous snake found in the UK, and its venom contains substances with anticoagulant and cardiotoxic properties.

Clinical Features. Local signs are swelling and oedema with bruising. General symptoms include diarrhoea and vomiting and sometimes urticaria. In severe cases there may be collapse with low blood pressure and loss of consciousness. Death is very rare.

Treatment. The immediate treatment consists of splinting the affected limb, analgesia for the pain and antihistamines if urticaria develops. Many patients are frightened and need reassurance. Most patients only require observation in hospital and symptomatic treatment for 48 hours.

Antivenom is available and the Zagreb antivenom is less likely to produce anaphylactic reaction than previous preparations. Indications for giving antivenom are:

(a) Hypotension and/or coma
(b) Systemic bleeding
(c) Leucocytosis $> 20\,000 \times 10^9$/litre
(d) Acidosis
(e) Markedly raised CPK.

Great care should be taken with atopic patients as reactions are common.

A further possible reason for giving antivenom is to reduce the local reaction which can be severe and persistent.

10.8 ml of antivenom is diluted in 100 ml of saline and infused intravenously over 1 hour.

Lead

Lead poisoning may occur in a number of industries including lead smelting and lead burning, the manufacture of white and red lead and the making of accumulators. Children may also develop lead poisoning from sucking lead-containing paint. Poisoning is infinitely more probable when lead is absorbed through the lungs as dust or fumes rather than when taken by mouth. If lead is absorbed slowly it is stored in the bones. The development of the symptoms of lead poisoning depends not so much on the total amount of lead in the body, but on its rate of absorption or mobilisation from the bones.

Acute Lead Poisoning

Lead salts are irritant and produce vomiting, diarrhoea and collapse. Organic lead compounds produce an acute confusional state with delusions and fits.

Chronic Lead Poisoning

Clinical Features

Lead Colic. Intestinal colic and constipation are the most common symptoms of lead poisoning. The pain is usually peri-umbilical and there are no abnormal signs in the abdomen.

Lead Neuropathy. In lead poisoning weakness develops in certain groups of muscles, usually the extensor muscles of the wrist and rarely of the foot. Sensory changes do not occur. The site of the lesion in lead neuropathy is not certain, but is probably in the muscles.

Lead Encephalopathy. This manifestation of lead poisoning is rare. The patient complains of severe headaches and may suddenly develop epileptic fits.

Anaemia. A normocytic hypochromic anaemia occurs in lead poisoning, usually with punctate basophilia.

Gums. Patients with lead poisoning may show a bluish stippled line on the gum margin. It is only found in association with gingivitis and is due to the deposition of lead sulphide in the gums. The lead line may be found in patients without other manifestations of lead poisoning.

Other symptoms consist of weakness, loss of weight, joint pains, and a metallic taste in the mouth.

Generally speaking, a blood level of 100 μg of lead per 100 ml of blood (5 μmol/litre) or 200 μg of lead per litre of urine are associated with symptoms of lead poisoning. Levels above 60 μg/100 ml (3.0 μmol/litre) in lead workers necessitates withdrawal from exposure.

Treatment. Lead colic can be relieved by intravenous injections of 10 ml of a 10 % solution of calcium gluconate. Lead can be cleared from the body by using a chelating agent. Certain of these substances form compounds with lead which are soluble and which are excreted by the kidneys. The agent of choice is sodium calcium edetate. The lead in the body displaces the calcium from this chelating agent and the resulting compound is excreted. The adult dose is 1 g twice daily, given by slow intravenous infusion in saline, at intervals of twelve hours. Such treatment may be carried out for five days and then repeated if necessary. A high calcium diet should be given after treatment.

Prophylaxis. Prophylactic measures include:

(1) Avoidance of exposure to lead dust or fumes by ventilation, hygiene, and by wearing masks.
(2) Avoidance of absorption from the intestine by personal cleanliness, including washing of the hands, etc., before meals.
(3) Regular medical examination of those exposed to lead.
(4) A high calcium diet helps to prevent lead poisoning.

Food Poisoning

Food poisoning may be due to bacteria or viruses, or their products, in the food, to poisonous substances or to allergy to something ingested.

Bacterial Food Poisoning

(1) Staphylococcal

Some strains of staphylococci produce an enterotoxin which is fairly stable to heat and will resist boiling. The chief symptoms which start abruptly in from one to six hours, are nausea, vomiting, intestinal colic, and diarrhoea. The attack is short-lived and is all over within a few hours. It is not usually serious, but rarely there may be collapse with dehydration and deaths have occurred, particularly in young children and the aged.

Treatment. In most cases rest in bed with frequent sips of fluid and mist. kaolin and morphine (BPC) 15 ml 4-hourly will control the symptoms. Rarely if there is collapse with severe dehydration and sodium chloride deficiency, intravenous fluids will be required.

(2) Salmonella

Certain of the salmonella group of organisms produce specific diseases such as typhoid and paratyphoid fevers. Others of the group, particularly *S. typhimurium*, *S. newport*, *S. St. Paul*, *S. thompson*, and *S. dublin*, produce an acute gastroenteritis which presents as a food poisoning.

Clinical Features. The onset is usually within 48 hours of eating infected food. The main symptoms are general malaise, headache, and fever combined with vomiting, intestinal colic, and diarrhoea. Occasionally there may be high fever with rigors, suggesting a septicaemia and the spleen may be palpable. The disease usually lasts several days.

The diagnosis is confirmed by culture of the pathogenic organism from the stools. This is important in indicating the most appropriate treatment and in helping to trace the source of infection.

Treatment. General measures include rest in bed and sips of fluid by mouth. If the diarrhoea has been severe, the oral fluids should consist of 0.3 % saline flavoured with fruit juice. Occasionally when vomiting is severe and prolonged, fluids and electrolytes must be given intravenously and this requires a daily estimation of the blood electrolytes and a full record of fluid balance. The diarrhoea and colic can be controlled by mist. kaolin and morphine 15 ml 4-hourly.

There is little evidence that antibiotic treatment modifies the course of salmonella gastroenteritis.

(3) Campylobacter Infections

This group of organisms usually causes an enteritis. *Campylobacter jejuni* and *Campylobacter coli* are associated with an illness characterised by diarrhoea, abdominal pain and sometimes fever. Rarely septicaemia can occur and the infection may involve other organs. It is commonest in the young child but may be seen at any age. In mild cases no treatment is required but more severe intestinal infection responds to oral erythromycin and the rare systemic infections to gentamicin.

(4) Pseudomembranous enterocolitis

Diarrhoea is common after a number of antibiotics but is not usually severe. However, occasionally a much more serious clinical picture emerges and is particularly associated with clindamycin and lincomycin. It is believed to be due to superinfection with *Clostridium difficile*. The diarrhoea is profuse and may be associated with toxaemia and shock. Sigmoidoscopy shows whitist membrane adhering to the bowel wall.

Treatment consists of rehydration and combating infection with metronidazole 400 mg three times daily or vancomycin orally 500 mg four times daily. Alternatively cholestyramine can be given which binds the toxin produced by the organism.

Virus

There is no doubt that certain outbreaks of gastroenteritis are due to a virus; they are usually mild and respond to symptomatic treatment.

Mushroom Poisoning

Mushroom poisoning is usually due to *Aminata phalloides*. This mushroom has a yellow or olive yellow cap with white gills and there is a volva (cup) at the base of the stem.

Clinical Features. There is often a delay of several hours before the onset of symptoms. This is followed by severe abdominal colic with bloody diarrhoea and vomiting. Death may occur from shock or collapse. If the patient survives this stage, acute liver necrosis may develop and prove fatal.

Treatment. The stomach should be washed out. Atropine 1 mg should be given intravenously and repeated as required. Fluid and electrolyte replacement will be necessary and this will have to be given intravenously. Antiphallinic serum should be given if available. It has been suggested that mashed rabbit stomach and brain should be given as these animals are resistant to mushroom poisoning. Otherwise, treatment is symptomatic.

Allergy to Food

Some patients are hypersensitive to certain articles of food and may suffer from urticarial rashes, vomiting, diarrhoea, and even attacks of asthma. It is best for them to avoid foods although desensitisation can be attempted.

Treatment. An attack due to allergy to food is treated as a sensitisation reaction (p. 740). If diarrhoea is a prominent symptom it can be relieved by a mixture containing morphine, such as mist. kaolin and morphine (NF) 15 ml 4-hourly.

FURTHER READING

Matthew, H. and Lawson, A. A. H., *Treatment of Common Acute Poisonings*, 4th edition, Churchill Livingstone, 1979.

CHAPTER 22

DISEASES DUE TO PHYSICAL AGENTS

DECOMPRESSION SICKNESS

Decompression sickness occurs when people who have been working at a high atmospheric pressure, such as workers in a caisson or diving bell, are suddenly decompressed. It may also occur in a subject who rises quickly to a height above 7500 m (25 000 ft). In both circumstances, nitrogen rapidly comes out of solution both in the blood and in the tissues and forms bubbles. Oxygen and carbon dioxide also come out of solution, but rapidly diffuse away. These bubbles occur particularly in the nervous system and in adipose tissue, as nitrogen is soluble in fat.

Clinical Features. Within a few hours of decompression the patient complains of severe pain in the muscles and joints. This may be followed by evidence of involvement of the central nervous system, including vertigo, weakness of the limbs, and sphincter disturbances. Various skin rashes may develop.

Treatment. *Preventive.* Where possible workers should not be exposed to pressures greater than 124 kPa (18 lbf/in^2), for below this pressure sickness does not occur. If they work under higher pressures they should be slowly decompressed. *Curative.* If decompression sickness develops the subject should be recompressed again and then very slowly decompressed.

MOTION SICKNESS

Motion sickness may occur as a result of sea, land, or air travel. Although the exact mechanism is not known it would seem that repetitive stimulation of the vestibular apparatus plays a large part; it is not possible to produce sickness in animals who have had their vestibular apparatus removed, nor are deaf mutes seasick. Susceptibility to motion sickness varies, but is particularly common in migrainous subjects.

Clinical Features. The victim of motion sickness complains of feeling unwell with nausea, headache, and sometimes faintness. Finally symptoms are such as to require a rapid withdrawal from company and terminate in severe vomiting. The duration of the attack is variable and may last only a few hours, although susceptible subjects may be prostrate for several days.

Treatment. People susceptible to motion sickness should avoid undue movement. When at sea they should remain near the centre of the ship and if possible lie down with the eyes closed. In an aeroplane the head should be rested back on the head rest. Some food should be taken and if this is not possible, barley sugar should be sucked.

Certain drugs diminish the liability to sea-sickness. They are the hyoscine group and the antihistamines. The most satisfactory drug is not decided, but there is a little evidence that hyoscine is better for short journeys and the antihistamines for longer ones. The doses are:

Hyoscine, 0.5–1 mg according to weight, taken 20 minutes before starting, is suitable for journeys lasting up to 4 hours. Side-effects include dry mouth and paralysis of accommodation.

Cyclizine, 50 mg three times daily or meclozine 50 mg daily, are suitable for longer journeys.

Cinnarizine 30 mg two hours before travelling and then 15 mg 8-hourly is also suitable but can cause drowsiness.

These drugs can be used for children in reduced dosage.

Anxiety even before the journey begins may upset some people and diazepam 2–5 mg taken before setting out is sometimes helpful.

DISORDERS DUE TO HEAT

A number of syndromes may appear in those exposed to heat. They are more liable to occur in subjects who have had no opportunity to become acclimatised, in the very young, the elderly and in association with heavy exertion.

Heat Stroke (Heat Hyperpyrexia)

Heat stroke is due to a failure of the heat-controlling mechanism. It may occur merely as a result of exposure to heat or may complicate some pyrexial illness such as malaria. The symptoms are mental confusion, headaches, and incoordination proceeding to delirium, convulsions, and death. The body temperature is raised and may be 41°C or higher. The skin is hot and dry, the sweating mechanism having failed.

Treatment. Heat stroke is a medical emergency and the body must be cooled as rapidly as possible until the rectal temperature is 39°C. This may be achieved by keeping the body surface moist by sponging or by sprays of water and encouraging evaporation by means of fans. The possibility of some complicating infection such as malaria must be remembered and appropriate treatment given.

Heat Exhaustion

Heat exhaustion may occur for a number of reasons and has to be subdivided on this basis:

(a) **Salt Deficiency Heat Exhaustion**

This is due to salt loss with inadequate replacement.

Clinical Features. The symptoms are those of salt deficiency, i.e. weakness, cramps, vomiting, and collapse with a low blood pressure. The plasma sodium and chloride levels are reduced and the urine may be low in chlorides.

Treatment is aimed at replacing the salt loss and this may be done by mouth, or by intravenous infusion if vomiting is troublesome.

(b) **Anhidrotic Heat Exhaustion**

Clinical Features. This form of heat exhaustion is usually associated with prickly heat. The symptoms are weakness and irritability and if exertion is attempted the patient may collapse. Examination shows that sweating is confined to localised areas, usually the face and axillae and sometimes the hands and feet. The condition may proceed to heat stroke.

Treatment is to remove the subject to a cooler environment.

In addition, heat exhaustion on effort may occur without clear evidence of either salt deficiency or anhidrosis.

Prickly Heat

Prickly heat is due to excessive sweating. It is a fine papular rash which sometimes becomes vesicular and usually gives a sensation of prickling (thus the name). It may become infected.

Treatment is removal to a cooler and less humid atmosphere.

Sunburn

Sunburn is due to the ultraviolet fraction of sunlight. It may be merely an erythema but if severe the erythema will be accompanied by some local oedema and sometimes headache and pyrexia.

Treatment. Sunburn may be prevented by graduated exposure to direct sunlight and by applying creams which exclude part of the ultraviolet end of the spectrum. If sunburn has occurred further exposure to sunlight should be avoided and some soothing lotion such as oily calamine applied.

DISORDERS DUE TO COLD

They may be either local or general. Local effects in temperate climates are commonly chilblains or Raynaud's phenomenon (p. 231). If cold is extreme, then the tissues of the extremities may freeze, and frostbite result. General effects result from the progressive cooling of the whole body, the syndrome of hypothermia.

Hypothermia

Immersion in cold water causes rapid heat loss and hypothermia, and in water near to freezing point death occurs within an hour.

Hypothermia in air in this country usually affects the elderly.

Old people may lose heat from their bodies faster than it can be generated, despite apparently adequate insulation with bedding or clothes, and so pass gradually into hypothermia. This occurs only when the external temperature is very cold.

Aggravating features are malnutrition, loss of mobility from arthritis or paralysis, urinary incontinence, dementia, and myxoedema.

Clinically, the patients become confused, then drowsy, and fall asleep, often in exposed positions. Unless rescued they pass into coma and ultimately die. On examination, their bodies are cold, and the rectal temperature low (usually 30°C). Respiration is slow and shallow, the pulse very slow, and the blood pressure low. The ECG is characteristic (Fig. 22.1).

Treatment. The elderly hypothermic patient should be placed under a space blanket in a warm environment and allowed to rewarm naturally. Water and electrolytes should be replaced if necessary and an antibiotic is usually given. Some authorities would give hydrocortisone 100 mg IV 4-hourly. Prognosis depends upon how cold the body is on discovery, how old and how frail the patient is, and on coincident disease. In general it is not good. For subjects who are hypothermic as a result of exposure rewarming can be carried out in a bath with the water just warm to the hand.

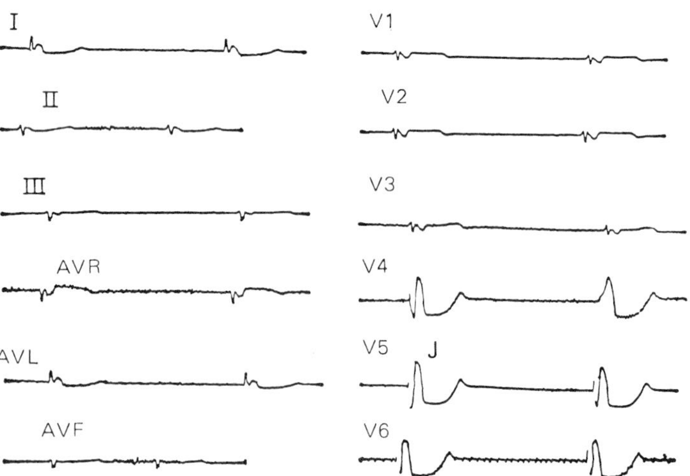

Fig. 22.1 ECG in hypothermia, showing J waves from male, aged 80, rectal temperature 24.5°C, pulse rate 16/min.

ALTITUDE SICKNESS

Altitude sickness is due to hypoxia occurring as a result of the decrease in the partial pressure of oxygen in the atmosphere at high altitudes. It may arise as a result of flying or mountain climbing. Up to 2400 m (8000 ft) no symptoms occur, but over 3000 m (10 000 ft) symptoms may begin to appear. The susceptibility of people varies considerably, being less in the young and healthy and more marked in the elderly and those with respiratory or cardiac disease.

Some acclimatisation can occur to high altitudes. This is brought about by increased respiration, by increase in the pulmonary vascular diffusing surface and by polycythaemia.

Clinical Features

The earliest symptoms are some blunting of mental acuity with motor incoordination and slurred speech. These may be followed by headache and weakness. If the degree of hypoxia is increased there will be loss of consciousness and convulsions and finally death.

FURTHER READING

Hunter, D., *Diseases of Occupations*, 6th edition, Hodder and Stoughton Educational, Sevenoaks, 1978.

Conversion Scales for SI Units

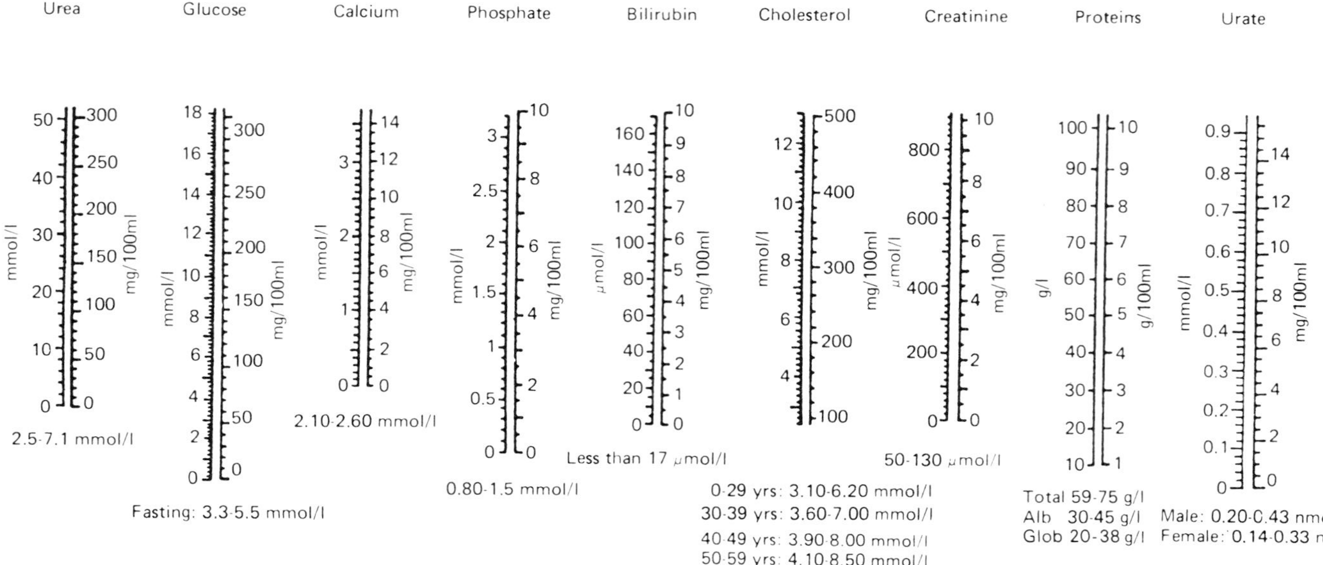

INDEX